T.M. Lotti · L.C. Parish · R.S. Rogers, III (Eds.)

ORAL DISEASES

Springer

Berlin
Heidelberg
New York
Barcelona
Hong Kong
London
Milan
Paris
Singapore
Tokyo

T.M. Lotti · L.C. Parish · R.S. Rogers, III
(Eds.)

ORAL DISEASES

Textbook and Atlas

With 485 Figures, mostly in Color, and 44 Tables

Springer

Prof. Torello M. Lotti, M.D.
Department of Dermatology
University of Florence
37, via Alfani
50121 Florence, Italy

Lawrence Charles Parish, M.D., F.A.C.P.
1819 J.F. Kennedy Boulevard
Suite 465
Philadelphia, PA 19103, USA

Roy Steele Rogers, III, M.D.
Mayo Clinic, Department of Dermatology
200 First Street SW
Rochester, MN 55905-0001, USA

ISBN 3-540-62416-3 Springer-Verlag Berlin Heidelberg New York

Library of Congress Cataloging-in-Publication Data
Oral diseases : textbook and atlas / T.M. Lotti, L.C. Parish, R.S. Rogers, III (eds.) p. cm. Includes bibliographical references and index.
ISBN 3-540-62416-3 (hard cover : alk. paper) 1. Mouth-Diseases. 2. Mouth-Diseases-Atlases. I. Lotti, T.M. (Torello M.), 1953- . II. Parish, Lawrence Charles. III. Rogers, III, Roy S., 1940- .
[DNLM: 1. Mouth Diseases. 2. Mouth Diseases atlases. WU 140 0626 1999]
RC815.06736 1999 616.3'1–dc21

Production: PRO EDIT GmbH, D-69126 Heidelberg
Cover design: Frido Steinen-Broo, Estudio Calamar, Spain
Typesetting: Mitterweger Werksatz, D-68723 Plankstadt

SPIN: 10475817 23/3134-5 4 3 2 1 0 – Printed on acid-free paper

Preface

The editors have planned the present volume primarily for the dermatologist, the dentist, the stomatologist, and otolaryngologist in practice or in training. They have also considered the requirements of specialists in other fields of medicine, as well as the needs of primary care physicians.

An attempt has been made throughout this comprehensive textbook and atlas to discuss succinctly but exhaustively all disorders of the oral mucosa, the jaw, and the salivary glands. The 24 chapters of this atlas book represent a multiple-authored, concise, and readable text, in which color photographs have been provided to illustrate nearly every disease and to amplify related diagnostic and technical procedures.

Each chapter is readable as an independent entity, making the repetition of some material necessary. In each chapter, an attempt has been made to integrate our growing knowledge about the biology of the oral cavity with the available information about the pathological processes and practical clinical problems. Detailed clinical descriptions, pathophysiology, and differential diagnoses are fully discussed, as are histopathology and therapeutics. The list of references has been selected to provide both a general guide to the current literature and a substantial and specific updated bibliography.

The editors hope that this volume will prove of value to the reader.

Torello M. Lotti, MD
Florence, Italy

Lawrence Charles Parish, MD
Philadelphia, Pennsylvania

Roy S. Rogers, III, MD
Rochester, Minnesota

Contents

List of Contributors

Antoniades, Demetris, M.D., D.D.S.
Aristotle University School of Dentistry
20, Neckle Kazazi Street
Thessaloniki, Greece

Argenta, M.
Clinica Dermatologica
II Università di Roma
"Tor Vergata"
Via O. Raimondi
00173 Rome, Italy

Ayala, Fabio, M.D.
Dipartimento di Dermatologia
Venereologia e Chirurgia Plastica
Università di Napoli "Federico II"
Naples, Italy

Poiares Baptista, A., M.D.
Department of Dermatology
University of Coimbra
Coimbra University Hospital
Coimbra, Portugal

Benci, Maurizio, M.D.
Department of Dermatology
University of Florence
37, via Alfani
50121 Florence, Italy

Bianchi, L.
Clinica Dermatologica
II Università di Roma
"Tor Vergata"
Via O. Raimondi
00173 Rome, Italy

Bialy-Golan, Anat, M.D.
Department of Dermatology
Tel Aviv-Sourasky Medical Center
Tel Aviv, Israel

Born, A., M.D.
Pathology Institute
Department of Oral Pathology
University of Heidelberg
69121 Heidelberg, Germany

Borroni, Giovanni, M.D.
Department of Human
and Hereditary Pathology
Institute of Dermatology
Policlinico S. Matteo
Piazzale Golgi, 25
27100 Pavia, Italy

Brazzelli, Valeria, M.D.
Department of Human
and Hereditary Pathology
Institute of Dermatology
Policlinico S. Matteo
Piazzale Golgi, 25
27100 Pavia, Italy

Brenner, Sarah, M.D.
Department of Dermatology
Tel Aviv-Sourasky Medical Center
Tel Aviv, Israel

Bucci, Eduardo
Cattedra di Patologia Speciale
Odontostomatologica
Istituto di Discipline
Odontostomatologiche
Università di Napoli "Federico II"
Naples, Italy

Cagnoni, Matteo, M.D.
Institute of di Dermatology
University of Siena
Siena, Italy

Camacho, Francisco M.
Department of Medical-Surgical Dermatology
and Venereology
University Hospital Virgen Macarena
University of Seville
Avda. Dr. Fedriani s/n
41009 Seville, Spain

Campanile, Grazia L., M.D.
Department of Dermatology
University of Florence
37, via Alfani
50121 Florence, Italy

Caproni, Marzia, M.D.
Department of Dermatology
University of Florence
37, via Alfani
50121 Florence, Italy

Caputo, Rugero, M.D.
Institute of Dermatologic Science
University of Milan
Milan, Italy

Çelebi, Celalettin R., M.D.
Ankara Training Hospital
Dermatology Clinic
Ankara, Turkey

Cerimele, Decio, M.D.
Clinica Dermatologica
Università Cattolica
Largo A. Gemelli, 8
00168 Rome, Italy

Cerinic, Marco Matucci, M.D.
Istituto di Medicina Interna
University of Florence
via P. Thouar 18
50122 Florence, Italy

Cortellini, Pierpaolo, M.D., D.D.S.
Department of Periodontology
and Fixed Prosthodontics
University of Bern
Bern, Switzerland

Cottoni, Francesca, M.D.
Department of Dermatology
University of Sassari
Sassari, Italy

De Pità Ornella, M.D.
Istituto Dermopatico dell'Immacolata
via Monti di Creta, 104
00187 Rome, Italy

Difonzo, Elisa M., M.D.
Department of Dermatology
University of Florence
37, via Alfani
50121 Florence, Italy

Fabbri, Paolo, M.D.
Department of Dermatology
University of Florence
37, via Alfani
50121 Florence, Italy

Falcini, F., M.D.
Department of Pediatrics
University of Florence
37, via Alfani
50121 Florence, Italy

Feletti, Stefano, M.D.
Dermatology Division
"M. Bufalini" Hospital
Cesena, Italy

Feliciani, Claudio, M.D.
Clinica Dermatologica
Policlinico SS, Annunziata
Via di Vestini
66031 Chieti Scalo, Italy

Ferranti, Giulio, M.D.
Istituto Dermopatico dell'Immacolata
Rome, Italy

Flint, Stephen R., M.D.
Dublin Dental Hospital
Lincoln Place
Dublin 2, Ireland

Gaeta, G.M., M.D.
Department of Oral Pathology
School of Dentistry
II University of Naples
Via S. Andrea Delle Dame, 7
80138 Naples, Italy

Ghersetich, Ilaria, M.D., Ph. D.
Department of Dermatology
University of Florence
37, via Alfani
50121 Florence, Italy

Giacomelli, Andrea, M.D.
Department of Dermatology
University of Florence
37, via Alfani
50121 Florence, Italy

Gollnick, A., M.D.
Klinik für Dermatologie und Venerologie
Otto von Guericke University
39104 Magdeburg, Germany

Hall, J. Michael, D.D.S.
Mayo Clinic
Department of Dermatology
Rochester, MN 55905-0001, USA

Hautmann, Giuseppe, M.D.
Department of Dermatology
University of Florence
37, via Alfani
50121 Florence, Italy

Humke, Stefanie, M.D.
Hautklinik
Heinrich Heine University
Moorenstraße 5
40225 Düsseldorf, Germany

Ioannides, Demetris, M.D.
3, P.P. Germanou Street
54622 Thessaloniki, Greece

Ippolito, V., M.D.
Specialist in Odontostomatology
Montecatini T. (PT), Italy

Jablonska, Stefania, M.D.
Department of Dermatology
Warsaw School of Medicine
Koszykowa 82 a
02-008 Warsaw, Poland

Jordan, Richard, M.D.
Departments of Dentistry
and Laboratory Medicine
Sunnybrook Health Science Centre
University of Toronto
Toronto, Canada

Katsambas, Andreas D., M.D.
Department of Dermatology
University of Athens
Athens, Greece

Landi, Giorgio, M.D.
Dermatology Division
"M. Bufalini" Hospital
Cesena, Italy

La Placa, Michelangelo, M.D.
Department of Dermatology
University of Bologna
Bologna, Italy

Lombardi, Arrigo, M.D.
Istituto di Clinica Medica IV
University of Florence
Florence, Italy

Lorusso, Bartolomeo, M.D., D.D.S.
Department of Periodontology
University of Florence
via Pier Capponi, 68
50132 Florence, Italy

Lotti, Torello M., M.D.
Department of Dermatology
University of Florence
37, via Alfani
50121 Florence, Italy

Micali, Giuseppe, M.D.
Department of Dermatology
University of Catania
Catania, Italy

Millikan, Larry E., M.D.
Tulane University School of Medicine
Department of Dermatology
New Orleans, LA, USA

Moritz, Trope, B., M.D.
HUCFF-UFRJ, School of Medicine
Federal University of Rio de Janeiro
Rio de Janeiro, Brazil

Mroczkowski, Tomasz F., M.D.
Department of Dermatology
Tulane University School of Medicine
New Orleans, LA, USA

Neri, Iria, M.D.
Department of Dermatology
University of Bologna
Bologna, Italy

Nini, L.
Clinica Dermatologica
II Università di Roma
"Tor Vergata"
Via O. Raimondi
00173 Rome, Italy

Orlandini, Zecchi Sandra, M.D.
Department of Human Anatomy and Histology
University of Florence
Florence, Italy

Ortega, Rosa M., M.D.
Department of Medical-Surgical Dermatology
and Venereology
Hospital Clinico San Cecilio
University of Granada
Granada, Spain

Palleschi, Giovanni Maria, M.D.
Department of Dermatology
University of Florence
37, via Alfani
50121 Florence, Italy

Panconesi, Emiliano, M.D.
Department of Dermatology
University of Florence
37, via Alfani
50121 Florence, Italy

Parrini, Stefano, D.D.S.
Department of Oral Surgery
University of Siena
Siena, Italy

Patrizi, Analisa, M.D.
Department of Dermatology
University of Bologna
Bologna, Italy

Pignone, Alberto, M.D.
Istituto di Clinical Medica IV
University of Florence
Florence, Italy

Powell, Frank C., F.R.C.P.
Regional Centre of Dermatology
Mater Hospital
Dublin 7, Ireland

Pinto, S.
Clinica Dermatologica
II University of Naples
via Pansini, 5
80100 Naples, Italy

Prato, Giovampaolo Pini, M.D., D.D.S.
Department of Periodontology
University of Siena
Siena, Italy

Ramos-e-Silva, Marcia, M.D., Ph.D.
HUCFF-UFRJ, School of Medicine
Federal University of Rio de Janeiro
Rio de Janeiro, Brazil

Rogers III, Roy Steele, M.D.
Mayo Clinic
Department of Dermatology
Rochester, MN 55905-0001, USA

Ruocco, Vincenzo, M.D.
Clinica Dermosifilopatica, II Ateneo
via S. Pansini, 5
80131 Naples, Italy

Ruzicka, Thomas, M.D.
Hautklinik
Medizinische Einrichtungen
Heinrich Heine University
Moorenstraße 5
40225 Düsseldorf, Germany

Saletta, Daniele, M.D., D.D.S.
Department of Periodontology
University of Siena
Siena, Italy

Sapuppo, Antonio, M.D.
Department of Dermatology
University of Catania,
Catania, Italy

Satriano, R.A., M.D.
Department of Dermatology
School of Medicine
II University of Naples
via Pansini, 5
80131 Naples, Italy

Seidenari, Stefania, M.D.
Department of Dermatology
University of Modena
via del Pozzo 71
41100 Modena, Italy

Stavropoulos, Panagiotis G., M.D.
Department of Dermatology
University Medical Center Benjamin Franklin
The Free University of Berlin
Hindenburgdamm 30
12200 Berlin, Germany

Vallecchi, Carlo, M.D.
Department of Dermatology
University of Florence
37, via Alfani
50121 Florence, Italy

Vierucci, S.
Clinica Pediatrica Università
Ospedale "Anna Mayer"
50100 Florence, Italy

Wolff, Klaus-Dietrich, M.D.
Oral and Maxillofacial Plastic Surgery
University Medical Center Benjamin Franklin
The Free University of Berlin
Hindenburgdamm 30
12200 Berlin, Germany

Yörükan, Selma, M.D.
Hacettepe University Faculty of Medicine
Physiology Department
Ankara, Turkey

Zaitz, Clarisse, M.D.
Department of Dermatology
Santa Casa de Misericórdia de São Paulo
School of Medicine
São Paulo, Brazil

Zouboulis, Christos C., M.D.
Department of Dermatology
University Medical Center Benjamin Franklin
The Free University of Berlin
Hindenburgdamm 30
12200 Berlin, Germany

Macroscopic Anatomy, Histology and Electron Microscopy of the Oral Cavity and Normal Anatomic Variants

G.L. Campanile, T.M. Lotti, and S. Zecchi Orlandini

1.1 Anatomy of the Oral Cavity

The oral cavity is a space bound anteriorly and laterally by the lips and cheeks, superiorly, by the palate and inferiorly by a muscular floor. It opens externally through the mouth, whereas posteriorly it is continuous with the pharynx through the isthmus of the fauces. The alveolar processes and the teeth divide the mouth into two parts: the vestibule, external to the teeth, and the oral cavity proper internal to the teeth.

From a general point of view, the oral cavity is composed primarily of the jaw bones, the facial and mastication musculature, the mucosal integument, and other specialized structures, including the teeth, tongue and salivary glands, which together constitute a regional physiologic unit.

A number of clinically distinct anatomic areas can be recognized: the lips, the labial and buccal mucosa, the floor of the mouth, the tongue, the palate, the tonsillar pillars and the gingivae [1].

The *lips* consist of superior and inferior fleshy folds limiting the mouth orifice. They are covered by mucosa internally and on their appositional surfaces, and by cutaneous tegument externally. The line of demarcation between them is the mucocutaneous junction, also named the vermilion area.

The *labial mucosa* extends from the vermilion area to the alveolar ridge, joining the gingiva at the mucogingival junction and incorporating the superior and inferior labial frenuli in the midline.

The *buccal mucosa* continues bilaterally from the labial mucosa anteriorly, to the pterygomandibular raphe posteriorly. Similarly, it forms the mucolabial fold and the alveolar ridges. The buccal mucosa lies in apposition to the bicuspid and molar teeth and covers the buccinator muscle. On the upper half of the buccal mucosa opposite the maxillary second molar tooth lies the opening of the parotid duct, marked by a triangular papilla (Stenon's papilla).

The color of the normal labial and buccal mucosa is pink, crossed by a fine capillary network.

The *floor of the mouth* extends from the mandibular lingual gingiva to the ventral surface of the tongue, from which it is demarcated by the submandibular (Wharton's) duct. The lingual frenulum runs from the midline of the mandible, across the floor of the mouth, up the midline of the ventral tongue surface to insert near the tip of the tongue. The sublingual duct orifices open along the sublingual fold on either side of the lingual frenulum.

The *ventral surface of the tongue* represents a continuation of the mucosa of the floor up to the lateral border of the tongue. With increasing age and cardiovascular decompensation, prominent venules may be noted under the tongue.

The *dorsum of the tongue* is lined by a specialized type of mucosa. The mucosa of the anterior two-thirds is rough and covered by three types of papillae: the filiform (evenly distributed), the fungiform (concentrated near the tip and sides) and the vallate (along the sulcus terminalis). The base of the tongue is covered by a smooth mucosa in which numerous aggregates of lymphoid tissue (lingual tonsilla) are present. These, together with the palatine tonsils and pharyngeal tonsils, constitute the so-called Waldeyer's ring.

The *palate* is divided into the hard and soft palatal regions.

The mucosa of the hard palate is firmly bound to the underlying bone. It blends into the palatal gingiva around the teeth-, and anteriorly, in the midline just posterior to the two central incisor teeth, the incisive papilla, a small soft tissue projection, can be seen. The palatine raphe, a firm whitish streak, extends along the midline from the incisive papilla to the soft palate. Radiating from it in the anterior hard palate are several firm, curved ridges of fibrous tissue, the palatine rugae.

The soft palate, having no bony support, is freely movable and demarcated from the hard palate by the "vibrating line." It contains numerous mucous glands and, in the pharyngeal region, some mixed glandular elements.

The *tonsillar area* is formed by the glossopalatine and pharyngopalatine arches, respectively the anterior and posterior pillars of the isthmus of the fauces. Inferiorly, they are bounded by the lateral aspect of the posterior third of the tongue and within these spaces lie the palatine tonsils.

The *gingiva* is a mucous membrane closely adapted to the alveolar process of the teeth. It is demarcated from the labial and buccal mucosa by a scalloped margin, the mucogingival junction.

Towards the neck of the tooth, the gingiva and the interdental papilla that fill the space between two contacting teeth are stippled except for a thin free margin, the marginal gingiva, which provides a knife-like collar or sulcus around the neck of the tooth. The epithelium dipping into this sulcus forms an attachment which, with age or disease, migrates apically along the root of the tooth [2].

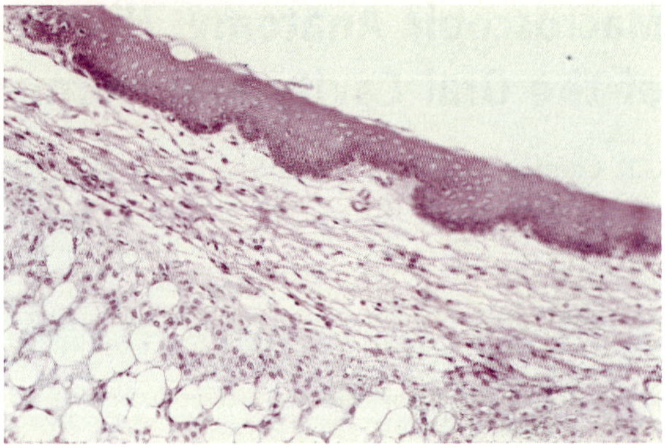

Fig. 1.1. Oral mucosa at human soft palate. 90

1.2 Microscopic Anatomy of the Oral Mucosa

The oral mucosa can be classified into three different types:

1. The lining mucosa, which allows movement and stretching and is provided with an elastic connective tissue stroma and a rather stretchable epithelium.
2. The masticatory mucosa, which has to sustain remarkable physical forces, covers the palatine and alveolar processes to which it adheres firmly and is supported by a dense fibrons connective stroma and a structurally "rigid" epithelium undergoing a moderate degree of keratinization.
3. The specialized mucosa, covering the dorsum of the tongue, is provided with specialized formations, the lingual papillae, capable of receiving even very weak stimuli, tactile and taste-related in nature.

The oral mucosa consists of a stratified squamous epithelium of 100–500 μm thickness separated by a continuous interface, the basement membrane, from a connective tissue stroma, the lamina propria. Except for the gingiva and the anterior hard palate, an additional connective tissue layer, the submucosa, is present.

The *stratified squamous epithelium* is normally nonkeratinized and it is composed of a stratum germinativum, or basal layer, consisting of cuboidal or columnar cells with a large, dark-staining nucleus, and a stratum spinosum, or prickle cell layer, in which large, polyhedral-cells have large, paler-staining nuclei. The stratum spinosum is sometimes divided into a lower "intermediate" layer and an upper "superficial" flattened layer of cells (Fig. 1.1).

The absence of a cornified layer and the prominence of the vascular network in the underlying connective tissue determine the normal intense pink color of the mucosa.

The masticatory mucosa, present on the gingiva and the anterior hard palate, contains a thin stratum granulosum with distinct keratohyaline granules, along with a thin stratum corneum. The basement membrane is more fully developed and the subjacent connective tissue is considerably more dense.

The *lamina propria* is a thin layer of more or less dense, collagenous connective tissue bundles and associated fibroblasts. Elastic fibers, lymphatics, blood vessels, sense receptors, and nerve fibers are also present. Particularly in masticatory mucosa, the connective tissue is thrown up into numerous ridges and papillae, providing a considerably increased area of contact between the epithelium and the stroma.

The *submucosa* is a variably loose connective tissue layer that allows for considerable distensibility and serves as an attachment to underlying structures. It provides a network of vascular and neural structures feeding the finer arborizations seen in the lamina propria. Most of the minor salivary glands and variable amounts of adipose tissue are found here.

In the submucosa of the mucogingival junction, in contrast to the attached gingiva, a considerable increase in elastic fibers has been observed.

The oral cavity contains numerous *neuroreceptors.* They are found more frequently in the anterior oral mucosa, especially in the lips, which are richly equipped with tactile corpuscles, both intra- and subepithelial, on the dorsal surface of the tongue as tactile and specialized sensorial receptors (taste buds), and in the hard palate. More generally, they are encountered in the lamina propria of the oral mucosa as encapsulated corpuscles (Meissner's, Krause's, Ruffini's, etc.) or as free nerve endings.

The *blood vessels* run through the submucosa. The arterioles that enter the lamina propria form a subepithelial capillary network in the papillae. The veins follow the course of the arteries.

A rich *lymphatic network* runs generally with the blood vessels and nerves. Lymphoid tissue can be found in almost any oral mucosa site [3].

The glands of the oral cavity are almost exclusively of the *tubulo-salivary*, merocrine type. They are classified according to size (major and minor), location (palate, floor of the mouth, tongue, etc.), or cell type (serous, mucinous, mixed secretory). The major salivary glands (parotid, submandibular, sublingual) are paired, while the minor salivary glands are scattered throughout the oral mucosa (Figs. 1.2, 1.3).

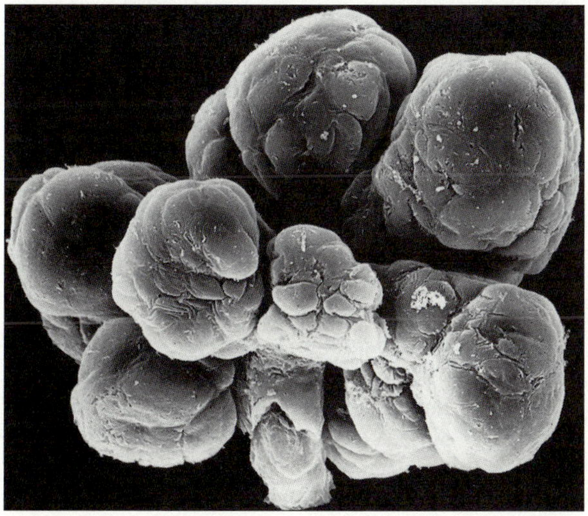

Fig. 1.2. Scanning electron microscopy of a serous lobule of human submandibular gland after removal of connective tissue and basement membrane. (Courtesy of Prof. A. Riva, Italy), 2000

The salivary glands are composed of a ductal system and a terminal acinar portion. Progressing from the mucosal surface, primary ducts, lobar ducts, interlobular ducts, and intralobular ducts can be recognized. The intralobular ducts consist of intercalated and striated (secretory) ducts. The acinar cells encompass a small lumen which drains into the ductal system. Mucous and/or serous cells (alone or in combination) form the acinar structure of the glands. The glandular cells are surrounded by cells of stellate shape (basal or basket cells) which are believed to act as smooth muscle cells aiding in the expulsion of the glandular content. They are called myoepithelial cells [4].

Melanocytes are present, occurring as groups or as isolated cells in the basal layer. They vary in number from 1 in 4 to 1 in 18 in proportion to basal keratinocytes. They are more numerous and tend to be aggregated in the mucosa adjacent to the dental lamina [5].

The density of *Langerhans cells* varies, being most abundant in the epithelium of the dorsum of the tongue, the hard palate, and the gingiva [6].

Nonspecific or indeterminate dendritic cells are also seen, but their identification is possible only by electron microscopy.

1.3 Electron Microscopy of the Oral Mucosa

The ultrastructural organization of the oral epithelium consists of basal, prickle, and successively superficial cell layers.

Basal cells are 15–20 μm in length and contain, in addition to the usual organelles, bundles of tonofibrils (Fig. 1.4). Migrating basal cells form prickle cells, larger and more irregular in shape and con-

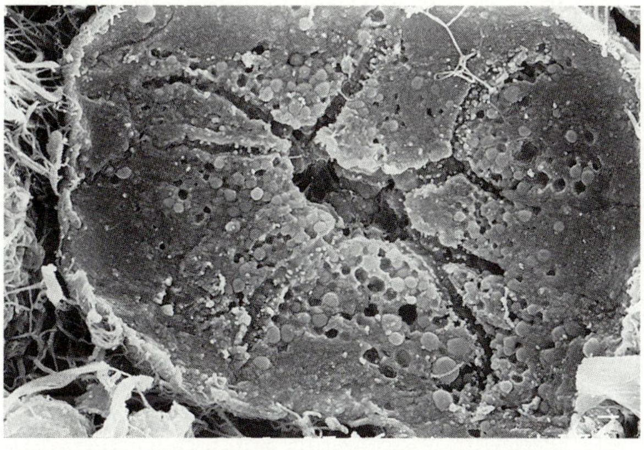

Fig. 1.3. SEM of a serous acinus of human submandibular gland following fracture. (Courtesy of Prof. A. Riva, Italy), 3600

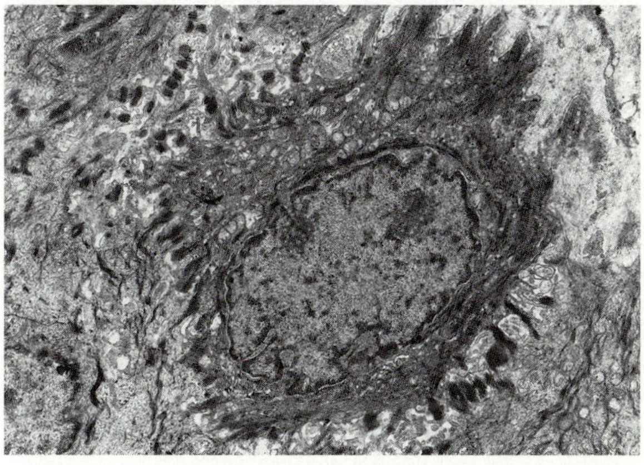

Fig. 1.4. Transmission electron microscopy of keratinizing epithelium of human hard palate. The basal layer cells contain numerous tonofibrils. (Courtesy of Prof. P. Romagnoli, Italy), 10 000

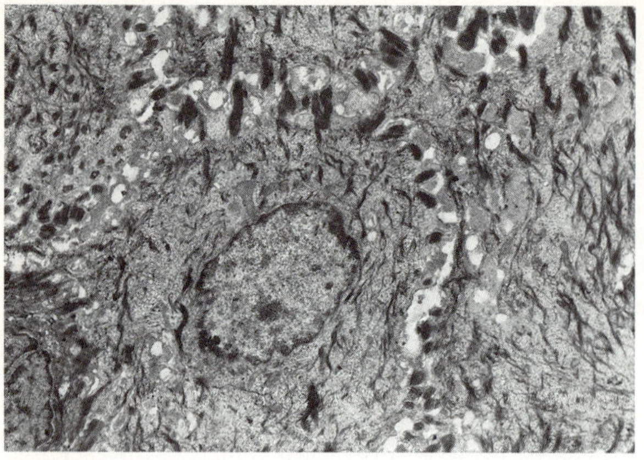

Fig. 1.5. TEM of keratinizing epithelium of human hard palate. Prickle cell layer. (Courtesy of Prof. P. Romagnoli, Italy), 10 000

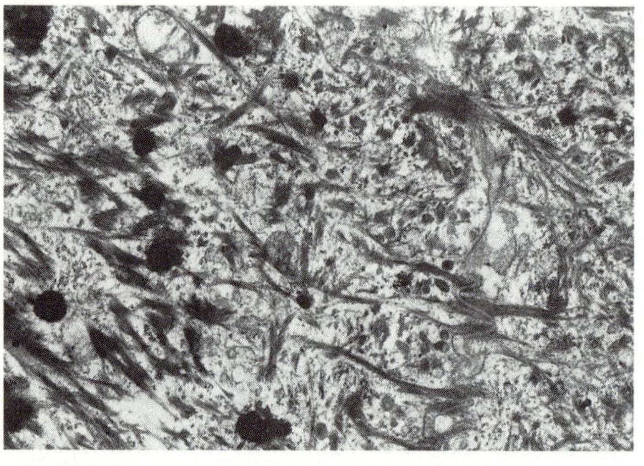

Fig. 1.6. TEM of keratinizing epithelium of human hard palate. Borderline between the upper prickle and granular layers. Many membrane coating granules and some keratohyalin granules are shown. (Courtesy of Prof. P. Romagnoli, Italy), 28 000

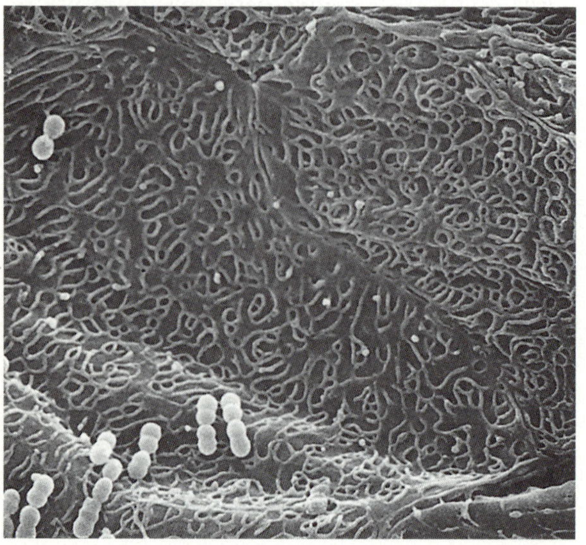

Fig. 1.7. SEM, higher magnification, of the superficial plasmalemma. Note the apical pattern characterized by a complicated labyrinth of microplicae. 5000

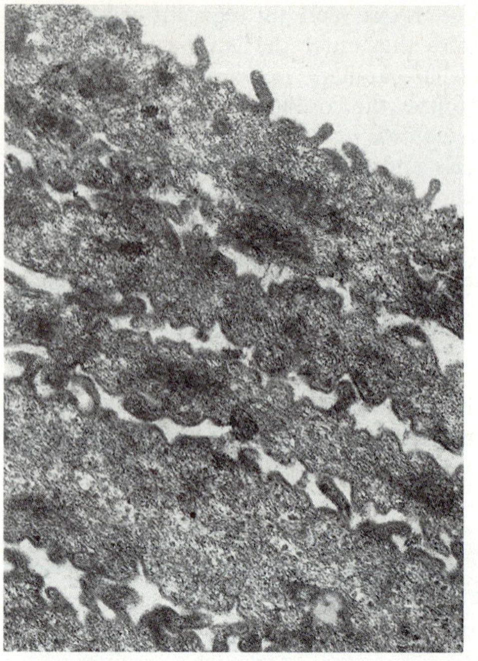

Fig. 1.8. TEM of the superficial layers of nonkeratinizing oral epithelium. Note the lack of desmosomes and the irregular projections from the cell surface (microplicae). (Courtesy of Prof. P. Romagnoli, Italy), 28 000

taining more conspicuous bundles of tonofibrils (Fig. 1.5). In the upper prickle cell region there is progressive flattening of the cells and tonofibrils appear more dense. Membrane-coating granules are noted in this region along the apical plasmalemma, where they discharge into the intercellular space, presumably to form an intercellular barrier to permeable substances. These granules are more numerous in keratinized oral epithelium (e.g., vestibular edge of gingiva, small areas of tongue) where keratohyaline granules occur in the granular layer, as irregular, electron-dense structures intermingled with tonofilaments (Fig. 1.6). The nuclei tend to persist through the upper prickle cell and superficial layers of nonkeratinized epithelia (Figs. 1.7, 1.8). On the contrary, they tend to flatten, shrink, and disappear, along with other organelles, in keratinizing areas. In these areas, the keratinized layer consists of flattened, amorphous cells usually devoid of nuclei in which compressed tonofilaments constitute the only identifiable cytoplasmic material.

Desmosomes are the most important intercellular junction, especially prominent in the basal and prickle cell regions where also gap junctions can occur. Hemidesmosomes, more numerous in nonkeratinizing mucosa, are arranged along the basal lamina and provide anchoring fibrils that are interlocked with the underlying collagen fibrils (Fig. 1.9).

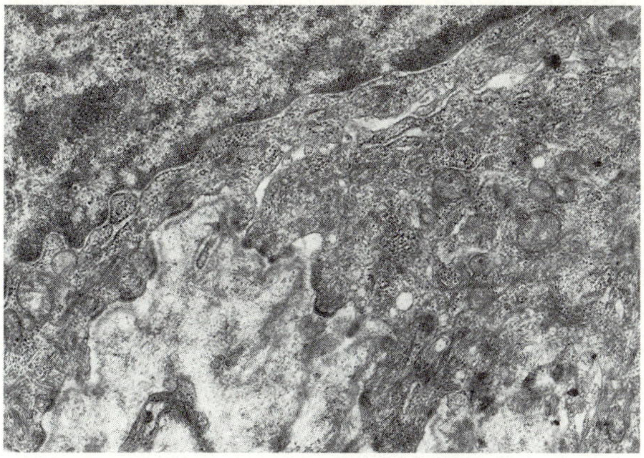

Fig. 1.9. TEM of nonkeratinizing oral epithelium. Basal layer: few tonofibrils insert to hemidesmosomes. (Courtesy of Prof. P. Romagnoli, Italy), 25 000

Isolated melanocytes are sometimes found in the lower portion of the folds characterizing the gingival mucosa. They are located among the keratinocytes of the basal and prickle layers. Active and nonactive melanocytes can be distinguished by the presence or absence of melanosomes.

Langerhans cells are predominantly located in a suprabasal position. They tend to be located mostly above the rete ridges areas in the palate and the gingiva [7].

Merkel cells are also found in the basal region as nondendritic cells. These cells have few desmosomes and tonofilaments, but numerous small, membrane-bound, electron-dense granules. Often they lie in direct contact with an intraepithelial nerve ending [8, 9].

1.4 Normal Anatomic Variants

1.4.1 Linea Alba

The linea alba or occlusal line is a delicate, slightly raised, white ridge, often seen where the teeth occlude along the buccal mucosa, extending mesiodistally from the labial commissure posteriorly to the molar region.

It occurs more often in obese subjects [10].

1.4.2 Leukoedema

The prickle cells do not normally go on to form a granular or keratinized layer in the labial and buccal mucosa. Occasionally, areas of the oral mucosa may contain a layer or two of tinctorially altered, plump or flattened, structureless cells in which nuclear material may or may not persist. If widespread, this variation may impart a diffuse, opaque whiteness to the mucosa, referred to as leukoedema. Leukoedema occurs bilaterally and has normal consistency on palpation. The differential diagnosis includes leukoplakia and lichen planus [11, 12].

1.4.3 Normal Oral Pigmentation

The presence of single or multiple circumscribed areas of hyperpigmentation in the oral mucosa is not always a pathological finding. It may be an idiotypic pigmentation (inverse ephelides, tattoos, ethnic characteristic in dark-skinned persons). Important factors in the differential diagnosis are the history (hereditary, congenital, or of spontaneous occurrence), the patient's general condition, the administration of drugs, dental procedures and occupational exposure. The histologic findings are helpful in cases of doubt [13].

References

1. Archard HO. Biology and pathology of the oral mucosa. In: Fitzpatrick TB, Wolff K, et al. (Eds). Dermatology in general medicine, 3rd Ed. New York, McGraw-Hill, 1987: 11–1239
2. Ten Cate AR. Oral histology: development, structure, and function, 3rd Ed. St. Louis, Mosby, 1989: 1–37
3. Autori vari. Anatomia Umana. Milano: Edi Ermes, 3rd Ed, 1990: 1–60
4. Palmer RM. The identification of myoepithelial cells in human salivary glands. A review and comparison of light microscopic methods. J Oral Pathol 1986: 15: 221
5. Axell T, Hedin CA. Epidemiologic study of excessive oral melanin pigmentation with special reference to the influence of tobacco habits. Scand J Dent Res 1982: 90: 434
6. Cruchley AT. Regional variation in Langerhans cell distribution and density in normal human oral mucosa determined using monoclonal antibodies against CD1, HLADR, HLADQ and HLADP. J Oral Pathol Med 1989: 18: 510
7. Daniels TE. Human mucosal Langerhans cells: postmortem identification of regional variations in oral mucosa. J Invest Dermatol 1984: 82: 21
8. Garant PR. Ultrastructure of Merkel cells in the hard palate of the squirrel monkey (*Saimiri sciures*). Am J Anat 1980; 157: 155
9. Hashimoto K. Fine structure of Merkel cells in human oral mucosa. J Invest Dermatol 1972; 58: 381
10. Shafer WG, Hine MK, Levy BM (Eds). A textbook of oral pathology, 4th Ed, Philadelphia, Saunders, 1983: 10–37
11. Archard HO. Leukoedema of the human oral mucosa. Oral Surg 1968; 25: 717
12. Van Wyk CW. Abnormal keratohyalin-like forms in leukoedema. J Oral Pathol 1984; 13: 271
13. Braun-Falco O, Plewig G, Wolff HH, Winkelmann RK (Eds). Dermatology, 4th Ed. Heidelberg, Springer-Verlag, 1991

CHAPTER 2

Physiology of the Oral Cavity

C. R. Çelebi, and S. Yörükan

The oral cavity or mouth is the first portion of the digestive tract and is bounded by the lips anteriorly, the fauces posteriorly, the cheeks laterally, the palate superiorly and a muscular floor inferiorly. The tongue fills the available space in the floor of the mouth within the arch of the lower teeth. The oral cavity can be divided into two regions: (1) *the vestibule,* which is the space between lips or cheeks and the teeth; and (2) *the oral cavity proper,* the region medial to the teeth. The oral cavity is lined with moist stratified epithelium which shows characteristic variations of the different regions [1].

2.1 Functions of the Oral Cavity Organs and Tissues

2.1.1 Lips and Cheeks

The lips or labia are fleshy muscular folds covered internally by mucosa and externally by skin. The epithelial covering tissue of the lips is a thin and transparent transitional zone of the two kinds of covering tissue. Thus the lips are not highly keratinized and this allows the color of the blood in the underlying vessels to be visible, giving a reddish-pink appearance.

The cheeks are muscular structures covered on the outside by skin and lined interiorly by moist non-keratinized stratified squamous epithelium. They are anteriorly terminated in the superior and inferior lips and are contributed to laterally by the buccinator muscles, which flatten the cheeks against the teeth, and the buccal fat, which gives the profile on the side of the face. The lips and cheeks function in mastication by manipulating the food within the mouth and holding the food in place while the teeth split it. They also assist the speech process by helping to form words. Muscles of facial expression are involved in movements of the lips. Closure of the lips allows retention of food and saliva in the mouth [1].

2.1.2 Tongue

The tongue is a muscular organ which occupies and forms the floor of the oral cavity. The muscles associated with the tongue are divided into two categories. The intrinsic muscles are within the tongue and are responsible for altering its shape and size for speech and swallowing. The extrinsic muscles are outside the tongue and move the tongue from side to side and forward and backward. The movements of both muscle types move food in the mouth and, in cooperation with the lips and gums, hold the food in place during mastication. Then the tongue maneuvers food for chewing, shapes it into a rounded mass, which is called a bolus, and transfers the bolus to the back of the mouth for swallowing [2].

The lingual frenulum is a short fold of mucous membrane which aids in limiting the movements of the tongue posteriorly and in facilitating normal speech.

The upper surface and sides of the tongue are covered by moist, stratified squamous epithelium. Functionally, the dorsum of the tongue is divided into two portions by a groove called the terminal sulcus. The anterior portion of the sulcus has papillae, some of which contain taste buds, and in the posterior region there are a few taste buds and small glands and a considerable amount of lymphoid tissue. The papillae on the posterior surface are called *circumvallate* papillae which contain taste buds and are arranged in an inverted V and are 10–12 in number, into each of which open the ducts of minor salivary glands known as the glands of Von Ebner. The whitish conical projections distributed in parallel rows over the anterior two-thirds of the tongue are called *filiform* papillae which do not contain taste buds.

Filiform papillae form a rough abrasive surface which is involved in compressing and breaking food when the tongue is apposed to the hard palate. In this way, the dorsal mucosa of the tongue functions as a masticatory mucosa. Mushroom-like red dots distributed among the filiform papillae are *fun-*

giform papillae, which are numerous near the tip of the tongue and contain taste buds. Leaf-like *foliate* papillae are sometimes present on the lateral margins of the posterior region of the tongue. They have a few taste buds [3].

2.1.3 Teeth and Gingiva

The types of teeth are shown in Fig. 2.1. They are incisors, canines, premolars, and molars. Their shapes and positions assist in their functions. The incisor teeth have a cutting function during mastication of the food. The canine teeth (cuspids) tear the food being eaten. Premolars (bicuspids) provide breakdown of the food by grinding between their large, flat surfaces. The tongue, cheeks, lips, and teeth together form the food into a bolus prior to being swallowed [4].

Each tooth has three portions: crown, neck, and root. The crown, which is visible and covered by enamel, is ideally located to withstand the grinding that occurs during the chewing of hard and brittle foods. There is dentine under the enamel in the crown and cementum in the neck. Embedded projectional root portions serve to anchor the tooth in the jaw.

The teeth play an important role in mastication and also have a role in speech.

The teeth are located in alveoli along the alveolar ridges of the mandible and maxilla. Alveolar processes are covered by the gingivae or gums, which extend slightly into each socket forming the gingival sulcus. The sockets are lined by the periodontal ligament, which consists of dense fibrous connective tissue and is attached to the socket walls and the cemental surface of the roots. Thus, it anchors the teeth in position and also acts as a shock absorber to dissipate the pressures produced by chewing.

2.1.4 Oral Mucosa

The moist lining of the oral cavity is called the oral mucus membrane or oral mucosa. Histologically, oral mucosa is of a transitional type and shows some of the properties of skin and intestinal mucosa. The oral mucosa has several functions. These are protection, sensation, thermal regulation, secretion, immunological activities, and absorption [3].

2.1.4.1 *Protection*

As a surface lining, the most important function of the oral mucosa is separating and protecting the deeper tissues and organs of the oral cavity from the environment. The normal activities of seizing, biting, and chewing food expose the oral soft tissues to mechanical forces such as compression, stretching, shearing, and surface abrasion by hard particles in the diet. Both the epithelium and the connective tissue of the oral mucosa adapt to withstand the possible trauma resulting from these functions. A high basal turnover of epithelial cells provides for losses due to friction. It also indirectly controls microbial colonization because adherence of microbial agents to the surface cells of mucosa does not occur due to

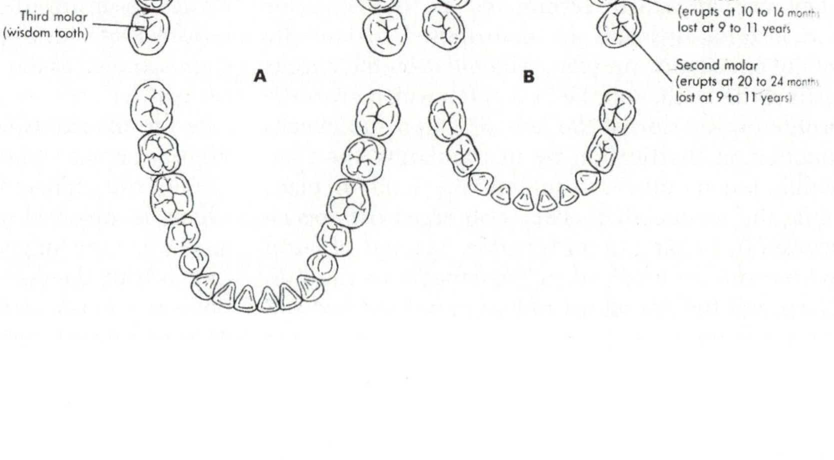

Fig. 2.1 A, B.
The deciduous (baby) teeth and adult teeth (**A**). In the deciduous set (**B**), there are no premolars and only two pairs of molars in each jaw. Generally, the lower teeth erupt before the corresponding upper teeth

rapid renewal of the surface. In addition, due to the high basal turnover, wound healing in the oral cavity is faster and more effective. The epithelium of the oral mucosa therefore acts as the major protective barrier against harmful factors.

2.1.4.2
Sensation

The oral mucosa provides information by its sensorial activity. There are receptors in the oral mucosa that respond to temperature, touch, pain and taste. Reflexes of swallowing, gagging, retching, and salivation also arise from these receptors. There are also specific receptors which respond to the taste of water and lead to the sensation of thirst.

2.1.4.3
Thermal regulation

Human oral mucosa plays a small role in the regulation of body temperature in contrast to other mammals such as dogs where mucosal regulation of temperature is important. This is due to the absence of specific receptors to control heat transfer in the blood vessels.

2.1.4.4
Secretion

The major secretion of the oral mucosa is saliva, which is produced by the salivary glands and ensures the maintenance of a moist surface.

In humans, there are three pairs of major salivary glands: the parotid, submandibular, and sublingual. These glands are located outside the oral cavity and are encapsulated and their secretions pass through the mucosa by long ducts. There is also a large group of smaller minor salivary glands, the labial, lingual, palatal, buccal, glossopalatine, and retromolar glands. These unencapsulated glands are located within the mucous membranes and have shorter ducts.

2.1.4.5
Immune Mucosal Network

Around the oral cavity, there are some components of the immune system. These are inflammatory cells in the gingival sulcus, Langerhans cells of the epithelium, and the oral tonsillar tissues.

Other elements of the immune system in the oral tissues of normal individuals which play a role in antigen processing and presentation, antibody production and secretion, and cell-mediated effector pathways also exist in mucosal-associated lymphoid tissue (Malt), etc. [5].

2.1.4.6
Absorption

Oral epithelium has no absorptive function; however, there are differences in permeability in different oral regions depending on the thickness of the epithelial barrier, pattern of maturation, and absence of the stratum corneum. One of the thinnest epithelial regions, the floor of the mouth, may be more permeable than other areas. This is perhaps the reason why certain drugs are successfully absorbed sublingually (salicylic acid, nitroglycerin, etc.). Blood drainage from the oral cavity directly into the systemic circulation optimizes this pathway of drug delivery [3].

2.2
Physiological Processes in the Oral Cavity

2.2.1
Salivary Secretion

2.2.1.1
Control of Salivary Secretion

Salivary secretion is under neural control. The salivary glands are controlled mainly by parasympathetic nervous signals from the salivatory nuclei. The salivatory nuclei are located at the juncture of the medulla and pons. They are excited by both taste and tactile stimuli from the tongue and other regions of the mouth. These stimuli elicit abundant secretion of saliva. While the presence of a smooth object in the mouth causes marked salivation, rough objects cause less salivation or even inhibit it.

Higher centers of the central nervous system can regulate the secretion of saliva. The appetite area of the brain which is located near the parasympathetic centers of the anterior hypothalamus partially regulates salivation via signals arising from the taste and smell areas of the cerebral cortex or amygdala.

Stimulation of parasympathetic cholinergic nerves causes copious secretion of watery, isotonic saliva with a low organic material content. Vasoactive intestinal polypeptide (VIP) is also locally released during this stimulation, which produces vasodilation in the gland. The accompanying increase in blood flow to the gland also stimulates glandular metabolism and growth [6].

Stimulation of the sympathetic nerve supply causes vasoconstriction and secretion of smaller amounts of saliva rich in organic contents such as ptyalin via primarily β-adrenergic receptors. The myoepithelial cells are also sympathetically innervated and the secretory response may be partially mediated by the contractions of these cells. Salivary secretion mostly occurs in the presence of both adrenergic and cholinergic stimuli and experiments with pharmacologic agonists and antagonists indicate that synergistic effects exist between the two systems. Salivation also occurs in response to reflexes arising from the stomach and upper intestines. This mechanism helps to dilute or neutralize any irritating substance present in the gastrointestinal tract [5, 7].

The smell, sight, touch, and sound of food preparation also stimulate salivary secretion. These stimuli constitute psychological activation and involve learned behavior. Memories stored in the cerebral cortex that associate the stimuli with food are stimulated. The cortex sends impulses to the nuclei in the brain stern via extrapyramidal pathways and the salivary glands are activated.

2.2.1.2
Saliva and Its Composition

The fluids secreted by the major and minor salivary glands constitute saliva. The volume of saliva secretion in humans is 1–1.5 l/day. Salivary flow is diurnal and is lowest during sleep, exhibiting a fairly constant basal level during waking hours, with exacerbations of stimulated flow. Basal rates in adults are approximately 0.3–0.5 ml/min.

Chemically, saliva is composed of 99.5 % water and 0.5 % solutes (electrolyte components, enzyme and other salivary proteins). The secretions of different glands vary markedly. The parotid glands secrete a watery serous saliva which is rich in amylase, the sublingual gland secretes a viscous saliva, and the submandibular gland secretes a mucinous saliva. The saliva in the mouth is a mixture of these various secretions and is known as mixed saliva; however, mixed saliva is not the simple additive sum of these secretions because many proteins in saliva are rapidly removed by adhering to the hydroxyapatite of teeth and to oral mucosal surfaces.

The pH of saliva ranges normally from about 5.8 to 7.4, but saliva becomes more isotonic and more alkaline the more rapidly it is secreted. Salivary flow rate is influenced by the type of taste stimulus. In general, sour taste elicited by citric acids or sour food induces the highest flow rate and Na^+ concentrations, while salt gives rise to high protein and Ca^{2+} concentrations [8].

Among the solutes in the saliva are salts such as chlorides, bicarbonates, and phosphates of sodium and potassium and calcium. Some dissolved gases and various organic substances including urea, uric acid, serum albumin, globulin, mucin, the bacteriolytic enzyme lysosyme, and the digestive enzyme salivary amylase (ptyalin) are normal constituents of saliva. Lactoperoxidase, blood group antigens, EGF, VIP, RNAase, DNAase, lingual lipase, kallikrein and lactoferrin are also present. Iodine is concentrated by the salivary glands and is also found in saliva [5].

2.2.1.3
Salivary Functions

Salivary secretion plays an important role in maintaining healthy oral tissues [5, 6, 7, 9]. The functions of this secretion are as follows:

1. Saliva provides moisture and lubrication to the oral tissues.
2. Saliva helps in speech by moistening the lips and oral cavity.
3. It facilitates the chewing and swallowing of food.
4. By acting as a solvent medium, it delivers chemical substances to taste buds, thus facilitating the sense of taste and enjoyment of food.
5. With its buffering capacity, mineral content, and antibacterial qualities, it protects the oral tissues.
6. The flow of saliva helps wash away pathogenic bacteria, food particles, and cast off cells of the oral tissues, keeping the mouth and teeth clean.
7. The wearing of removable dental prostheses is facilitated by the presence of saliva.
8. The major digestive function of saliva results from the action of salivary amylase on starch. It cleaves the internal α1,4-glycocidic linkage in starch leading to production of disaccharides. The pH of the saliva is optimum for amylase activity. Lingual lipase, produced by the Von Ebner glands on the tongue, is active on fats and is responsible for the digestion of up to 30 % dietary triglycerides.
9. The buffers in saliva help maintain a constant oral pH and neutralize regurgitated gastric acid in the esophagus.
10. Major human salivary histatins, histatin-rich proteins, present in human parotid and submandibular secretions have recently been shown to have anticandidal activity [10].
11. Mercury, lead, sulfur, iodides, morphines, many antibiotics, and several viruses such as rabies, poliomyelitis, and HCV can be excreted from the body by secretion into saliva.

2.2.2
Mastication (Chewing)

Mastication is the process whereby ingested food is cut or crushed into small pieces, mixed with saliva, and formed into a bolus in preparation for swallowing. Various functions listed below have been ascribed to mastication:

1. It forms the food into a bolus which is easily swallowed.
2. It enhances the digestibility of food by:
   - Mechanically decreasing the size of particles thus increasing the surface area for enzyme activity.
   - Reflexly stimulating the secretion of saliva and gastric juice for chemical digestion.
3. It mixes the food with saliva and initiates digestion by the activity of salivary amylase.
4. It prevents irritation of the gastrointestinal system by large food masses.
5. It ensures healthy growth and development of the oral tissues.
6. It contributes to the drainage of the lymphatic and venous vessels of facial skin and muscles.

Mastication is dependent upon a complex chain of events which produce rhythmic opening and closing movements of the jaws and significant tongue movement. A diagrammatic representation of the movements of mastication and their neural control is presented in Fig. 2.2 [11].

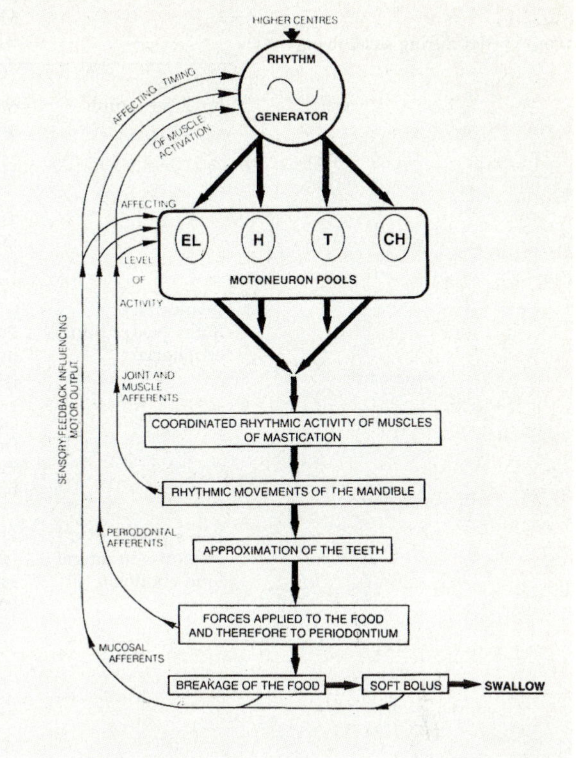

Fig. 2.2. An oral rhythm/pattern generator is situated in the brain stem and is activated by drive from the higher centers and from peripheral sensory input. The pattern of activity is then distributed to the motor neuron pools, which also receive excitatory or inhibitory sensory inputs from a variety of peripheral structures. The hypothesis is that the sensory input generated by closing on hard food supports the generation of rhythmic activity whereas closure on a softened bolus elicits a swallow, and may consequently terminate the rhythmic activity. *EL*, jaw elevator muscle; *H*, hyoid and associated muscles; *T*, tongue and associated musculature; *CH* cheeks and associated musculature

2.2.3 Swallowing (Deglutition)

Swallowing involves an ordered sequence of events that carry food and saliva from the mouth into the stomach. The main events and stages of this process are presented in Table 2.1.

Swallowing is a complex reflex response that is triggered by afferent impulses in the trigeminal, glossopharyngeal, and vagus nerves. These impulses are integrated in the nucleus of the tractus solitarius and the nucleus ambiguous. The efferent fibers pass to the pharyngeal musculature and the tongue via the trigeminal, facial, and hypoglossal nerves. Swallowing is initiated by the voluntary action of collecting the oral contents on the tongue and propelling them backward into the pharynx. The subsequent phases of swallowing are involuntary.

2.2.4 Speech

The acquisition of speech ability is probably the most complex sensorimotor developmental process in humans. Sounds are produced initially in the larynx (phonation) by the coordinated movements of abdominal, thoracic, and laryngeal muscles. Subsequent modification of laryngeal sound to produce meaningful speech (articulation) occurs principally within the pharyngeal, oral, and nasal cavities. The principal sensory and motor mechanisms during speech are presented in Fig. 2.3 [11].

The fundamental laryngeal note has a thin and reedy quality. This sound therefore contains a limited amount of speech information and is later modified within resonating chambers and by the activity of organs such as the lips, tongue, and soft palate by a process of sympathetic vibration. The resonators act as acoustic filters, amplifying selected frequencies and alternating others.

Motor refinements of speech articulation are the product of sensorimotor mechanisms analogous to those employed in oral feeding and in fine coordination elsewhere in the body. The effectors of speech, however, are more heterogeneous and are anatomically dispersed, performing in a greater variety of patterns and schedules with greater relevance to the environmental circumstances and/or context than is true of any other sensorimotor coordination. Speech is clearly the ultimate externalized human performance.

Table 2.1.
Main events during swallowing

Stage	Mechanism associated with passage of bolus	Mechanisms associated with protecting airway
1. Voluntary		
Bolus in mouth	Mouth closed (temporalis, masseter, medial pterygoid)	Airway open
	Lips closed (orbicularis oris)	Pillars of fauces contracted against posterior surface of tongue (palatoglossus, palatopharyngeus)
	Tongue grooved, anterior part raised against palate (intrinsic tongue muscles, genioglossus)	
2. Involuntary		
Bolus passes into oropharynx	Posterior part of tongue moves upward and backwards (styloglossus, mylohyoid)	Nasopharynx closed off
	Groove in tongue flattened out (intrinsic tongue muscles). Pillars of fauces contract behind bolus	Soft palate tensed and elevated (tensor veli palatini, levator vile palatini, Passavant's muscle
Bolus passes over epiglottis to lateral food channels	Pharynx elevated (stylopharyngeus, salpingopharyngeus, palatopharyngeus)	Inlet of larynx closed off and respiration interrupted
		Larynx elevated beneath epiglottis and posterior part of tongue (stylopharyngeus, salpingopharyngeus, palatopharyngeus, thyrohyoid)
		Laryngeal inlet reduced by approximation (interarytenoid, thyroarytenoid) and tension (lateral cricoarytenoid interarytenoid) of aryepiglottic folds
Bolus passes into esophagus	Relaxation of cricopharyngeus	Airway reestablished
		Soft palate and larynx return to original positions

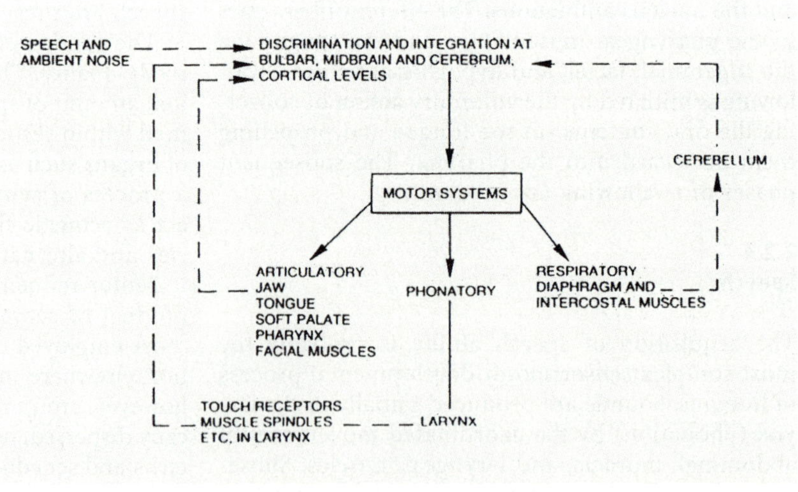

Fig. 2.3. The main speech area of the brain is located within the temporoparietal region of the dominant cerebral hemisphere. The diagram indicates the many monitoring systems which are involved in the control of speech. Note that there has to be coordinated activity of respiration, laryngeal behavior, and oral structures to produce effective speech

2.2.5 Sensation

The sensory function of the oral mucosa is important because it provides considerable information about events in the oral cavity, while the lips and tongue can also perceive stimuli outside the mouth. In the mouth, there are receptors that respond to temperature, touch, and pain as well as the taste buds which are not found elsewhere in the body. Certain receptors in the oral mucosa probably respond to the taste of water and signal the satiation of thirst. Reflexes such as swallowing, gagging, retching, and salivation are also initiated by receptors in the oral mucosa.

The sense of taste is an oral chemical sense involved in the choice of food in mammals. Initial transduction of taste stimuli occurs in taste buds which are distributed in four discrete fields in the oral cavity. Medications can affect the taste buds, and ion channels in taste bud cell membranes are involved in stimulus transduction. The sense of taste gradually declines with aging due to a decrease in the number of taste buds, with bitter taste being most affected. The neural circuits that mediate taste in primates include cranial nerves VII, IX, X, the solitary nucleus in the brain stem, the ventroposteromedial nucleus of the thalamus, and the insular opercular cortex. The central taste pathways process taste information about sweet, salty, sour, and bitter stimuli serially and in parallel [12].

2.2.6 Suckle Feeding

Suckle feeding is a sensorimotor performance that is mature at term and becomes fully competent within 2 h of birth of a normal infant. Suckling is an infant's principal behavior during the first post-term weeks. As the infant matures, suckling becomes stronger and more rhythmic and finally the gestures of latching and rooting are acquired. Suckling is accomplished by motions of the tongue, lower lip, and lower jaw in relation to the palate [13].

2.3 Some Other Functions and Activities of the Oral Cavity

The mouth has several other functions, most of which are shared with the pharynx. The mouth and pharynx are continuously active during periods of sleep and consciousness, both as a sensory source and in sensorimotor performance. During sleep, the mouth is actively held in a stable position, except for non-nutritional suckling in infancy, which indicates periodic thalamic activation. In the awake state the mouth and pharynx actively participate in maintaining the posture of the neck as well as the position of the structures around the pharyngeal airway. The positional function is thus considered to be a major activity of the mouth and pharynx by some authors [13].

Motor stabilization of oral and pharyngeal position is continued during quiet tidal respiration; this positioning around the pharynx is the basic mechanism in maintaining the pharyngeal airway during nasal portal respiration. The oral cavity plays a role during both nasal and oral respiratory procedures. The genioglossus muscle of the tongue, in particular, is continuously active during inspiration.

In crying, the oral actions are also coordinated with those of the pharynx. During phonated expiration, the mouth opens by downward and forward displacement of the jaw. The tip of the tongue is commonly protruded forward and upward and the body of the tongue is medially grooved. These general activities of the mouth, pharynx, and larynx are achieved with the reciprocal coordination of forced expiration and inspiration. During the inspirations between cries, the tongue becomes partially flattened and rises toward the palate; and inspirations are achieved partially through the nose. External observation shows that the oral gestures of coughing are similar to those of crying. In addition, the gestures of emesis are grossly similar to those of crying expirations.

The mouth is an important erogenous area as its stimulation during sexual contact elicits psychological and endocrine responses. The mouth itself responds to sexual stimulation in other areas by an increase in sensitivity, vascularity, and salivation [13].

References

1. Seeley RR, Stephens TD, Tate P (Eds). Digestive system. In: Anatomy and physiology. 2nd Ed. St. Louis: Mosby Year Book, 1992: 773–781
2. Tortora GJ, Anagnostakos NP (Eds). The digestive system. In: Principles of anatomy and physiology. 5th Ed. New York: Harper and Row, 1987: 595–600
3. Cate TAR (Ed.). Oral mucosa. In: Oral histology. 3rd Ed. St. Louis: Mosby, 1989: 341–381
4. Thibodeau GA, Patton KT (Eds). The digestive system. In: The human body in health and disease. 1st Ed. St. Louis: Mosby, 1992: 405–411
5. Fitzpatrick TB, Eisen AZ, Wolff K, et al. (Eds). Disorders of the mucocutaneous integument. In: Dermatology in general medicine. 4th Ed. New York: McGraw Hill, 1993: 1355–1417
6. Ganong WF (Ed). Regulation of gastrointestinal function. In: Review of medical physiology. 15th Ed. London: Lange, 1993: 444–445
7. Guyton AC (Ed). Secretory functions of the alimentary tract. In: Textbook of medical physiology. 8th Ed. Philadelphia: WB Saunders, 1991: 711–713

8. Spielman AI. Interaction of saliva and taste. J Dent Res 1990: 69: 838–843
9. Berne RM, Levy MN (Eds). Gastrointestinal secretions. In: Physiology. 3rd Ed. St. Louis: Mosby, 1993: 652–658
10. XU T, Levitz SM, Diamond RD, Oppenheim FG. Anticandidal activity of major human salivary histatins. Infect Immun 1991; 59: 2549–2554
11. Berkovitz BKB, Holland GR, Moxham BJ. Color atlas and textbook of oral anatomy, histology and embryology. 2nd Ed. St. Louis: Mosby, 1992: 96–107
12. Frank ME, Hettinger TP, Mott AE. The sense of taste: Neurobiology, aging and medication effects. Crit Rev Oral Biol Med 1992; 3: 371–391
13. Paparella MM, Shumrick DA, Gluckman JL, Meyerhaff WL (Eds). Physiology. In: Otolaryngology. 3rd Ed. St. Louis: Mosby, 1991: 361–391

CHAPTER 3

Morphology of the Oral Cavity

G.L. Campanile, V. Ippolito, and T.M. Lotti

3.1 Generalities

The oral cavity includes lips, labial and buccal mucosa, floor of the mouth, tongue, palate, tonsillar pillars, and gingivae. There are many different diseases of the oral cavity that can only be diagnosed through microscopic examination; however, the clinical appearance of oral lesions can give the clinician a reliable provisional diagnosis on which to plan further management of the patient. Oral diagnosis is based upon a close examination and careful study of the individual lesions, their location, extent, and their pattern of evolution [1–3].

3.2 Types of Dermatological Individual Lesions

3.2.1 Macule

A macule is a flat, circumscribed area of change in normal skin color. It can result from pigmentary abnormalities, such as hypopigmentation (e.g., vitiligo) or hyperpigmentation (melanin or hemosiderin) (Fig. 3.1), permanent vascular abnormalities (Fig. 3.2) of the skin (e.g., capillary hemangioma) or transient capillary dilatation (erythema) (Fig. 3.3), deposits of endogenous products (bile pigments, carotene) or exogenous pigments (by tattooing or drugs).

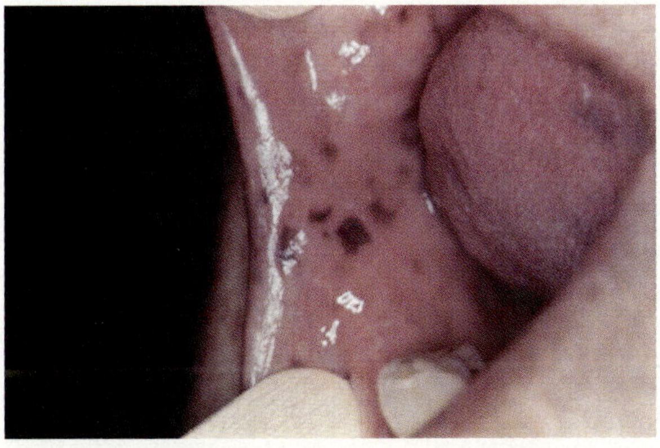

Fig. 3.1. Hypermigmented lesions on the oral mucosa (Courtesy of Prof. A. Kastsambas, Greece)

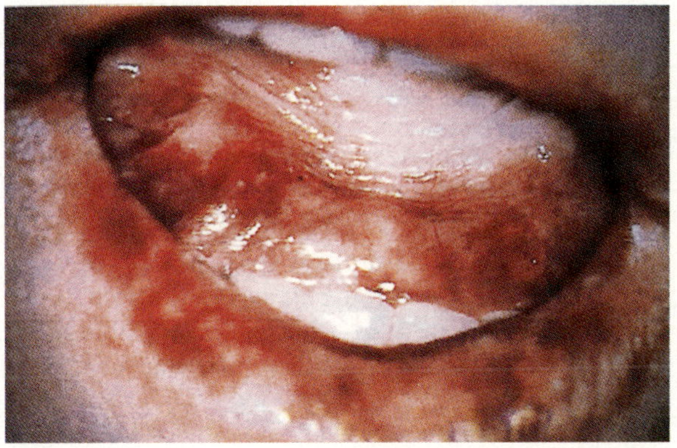

Fig. 3.2. Presence of several hemorrhagic lesions on the lips and oral mucosa

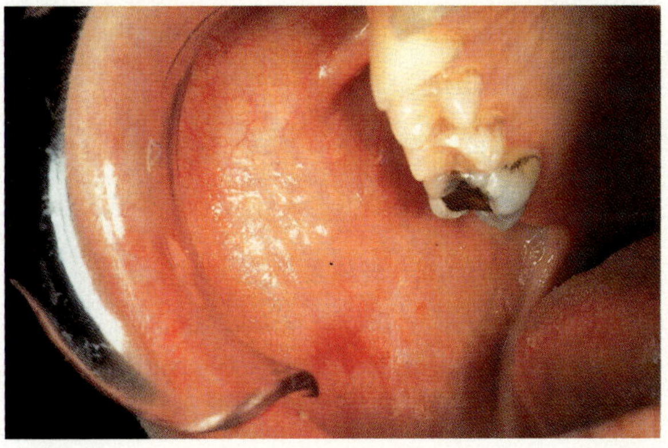

Fig. 3.3. Erythematous lesion on oral mucosa

3.2.2 Papule

A papule is a solid, elevated lesion up to 1 cm in diameter (Fig. 3.4). Epidermal papules result from circumscribed thickening of the epidermis (e.g., verruca vulgaris). Dermal papules are due to metabolic deposits in the dermis (e.g., lichen amyloidosus)

or to localized infiltrates in the dermis (e.g., lichen nitidus).

3.2.3 Plaque

A plaque is a flat, solid, elevated lesion more than 1 cm in diameter (Fig. 3.5). They are formed either by extension or coalescence of papules.

Lichenification is an inflammatory thickening of the skin with an exaggeration of the normal skin relief and deepening of the natural creases.

3.2.4 Wheal

A wheal is an evanescent pinkish plaque that often has pseudopods at its periphery. It consists of abundant edema and near absence of inflammatory cells. Wheals that do not disappear in 72 h are typical of urticarial vasculitis and a biopsy is indicated.

Angioedema is a huge wheal in distensible sites, such as the lips, tongue and eyelids (Fig. 3.6).

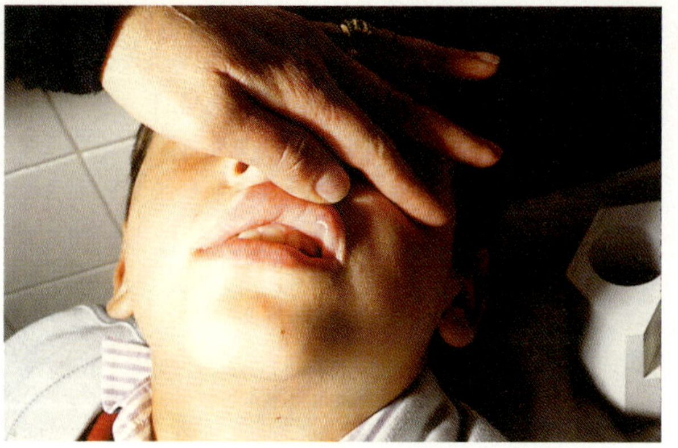

Fig. 3.6. A huge wheal in the superior lip

3.2.5 Nodule

A nodule is a palpable, round, or ellipsoidal elevated lesion greater than 1 cm in diameter. They usually result from massive infiltrates, neoplasms, or metabolic deposits in the dermis or subcutaneous tissue and often indicate systemic disease (Figs. 3.7, 3.8).

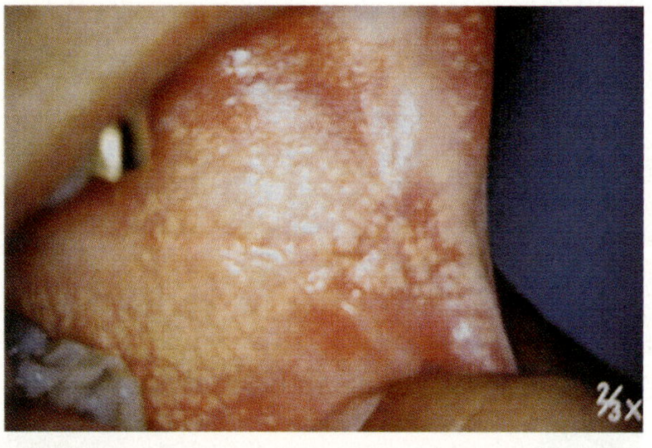

Fig. 3.4. Numerous papules localized on the oral mucosa

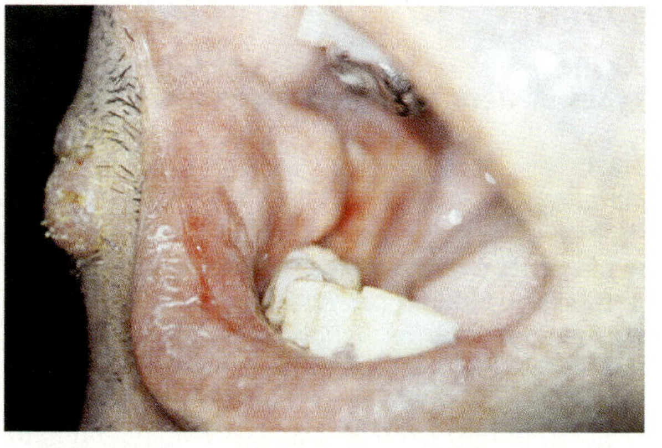

Fig. 3.7. A large nodule on the oral mucosa

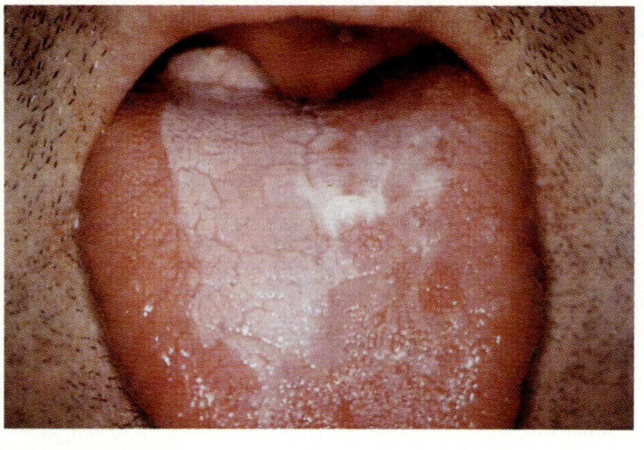

Fig. 3.5. A large plaque on the tongue

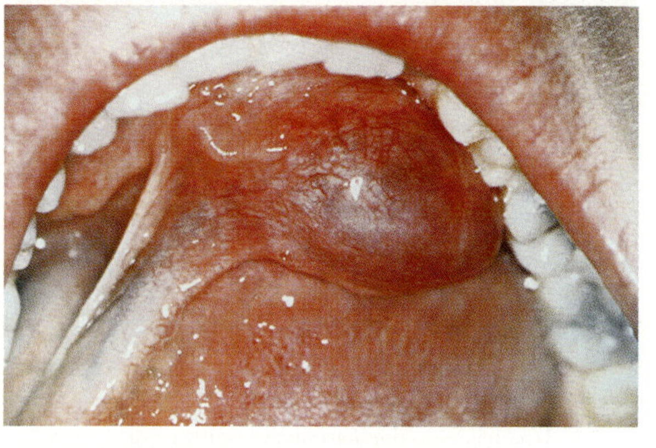

Fig. 3.8. An elevated lesion in the mouth

3.2.6 Papilloma

A papilloma is a finger-like projection above the skin surface due to upward extensions of the dermal papillae, which are usually covered by hyperplastic epidermis.

3.2.7 Pustule

A pustule is a circumscribed elevation of the skin that contains a collection of pus (neutrophils and necrotic debris). Most pustules are intraepidermal in location and they may be intracorneal (e.g., in candidiasis), subcorneal (e.g., in subcorneal pustular dermatosis), or spongiform (e.g., in pustular psoriasis). Follicular pustules are seen in acne. Bacterially caused pustules are seen in impetigo and furunculosis.

3.2.8 Vesicle

A vesicle is a fluid-filled circumscribed elevated lesion up to 1 cm in diameter. The walls are often so thin they are translucent, and the serum, lymph fluid, or extracellular fluid can be seen (Fig. 3.9). Vesicles arise from a cleavage at various levels of the skin; the cleavage may be within the epidermis (e.g., intraepidermal vesication of allergic contact dermatitis), or at the epidermal-dermal interface (e.g., subepidermal vesicles in dermatitis herpetiformis).

3.2.9 Bulla

A bulla is a fluid-filled circumscribed elevated lesion greater than 1 cm in diameter (Fig. 3.10). Bullae can also be divided into intraepidermal (e.g., pemphigus vulgaris) and subepidermal (e.g., pemphigoid) types. *Acantholysis* is a type of intraepidermal vesication due to the loss of intercellular bridges, or desmosomes. It is seen in the vesicles or bullae of pemphigus vulgaris (Fig. 3.11).

Viruses cause a curious *ballooning degeneration* of epidermal cells, as in herpes simplex, herpes zoster, and varicella.

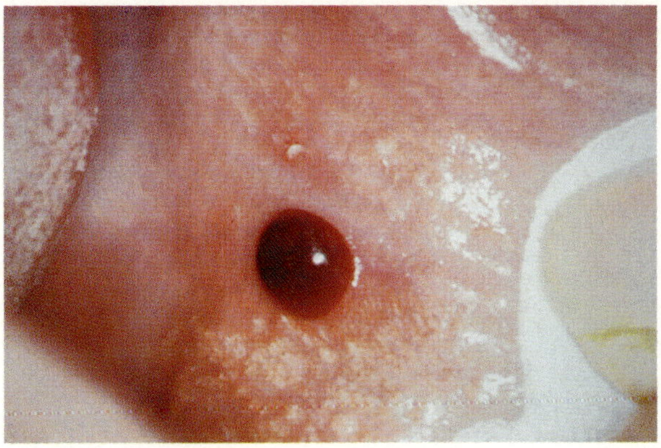

Fig. 3.10. A large hemorrhagic bulla on the oral mucosa

3.2.10 Crust

Crust develops when serum, blood, or purulent exudate dries on the skin surface. They are yellow when formed from dried serum, green or yellow-green when formed from purulent exudate, or brown or dark red when formed from blood. The typical crust is not usually evident in the oral cavity while it is an obvious sign on the lips.

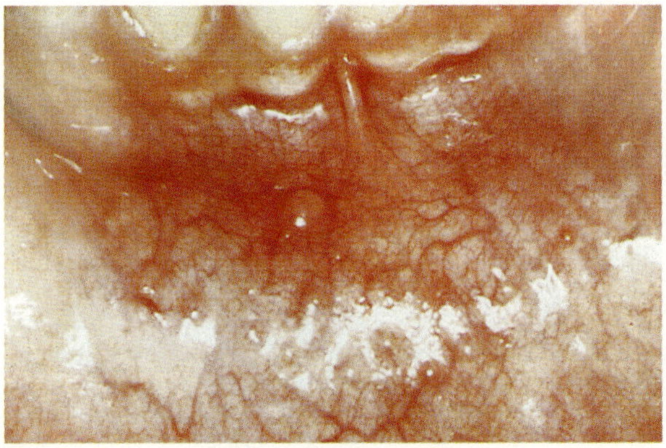

Fig. 3.9. Some vesicles on the oral mucosa

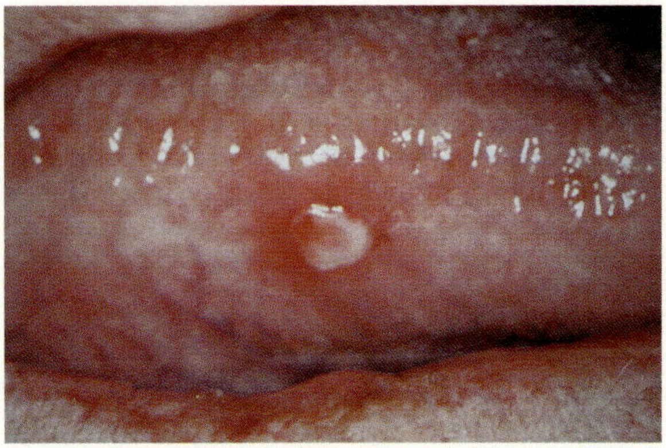

Fig. 3.11. A bulla due to acantholytic process in a patient with pemphigus vulgaris

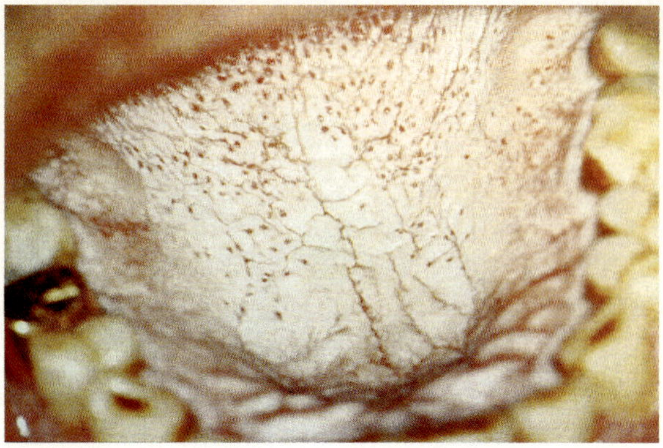

Fig. 3.12. Large desquamation of the oral cavity

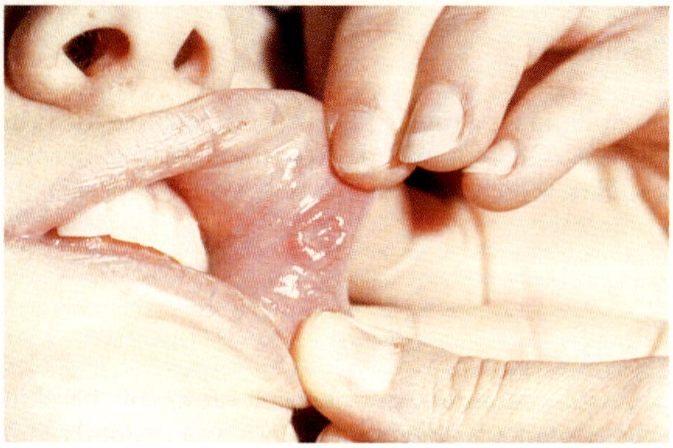

Fig. 3.13. A large erosion of the oral mucosa

3.2.11 Scale

Scales are cornified cells that have become visible on the skin surface. Scale is described as pityriasiform (fine, bran-like scales), psoriasiform (white, noncoherent scales, as in psoriasis), small-lamellar (shedding of small lamellae, as in eczema), ichthyosiform (large scales, as in ichthyosis), exfoliative (large, sheet-like, as after scarlet fever) or collarette desquamation (scales surrounding lesion, as in pityriasis rosea). Scale is an unusual finding in the oral cavity, while it may be evident in the lips (Fig. 3.12).

3.2.12 Keratosis

Keratosis is a horny growth that adheres firmly to the skin and is very difficult to remove. It may indicate a genetic impairment of keratinization or a long-term exposure to light. Follicular keratosis is typical of discoid lupus erythematosus.

3.2.13 Erosion

This is due to the loss of epithelium down to the basement membrane. It heals by reepithelization without scarring. The prototypic erosion is the denuded lesion of pemphigus vulgaris where a blister has occurred (Fig. 3.13).

3.2.14 Ulcer

An ulcer may involve tissue loss extending into the dermis or even the subcutis. An ulcer is slow to heal and inevitably leaves a scar (Fig. 3.14). It can be caused by venous insufficiency, vasculitis, chronic infection, or neoplasm. It can also be factitial, i.e., self-induced by caustics, instruments, or by the patient's own fingernails.

3.2.15 Fissure

This is a linear defect that extends from the skin surface into the dermis, especially over flexural areas (i.e., psoriasis of palms, soles, and intergluteal cleft) (Fig. 3.15).

3.2.16 Scar

A scar is a permanent fibrous secondary skin lesion and represents the end stage of an inflammatory process. A scar should be level with the skin surface. Excessive connective tissue proliferation results in a protruding *hypertrophic scar,* whereas inadequate regeneration results in an *atrophic scar* below the level of the surrounding skin.

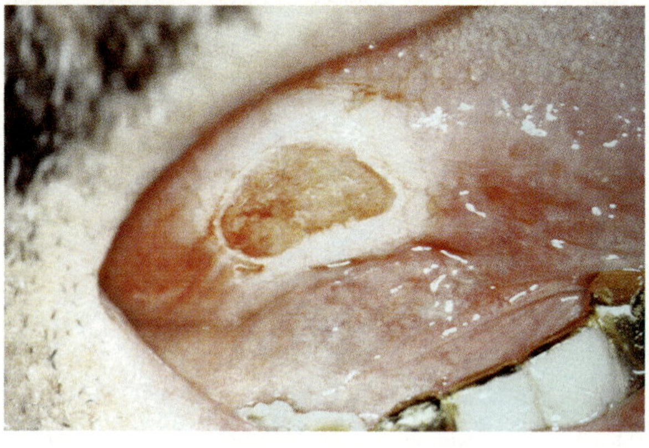

Fig. 3.14. Ulcer on the oral mucosa

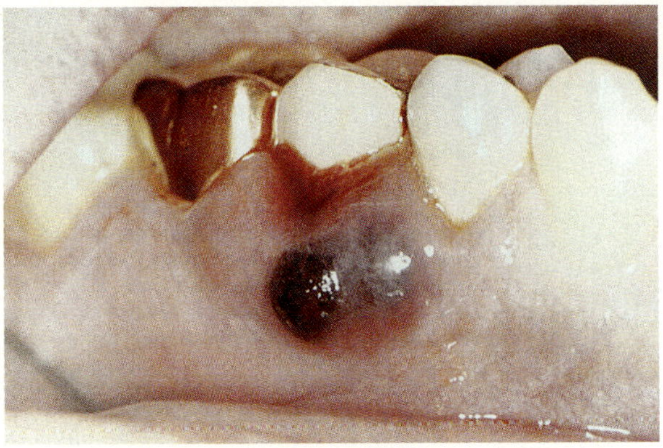

Fig. 3.15. A fissure in the oral mucosa surrounding a nodule

3.2.17
Atrophy

This is a decrease in the skin substance due usually to decreased thickness of the dermis and less commonly of the subcutaneous fat. Clinically, the characteristics are shininess, whiteness, loss of the normal skin surface markings, wrinklings, and loss of cutaneous adnexa, especially hair follicles. The best-known example is senile or actinic atrophy of the skin of the back of the hand.

3.2.18
Sclerosis

This is a circumscribed area of diffuse induration of the skin, detectable only by palpation. Hardening of the skin is seen in scleroderma, scleredema, and scleromyxedema.

3.3
Individual Lesions of Oral Mucosa

The lesions of the oral cavity are classified according to their clinical appearance and are presented in tabular form. This schematic manner of illustrating these can be helpful to clinicians in making a rational assessment of a given lesion.

3.3.1
White Lesions of Oral Mucosa

They usually appear as white or whitish surface lesions of the oral mucosa:

Desquamative gingivitis
Leukoplakia
Allergic reactions
Hereditary benign intraepithelial dyskeratosis
Stomatitis nicotina
Candidiasis
Chemical burn
Epstein's pearl
Benign hyperkeratosis
(pachyderma oris, pachyderma oralis, focal keratosis)
Carcinoma in situ
Squamous cell carcinoma
White sponge nevus
Lichen planus
White hairy tongue
Fordyce's disease
Geographic tongue

3.3.2
Vesicular or Bullous Lesions of Oral Mucosa

These are short-lived because they rupture soon after formation and leave superficial ulcers:

Primary herpetic gingivostomatitis
Aphthous ulcer
Herpes zoster
Behcet's syndrome
Pemphigus vulgaris
Smallpox and chickenpox
Hand-foot-and-mouth disease
Allergic reactions
Secondary herpetic lesion
Periadenitis mucosa necrotica recurrens
(Sutton's disease, Mikulicz's ulcer)
Erythema multiforme
Reiter's syndrome
Pemphigoid
Herpangina
Epidermolysis bullosa
Mucocele

3.3.3
Ulcerations of Oral Mucosa

In the presence of an ulcer, a number of possibilities should be considered. It should be noted that all vesicular lesions of the oral mucosa terminating in ulcers are not included among the following:

Traumatic ulcer
Eosinophilic granuloma
Candidiosis
Lymphomas and leukemias
Tuberculosis
Infectious mononucleosis
Riga-Fede disease
Vincent's stomatitis
Erosive lichen planus
Squamous cell carcinoma and other malignant epithelial tumors

Syphilitic chancre
Histoplasmosis
Lupus erythematosus
Pterygoid ulcer (Bednar's aphtha)

3.3.4 Pigmented Lesions of Oral Mucosa

Pigmentation of the oral mucosa is produced by one of the following conditions:

Black hairy tongue
Heavy metal poisoning
Amalgam tattoo
Postmenopausal state
Addison's disease
Nevus
Melanoma
Drug ingestion
Normal pigmented patches
Varicosity
Jegher's syndrome
Malnutrition
Melanotic macule

3.3.5 Soft Tissue Growths of Oral Cavity

These are divided into nonhemorrhagic, hemorrhagic, and compressible:

Firm, nonhemorrhagic
Schwannoma
Granular cell myoblastoma
Peripheral fibroma
Squamous cell carcinoma
Periodontal abscess
Pyogenic granuloma
Compressible
Mucous cyst
Lymphangioma
Cystic hygroma
Neurofibroma
Eosinophilic granuloma
Giant cell granuloma
Other malignant tumors
Eruption cyst
Ranula
Hemangioma
Lipoma
Salivary gland tumor
Irritation fibroma
Hemorrhagic
Epulis fissuratum
Pregnancy tumor
Lymphomas and leukemias
Mucocele

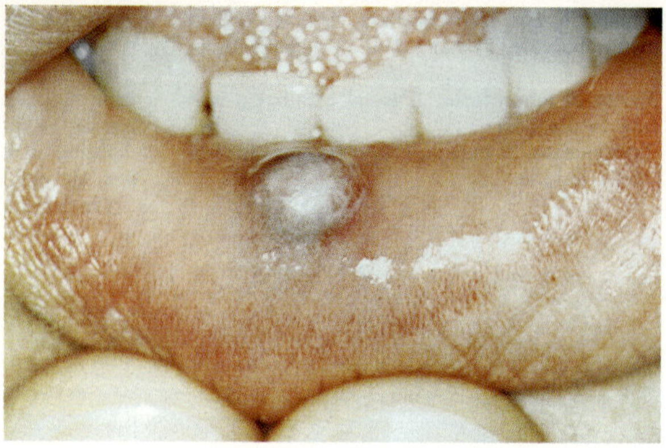

Fig. 3.16. Mucocele

Gingival cyst
Epidermoid cyst

3.3.6 Papillary or Cauliflower-Like Lesions of Oral Cavity

Verrucous leukoplakia
Condyloma acuminatum
Keratoacanthoma
Verrucous carcinoma
Verruca vulgaris
Papilloma
Inflammatory papillary hyperplasia

3.3.7 Swelling of Salivary Glands

Mucocele (Fig. 3.16)
Infectious parotitis
Sarcoidosis
Sjogren's disease
Hypertrophy
Benign tumor
Ranula
Cat-scratch-disease
Mikulicz's disease
Fatty infiltration
Sialadenitis
Malignant tumor

3.4 Laboratory Tests

Special laboratory tests are frequently required in oral pathology diagnosis. The methods of investigation important for the diagnosis of specific diseases and their indications, principles, and informational value will be discussed in greater detail in the chapters on the relevant conditions.

Patch testing is used to document and validate a diagnosis of allergic contact sensitization and identify the causative agent. It is a unique means of in vivo reproduction of disease in diminutive proportions, for sensitization affects all the skin and may therefore be elicited at any cutaneous site.

Gram stain and culture of an exudate and of a tissue specimen should be made in lesions suspected of being bacterial or yeast infection.

Microscope examination for mycelia should be made from the roof of a vesicle or of the scale. The tissue is cleared with 10 % KOH and warmed gently. Fungal cultures with Sabouraud's medium should be made.

Tzanck preparation consists of a microscopic examination of cells obtained from the base of vesicles. It may reveal the presence of giant epithelial cells and multinucleated giant cells in herpes simplex, herpes zoster, varicella, and pemphigus.

Direct and indirect immunofluorescence tests are essential for diagnosis of some autoimmune diseases (lupus erythematosus pemphigus, pemphigoid, vasculitis).

3.5 Biopsy and Histopathological Examination

Biopsy of the oral mucosa is one of the most rewarding diagnostic techniques in medical practice for the relatively easy accessibility of the oral mucosa and the variety of techniques for study of the excised specimen (e.g., immunofluorescence, electron microscopy).

The selection of the site of the biopsy is based primarily on the stage of the eruption (early lesions are usually more typical). This is especially important in vesiculo-bullous eruptions (e.g., pemphigus), in which the lesion should be no more than 24 h old. However, older lesions (2–6 weeks) are often more characteristic in discoid lupus erythematosus.

A common technique for diagnostic biopsy is the use of a 3.0–4.0-mm punch which by rotating movements cuts through the epidermis, dermis, and subcutaneous tissue; the base is cut off with scissors.

Specimens for light microscopy should be fixed immediately in buffered neutral formalin. A brief but detailed summary of the clinical history and description of the lesions should accompany the specimen.

Some limitations of histopathological diagnosis are technical and may be due to failure to adhere to the principles outlined above. However, even an ideal preparation, good clinical information, and an experienced dermatohistopathologist do not always guarantee an unequivocal diagnosis. Only certain reactive patterns are sometimes discernible in inflammatory diseases that can be assessed only in conjunction with the clinical data. Problems of differential histopathological diagnosis occur in granulomatous inflammation (sarcoidosis, leprosy, tertiary syphilis, deep fungus infection) or between keratoacanthoma and squamous cell carcinoma [1, 3].

References

1. Archard HO. Biology and pathology of the oral mucosa. In: Fitzpatrick TB, Eisen, AZ, Wolff K et al. (eds). Dermatology in general medicine. 3rd Ed., New York: McGraw-Hill; 1987: pp 1152–1239
2. Shafer WG, Hine MK, Levy BM (Eds). A textbook of oral pathology, 4th Ed., Philadelphia: Saunders; 1983
3. Braun-Falco O, Plewig G, Wolff HH, Winkelmann RK (Eds). Dermatology, 4th Ed., Heidelberg: Springer-Verlag, 1991

CHAPTER 4

Cytodiagnosis for Oral Disorders

V. Ruocco and F. Pinto

4.1 Introduction

Exfoliative cytology of the oral cavity has been clinically used for years as an important diagnostic means [1–4] because the oral mucosa is particularly suitable for making cytologic diagnoses for anatomical reasons (easy and immediate access) and due to biological conditions. In fact, the continuous epitheliocyte turnover and the presence of saliva, which represents a real physiological dispersion medium, allow the harvesting of cells in a satisfactory manner most of the time.

4.2 Procedure for Smear Taking

The method used for taking cytological smears is of great importance to the diagnosis and some experience is essential. Before preparing a cytological smear, the oral mucosa should be cleaned with a non-irritant antiseptic collutory; for keratotic and leukoplakic lesions we use compresses of sodium bicarbonate (3 %) for a keratolytic effect. The smear is taken from the active edge of the lesion and from fresh, untreated lesions.

A straight-bladed scalpel is used for papular, nodular and infiltrative lesions and for unruptured vesicles and bullae. A blunt-ended spatula, of wood or steel, is used for erosions or ulcerations. An aspirating needle may be used for some carcinomas and deep lesions.

4.3 Technical Hints on Fixation and Staining; Observation of Cytological Preparations from the Oral Mucosa

The material obtained is spread uniformly. Smears must be fixed and stained before they can be examined microscopically. The stain most frequently used in oral mucosa cytodiagnosis is the May Grünwald-Giemsa dye, which does not involve pretreatment with a fixative. The slides are simply air-dried, or dried in an incubator at 37 °C. For Papanicolaou's stain, particularly employed for the diagnosis of carcinoma, the most frequently used fixative is a mixture of equal parts of 95 % ethyl alcohol with ethyl ether. For bullous autoimmune diseases (e.g. pemphigus), we also use the technique of immunocytofluorescence that requires fluorescein-conjugated antiserum and UV microscopy.

4.4 Use of Cytological Smears for Oral Disorders

In this chapter we describe the cytological pictures of dermatological disorders with oral involvement for which cytodiagnosis may be useful [5]. For practical purposes we divided them into infectious, immunological and neoplastic diseases. We also hint at the cytological features of topical disorders of oral mucosa (herpangina) involved in the differential diagnosis with dermatological diseases (Table 4.1). For a correct interpretation of the cytological test we first describe the normal cell pattern from the oral cavity.

4.4.1 Normal Cell Pattern from the Oral Cavity

Smears from the oral cavity usually contain a fair number of cells. The epithelial cells of the buccal mucosa do not differ essentially from those of the skin. These cells have a laminar and polygonal or circular cytoplasm which stains variably according to the degree of maturity of the cells. The nucleus appears round and single, small and dark (pycnotic in the superficial layers) (Fig. 4.1). In some areas (lip, cheek mucosa, soft palate, crevicular epithelium, alveolar mucosa, sublingual mucosa), the stratum granulosum is lacking and physiological parakeratosis occurs forming nucleated epitheliocytes. In other areas (gingiva, hard palate, dorsum of tongue), like the skin, the stratum granulosum is present and

Table 4.1. Usefulness of cytodiagnosis for oral disorders

Disease	Cytological pattern	Validity of the test
Herpes simplex (primary herpetic gingivostomatitis, recurrent herpes labialis, secondary herpetic stomatitis)	Ballooning cells, hypertrophic and multinucleate cells, viral nuclear inclusion bodies	Diagnostic for viral group
Herpes zoster	Ballooning cells, hypertrophic and multinucleate cells, viral nuclear inclusion bodies	Diagnostic for viral group
Hand-foot-mouth disease	Multinucleate epitheliocytes, syncytial moderately hypertrophic nuclei	Diagnostic for viral group
Herpangina	Multinucleate epitheliocytes, syncytial moderately hypertrophic nuclei	Diagnostic for viral group
Oral molluscum contagiosum	Henderson-Patterson's bodies	Diagnostic
Mucocutaneous leishmaniasis	*Leishmania* organisms (Leishman-Donovan bodies) within macrophages (Wright's cells) or extracellulary	Diagnostic
Pemphigus vulgaris	Acantholytic cells, Sertoli's rosette phenomenon, leukocyte adherence, IgG and C3 on the epithelial cell membrane with DIF	Diagnostic (if performed by DIF also)
Bullous pemphigoid	Scarcity of epithelial cells, leukocyte adherence	Orientative for pemphigoid group
Cicatricial pemphigoid	Scarcity of epithelial cells, leukocyte adherence	Orientative for pemphigoid group
Stevens-Johnson syndrome	Leukocytes, fibrin filaments, necrotic epitheliocytes, fibroblasts	Useful to rule out pemphigus
Erosive lichen planus	Leukocytes, fibrin filaments, necrotic epitheliocytes, fibroblasts	Useful to rule out pemphigus
Recurrent aphthous stomatitis	Leukocytes, fibrin filaments, necrotic epitheliocytes, fibroblasts	Useful to rule out herpetic infections
Squamous cell carcinoma	Epithelial cells with nuclear dysplasia, alterations of cytoplasm staining properties	Orientative
Oral malignant melanoma	Atypical melanocytes ("fly-eye" nuclei), macronuclealization	Diagnostic (in most cases)

anuclear epitheliocytes are produced. In addition to epithelial cells, there may be neutrophilic leukocytes, sometimes histiocytes and, frequently, contamination by bacteria or fungi.

4.5 Infectious Diseases

4.5.1 Herpes Group

Herpes simplex virus (HSV) infection is common. In the oral cavity, HSV1 causes both primary herpetic stomatitis and secondary infections (recurrent herpes labialis or, rarely, secondary herpetic stomatitis). Oral infection by HSV2 may also be seen. In varicella, oral lesions are common and show a predilection for the palate and the lips. Herpes zoster can affect maxillary or mandibular branches of the trigeminal nerve and causes mouth ulcers surrounded by a broad erythematous zone.

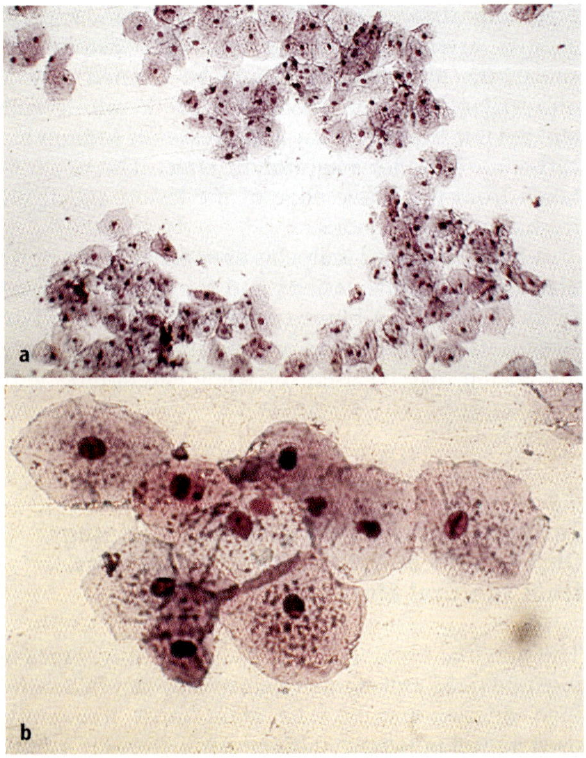

Fig. 4.1 a, b. Normal epitheliocytes from the oral cavity. May Grünwald-Giemsa. **a**, ×100; **b**, ×1000 ►

Clinical recognition of these diseases is usually easy, but diagnostic problems may arise with atypical cases of recurrent herpes labialis vs oral fixed drug eruption or vs aphthous ulcers of the herpetiform type. All doubts can easily be resolved by cytologic examination, which, in case of herpes infection, shows virally modified epithelial cells. The cytological features of herpes simplex (types I and II) and varicella-zoster are basically indistinguishable, so that monoclonal antibodies are needed to characterize the group (HZV or HVS) and the type (HSV1 or HSV2) of the virus involved. Cytologically, herpes infection is characterized by hypertrophic epitheliocytes (ballooning cells) having different sizes and a round or oval shape. The cytoplasm appears hyperbasophilic, the nucleus is bulky (sometimes dramatically enlarged) and the chromatin structure is poorly defined (Figs. 4.2, 4.3). There are many multinucleate cells (multinucleate giant cells). The presence of characteristic intranuclear inclusion bodies is pathognomonic of viral infection.

4.5.2 Infections by Coxsackie Viruses (Hand-Footh-Mouth Disease, Herpangina)

Hand-footh-mouth disease is mainly caused by Coxsackie A viruses, sometimes by Coxsackie B viruses or other enteroviruses. The incubation period is 3–10 days and the clinical features are characterized by round or ovoid mouth ulcers, which are usually sparse and affecting any site of the oral cavity.

Herpangina is mostly caused by Coxsackie viruses. The incubation period is 3–7 days and it predominantly affects young children. Clinically, mouth ulcers, mostly on the soft palate, are present.

In both infections the affected epitheliocytes show a distinctive cytopathic effect that is useful for the diagnosis. The cells appear moderately hypertrophic, with a large and basophilic cytoplasm, an enlarged – often multiple – nucleus: in multinucleated elements the size of individual nuclei are quite uniform and this gives the cells a typical syncytial appearance (Fig. 4.4).

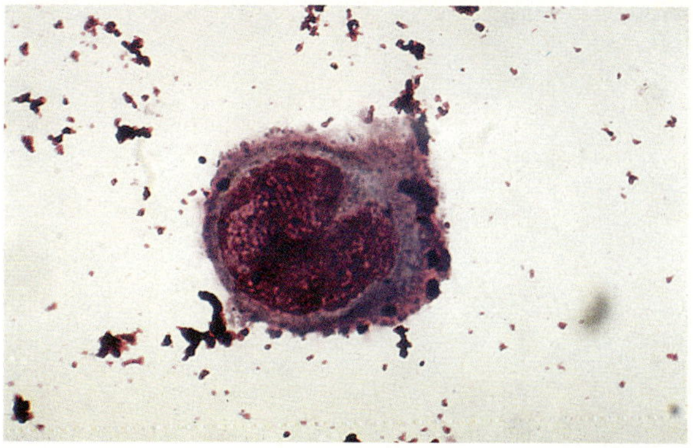

Fig. 4.3. Herpes zoster: ballooning cell with hypertrophic, bilobated nucleus. May Grünwald-Giemsa, ×1000

4.5.3 Molluscum Contagiosum

Molluscum contagiosum is an infectious disease caused by poxviruses. The oral involvement is rare and it presents some difficulty for clinical diagnosis. The cytological picture is characterized by Malpighian cells that appear large, round or oval in shape and homogeneous in structure. They are hyperbasophilic, with no visible nucleus, and contain intracytoplasmic inclusions (molluscum bodies or Henderson-Patterson's bodies) (Fig. 4.5). These cells represent epitheliocytes which are profoundly altered by the presence of viruses.

4.5.4 Mucocutaneous Leishmaniasis

The clinical diagnosis of leishmaniasis with labial or oral localizations is very difficult. In the initial stages cytological techniques can demonstrate the presence

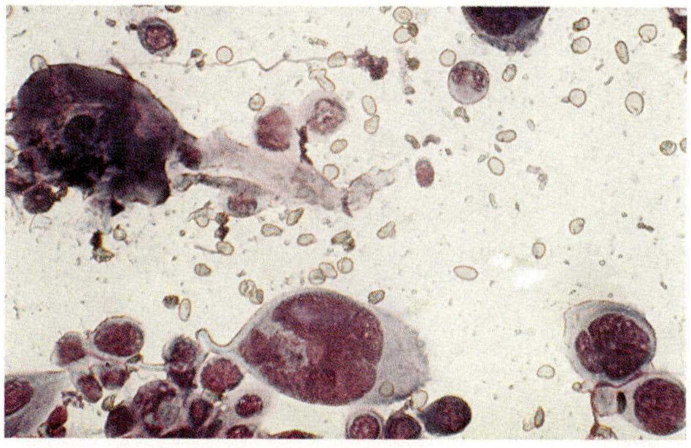

Fig. 4.2. Herpes simplex: ballooning cells with remarkable hypertrophic nuclei. May Grünwald-Giemsa, ×200

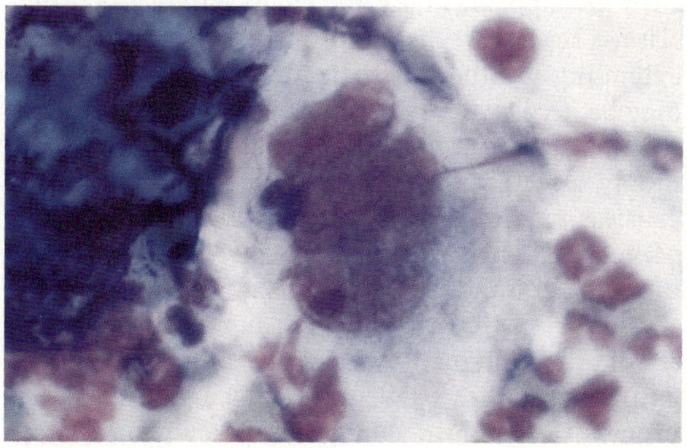

Fig. 4.4. Hand-footh-mouth disease: syncytial nuclei. May Grünwald-Giemsa, ×1000

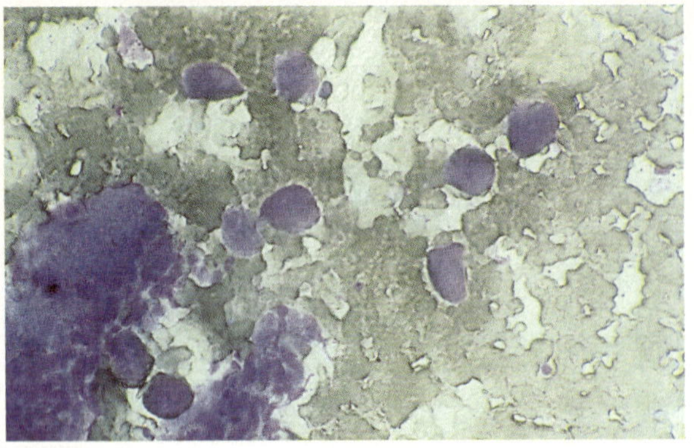

Fig. 4.5. Oral molluscum contagiosum: Henderson-Patterson's bodies. May Grünwald-Giemsa, ×400

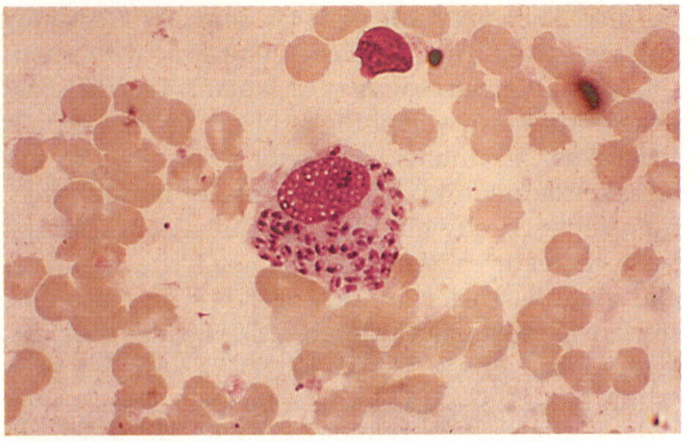

Fig. 4.6. Perioral cutaneous leishmaniasis: *Leishmania* organisms within Wright's cell. May Grünwald-Giemsa, ×1000

of causative organisms (Leishman-Donovan bodies or *Leishmaniae*), a finding which is obviously diagnostic.

In the smears, *Leishmaniae*, which are amastigote protozoa, appear as small (2–4 µm long) blue, ovoid, ellipsoid or pyriform bodies, with a basophilic cytoplasm, an eccentric true nucleus (trophonucleus) and a smaller paranuclear formation (kinetoplast) that gives rise to a very small endocytoplasmic flagellum; both trophonucleus and kinetoplast stain bright red.

Several parasites (about 20–40) are usually found within large (20–30 µm) macrophagic histiocytes (Wright's cells) (Fig. 4.6), where protozoa are often grouped together with the characteristic "swarm of bees" appearance. Isolated extracellular *Leishmaniae* are sometimes detected.

4.6 Immunological Diseases

4.6.1 Pemphigus Vulgaris

In more than two-thirds of cases, pemphigus vulgaris first appears in the oral cavity where it may persist for several weeks, months, or even years before extending to other sites. In the oral cavity any site may be involved, but the soft palate, the buccal mucosa and the lower lip are usually the most commonly affected areas. Oral bullae rapidly rupture causing painful erosions that show little evidence of healing. The oral erosions, therefore, represent the most common presenting signs of pemphigus.

The cytological diagnosis of pemphigus vulgaris should be obtained both from light microscopy and from studies using ultraviolet light [1, 3]. The procedure for smear taking requires a gentle scraping that permits the easy harvesting of the cells involved in the acantholytic process.

On light microscopy the cytological pattern of pemphigus vulgaris is characterized by epithelial cells that retain those particular morphological features (acantholytic changes) which were originally due to the pathogenetic mechanism (acantholysis). The acantholytic cells (or Tzanck's cells) (Fig. 4.7) appear either isolated or clustered in small groups which maintain a certain cohesion. They are round in shape and usually have a basophilic cytoplasm, especially at their periphery (hyperchromatic ring). The nucleus appears hypertrophic and shows very atypical neoplastic-like changes (double or multiple nuclei, mitotic and amitotic divisions), but the nucleoli look "hazy" and do not stand out from the other nuclear structures. Phenomena of cell adherence represent other characteristic, but not pathognomonic, signs of pemphigus. Sertoli's rosette phenomenon consists of cell aggregates with an epithelial cell at the center surrounded by a ring of leukocytes (Fig. 4.8). Leukocyte adherence is characterized by several cells ("streptocytes") that are joined by a filamentous, fibrinoid, glue-like substance [1].

By the immunocytofluorescence technique (using anti-IgG serum and anti-C3 serum) isolated

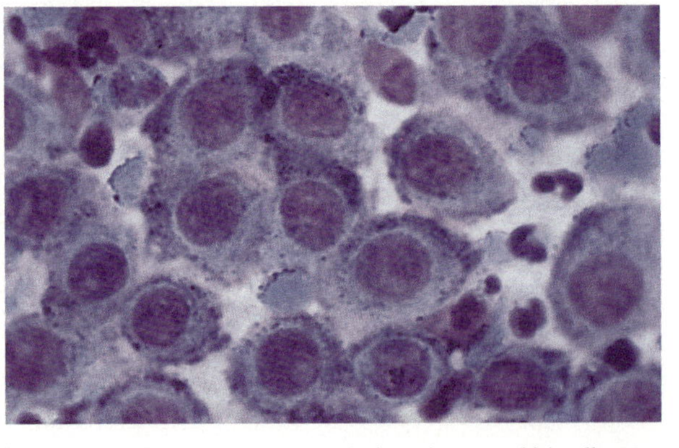

Fig. 4.7. Pemphigus vulgaris: acantholytic (or Tzanck's) cells. May Grünwald-Giemsa, ×1000

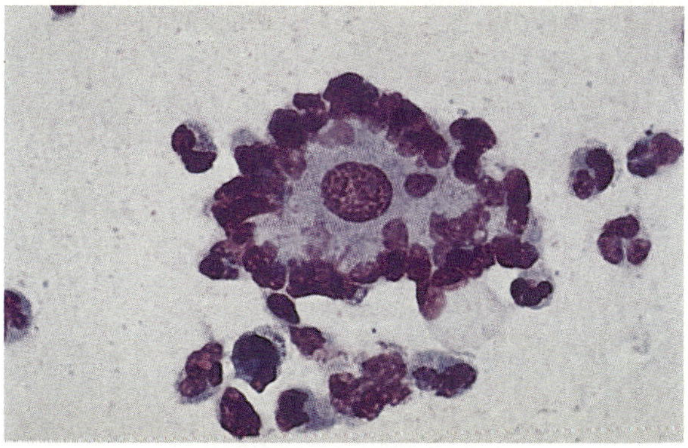

Fig. 4.8. Pemphigus vulgaris: Sertoli's rosette phenomenon. May Grünwald-Giemsa, ×1000

acantholytic cells show a typical fluorescence of the membranes (Fig. 4.9). When the cells are grouped together, the fluorescence has a network-like appearance, the same as histological preparations. These patterns are typical of pemphigus.

4.6.2 Pemphigoid Group: Bullous Pemphigoid and Cicatricial Pemphigoid

Bullous pemphigoid is a chronic autoimmune mucocutaneous bullous disease that prevalently affects elderly persons. Its onset is characterized by a nonspecific, generalized, often pruritic rash (a mixture of erythema and wheals). Later on, large, tense bullae develop that rupture, leaving denuded areas on the trunk, arms and legs. The oral involvement occurs in about one-third of cases, but it is usually delayed. Bullae and, ultimately, erosions develop most frequently on the buccal mucosa, palate, tongue and lower lip. A gingival involvement, such as "desquamative gingivitis," is also possible.

The cytological pattern is characterized by lack of acantholytic cells, scarcity of epithelial cells, abundance of blood cells (neutropus and eosinophils)

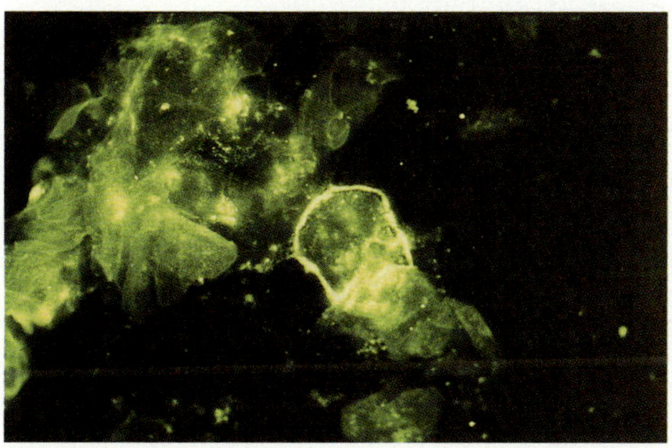

Fig. 4.9. Pemphigus vulgaris: IgG on an isolated epithelial cell membrane. DIF: anti-IgG serum with fluorescein, ×400

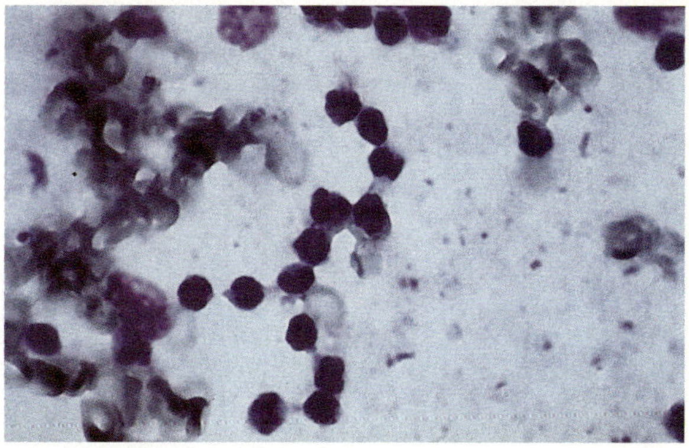

Fig. 4.10. Bullous pemphigoid: leucocyte adherence ("streptocytes"). May Grünwald- Giemsa, ×1000

and by leukocyte adherence (Fig. 4.10). In bullous pemphigoid, immunocytofluorescence, using anti-IgG serum and anti-C3 serum, can show a linear, fluorescent band confined to one of the cellular poles [1].

4.6.3 Stevens-Johnson Syndrome, Erosive Lichen Planus, Recurrent Aphthous Stomatitis

Although completely different from the clinical-pathogenic standpoint, these three disorders exhibit a quite similar and rather aspecific cytological picture, which is characterized by leukocytes, mostly neutrophils and lymphocytes, fibrin filaments, more or less altered, and frankly necrotic epitheliocytes and fibroblasts (Fig. 4.11). Though trivial, such a finding can be equally useful to rule out other oral disorders which may clinically mimic the above pictures, but the cytology of which is completely different. This is the case of pemphigus vulgaris, which is often the object of differential diagnosis from both Stevens-Johnson syndrome and erosive lichen planus. The same is true for some vesicular viral diseases (oral herpes simplex, hand-footh-mouth disease) with isolated lesions, which can be mistaken for recurrent aphthous stomatitis. In such circumstances, the absence of acantholytic cells is a finding that excludes the suspicion of pemphigus, while the absence of ballooning cells and multinucleated syncytial elements rules out the diagnoses of herpes or Coxsackie virus infections, respectively.

4.7 Neoplastic Diseases

4.7.1 Squamous Cell Carcinoma

More than 90% of malignant neoplasms in the mouth are squamous cell carcinomas. Nearly 30% of all oral cancers affect the lips, and about 25% af-

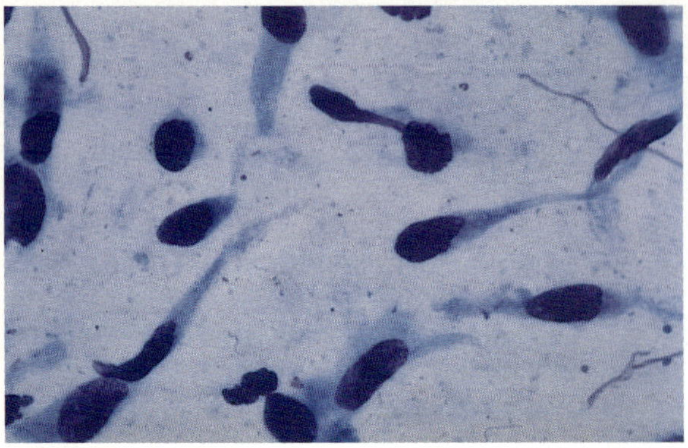

Fig. 4.11. Stevens-Johnson syndrome: fibroblasts and few lymphocytes. May Grünwald-Giemsa, ×1000

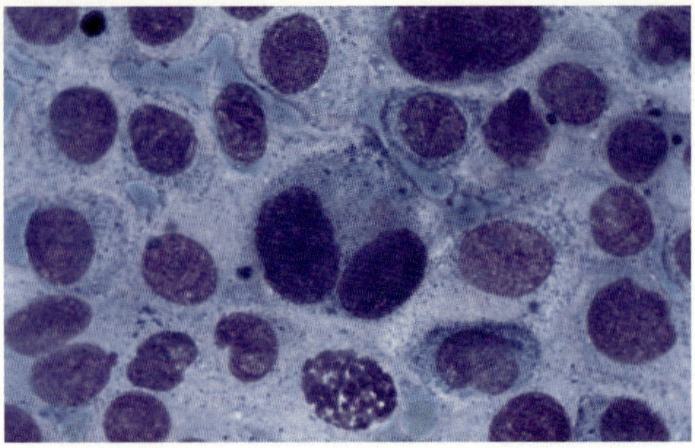

Fig. 4.13. Oral malignant melanoma: atypical melanocytes, one of them (centre) with "fly-eye" nuclei. May Grünwald-Giemsa, ×1000

fect the tongue, the common intraoral site. Most intraoral cancers involve the lateral edge of the tongue and/or the floor of the mouth (the "graveyard area"), though the reason why this site appears predisposed to tumour development is unclear. In some patients who develop oral cancer, the tumour arises from clinically definable premalignant lesions such as erythroplasia, some types of leukoplakia, oral submucous fibrosis or erosive lichen planus. The most demonstrative cytological patterns can be obtained by nodular, ulcerated, non-keratotic lesions.

Distinguishing cytological features of a squamous cell carcinoma at low magnification are paucity of cells, absence of clusters of cells and cellular pleomorphism. At higher magnification the squamous cells show nuclear alterations (hypertrophic, hyperchromic, lobated or multiple nuclei, abnormal mitoses) and a more basophilic cytoplasm than is normal (Fig. 4.12). The cytology of squamous cell carcinoma is only preliminary and it is always wiser to complete the examination by histological studies.

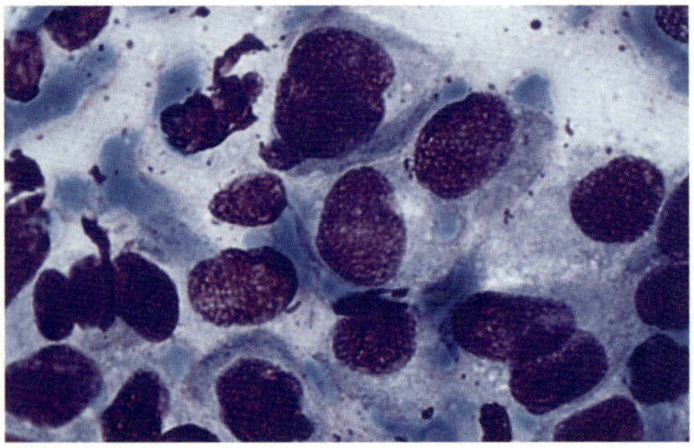

Fig. 4.12. Squamous cell carcinoma: epitheliocytes with severe nuclear dysplasia. May Grünwald-Giemsa, ×1000

4.7.2 Oral Malignant Melanoma

Oral malignant melanoma is rare. Most patients are over 50 years of age and men. Malignant melanoma may arise in an apparently normal oral mucosa or in a pre-existent pigmented naevus. The most common site of oral melanoma is the palate or the maxillary alveolus.

The cytodiagnosis of melanoma is allowed only for ulcerated lesions, where a very gentle scraping can immediately clinch the clinical suspicion of this neoplasm. The microscopic picture is characterized by atypical melanocytes that show marked variations in shape (round, oval, elongated, spindle-shaped cells). The cytoplasm contains melanin granules, which are very important for the diagnosis, and a highly atypical nucleus. Pathognomonic features are cells with "fly-eye" nuclei and the presence of a large nucleolus (macro-nucleolization (Fig. 4.13). In any case, histological confirmation is mandatory.

4.8 Conclusions

The use of oral mucosa cytology as an immediate aid in helping to establish a precise clinical diagnosis in certain diseases should be stressed. In this note we have treated the most important cytological patterns of some oral disorders which also involve the skin. The technique for this methodology is practical, useful, simple and quick. The test proves to be demonstrative for some infections like leishmaniasis, viral diseases as well as for pemphigus vulgaris, while it is only orientative for bullous pemphigoid and squamous cell carcinoma. Notwithstanding its advantages, cytodiagnosis is not intended to be a substitute for standard histology.

References

1. Ruocco V. Cytodiagnosis in dermatology. Napoli: CLU (Ed), 1980
2. Barr RJ. Cutaneous cytology. J Am Acad Dermatol 1984, 10: 163–180
3. Ruocco V, Coscia-Porrazzi L, Pisani M. Reliability of cytodiagnosis in oral pemphigus vulgaris. A study of 30 cases. J Dermatol 1984; 11: 535–540
4. Gombos F, Ruocco V. Stomatologia: la citodiagnosi. In: Coppo M, Gibertini P (Eds) Dizionario delle analisi e ricerche cliniche d'uso corrente. Padova: Piccin Nuova Libraria S.p.a. (Ed), 1991: 1331–1342
5. Scully C. The oral cavity. In: Rook/Wilkinson/Ebling. Textbook of dermatology, 5th Ed. Oxford: Blackwell Scientific Publications, 1992: 2689–2760

Development and Embryology of Oral Mucosa and Structures: Developmental Disturbances

C. Feliciani and R. Jordan

5.1 Developmental Disorders

Disordered embryonic development can lead to a wide range of developmental disorders in the oral cavity. Many of these are related to the disordered or incomplete fusion of separate developmental lines of the face. Whilst some are relatively common and often trivial, others are rare and can be more serious. For example, small developmental cysts are commonly found on the palate of newborns. It is believed, by some, that these are the result of epithelial entrapment in the median palatal raphe. Others hold that they are the result of epithelial remnants of developing salivary glands. These cysts are termed Epstein's pearls when they occur in the midline of the palate and Bohn's nodules when they occur scattered on the palate. Ectopic sebaceous glands are common and termed Fordyce's granules. They can be found in 80 % of the population and hence are not generally considered a true developmental abnormality but rather a variant of normal development. It was long held that median rhomboid glossitis (central papillary atrophy) was a developmental abnormality due to failure of the tuberculum impar to retract or withdraw before the fusion of the lateral halves of the tongue. In this condition there is a red, rhomboid-shaped flattening of the filliform papillae on the dorsum of the tongue, immediately anterior to the circumvalate papillae. Its absence in children and histological features now support a strong aetiological relationship with *Candida albicans* rather than as a developmental disturbance. Failure of the fusion of developmental fissures of the face can lead to more serious facial clefting such as the cleft lip and palate and the cleft palate alone. Uncorrected, these conditions can be associated potentially with significant morbidity. A very rare developmental disorder is the lack of fungiform and circumvallate papillae which is found in the dysautonomia syndrome. This condition is also associated with other systemic manifestations related to altered autonomic nerve function [1–8].

5.2 Embryological Development of the Oral Cavity (Figs. 5.1–5.5)

The embryological development of the head, face and oral cavity is a complicated process characterised by the proliferation, migration and fusion of a number of different embryological tissues. The primitive mouth develops as a head fold that is lined by ectoderm and is separated from the gut by the buccopharyngeal membrane. The proliferation of the branchial arches together with migra-

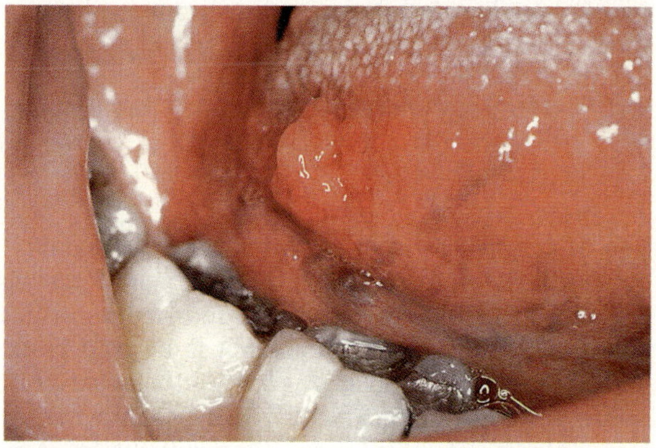

Fig. 5.1. Lingual tonsil

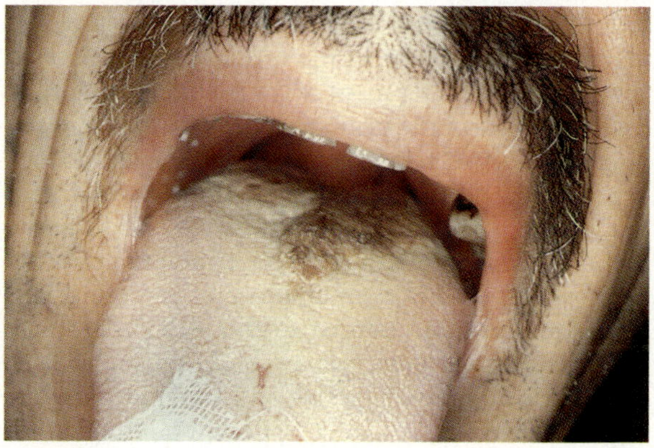

Fig. 5.2. Small median rhomboid glossitis in a patient with black hairy tongue

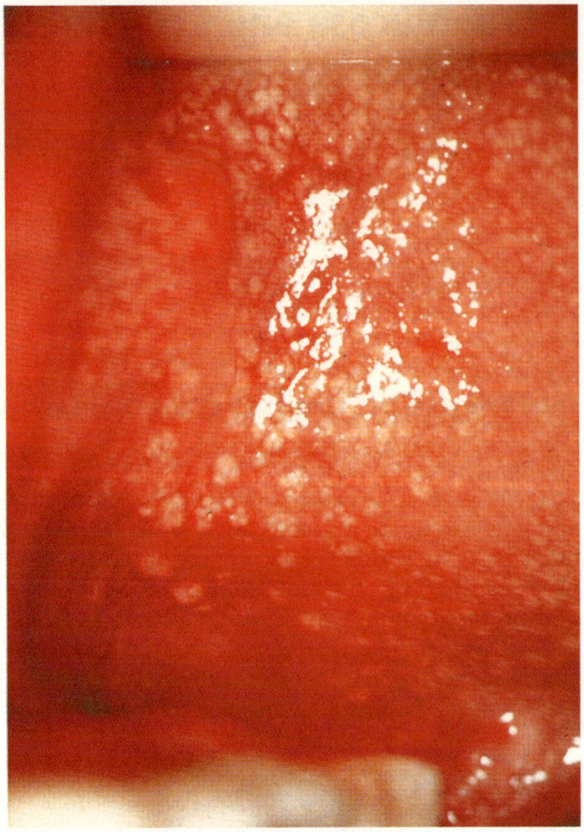

Fig. 5.3. Fordyce's granules on the inner side of the buccal mucosa

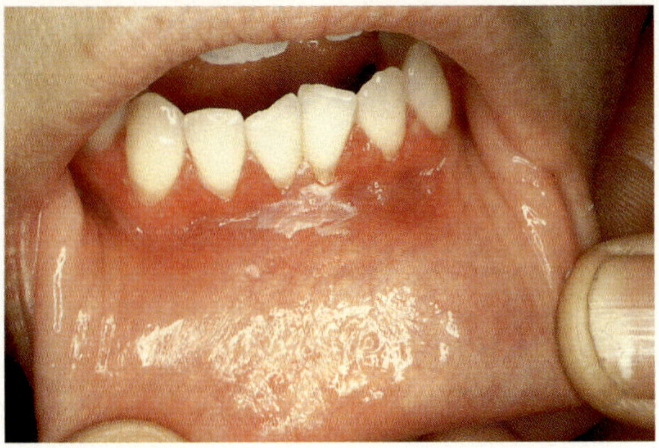

Fig. 5.4. Fordyce's granules in a patient with cicatricial pemphigoid

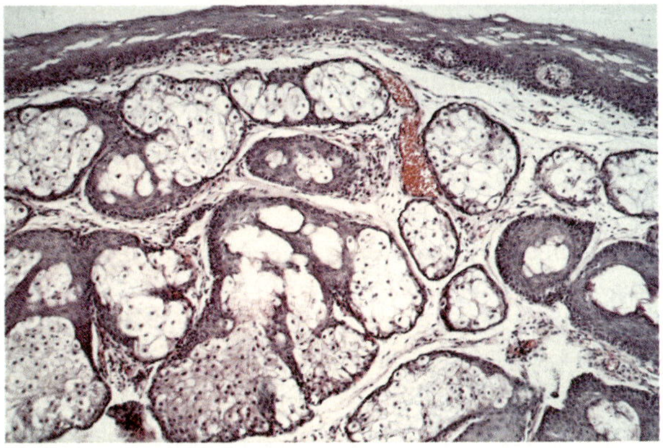

Fig. 5.5. Fordyce's granules. Histology

tion of neural crest cells form fundamental components of the facial structures. Early development of the face, in days 24–28, is dominated by the proliferation of ectomesenchyme which is derived from neural crest tissues. At about day 28 the nasal processes develop as bulges in the head. The upper lip is formed from the paired maxillary processes on each side and the medial nasal processes. Failure of these structures to fuse results in a cleft upper lip. The lower lip is formed from the fusion of the two mandibular processes. Fusion of the medial nasal processes results in the development of the premaxilla which is destined to form the primary palate and contain the maxillary incisor teeth. Separation of the nasal from oral cavities occurs at between 7 and 8 weeks with the formation of the secondary palate. The tongue withdraws down into the oral cavity and the palatine shelves rotate to a horizontal position and then close in the midline. In contrast to the closure of facial bulges that form the face, union of the palatal shelves is a true fusion requiring the epithelial lining covering the two processes to disappear. The tongue begins to develop at about 4 weeks and is the result of the local proliferation of a number of swellings in the floor of the mouth. The tuberculum impar arises in the midline and is flanked by two lateral swellings which fuse to form the anterior portion of the tongue. The posterior portion of the tongue is formed from the hypobranchial eminence, a large midline swelling arising from the third branchial arch mesenchyme. Hence, the composition of the tongue from different embryological tissues explains the differing cranial nerve supply of the anterior and posterior portions.

5.2.1 Cleft Lip and Palate (Figs. 5.6, 5.7)

Cleft lip and palate results from the fusion failure of the median nasal prominence and the maxillary process during the embryological development of the face. The aetiologies of cleft lip, cleft lip and palate, or cleft palate alone are not known. Some occur as components of one of the approximately 250 syndromes that are associated with clefting of the face. In these instances cleft lip and palate can be inherited in autosomal dominant, autosomal recessive or X-linked fashions. A number of genetic and/

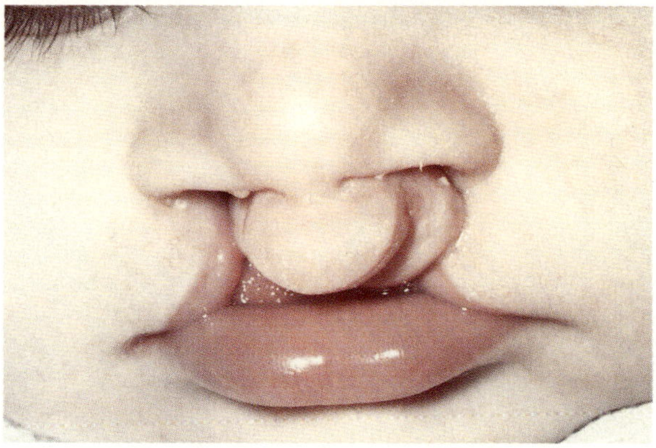

Fig. 5.6. Cleft lip. (Courtesy of Dr. Gianfranco Favia, University of Bari, Dental School, Bari, Italy)

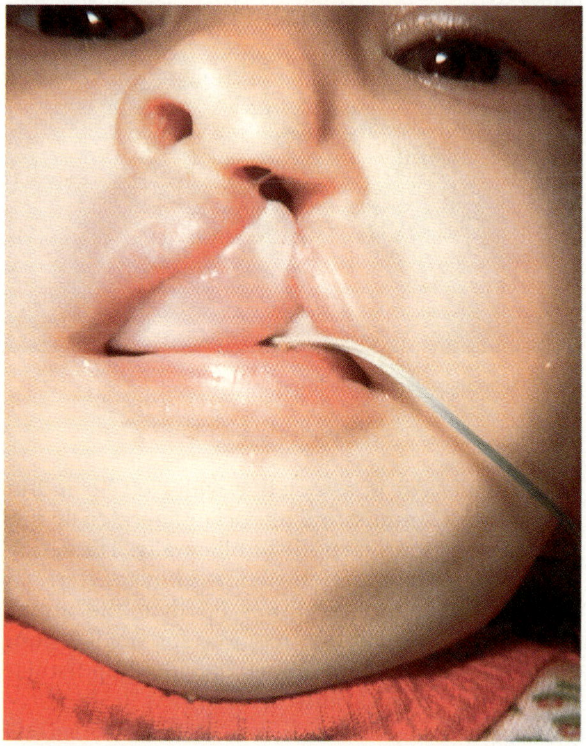

Fig. 5.7. Cleft lip and palate. (Courtesy of Dr. Gianfranco Favia, University of Bari, Dental School, Bari, Italy)

or environmental factors may contribute to those cases of facial clefting not associated with a recognised syndrome.

Common to all is the inhibition of neural crest cell migration and fusion of mesenchyme at the junction between developmental processes of the face. Most commonly, cleft lip occurs together with cleft palate, accounting for 45 % of these facial clefting conditions. Cleft lip alone accounts for 30 % of cases and one-quarter occur as cleft palate alone. Cleft lip alone and cleft lip and palate are aetiologically related and distinct from isolated cleft palate. There are considerable racial differences in the incidence of cleft lip and palate. In whites the prevalence is 1:660–1:1000 births. In Asians the incidence is 1.5 times higher. Blacks have a low prevalence of cleft lip and palate at 0.4 per 1000 in contrast to the prevalence in Native Americas which is 3.6 per 1000 births. Both cleft lip alone and cleft lip and palate are more common in male babies than females and this difference is greater with the combined defect. Cleft lip is unilateral in over 80 % of cases with two-thirds occurring on the left side. An affected woman has a greater chance of having an affected offspring than an affected male. The risk for a second child to be affected increases rapidly if one child already has the condition. This risk is 4 % for one affected child rising to 9 % for two affected children. The risk when one adult is affect with one affected offspring is 17 %. In the rare case where both parents are affected then the risk of an offspring also having the condition is 25 %–50 %. The treatment of cleft lip and palate is complex, requiring the early intervention of a team of surgeons, dentists, prosthodontists, orthodontists and speech therapists. Timing of surgical treatment depends on the site and extent of the cleft [9–14].

5.2.2
Cleft Palate (Figs. 5.8, 5.9)

Cleft palate is a congenital malformation due to the fusion failure of the palatal processes during embryonic growth. Cleft palate alone is distinct from cleft lip and palate and less common with a frequency of approximately 1 in 2500 births. In contrast to cleft lip and palate, the condition is two times more common in female infants than males. The severity of cleft palate varies from complete absence of the palate to clefting of just the uvula. The prevalence of bifid uvula in the general population, the

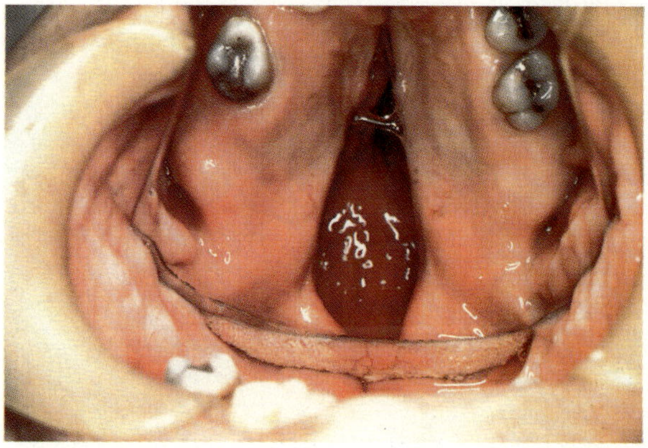

Fig. 5.8. Cleft palate

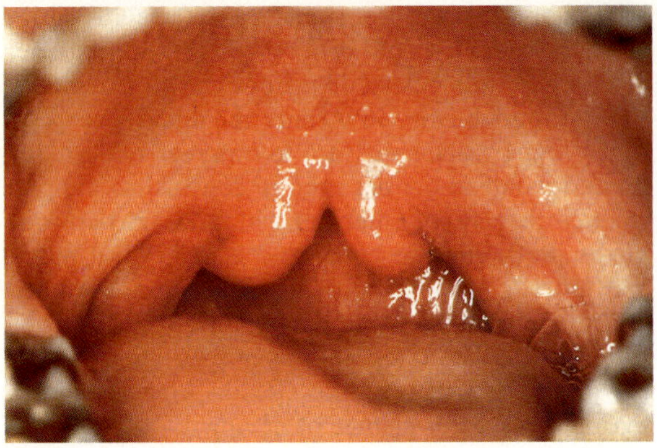

Fig. 5.9. Bifid uvula

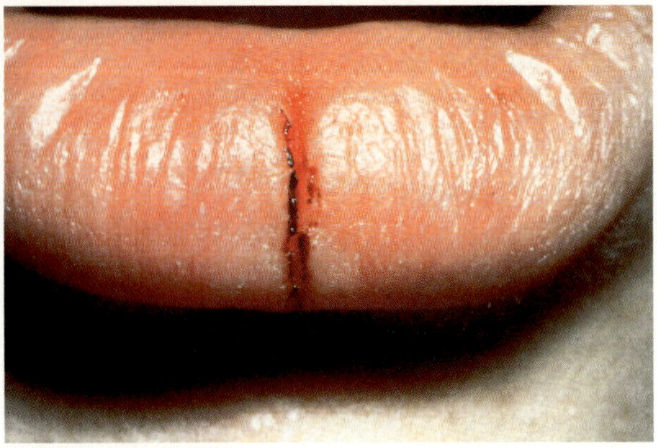

Fig. 5.11. Lip fissure

least severe manifestation of the condition, is 1 in 80 persons. This condition is also common in blacks but less so, occurring in 1 in 250 individuals. Similar to cleft lip and palate, the treatment of isolated cleft palate is complicated [15–24].

5.2.3 Bifid Tongue

A completely cleft or bifid tongue is an uncommon developmental abnormality frequently associated with other abnormalities of the skull and face including cleft lip and cleft palate. More common is the partial bifid tongue, which is manifested as a deep groove in the midline dorsum of the tongue. Apart from collecting food and debris, the condition is asymptomatic and rarely requires surgical correction [25].

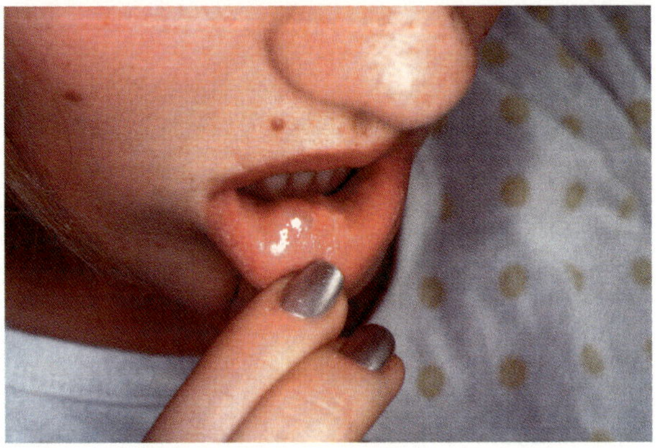

Fig. 5.12. Solitary cyst of the lower lip

5.2.4 Depressions, Cysts and Fistulae of the Lower Lip (Figs. 5.10–5.15)

Congenital pits and fistulae of the lip are often hereditary and can occur as solitary defects or together with a recognised syndrome. Up to three-quarters of lip fistulae occur in association with cleft lip and/or cleft palate. Commissural pits occur lateral to lip pits and may occur unilaterally or bilaterally. The aetiology of these defects is not known but they are far more common on the lower lip than the upper. Treatment is usually not required for small lesions but more extensive lip lesions including lip fistulae may require surgical intervention [26].

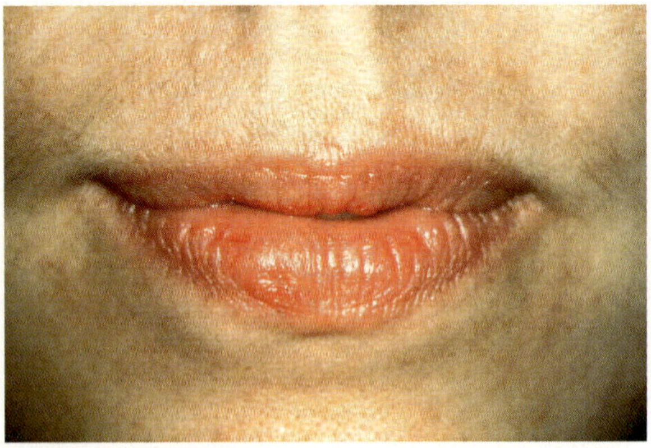

Fig. 5.10. Lip pits

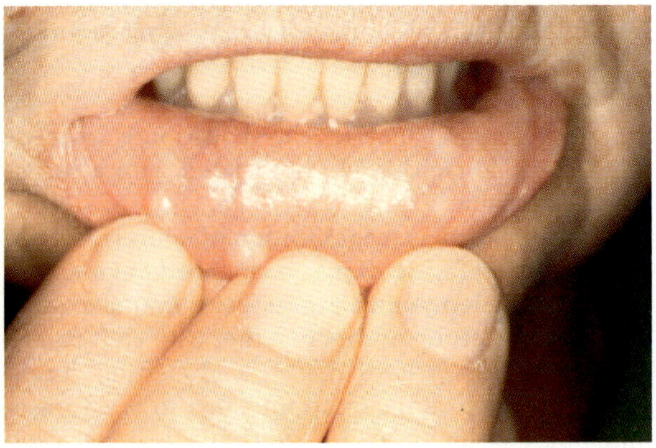

Fig. 5.13. Multipie cysts on the lower lip

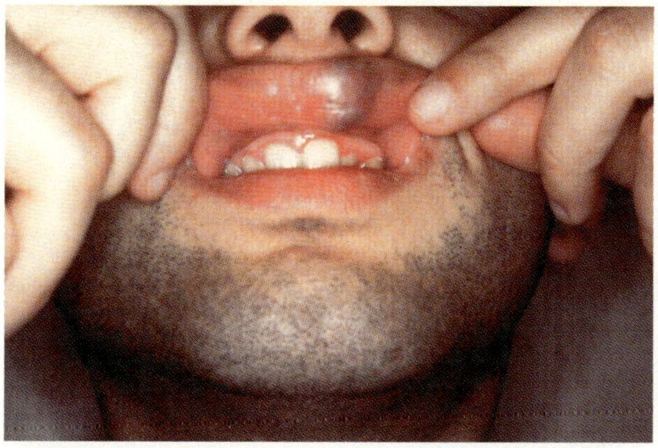

Fig. 5.14. Angioma of the lip

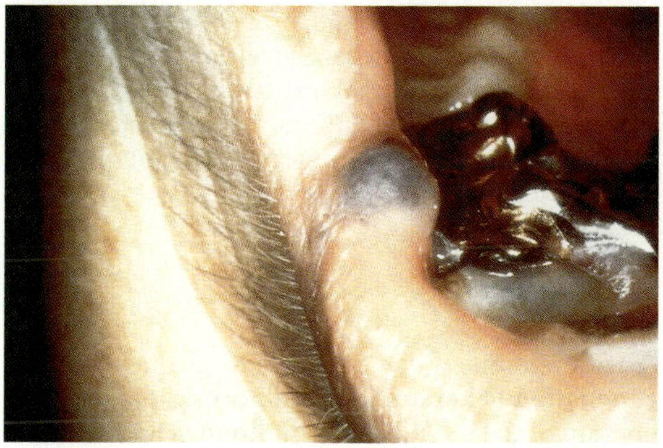

Fig. 5.15. Angioma of the lip

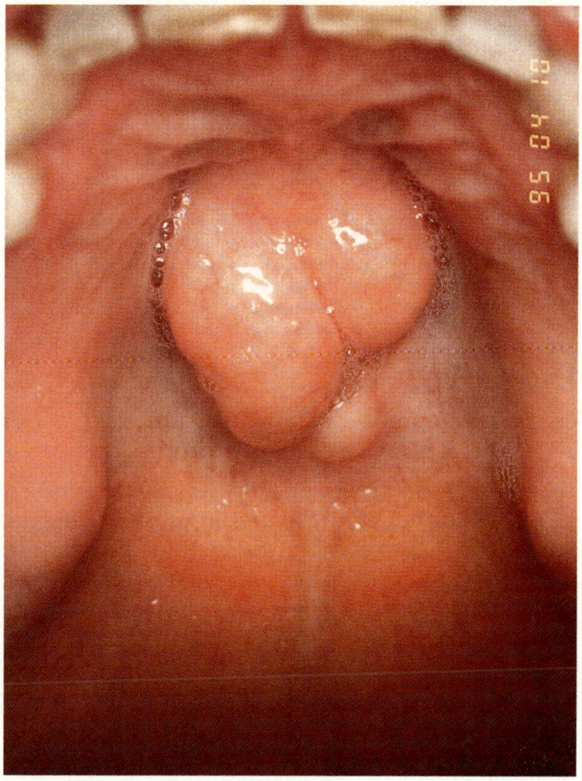

Fig. 5.17. Torus palatinus. (Courtesy of Dr. Gianfranco Favia, Dental School University of Bari, Bari, Italy)

5.2.5 Torus Palatinus

Torus palatinus is a common, slow-growing hyperostosis occurring in the midline of the hard palate. Commonly it is diagnosed after the age of 30 years and generally increases in size with age. Regression has been noted in some individuals and this suggests a dynamic process. The aetiology of the condition is not known but likely has a hereditary component. Tori can vary in both size and shape, ranging from a few millimetres to a few centimetres in greatest dimension and can be flat, spindled, nodular or lobulated in shape. The diagnosis is made by its location and clinical appearance. The mucosa overlying a torus palatinus is typically thin and readily susceptible to trauma and hence ulceration. Treatment of a torus palatinus is rarely required except in those instances where its presence interferes with prosthetic intervention. In these cases surgical removal of the condition is indicated [27].

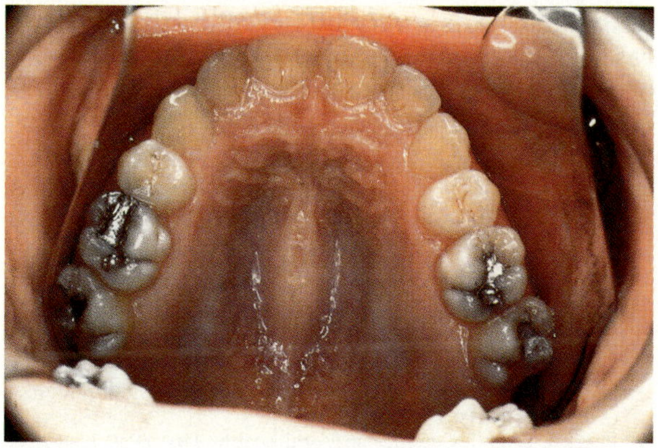

Fig. 5.16. A small torus palatinus

5.2.6 Torus Mandibularis (Fig. 5.18)

Similar to its counterpart on the hard palate, the torus mandibularis is a slow-growing hyperostosis of the lingual mandibular cortex, above the mylohyoid line. It occurs with a frequency of 2.7 % in the general population and there is no predilection for either sex. Curiously, there is no correlation with the presence of a torus palatinus and the conditions generally occur separately. Mandibular tori are usually symmetrical, but occasionally asymmetrical

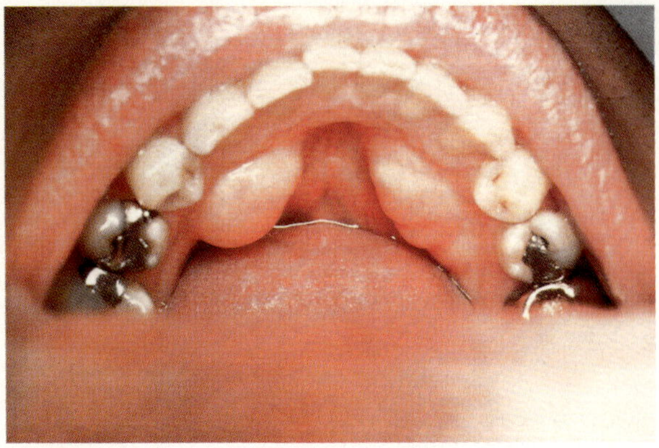

Fig. 5.18. Torus mandibularis

enlargement can be striking. The diagnosis is based on the clinical appearance and location. Radiographically, the condition can be seen as a uniformly dense radio-opacity in the premolar region of the mandible. Histologically, tori consist of dense lamellar bone. Similar to a torus palatinus, surgical excision is only required when there are problems related to the placement of a mandibular denture [28, 29].

5.27 Multiple Exostoses (Fig. 5.19)

Exostoses are usually diffuse, bilateral, multiple and symmetrical. Skull and face are the most affected areas from exostoses; they can be found mostly on the maxilla or external auditory canal. Differential diagnosis include osteomas that are unilateral and solitary. Inherited multiple exostoses is an autosomal dominant disorder characterized by the presence of multiple cartilage-capped exostoses in the juxta-epiphyseal regions of the long bones. Most patients are men under 30 years of age; family history is positive in 60 % of cases. Genetic linkage of this disorder has been described to three independent loci

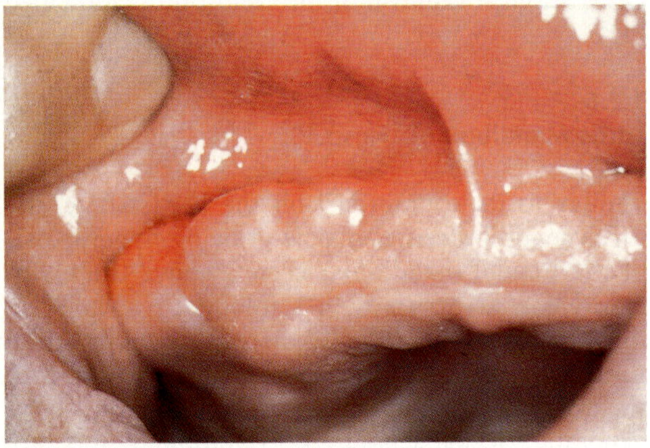

Fig. 5.19. Exostoses

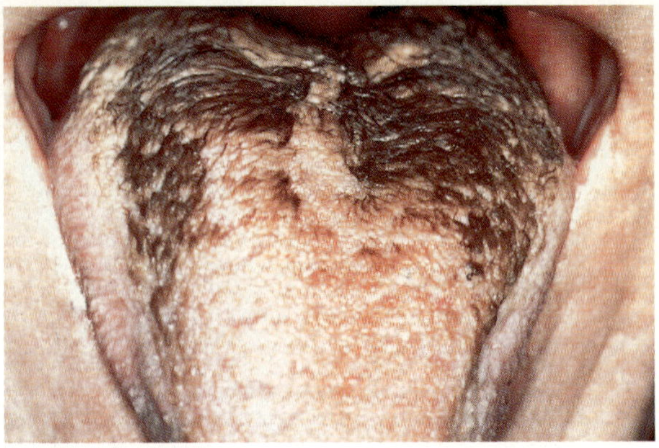

Fig. 5.20. Black hairy tongue

on chromosomes 8, 11 and probably 19. Genes related to multiple exostoses show significant homology with one additional expressed sequence tag, suggesting a potential tumour suppressor activity. Rarely these exostoses progress to malignant chondrosarcomas [30–35].

5.2.8 Oral Hair

The development of a hairy tongue is due to the accumulation of keratin in the filliform papillae on the dorsum of the tongue. The condition is found on the midline dorsum of the tongue anterior to the circumvalate papilla. It has a characteristic yellow to black colour with matting together of the "hairs". This finding is associated with heavy smoking, antibiotic use or radiation therapy. No treatment apart from local hygiene measures is required since the condition is mainly an aesthetic problem. The condition should not be confused with oral hairy leukoplakia, which is an Epstein-Barr virus infection producing hyperkeratosis along the lateral borders of the tongue. Underlying immunosuppression such as HIV infection is frequently associated with hair leukoplakia. The appearance of true hair occurring in the mucosa is a very rare event, with only three cases of congenital hair on the mucosa having been described and the authors suggesting that it is an ectodermal disorder [36, 37].

References

1. Bottomley WK. Physiology of the oral mucosa. Otolaryngol Clin North Am 1979; 12: 15–20
2. Nakata M. Genetics in oral-facial growth and diseases. Int Dent J 1995; 45: 227–244
3. Gafar M, Klein A, Genetic problems in dentistry. Stomatologia (Bucur) 1968; 15: 295–298
4. Pearn J, Gage J. Genetics and oral health. Aust Dent J 1987; 32: 1–10

5. Sloan P, Picardo M, Schor SL. The structure and function of oral mucosa. Dent Update 1991; 18: 208–212
6. Pitaru S, McCulloch CA, Narayanan SA. Cellular origins and differentiation control mechanisms during periodontal development and wound healing. J Periodontal Res 1994; 29: 81–94
7. Ferguson MW, Palate development. Development 1988; 103 Suppl: 41–60
8. Sharpe PM, Ferguson MW. Mesenchymal influences on epithelial differentiation in developing systems. J Cell Sci 1988; Suppl 10: 195–230 (1988)
9. Pelz L, Amling A. Informative morphogenetic and phenogenetic variants in children with cleft lip/cleft palate. Am J Med Genet 1996, 3; 63: 305–9
10. Rowan DM. Scalp dermatitis, ectodermal dysplasia and cleft lip and palate: rapp-hodgkin or AEC syndrome. Australas. J Dermatol 1996, 37: 102–3
11. Johnston MC, Bronsky PT. Prenatal craniofacial development: new insights on normal and abnormal mechanisms. Crit Rev Oral Biol. Med 1995; 6: 368–422
12. Kjaer I. Human prenatal craniofacial development related to brain development under normal and pathologic conditions. Acta Odontol Scand 1995; 53: 135–43
13. Johnston MC, Bronsky PT. Prenatal craniofacial development: new insights on normal and abnormal mechanisms. Crit Rev Oral Biol Med 1995; 6: 25–79
14. Richman JM. Head development. Craniofacial genetics makes headway. Curr Biol 1995; 5: 345–8
15. Roelfsema NM, Cobben JM. The EEC syndrome: a literature study. Clin Dysmorphol 1996; 5: 115–27
16. Wyatt R, Sell D, Russell J, Harding A, Harland K, Albery E. Cleft palate speech dissected: a review of current knowledge and analysis. Br J Plast Surg 1996; 49: 143–9
17. Sullivan G. Parental bonding in cleft lip and palate repair. Paediatr Nurs 1996; 8: 21–4
18. Johnston MC, Bronsky PT. Prenatal craniofacial development: new insights on normal and abnormal mechanisms. Crit Rev Oral Biol Med 1995; 6: 368–422
19. Mulliken JB, Warman ML. Molecular genetics and craniofacial surgery. Plast Reconstr Surg 1996; 97: 666–75
20. Snijders RJ, Sebire NJ, Psara N, Souka A, Nicolaides KH. Prevalence of fetal facial cleft at different stages of pregnancy. Ultrasound Obstet Gynecol 1995; 6: 327–9
21. Friede H. Abnormal craniofacial growth. Acta Odontol Scand 1995; 53: 203–9
22. Huggare J. Craniocervical junction as a focus for craniofacial growth studies. Acta Odontol Scand 1995; 53: 186–91
23. Smahel Z, Mullerova Z. Craniofacial growth and development in unilateral cleft lip and palate: clinical implications (a review). Acta Chir Plast 1995; 37: 29–32
24. Johnston MC, Bronsky PT. Prenatal craniofacial development: new insights on normal and abnormal mechanisms. Crit Rev Oral Biol Med 1995; 6: 25–79
25. Nocini PF, Urbani G, Manfrini F, Cavalleri G. Lingua bifida in associazione ad altre patologie maxillo-facciali. Min Stom 1987; 36: 511–515
26. Kretzschmar JL, Kretzschmar DP. Common oral conditions. Am Fam Physician 1996; 54: 225–34
27. Kretzschmar JL, Kretzschmar DP. Common oral conditions. Am Fam Physician 1996; 54: 225–34
28. Wang KY, Juriloff DM, Diewert VM. Deficient and delayed primary palatal fusion and mesenchymal bridge formation in cleft lip-liable strains of mice. J Craniofac Genet Dev Biol 1995; 15: 99–116
29. Seah YH. Torus palatinus and torus mandibularis: a review of the literature. Aust Dent J 1995; 40: 318–21
30. Legeai-Mallet L, Margaritte-Jeannin P, Lemdani M, Le Merrer M, Plauchu H, Maroteaux P, Munnich A, Clerget-Darpoux F. An extension of the admixture test for the study of genetic heterogeneity in hereditary multiple exostoses. Hum Genet 1997, 99: 298–302
31. Wise CA, Clines GA, Massa H, Trask BJ, Lovett M. Identification and localization of the gene for EXTL, a third member of the multiple exostoses gene family. Genome Res 1997; 7: 10–16
32. Mikawa Y, Watanabe R, Nakashima Y, Hayashida T. Cervical spinal cord compression in hereditary multiple exostoses. Report of a case and a review of the literature. Arch Orthop Trauma Surg 1997; 116: 112–115
33. Hecht JT, Hogue D, Wang Y, Blanton SH, Wagner M, Strong LC, Raskind W, Hansen MF, Wells D. Hereditary multiple exostoses (EXT): mutational studies of familial EXT1 cases and EXT-associated malignancies. Am J Hum Genet 1997; 60: 80–86
34. Stickens D, Clines G, Burbee D, Ramos P, Thomas S, Hogue D, Hecht JT, Lovett M, Evans GA. The EXT2 multiple exostoses gene defines a family of putative tumour suppressor genes. Nat Genet 1996; 14: 25–32
35. Blanton SH, Hogue D, Wagner M, Wells D, Young ID, Hecht JT. Hereditary multiple exostoses: confirmation of linkage to chromosomes 8 and 11. Am J Med Genet 1996; 62: 150–159
36. Baughman RA, Heidrich PD Jr. The oral hair: an extremely rare phenomenon. Oral Surg Oral Med Oral Pathol 1980; 49: 530–531
37. Humeniuk HM, Burns RA, Shelley ED, Weaver JR. Oral Mucosal hair: an ectodermal anomaly. J Am Acad Dermatol 1986; 15: 1301–1302

Genetic Diseases of Oral Mucosa

6.1 Introduction

A. D. Katsambas

A number of genetic or systemic diseases have characteristic manifestations of the oral mucosa. In the majority of these disorders, the oral lesions follow the onset of the skin or systemic disease and in some they appear simultaneously; however, there are few genetic diseases where the oral manifestations represent the first clinical sign of the generalized disease. Although the oral manifestation only rarely is necessary for the diagnosis, it sometimes represents the key point without which the diagnosis would be very difficult.

This chapter includes well established diseases of genetic origin that are mainly of integumental nature and have oral mucosa manifestations. These disorders are categorized into the following groups:

1. Disorders of melanin pigmentation
2. Disorders of keratinization
3. Hyperplasia – aplasia – dysplasia – atrophia
4. Bullous diseases
5. Diseases of connective elastic tissue
6. Neurocutaneous syndromes
7. Hereditary neoplasms
8. Hereditary diseases caused by disorders of metabolism

6.2 Disorders of Melanin Pigmentation

6.2.1 Peutz-Jeghers Syndrome (Synonyms: Mucocutaneous Melanosis and Gastrointestinal Polyposis)

Since 1921, when Peutz described the disease [1], more than 600 cases have been reported. The syndrome is characterized by mucocutaneous pigmented spots and gastrointestinal polyposis with a familial incidence and is transmitted as an autosomal dominant disorder with a high degree of penetrance [2]. There is no sex predilection, and it is diagnosed at any age but usually after puberty.

The oral pigmentation is almost constantly found and consists of pigmented macules that vary in size, color and shape. The pigmented spots, 1–10 mm in diameter, can be observed in any oral region, but more often on the lower lip and the buccal mucosa (Fig. 6.1). The shape is often oval or round, the color varies between dark and light brown, blue and black, and the spots are sometimes confluent.

Almost 50 % of patients have pigmented spots periorally, and less often around the other facial orifices (36 %). In certain cases similar spots may be observed on the extremities and other regions [3].

The most frequent manifestation, other than oral and skin pigmentation, is repeated attacks of colicky, abdominal pain due to the gastrointestinal polyps. The colicky pain may occur in early childhood or be delayed until later, but usually starts between 10–30 years of age. Melena, hematemesis, anemia, and prolapsed rectal polyps may also appear. The polyps (hamartomas and microadenomas) are 0.5–7 cm in diameter and are usually found in the jejunum and ileum, and less frequently in other parts of the intestine and the stomach. The malignant potential of the polyps, although not very significant, is not negligible [4, 5].

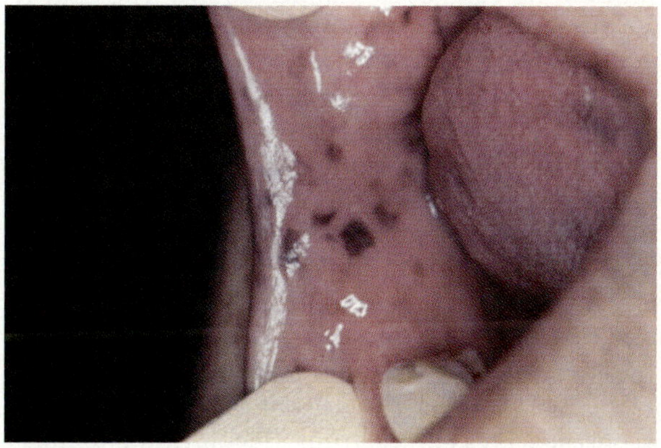

Fig. 6.1. Peutz-Jeghers syndrome. Pigmented spots (buccal mucosa)

Microscopic Findings. There is an increase of melanin in the basal layer, without an increase in the number of melanocytes, particularly at the tips of the rete pegs and in the melanophores in the upper dermis.

Diagnosis. This is based on the clinical signs. Oral pigmentation is the most important diagnostic finding and when it is associated with perioral pigmentation an investigation for gastrointestinal polyps is advised. Radiologic evaluation of the gastrointestinal tract is helpful to detect developing polyps.

Differential Diagnosis. This includes Addison's disease, Albright's syndrome, Gardner's syndrome, simple freckles, normal racial pigmentation, and other pigmentation of exogenous and other endogenous sources. The type of oral pigmentation, the gastrointestinal symptoms, and probably the gastrointestinal roentgenograms will distinguish Peutz-Jeghers syndrome from the above conditions.

Treatment. There is no treatment for the pigmented oral and skin lesions. Supportive treatment of the gastrointestinal bleeding is required. Endoscopic or surgical removal of some polyps is sometimes warranted.

6.3 Disorders of Keratinization

6.3.1 Darier's Disease (Synonyms: Dyskeratosis Follicularis/Darier-White Disease)

Darier's disease is an uncommon autosomal dominant genodermatosis, more common in men, the onset of which appears during childhood or early adolescence. Oral involvement occurs in 20%–50% of cases, not necessarily parallel in severity with the skin changes [7]. The onset of oral lesions follows the cutaneous manifestations. The oral lesions are minute, red papules that eventually turn whitish and may coalesce into hypertrophic plaques with a "cobblestone" appearance and a rough feeling to palpation. The whole picture in the oral mucosa resembles clinically nicotinic stomatitis with a characteristic lacy network (Fig. 6.2). The gingiva, palate, buccal mucosa, and tongue are the most frequent sites of involvement [8, 9].

The skin lesions are multiple skin-colored or yellow-brown firm papules that commonly coalesce into irregular warty plaques which in the flexures become malodorous. The sites of localization are the seborrheic areas of the trunk (Fig. 6.3), the temples, the flanks, ears, nasolabial furrows, the scalp, and the groin. The nails are usually abnormal and show subungual hyperkeratosis with longitudinal ridges and lines. Other mucosae may also be involved.

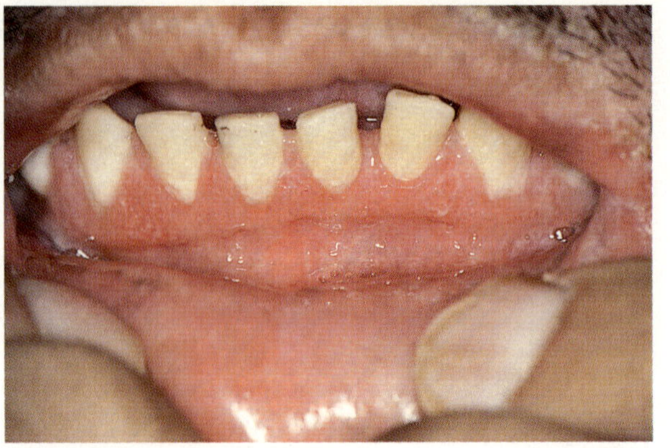

Fig. 6.2. Darier's disease. Lacy network gingivae

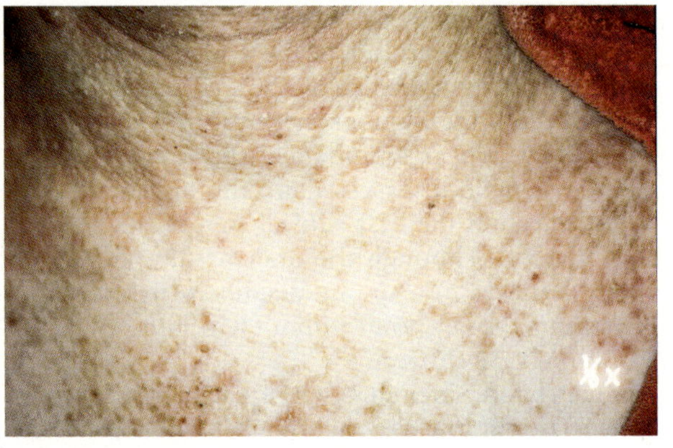

Fig. 6.3. Darier's disease. Follicular papules (trunk)

Microscopic Findings. The oral lesions show fissures (lacunae) above the basal layer and the characteristic "corps ronds", that is cells showing premature keratinization (dyskeratosis); however, the dyskeratotic cells are fewer than in the skin.

Diagnosis. This is based on the clinical picture of the skin and oral lesions and should always be confirmed by a biopsy.

Differential Diagnosis. This includes seborrheic dermatitis, acanthosis nigricans (the lesions are pigmented), familial benign pemphigus, and solitary warty dyskeratoma that has an indistinguishable histological picture.

Treatment. Oral and topical retinoids are very helpful.

6.3.2
Hyperkeratosis Palmaris et Plantaris with Periodontosis (Synonyms: Hyperkeratosis Palmoplantaris and Premature Periodontoclasia-Papillon-Lefevre Syndrome)

The syndrome was described in 1924 by Papillon and Lefevre [10] and is characterized by hyperkeratosis of the palms and soles, severe destruction of the periodontal tissue, leading to premature loss of the deciduous and permanent teeth, and meningeal calcifications. The syndrome is inherited as an antosomal recessive trait and consanguinity of the parents has been reported [11].

The periodontal inflammation appears simultaneously or just follows the appearance of the palmar and plantar hyperkeratosis.

The deciduous teeth erupt normally but the gingivae become red and swollen and bleed earily. Periodontal pockets form and bone destruction occurs. The teeth become mobile and exfoliate by themselves by about 4–5 years of age (Fig. 6.4). When the child is edentulous, the gingiva returns to its normal appearance. By the time the permanent teeth erupt, the disease process relapses and by the age of 14, all permanent teeth are lost. The oral mucosa remains normal during all the above described phases [12].

The manifestations of the palms and soles usually precede the periodontal involvement and appear around the third year of life (Fig. 6.5). The lesions consist of discrete, red, and scaly hyperkeratosis of the palms and especially the soles, although the overall degree of keratosis is usually not marked. The dorsum of the fingers and toes are often affected by similar lesions [12].

Diagnosis. This is based on the clinical characteristics and possibly on the family history. Panoramic radiography discloses severe periodontal destruction and bone loss.

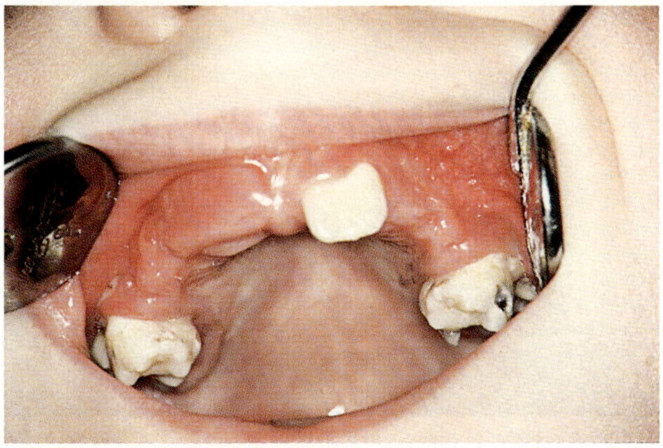

Fig. 6.4. Papillon-Lefevre syndrome. Exfoliation of the teeth

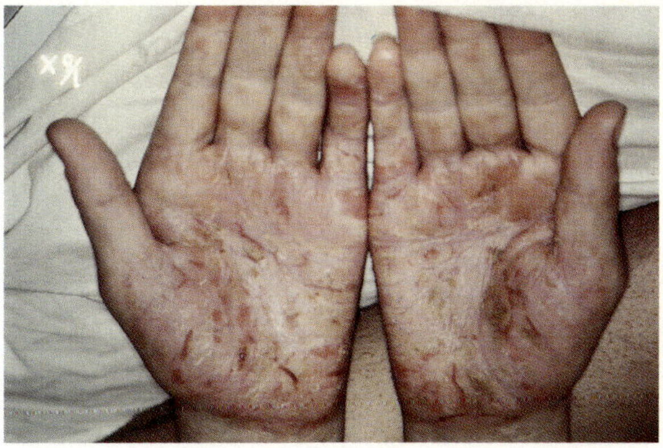

Fig. 6.5. Hyperkeratosis palmaris. Papillon-Lefevre syndrome

Differential Diagnosis. In periodontal lesions, this should include juvenile periodontitis, histiocytosis X, acatalasia, hypothosphatasia, hypohidrotic ectodermal dysplasia, agranulocytosis, diabetes mellitus, leukemia, Chediak-Higashi syndrome, etc. In addition, differential diagnosis of palmoplantar hyperkeratosis should include mal de Meleda, pachyonychiacongenita, focal palmoplantar, and oral mucosa hyperkeratosis syndrome, etc. [13].

Treatment. Periodontal disease cannot be treated successfully by any pharmacological agent; however, plaque control, scaling, and oral hygiene are advised. Eventually the patients lose their teeth and complete dentures will be the treatment of choice. Recently, oral retinoids (etretinate, isotretinoin, acitretin) have been very helpful in diminishing the cutaneous eruption, lessening the gingival inflammation, and in some cases saving the teeth [14–16].

6.3.3
Dyskeratosis Congenita (Synonyms: Zinsser-Engman-Cole Syndrome)

Dyskeratosis congenita is a rare disease characterized mainly by cutaneous hyperpigmentation, dystrophic nails, and dermal and mucosal bullae leading to oral leukokeratosis, blepharitis, and ectropion. The disease is probably inherited as a recessive autosomal and X-linked trait [17].

The oral lesions occur at between 5 and 10 years of age and are the first manifestation of the disease. They involve usually tongue, buccal mucosa, and less often gingiva, and they consist of blisters that rupture, leaving painful ulcers. The lesions tend to recur as the patient grows older. Atrophy and leukoplakia are the result of the repeated recurrence of the disease. Oral leukoplakias are a constant characteristic in all patients, from adolescence onward (Fig. 6.6). Finally, squamous cell carcinoma may occur [18].

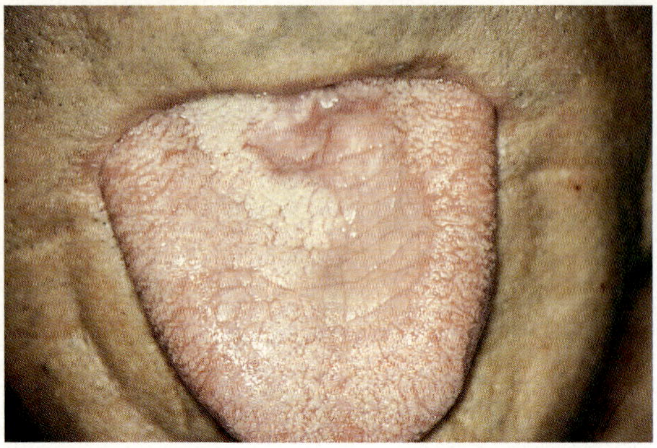

Fig. 6.6. Dyskeratosis congenita. Leukoplakia of the tongue

The nails become dystrophic and are shed in early childhood. Pigmentary changes, in the form of fine reticulate grey-brown pigmentation, most evident on the neck, appear simultaneously with the nail changes or 2–3 years later. Intracranial calcifications may occur and mental growth is sometimes retarded [19].

Diagnosis. This is based on the clinical picture and is supported by the presence of oral leukoplakia in heterozygous relatives [20].

Differential Diagnosis. This includes leukoplakia, lichen planus, pachyonychia congenita, and epidermolysis bullosa.

Treatment. Oral retinoids may inhibit the development of leukoplakia and reduce the incidence of malignancy [21].

6.3.4 Pachyonychia Congenita (Synonyms: Jadassohn-Lewandowsky Syndrome)

Pachyonychia congenita is characterized by symmetrical dystrophic thickening of the nails, hyperkeratosis and hyperhidrosis of the palms and soles, follicular keratosis of the elbows and knees, and hyperkeratosis of the oral mucosa [22]. The disease is transmitted by an autosomal dominant trait, although cases inherited by an autosomal recessive form have been reported [23].

The oral lesions appear at birth or shortly thereafter, and are located usually on the palate, buccal mucosa, the tongue, the lips, and the gingiva. These lesions consist of focal or diffuse, white or greyish-white areas with a thick, striate or spotted appearance. The variability and severity of nail changes categorize pachyonychia congenita into four types. In one case convulvions and fundal phacomas have been described [24].

Microscopic Findings. There is hyperparakeratosis and acanthosis with intracellular vacuolization and edema in the prickle cell and superficial layers [25].

Diagnosis. This is based on the age of the patient, the symmetric thickening of the nails, the palmoplantar hyperkeratosis, and the oral lesions.

Differential Diagnosis. This includes lichen planus, leukoplakia, dyskeratosis congenita, white sponge nevus, hereditary benign intraepithelial dyskeratosis and focal palmoplantar, and oral mucosa hyperkeratosis syndrome.

Treatment. No therapy is necessary.

6.3.5 Psoriasis

Psoriasis is a chronic inflammatory, non-infectious disease of the skin which affects 1 %–3 % of most populations. It may start at any age but most commonly during the second and third decades of life. The cause of the disease is unknown; however, there is often a genetic predisposition, and there are tables to predict the risk of a child having psoriasis when other persons in the family have the disease [26]:

Family condition	Risk of psoriasis in child
Psoriasis in both parents	60 %
Psoriasis in one parent	25 %
Psoriasis only in one brother/sister	17–20 %

Clinically, psoriasis is characterized by circumscribed erythematous plaques with loose silvery scales most commonly located over the elbows, knees, scalp, and the lower aspect of the back

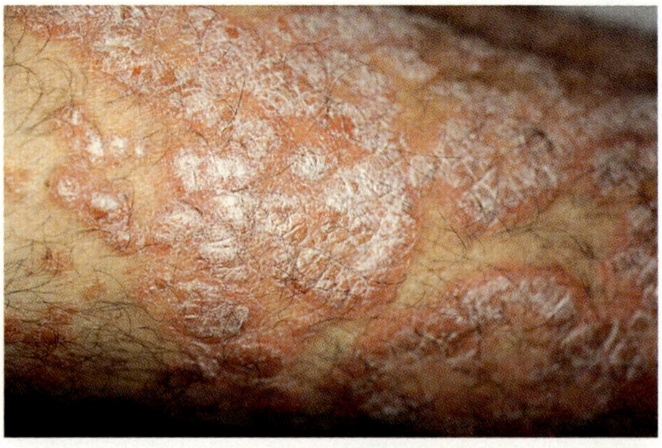

Fig. 6.7. Psoriasis of the skin. Silvery scales over erythematous plaques

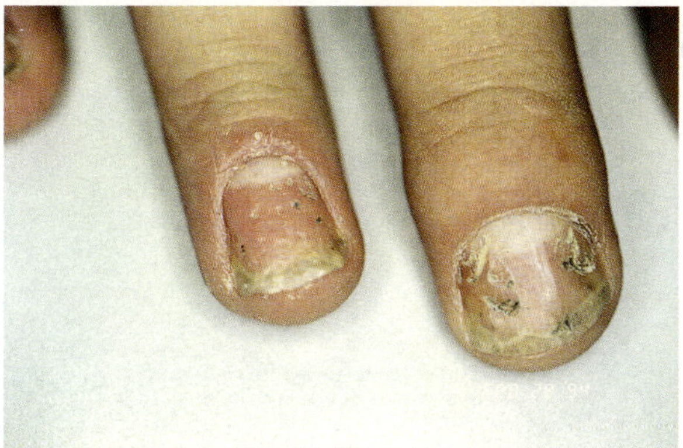

Fig. 6.8. Psoriasis of the nails

(Fig. 6.7). The nails are also very commonly affected (Fig. 6.8). Plaque type psoriasis is the most variant form of the disease. Other variants include annular, guttate, pustular, erythrodermarthritic, arthritic, etc. forms. The disease usually follows a chronic course with exacerbations and remissions.

Psoriasis of the oral mucosa is very rare and usually does not occur in psoriasis vulgaris but in the generalized pustular form of the disease [27–30].

The clinical appearance of oral psoriasis is characterized by white or grayish plaques or striae papules, erythematous patches, or lesions similar to geographic tongue (Fig. 6.9). Recently, it was reported that geographic tongue may be one of the manifestations of oral psoriasis [28].

The oral psoriatic lesions involve mainly the tongue and less often the gingiva, buccal mucosa, floor of the mouth, and lips.

Microscopic Findings. There is hyperparakeratosis, elongation, and thickness of the rete pegs, thinning of the suprapapillary epithelial layers (Fig. 6.10), and infiltration of polymorphonuclear leukocytes in the epithelium. Microabscesses of Munro may occasionally be seen [29].

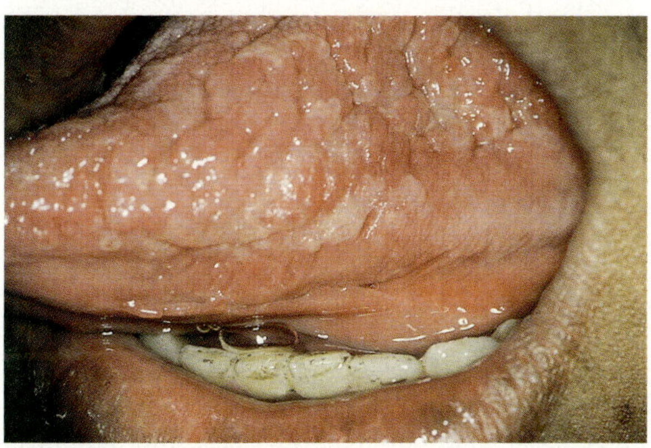

Fig. 6.9. Psoriasis of the tongue (lesions like geographic tongue)

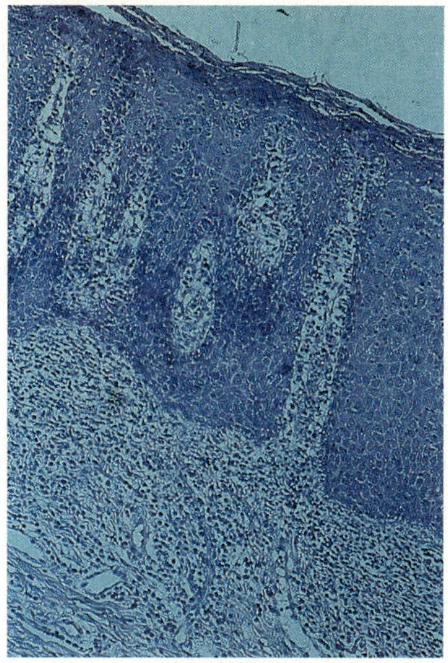

Fig. 6.10. Psoriasis of the tongue. Histology

Diagnosis. The diagnosis of oral psoriasis is facilitated when parallel psoriatic skin lesions exist and is supported by histologic confirmation and HLA typing [29].

Differential Diagnosis. This includes geographic tongue, lichen planus, geographic stomatitis, leukoplakia, etc.

Treatment. Aromatic retinoids, methotrexate, and cyclosporine have been tried for the treatment of skin lesions. For the treatment of oral lesions, the direct injection of corticosteroids, diluted in anesthetic solutions, is the most common therapy. Like the skin, oral lesions always have the possibility of recurrence [31].

6.3.6 Focal Palmoplantar and Oral Mucosa Hyperkeratosis Syndrome (Synonyms: Hyperkeratosis Palmoplantaris and Attached Gingivae Hyperkeratosis)

This syndrome is rare and is characterized by a combination of hyperkeratosis of the palms and soles and attached gingival hyperkeratosis. It is inherited as an autosomal dominant trait [32, 33]. Oral lesions appear in early childhood and are located constantly in the attached gingivae as sharply marginated hyperkeratosis. Other areas such as the hard palate and the lateral border of the tongue beneath denture bearing areas may also be affected by hyperkeratosis mimicking leukoplakia.

The weight-bearing areas of soles and pressure related areas of the palms present with focal to widespread hyperkeratosis. The toes are involved first at the age of 4–5 years and the fingers follow 3–5 years later. In a few cases, hyperhidrosis is observed in the hyperkeratotis lesions and rarely hyperkeratosis and thickening of the nails may be observed. The severity of the lesions increases with age [34].

Diagnosis. This is based on the clinical features.

Differential Diagnosis. This includes dyskeratosis congenita, pachyonchychia congenita, Papillon-Lefevre syndrome, inherited tylosis and carcinoma, and esophageal carcinoma syndrome.

Treatment. Systemic aromatic retonoids may occasionally be considerably helpful [35].

6.4 Hyperplasia, Aplasia, Dysplasia, Atrophy

C. Feliciani and R. Jordan

6.4.1 Anhidrotic Ectodermal Dysplasia (Hypohidrotic Ectodermal Dysplasia)

Ectodermal dysplasias (ED) are a group of inherited disorders affecting tissues of ectodermal origin including the skin, teeth, nails, and eccrine glands. Diagnosis requires the presence of defects at two or more of these sites. These disorders can be inherited in autosomal dominant, recessive and C-linked patterns. This group of conditions is rare, occurring in 1:10 000–1:100 000 births. Ectodermal dysplasia is characterized by heat intolerance, fine or sparse hair (atrichosis or hypotrichosis), abnormal or missing teeth (anodontia or hypodontia), inability to sweat

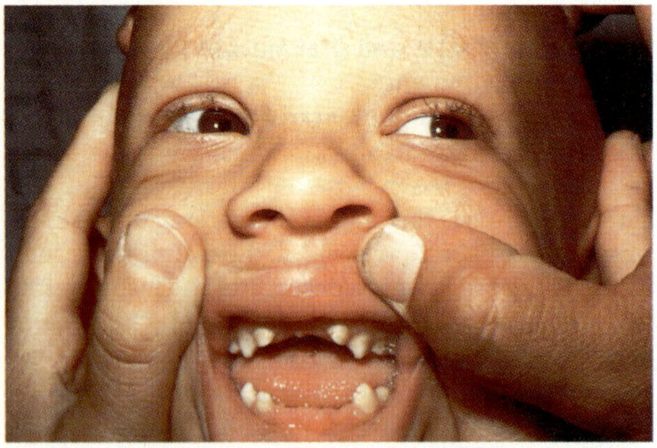

Fig. 6.11. Ectodermal dysplasia. (Courtesy of Dr. Robert Lester Dept. of Dermatology, Sunnybrook Health Science Center, Toronto, Ontario, Canada)

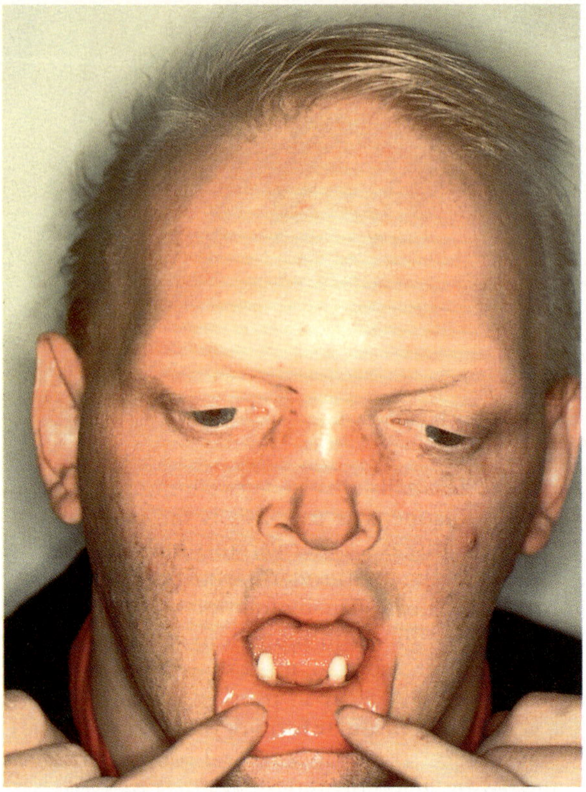

Fig. 6.12. Anhidrotic ectodermal dysplasia. (Courtesy of Dr. Benjamin K. Fisher, Dept. of Dermatology, Women's College, Toronto, Ontario, Canada)

due to absent sweat glands (anhidrosis or hydrochidrosis), and fine wrinkling with hyperpigmentation around the eyes (Figs. 6.11, 6.12). Affected individuals have dry skin due to the lack of sweat glands with dystrophic and brittle nails. Within the mouth, teeth are absent or defective incisors, canines, and bicuspids are conical and curved and molars have hooked cusps. The ED gene is located on the X-chromosome (Xq12–q13). Clouston syndrome is another rare form of ED and is characterized by dystrophic nails, palmoplantar hyperkeratosis, sparse, slow-growing hair, thin eyebrows, but normal sweating and normal teeth. Hence, Clouston syndrome can be considered a hair-nail dysplasia without oral involvement [36–38].

6.4.2 Acanthosis Nigricans

Acanthosis nigricans is a hypermelanotic disorder characterized by brown, velvety, cutaneous thickenings (Fig. 6.13). The usual sites of involvement are the axillae, nape and sides of the neck, the groin, antecubital and popliteal surfaces, and umbilical area. The oral cavity, including the tongue, buccal

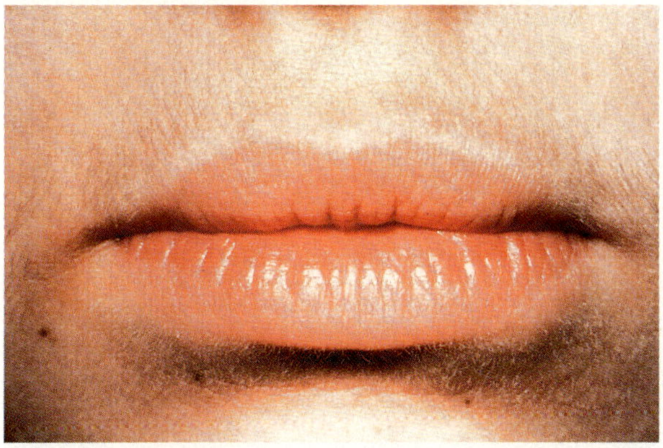

Fig. 6.13. Acanthosis nigricans with mild involvement of the lower lip. (Courtesy of Dept. of Dermatology, Sunnybrook Health Science Center, Toronto, Canada)

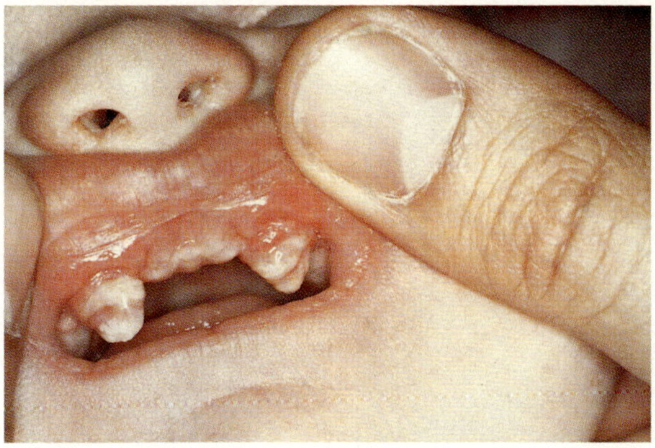

Fig. 6.14. Chondroectodermal dysplasia or Ellis-Van-Creveld syndrome. (Courtesy of Dr. Gianfranco Favia, Dental School University of Bari, Bari, Italy)

mucosa, and lips can be affected by florid papillary growths, normally without pigmentation. Acanthosis nigricans can be divided into many types, essentially three of which are the most common forms of the disease:

1. Benign acanthosis nigricans is inherited as an autosomal dominant trait with variable expressivity. The disorder becomes apparent at birth or in early childhood and increases in severity until puberty, after which it remains stationary or regresses.
2. Obesity-associated acanthosis nigricans, also called pseudoacanthosis nigricans, is the most common type. It is usually weight-dependent, appears at any age, and regresses with weight loss.
3. Malignant acanthosis nigricans is characterized by the presence of lesions that develop rapidly and tend to be more severe and extensive. Mucous membrane involvement and thickening of the palms and soles occur more frequently. Pruritus is common. Malignant acanthosis nigricans is much rarer than both benign and obesity-associated acanthosis nigricans. The most common cancer responsible for malignant acanthosis is gastric cancer but others reported include carcinoma of the uterus, liver, intestines, colon, rectum, or ovary. Commonly, malignant acanthosis nigricans regresses after tumor removal.

Other forms of acanthosis nigricans are rare and associated with a number of syndromes such as insulin resistance syndrome, Hirschowitz syndrome, Lawrence-Seip syndrome, Wilson's disease, Crouzon's syndrome, Bloom's syndrome, Prader-Willi syndrome, gigantism, acromegaly, and polycystic ovary disease.

In healthy, dark-skinned individuals, a form of the disease termed pseudo-acanthosis or acral-acanthosis nigricans may develop because the condition occurs on the plantar surface of the hands and feet. Drug-induced acanthosis nigricans is another rare form typically caused by steroids, nicotinic acid, fusidic acid, diethylstilbestrol, or subcutaneous insulin [39–42].

6.4.3 Chondroectodermal Dysplasia (Ellis-Van-Creveld)

Chondroectodermal dysplasia is an unusual congenital disease, inherited in an autosomal recessive fashion and involving the skeletal system and the ectodermal tissues (Fig. 6.14). The frequency of the disorder is estimated at 7:1 000 000 births, but it has an increased frequency amongst the Amish community in Lancaster County, Pennsylvania. The clinical features of Ellis-Van-Creveld syndrome include disproportionate dwarfism, polydactyly, and congential heart disease (single atrium, large atrial septal defect, ostium primum type). The affected individuals are dwarfed, with an average height from 110 to 155 cm. Affected individuals also have post-axial polydactyly of the hands and feet, thoracic dysplasia, small and natal teeth, hypodontia, and altered upper lip. The major striking finding is the absence of the mucobuccal folds. Other features include fusion of the hamate and capitate bones of the wrist, hypo/epispadia, and dysplastic finger nails. The gene for EVC syndrome is located on chromosome 4p16.1 [43–45].

6.4.4 Cleidocranial Dysplasia

Cleidocranial dysplasia (CCD) is a hereditary bone dysplasia presenting with a variety of dental abnormalities (Fig. 6.15). Recently, the locus for the CCD gene has been localized to between the 23

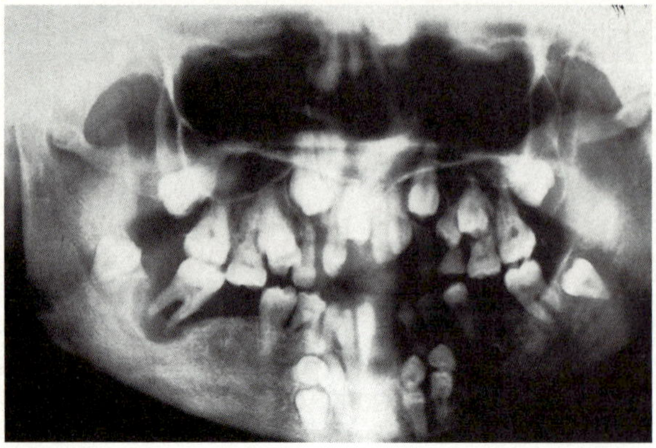

Fig. 6.15. Cleidocranial dysplasia. X-ray appearance. (Courtesy of Professor Adriano Piattelli, University "G.d'Annuzio", Dental School, Chieti, Italy)

and 17cM regions of the chromosome band 6p21. It is fully penetrant with widely variable expressivity. The classical phenotype includes mild to moderate short stature, clavicular aplasia or hypoplasia and a variety of dental abnormalities including supernumerary and ectopic teeth, crown and root abnormalities, and delayed eruption of secondary teeth. The skeletal features include brachycephalic skull with a wide, prominent forehead, frontal and parietal bossing, delayed ossification of anterior fontanel, hypertelorism, mid-facial hypoplasia, and a broad nasal base with a depressed nasal bridge [46–54].

6.4.5 Focal Dermal Hypoplasia (Goltz Syndrome; Goltz-Gorlin Syndrome)

Focal dermal hypoplasia, first reported in 1962, is a rare, hereditary mesoectodermal disorder (Fig. 6.16). Approximately 200 cases have been reported to date. The precise mode of inheritance is still unknown; however, an X-linked dominant fashion is presumed with lethality in hemizygote males. The pathogenic mechanism that produces this widespread mesoectodermal defect is not well understood although a compromised growth potential of dermal fibroblasts and defective formation of collagen fibers have been demonstrated, probably caused by a mutation of an X-chromosome gene. The affected individuals show anomalies of both mesodermal- and ectodermal-derived tissues including teeth, skin, and skeletal. Intraoral examination reveals a high arched palate, irregular spaced, conical teeth of varying size with enamel defects and caries, microdontia and papillomas of mucosa. Hypo- and oligodontia are the most frequent anomalies. Scoliosis, asymmetric limbs, syndactyly or clinodactyly, and hypoplastic thenar and hypothenar eminences

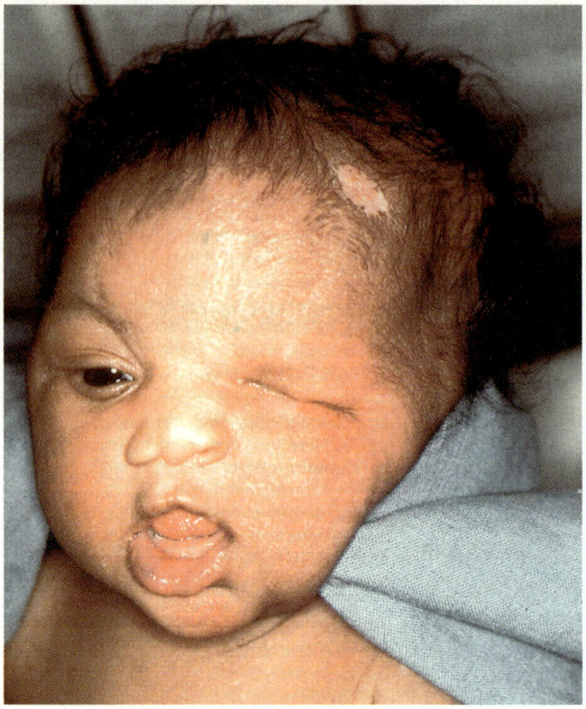

Fig. 6.16. Focal dermal hypoplasia. (Courtesy of Dr. Benjamin K. Fisher, Dept. of Dermatology, Women's College Hospital, Toronto, Ontario, Canada)

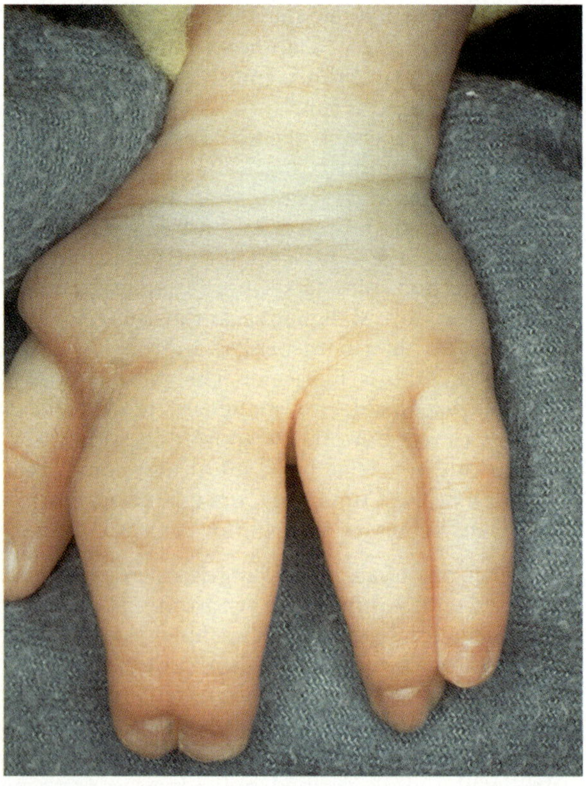

Fig. 6.17. Syndactyly in a patient with focal dermal hypoplasia. (Courtesy of Dr. Bejamin K. Fisher, Dept. of Dermatology, Women's College Hospital, Toronto, Ontario, Canada)

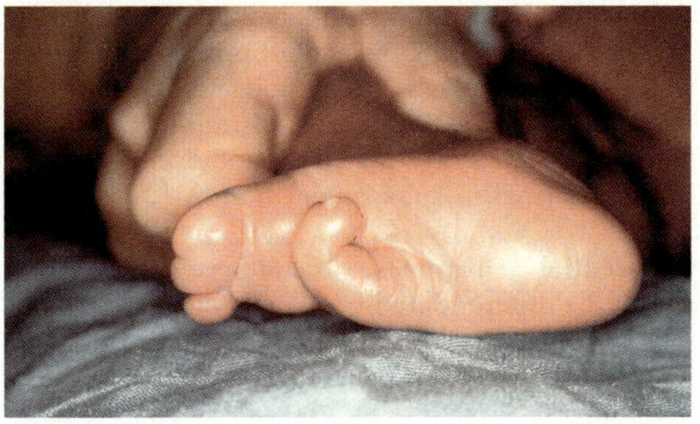

Fig. 6.18. Abnormal foot in focal dermal hypoplasia. (Courtesy of Dr. Benjamin K. Fisher, Dept. of Dermatology, Women's College Hospital, Toronto, Ontario, Canada)

are the most common skeletal abnormalities (Figs. 6.17, 6.18). Skin involvement is regarded as essential for diagnosis, and atrophic hypopigmented lesions following Blascko's lines are characteristic of this syndrome. Fat herniation and protrusion of adipose tissue occur frequently. The dental abnormalities are correctable by combined surgical and orthodontic therapy [55–57].

6.4.6 Orofacial Digital Syndrome

G. Hautmann, G.L. Campanile, and T.M. Lotti

Definition. There are four distinct clinical variants of this syndrome which is a genetic disorder [58–61].

Type I, also called Papillon-Léage syndrome, is present in 1.5% of children with cleft lip or palate. The familial incidence suggests X-linked dominant inheritance, lethal to males. Type II, also called Mohr syndrome, is inherited as an autosomal recessive trait. Type III has been described in two sisters by Sugarman and coworkers [60], and the inheritance is presumed autosomal recessive. Type IV is autosomal recessive, and its existence has been hypothesized by Baraister [61].

Oral Manifestations. Type I orofacial digital syndrome patients present a short upper lip and hypoplastic alae nasi on a hooked pug nose. The frenulae of upper and lower lips and tongue are usually hypertrophied. The tongue is bifid or multilobed and often shows small tumors within the clefts that contain aberrant mucous glands and nests of smooth muscle. Sometimes there are clefts of the hard and soft palates. The teeth may be widely separated and misplaced, and may develop early and atypical caries.

Type II patients present with lobate tongue, cleft palate, a normal or flaring alveolar ridge, and a broad bifid nasal tip. In type III there is a lobulated hamartomatous tongue, dental abnormalities, bifid uvula, whereas in type IV the oral manifestations are similar to type I [58–61].

Associated Findings. In type I, there are always deformities of the hands that represent the cardinal clinical manifestations: brachydactyly, syndactyly, clinodactyly, and polydactyly. There are often other skeletal disorders, associated with cutaneous anormalities: the hair is often dry, coarse, lustreless, and brittle. Alopecia may be present. On the face, ears, and backs of the hands there are numerous milia, sometimes exiting in scars. About 50% of patients present mental retardation.

Type II patients may present conductive hearing loss and bilateral polysyndactyly of the halluces.

Type III consists of mental retardation, eye abnormalities, postaxial hexadactyly of hands and feet, pectus excavatum, short sternum, and kyphosis.

Type IV differs from type I in terms of severe tibial dysplasia [58–61].

Diagnosis. In type I, dermatoglyphic studies are of value in diagnosis. Irregular mineralization of the bones of the hands and feet is an important feature of type I, distinguishing it from type II.

Differential Diagnosis. This disease must be differentiated from chondroectodermal dysplasia and oculo-dento-digital syndrome.

Treatment. The oral problems require dental care, but no treatment is available for this genetic disorder.

6.4.7 Incontinentia Pigmenti

Definition. Incontinentia pigmenti (or Bloch-Sulzberger's syndrome or Bloch-Siemens' syndrome) is a complex, X-linked dominant disease characterized by numerous ectodermal and mesodermal defects. Vesicular, verrucous, and pigmented cutaneous lesions are associated with developmental defects of the eye, skeletal system, and central nervous system. It is lethal to males [62–67].

Oral Manifestations. The oral manifestations mainly consist of dental defects that are frequent. Delayed dentition, partial anodontia, cone- or peg-shaped teeth are the most usual. Impacted teeth and dysplastic enamel may be present. The absence of teeth, especially the upper lateral incisors and premolars, has been reported in otherwise unaffected siblings and in the mother, who may likewise appear normal.

Associated Findings. The skin changes are often present at birth, have usually developed before the end of the first week, and rarely appear after the first 2 months. The roughly four stages in the evolution of cutaneous lesions frequently overlap. The first stage begins with erythema from which vesicles and, in time, bullae emerge (stage 1: erythematous-bullous). In the beginning, the blisters are filled with serum that become turbid because of the incursion and disintegration of eosinophils. All the lesions follow the whorled distribution of Blaschko's lines. As the vesicular lesions slowly heal, they are replaced in the course of a few weeks by verrucous crusts and keratoses (stage 2: verrucous stage). The verrucous lesions thicken progressively and affect mainly the limbs, especially the fingers and toes. Subungual keratoses may be painful. As the verrucous lesions involve, whorled and linear zones of hyperpigmentation following Blaschko's lines appear (stage 3: pigmentary stage), mainly on the trunk. These hyperpigmented lesions represent post-inflammatory changes and usually fade gradually during late childhood or adolescence. The fourth stage (stage 4: hypopigmented and atrophic stage) consists of hypopigmented and atrophic skin lesions. In addition to these lesions, in about 25 % of patients, other cutaneous anomalies may be found, including cicatricial alopecia, dystrophy of nails, and difficulties in sweating.

Neurologic disturbances (convulsions and paresis) and mental retardation are frequently reported.

Ocular abnormalities consist of cataracts, atrophy of optical nerves, strabismus, nystagmus, and chorioretinitis [62–67].

Diagnosis. The combination of bullae with linear nodular or warty lesions in a girl is pathognomonic. Many affected subjects have blood leukocytosis early in infancy. Notable is a relative eosinophilia of 25 %–30 % that peaks at age 3–4 weeks and declines slowly toward normal in subsequent months [62–67].

Differential Diagnosis. Incontinentia pigmenti should be differentiated from infantile pemphigoid, epidermolysis bullosa, congenital syphilis, and hypohidrotic ectodermal dysplasia.

Treatment. Usually no treatment is required other than the control of secondary infection. Systemic corticosteroids and sulfapyridine are unsuccessful. Skilled dental supervision is required to minimize the cosmetic disability.

6.5 Bullous Diseases

R. A. Satriano and G. M. Gaeta

6.5.1 Epidermolysis Bullosa (Figs. 6.19–6.25)

Epidermolysis bullosa (EB) is a heterogeneous group of genetically determined disorders where the hallmark is fragile skin and mucosae. It is characterized by a tendency to form blisters on the skin and mucosae, especially in the *aero*-digestive upper tract (mouth and esophagus). The blisters may either result from minor trauma or apparently arise spontaneously. Variants have been classified by electron microscopy and distinguished as an epidermolytic or simple type, a junctional type and a dermolytic or dystrophic type in relation to the plane of

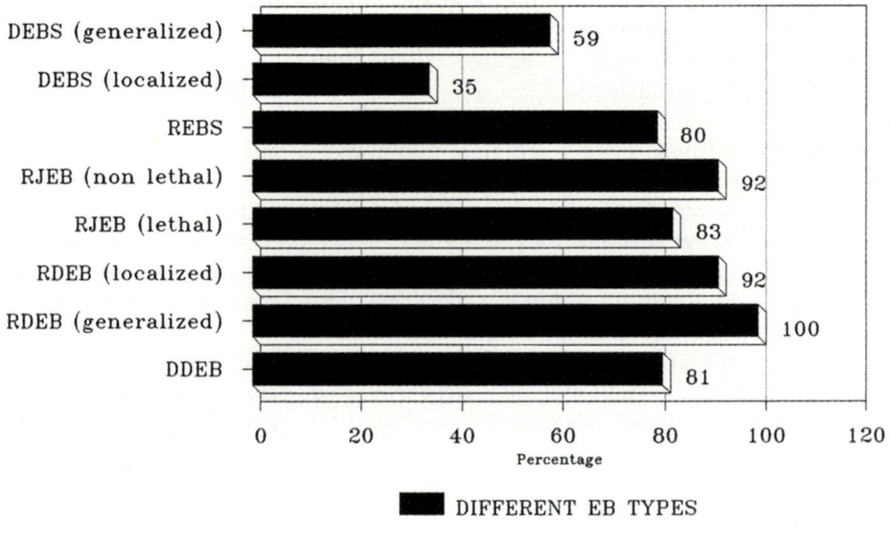

Fig. 6.19. Oral lesions in EB patients: percentage incidence. (From Wright et al. [80])

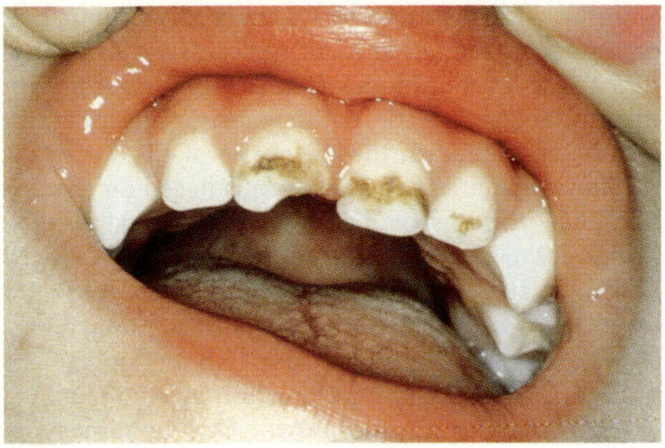

Fig. 6.20. Junctional epidermolysis bullosa

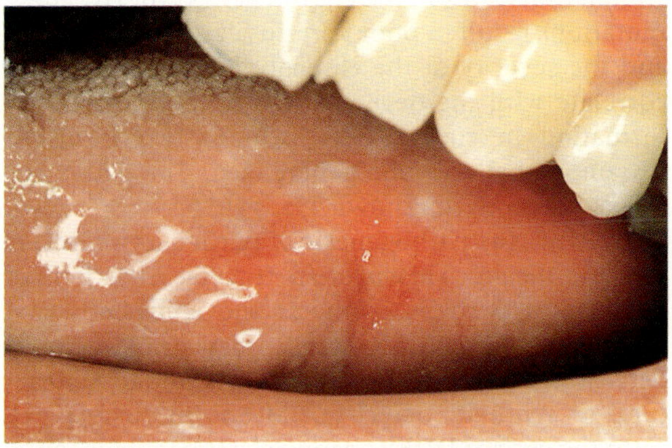

Fig. 6.21. Junctional epidermolysis bullosa: erosive lesion of the tongue

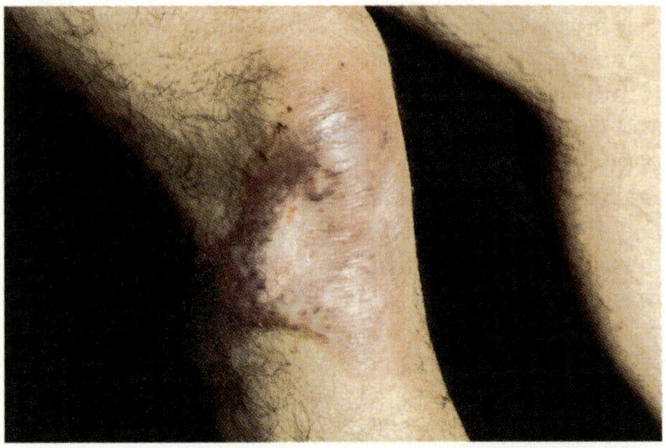

Fig. 6.22. Dystrophic epidermolysis bullosa: cicatricial lesion

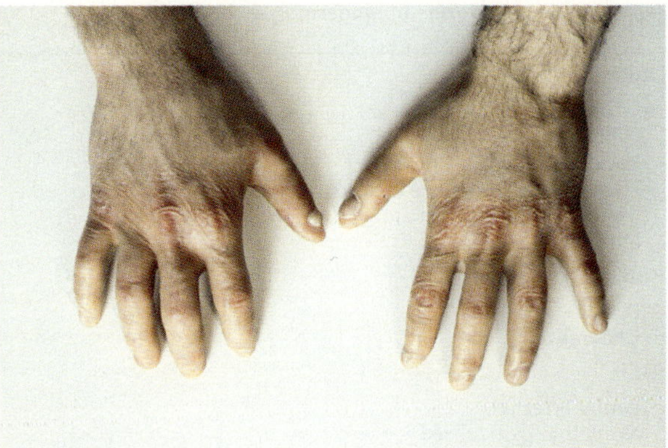

Fig. 6.23. Dystrophic epidermolysis bullosa: cicatricial lesion with onychodystrophy

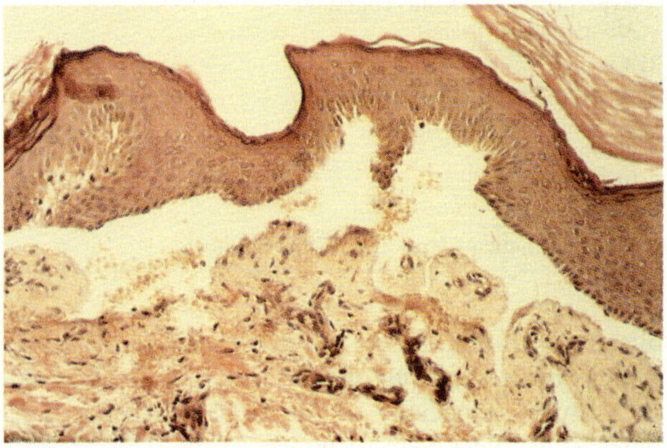

Fig. 6.24. Epidermolysis bullosa: histology, x 200

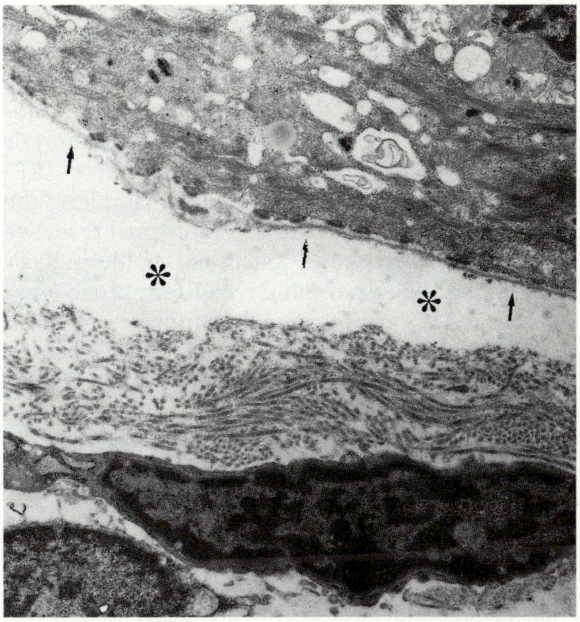

Fig. 6.25. Dystrophic epidermolysis bullosa: electron microscopy, dermoepidermal attachment (Centro Malattie Cutanee Ereditarie, Istituto di Scienze Dermatologiche, Milan, Italy), x 14900

Table 6.1. Genetic forms of epidermolysis bullosa

DEBS
Generalized (Köbner)
Ogna
Localized (Weber-Cockayne)
Herpetiform (Dowling-Meara)
Mottled pigmentation
Superficial
REBS
Lethal
Generalized
RJEB
Lethal (Herliz)
Nonlethal generalized
Nonlethal localized
Nonlethal inverse
Progressive cicatricial
DDEB
Hyperplastic (Cockaine-Touraine)
Albopapuloid (Pasini)
RDEB
Generalized (Hallopeau-Simens)
Generalized nonmutilating
Localized
Inverse
DDEB or RDEB
Transient bullous dermolysis of the newborn

blister separation. By the use of electron microscopy and an understanding of the same biochemical abnormalities, especially of the skin collagenase, 20 types of EB have been recognized [68]. The classification is reported in Table 6.1. It is clear that these variants described as EB represent a genetically distinct disease, mediated by different mechanisms.

Etiology. The inheritance patterns in EB are autosomat, both dominant and recessive. The simple type (epidermolytic type) and its variants are autosomal dominant (DEBS = dominant epidermolysis bullosa simplex) and autosomal recessive (REBS = recessive epidermolysis bullosa simplex); the junctional type and variants are autosomal recessive traits (RJEB = recessive junctional epidermolysis bullosa); and the dystrophic type (dermolytic type) is inherited as an autosomal dominant trait and as autosomal recessive (dystrophic epidermolysis bullosa – dominant and recessive = DDEB, RDEB).

Pathogenesis. It has been possible to address the molecular pathology of major types of EB using two different research approaches: the development of specific antibodies to various components of basement membrane zone (BMZ) and studies of the so-called candidate gene approach. For example, GB3 antibody defines the BM-600/nicein protein complex and localizes it to the lower portion of the lamina lucida with immunoelectron microscopy. Staining with the antibody is markedly diminished or absent in the lethal form of recessive junctional EB. These immunologic probes are important in the understanding of pathogenesis, but they can also be employed in the diagnosis of EB.

The candidate gene approach is based on the notion that proteins or antigens that are in physical proximity to the pathology, or play a key role in abnormal features, represent a candidate protein of importance in the pathogenesis of EB. The currently studied genes in various forms of EB are reported in Table 6.2. In DEBS the pathogenic mechanisms involved are currently unknown. One hypothesis is the activation of cytolytic enzymes, temperature-sensitive, in this group of disorders [69]. The most important observation in DEBS is the demonstrated mutations in the keratin genes [70, 71]. These mutations result in poor keratin filament formation, and the severity of the clinical disease appeared to correlate with the degree of disruption of filament formation in vitro. REBS includes two forms of EB: one lethal and one generalized. The pathogenesis is currently unknown [72, 73].

In RJEB, the pathogenesis of particular interest is BM-600/nicein. This protein traverses the lamina lucida and perhaps connects the epidesmosomal structure to the lamina densa; it has not yet been determined if the faulty adhesion is due to a structural or synthetic defect in BM-600/nicein [74, 75].

In the case of DDEB, strong genetic linkage to the type VII collagene gene locus has been demonstrated [76]. The cause of blistering in this variety may be a primary defect in anchoring fibrils [77].

The pathogenesis of REDB has not been defined. Consistent ultrastructural features include a profound decrease or absence of anchoring fibrils and the presence of collagenolysis. Two possible mechanisms have been proposed: destruction of dermal connective tissue by an excessive amount of collagenase and/or a defective structural protein in the dermis that is responsible for the integrity of the epidermal-dermal junction [78, 79].

Oral Manifestations. Oral mucous membrane involvement ranges from 35% to 59 % in the simple

Table 6.2. Candidate genes in various types of EB. (From Uitto, J Invest Dermatol 1992; 98: 391)

Type of EB	Candidate
Simplex	Keratins and other cytoskeletal proteins, linking proteins, cell-to-cell adhesion molecules
Junctional	Hemidesmosomal proteins, α 6/β 4 integrin, anchoring filament protein (type VII col)
Dystrophic	Enzymes that degrade BMZ structural proteins

type and is seen in 81 %–100 % of junctional and dermolytic types (Fig. 6.19). Bullae appear early in life, often precipitated by suckling, and rapidly evolve into erosions and ulcers because of maceration and mastication. Scarring is a common sequela of blisters and erosions on mucosa as it is in the skin. When the scarring is diffused in the whole oral cavity, it may produce significant functional disability for the obliteration of the oral vestibule, ankyloglossia and microstomia. Oral milia have been reported in patients with dominant dystrophic EB, but have not been described in other forms of EB [80]. Probably, oral milia are due to the entrapment of epithelial cells during the stages of blister formation and healing. The contracture due to minor trauma such as toothbrushing can lead to tongue-tie, obliteration of the sulci, and limited opening. The tongue becomes depapillated and scarred. Enamel hypoplasia is seen in all junctional EB subtypes and often leads to a rapid breakdown of the dentition. Dental treatment is difficult because of the ease with which the mucosa can be damaged; oral hygiene tends to be neglected with subsequent caries and periodontal diseases. Squamous cell carcinoma is a rare complication. In Fig. 6.19 the percentages of oral mucosa involvement in various types of EB are shown.

Associated Findings

Dominant Epidermolysis Bullosa Simplex (DEBS). In the simple types, the blisters, although widespread, have a predilection for the hands and feet. Mucosae, teeth, and nails are normally spared. In the herpetiform, simple type severe blistering is present at birth and tends to involve trunk, face, and extremities. Hands and feet are affected most markedly. Nails are involved with dystrophy. Mucous membranes are involved in some patients and it is possible to find enamel hypoplasia. In the simple type with mottled pigmentation, bullae resolves with hyper- or hypopigmented macules.

Recessive Epidermolysis Bullosa Simplex (REBS). In the lethal type, the onset of blistering is normally present at birth and is generalized with a predilection for the more distal portions of the limbs. Nails, teeth, and hair are unaffected. Oral mucosa is only mildly involved without scarring and milia. Normally, infants die during the first 2 years of life. In the generalized type the blistering is severe and is associated with scarring, nail dystrophy, milia, and significant involvement of oral mucosa. This type appears to be associated with myasthenia gravis or muscular dystrophy [81].

Recessive Junctional Epidermolysis Bullosa (RJEB). Severe generalized blistering that usually heals without scarring is present at birth. Mild atrophy may result. The nails show paronychia, and chronic plaques of nonhealing granulation tissue are found in the perioral region. The teeth show hypoplasia.

Dystrophic Epidermolysis Bullosa – Dominant and Recessive (DDEB, RDEB). Clinically, the dystrophic forms are characterized by severe generalized blistering with subsequent scarring, contractures, and milia formation, resulting in nail dystrophy, mitten-like encasement of the digits, and flexural contractures of the major joints. The involvement of the mouth, esophagus, pharynx, and anus is common. Esophageal scarring may cause strictures. It is possible to find conjunctival and corneal erosion. DDEB almost always remains limited to hands, feet, elbows, and knees. The clinical severity of the disease makes patients with DDEB indistinguishable from those with RDEB.

Microscopic Findings

DEBS and REBS. In DEBS the primary separation occurs within the basal cell layer. In bullae of more than 1 day's duration, the cleavage may be found intraepidermally or subcorneally as a result of epidermal regeneration. Electron microscopy data demonstrate that the initial sign is edema of subnuclear cytoplasm which progresses to form a cavity. When the cavity reaches the cell membrane, it causes the ruptures and a blister forms [82]. In the herpetiform type, the ultrastructural difference from localized and widespread types is that the basal cell cytolysis is preceded by clumping of tonofilaments and their attachment to hemidesomosomes.

RJEB. The separation is located between the epidermis and dermis. Dermal papillae tend to retain their size and shape. Little or no infiltrate of inflammatory cells can be observed. Electron microscopy shows a reduction in size and numbers of hemidesomosomes [83].

DDEB and RDEB. Light microscopy shows a dermal-epidermal separation. A subepidermal blister extends down along the epithelial structures and adnexa. Dermal papillae tend to be preserved. Fibrosing granulation tissue may occur beneath the subepidermal blisters. Milia and follicular cysts of the infundibula type are a consequence of subepidermal blistering. Albopapuloid lesions are slightly dome-shaped and characterized by fibrosis in the upper half of the epidermis. Electron microscopy studies demonstrate that blister formation occurs below the basal lamina [84].

In REBD, degeneration of connective tissue, observed by electron microscopy, is limited to the upper part of the papillary dermis as a result of a decrease in anchoring fibrils.

Diagnosis. The current diagnostic standard is ultrastructural analysis. Electron microscopy remains the method of choice for defining the level of cleavage and detecting other ultrastructural abnormalities. Also, the use of specific antibody probes has become an essential adjunct to accurate diagnosis.

Differential Diganosis. In infancy, differentiation of EB from other bullous diseases is rarely a problem. X-linked incontinentia pigmenti is characterized by streaky blistering which results in swirly patterns of pigmentation, especially over the trunk. Dominant bullous ichthyosiform erythroderma presents with flaccid bullae, but erythroderma and hyperkeratosis dominate especially over skin folds. Benign chronic bullous disease in childhood may mimic EB (inverse type), since the blistering involves genitalia, perineum, and buttocks. In these conditions, the presence of linear IgA on direct immunofluorescence confirms the diagnosis.

Treatment. Therapy is unsatisfactory and largely symptomatic. Families at risk must be given adequate genetic counselling. Because prenatal diagnosis has become possible, pregnancies in these families can be screened for the disease.

DEBS. Avoidance of trauma and heat are helpful but only palliative. Once blistering has occurred, saline soaks and topical steroids may produce relief. Topical antibiotics can minimize the risk of bacterial infections. The herpetiform type may improve with an increase in ambient temperature. Low doses of systematically administered steroids are beneficial [85].

RJEB. The treatment of the Herlitz variant (severe atrophic type) is only supportive. The systemic high dosage of corticosteroids is the treatment of choice during the life-threatening period. One promising form of therapy to address the problem of ulceration and chronic granulation tissue is the use of autografts [86]. In the other variants, treatment is palliative (topical steroids and topical antibiotics). Phenytoin may be useful in some patients [87].

DDEB. The treatment is palliative. Compresses and topical antibiotics for blistered areas are beneficial and avoidance of unnecessary trauma is advised.

RDEB. No effective treatment is available. Antisepsis of the eroded areas is necessary. The lesions should be covered with petrolatum and semipermeable dressing. Topical antibiotics may be used if there is evidence of local infections. Systemically administered antibiotics are required when more than minor infection occurs. Nutritional management is important. Vitamin, iron, and protein supplements are advised [88]. Surgical procedures are recommended for the treatment of esophageal strictures [59]. Low doses of systemic steroids given for a short period of time can be helpful to patients with serious problems with feeding. Phenytoin, which inhibits synthesis of collagenase by fibroblasts, has been reported to reduce blistering [90], but a recent multicenter double-blind trial of phenytoin in RDEB failed to confirm its efficacy, but could not exclude that occasionally patients benefit by its use [91]. Also, retinoids, because of their ability to inhibit collagenase production by fibrocytes, are proposed in RDEB treatment [92].

Oral Management of Epidermolysis Bullosa Patients. Because of the fragility of the oral mucosa and frequency of extensive dental involvement, many patients with severe EB require general anaesthesia to receive dental treatment [93]. Oral hygiene is necessary with use of chlorexidine gluconate mouthwash 0.2 %. Sometimes in the severe forms the use of a local anesthetic such as benzocaine 20 % or a eutectic mixture of local anesthetics (EMLA) can help patients during the food intake. The use of topical steroids like clobetasol propionate (0.05 % ointment) or bethamethasone valerate (0.01 % gel) leads to rapid healing of the oral mucosa erosions [94].

6.5.2 Acrodermatitis Enteropathica (Fig. 6.26)

Acrodermatitis enteropathica is a rare genetic disorder transmitted as an autosomal recessive trait. It is caused by the selective deficiency of zinc and is characterized by orofacial, perirectal, and acral dermatitis (vesiculobullous, pustular, and eczematous lesions), diarrhea, and alopecia. Growth retardation and recurrent infections develop if the disease is not diagnosed and treated.

Etiology. Acrodermatitis enteropathica is due to malabsorption of zinc. In these patients the absorption of dietary zinc is limited to 3 % of intake, although the biochemical mechanism of malabsorption is not yet correctly known. One hypothesis holds that exocrine pancreas that normally secretes a ligand that binds to zinc in the intestinal lumen

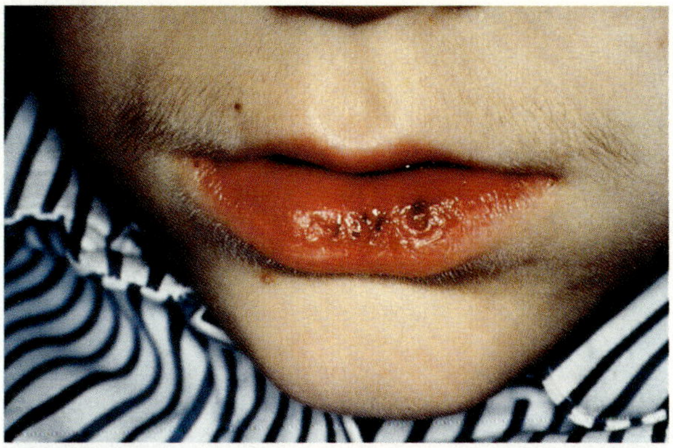

Fig. 6.26. Acrodermatitis enteropathica: lips lesions

and transports it into mucosa is not functioning adequately [95, 96]. This hypothesis has been confirmed by the occurrence of acrodermatitis enteropathica in laboratory animals. The onset of symptoms usually occurs within the first few months of life, and is associated with the change from breast feeding to cow's milk. Human colostrum is rich in zinc and contains a zinc-binding ligand similar to that secreted by the pancreas. When the newborn switches to cow's milk, the deficiency of zinc-binding ligand becomes clinically evident, because bovine milk contains a different ligand [97, 98]. Probably, the different molecular weight of two ligands (Mr 10 000 for mother's milk and about 50 000 for cow's milk) is the reason for malabsorption when the change starts in infants. Another hypothesis is that bovine milk is higher in protein concentration compared to human milk (29.0 ng/ml compared to 5.3 ng/ml), which reduces the availability of zinc [99]. Moreover, human milk contains about 8 times more essential fatty acids, which are able to increase zinc absorption [100].

Etiology. Zinc is needed in more than 200 metalloenzymes for DNA and protein synthesis and for cell division. So it plays a key role in many body functions. Zinc is found in all body tissue. Bone, muscle, and prostate are the major areas of deposit. Also, the skin concentration is high, and it is 5/6 times greater in the epidermis than in the dermis. The role of zinc in the skin is not yet understood, but it is known that histadine, a marker of epidermal differentiation, binds to zinc [101]. Zinc is also essential for thymic function. In the presence of a reduction of dietary zinc intake, thymulin and thymic hormone are reduced. As a result, cellular immunofunctions are depressed. Also, neutrophilis, monocytes, macrophage tissues, and mast cells are sensitive to a reduction in zinc [102]. Probably the candidal and bacterial infections of patients with AE are a consequence of the immunological pathway mediated by zinc. For these reasons, also severe erosive and infected lesions heal with zinc dietary supplementation without additional topical therapy.

Oral Manifestations. Acral dermatitis involving the face begins slowly with dry, scaly, and eczematous plaque formation. Angular cheilitis is a common and early lesion. Successively, the patient develops vesiculobullous, pustular, and erosive lesions, which involve the whole lip and face. In the oral cavity, it is possible to find aphthous-like lesions localized on keratinized and non-keratinized mucous membrane. In this stage, secondary infections are common, especially *Candida albicans* and bacteria. Over weeks the patients develop diminished sensations of taste (hypogeusia).

Associated Findings. The earliest signs of AE in an infant are apathy and irritability. The skin lesions involve the areas around the orifices: eyes, mouth, nose, ears, and neck. These lesions develop also on the perirectal areas, on the genitalia, and on elbows, knees, hands, and feet. The lesions range from dry scaly, eczematous plaques to vesiculobullous, pustular, and erosive. It is also possible to find *Candida albicans* and bacterial infections. Associated with these skin signs, the patients develop alopecia involving scalp, eyelashes and eyebrows. Other systemic findings are diarrhea (this being the most variable manifestation and which may be present or completely absent), cachexia, and anemia, which do not respond to iron. Nail changes are onycholysis, onychodystrophy, and paronychia. Photophobia is gradual and is probably due to the malfunction of zinc-dependent retinal binding protein. Blepharitis conjunctivitis may be complicated by scarring of the cornea. Mental retardation, hypogonadism, and retardation of growth may develop in time if the disorder goes unrecognized.

Microscopic Findings. Histologically, the bullous lesions are characterized by intraepidermal vacuolar change with massive ballooning, leading to intraepidermal vesiculation and blistering, with epidermal necrosis. Diffuse parakeratosis and acanthosis of varying degrees are seen associated with considerable mixed dermal infiltrate. The necrosis of keratinocytes chemotactically attracts neutrophilos to the epidermis, especially to intraepidermal blisters that then become vesiculopustules. The bullous lesions do not arise on erythematous patchy lesions but develop on unaffected skin.

Diagnosis. The patients with AE have lowered levels of zinc in their blood. In fact, the evaluation of levels of zinc in plasma or serum is the best and most common method for assessing zinc status. Normal zinc levels in serum levels are 80–120 μg/dl; low levels must be demonstrated for AE diagnosis. It is important to consider that the zinc blood levels fluctuate during injury, infections, and burns for the redistribution to other body compartments. Also, the hair zinc levels are of interest for diagnosis, but they reflect only long-term zinc status. Serum alkaline phosphatase is sensitive to zinc deficiency, although it is not an early marker of disease. Carboxypeptidase and thymidine kinase may have the same depression of alkaline phosphatase in zinc-deficient subjects, but they are less easily measured. It is possible to evaluate leukocyte zinc, which is probably the most sensitive and precise method. It is very expensive and difficult to perform [103]. To prevent contamination from environmental zinc in collecting containers and to obtain comparable results, blood samples should be collected in special plastic tubes that have been washed in acid.

Differential Diagnosis. AE must be distinguished from pustular psoriasis, epidermolysis bullosa, candidosis, and glucagonoma syndrome. The presence of additional findings of alopecia and diarrhea in zinc deficiency minimizes the clinical confusion. Also, biotin deficiency may present as perifacial dermatitis and alopecia, but normally it occurs in subjects who consume excessive raw egg whites, because biotin binds to avidin, which is found in egg whites, resulting in malabsorption of biotin in the intestinal tract. Lesions indistinguishable from those of acrodermatitis enteropathica may be seen in acquired zinc deficiency that occurs as a consequence of chronic inflammatory bowel disease with diarrhea and malabsorption, pancreatic insufficiency, Crohn's disease, cirrhosis, surgically-induced conditions, total parenteral nutrition for a very long time, extensive burns, and internal malignancies.

Treatment. Acrodermatitis enteropathica responds dramatically to elemental zinc administered as dietary or intravenous supplementation. The normal dosage is 3–5 mg/kg/day given as zinc sulfate, gluconate, acetate, or chloride. No differences between compounds are noted. Zinc sulfate has been recommended for oral administration and zinc chloride for intravenous therapy. The manifestation disappear in a few days. The oral associated lesions including infection (candidal or bacterial) do not need any different topical or systemic treatment. Higher zinc dosages can induce a state of low copper status and immunodysfunction that switch to normal when the zinc dosage is lowered. Copper status and immune functions should be regularly monitored in patients with acrodermatitis enteropathica [104].

6.5.3 Familial Benign Chronic Pemphigus (Familial Benign Pemphigus Hailey-Hailey Disease)

(Figs. 6.27–6.29)

Familial benign chronic pemphigus (FBCP) is a rare genodermatosis characterized by recurrent blister-

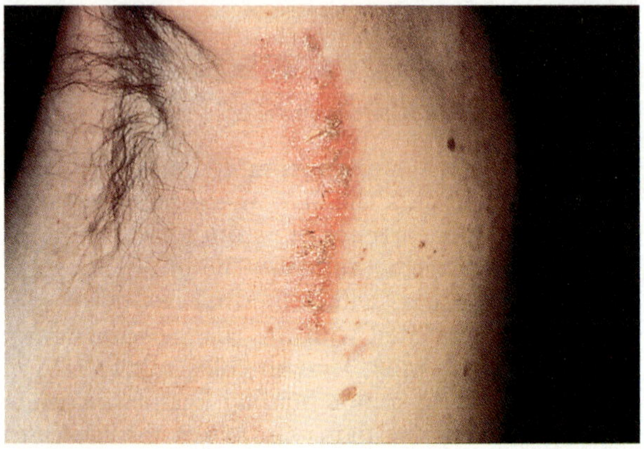

Fig. 6.27. Familial benign chronic pemphigus: skin lesions

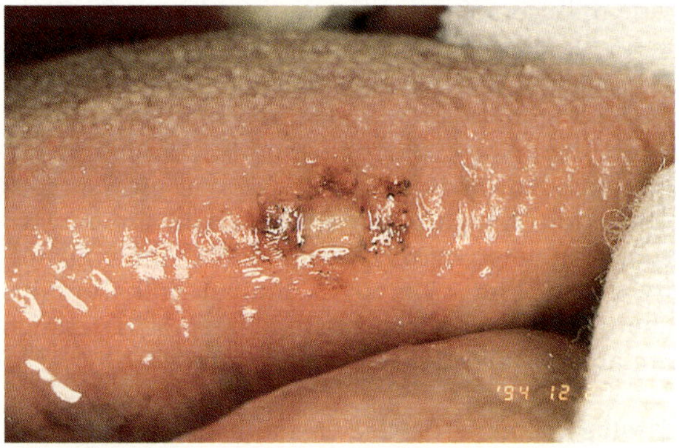

Fig. 6.28. Familial benign chronic pemphigus: bullous lesion of the tongue

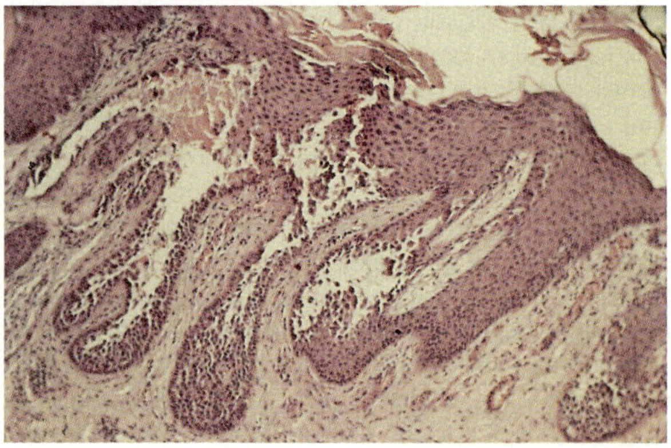

Fig. 6.29. Familial benign chronic pemphigus: histology, × 200

ing lesions on an erythematous base. Usually, the lesions are localized on the nape and the sides of the neck and in the intertriginous areas (axillae, groins, perianal, and inframammary regions). The mouth and other mucosae are affected by the lesions only in very few instances. A family history is obtainable in about two-thirds of patients [105].

Etiology. FBCP is an autosomal dominant disease with an irregular penetrance, characterized by an alteration of keratinocyte cohesion due to proteolysis of epidermal intercellular material [106]. The skin and mucosal lesions related to the disease occur sometimes spontaneously and sometimes as a result of friction produced by pressure from rubber bands, belts, or collars. Also heat, sweat, and ultraviolet radiation can trigger the lesions [107]. Often herpes simplex virus, *Candida albicans*, and bacteria can precipitate or exacerbate lesions [108, 109]. One study reports the presence of HLA-B 16 antigen in 55.5% of patients with FBCP compared to 8.2% in healthy controls [110]. Recent research suggests the presence of a gene not previously known to be involved in keratinocyte cohesion of FBCP in 3q chromosome, between D3S1589 and D3S1316 regions [111].

Pathogenesis. The results of keratinocyte coadhesion defect is a suprabasal epidermal acantholysis, causing blisters largely in a suprabasal location. In the acantholytic epidermal segments of the involved FBCP skin, some of the lower superbasal acantholytic cells fail to express keratin polypeptides 10 and 11 (Moll's catalog). This delay in expression of keratins is not accompained by an expression of hyperproliferative keratin polypeptide 16. Also, some of the FBCP lower suprabasal acantholytic cells retained staining by antikeratin KS-1A3 antibody, which in uninvolved epidermis is limited to the basal cell layer [112]. Probably, the delay in suprabasal keratin expression is related to an "arrest of differentiation," due to acantholysis. The pathogenesis of FBCP is not due to a primary defect in keratin expression, but secondary to the acantholysis. One hypothesis is that acantholysis in FBCP is not a result of a faulty synthesis of the intercellular substance that causes the desmosome disappearance, but is a consequence of a primary defect in the tonofilament-desmosome complex, resulting in separation between tonofilament and desmosomes with dissolution of desmosomes and subsequent acantholysis [113]. The two processes may have a common origin in a defect of the plasma membrane.

Oral Manifestations. Involvement of the oral mucosa is rare. The lips and hard palate are sometimes involved with numerous papular lesions. On the lips, the lesions can ulcerate with subsequent crust formation. The erosive oral lesions on non-keratinized epithelium are infrequent and wide.

Associated Findings. Often the disease is limited to one or a few areas like the perianal region. The predilection sites are the neck and intertriginous areas (axilla, groin, and inframammary regions). Sometimes, the lesions appear on the trunk. The involvement of mucosa (esophagus, larynx, and genital mucosa) is exceptional. In the early stage, the lesions of FBCP consist of small vesicles that easily break, becoming small areas of erosion. Successively, the denuded areas spread, assuming a serpiginous form with a border formed by vesicles and crusts. The lesions normally heal in several months without scarring. Symptoms include burning and pain due to friction and maceration of tissues in the intertriginous sites.

Microscopic Findings. Early lesions of FBCP may show small suprabasal separations which develop into large intraepidermal vesicles and bullae larger than pemphigus vulgaris. Acantholysis affects large portions of epidermis so that many cells show loss of their intracellular bridges. The cells of detached epidermis show only a slight separation from one another and are gathered in packets. This typical feature gives the detached epidermis the appearance of a "dilapidated brick wall" [114], but differs from pemphigus vulgaris in that these acantholytic cells can show normal mitotic activity and are not monstrous. It is possible to find a large number of cells within the blisters. Sometimes, a few corps ronds are present in the granular layer.

Diganosis. Diagnosis is essentially clinical and histological. The typical disposition of the lesions involving the intertriginous areas, the frequent presence of a family history, the recurrence of disease, and the microscopic findings described favor a diagnosis of FBCP.

Differential Diagnosis. FBCP may be distinguished from pemphigus vulgaris, Darier's disease, impetigo, and mycotic lesions of intertriginous areas. In pemphigus vulgaris, the bullae are larger and the oral cavity is often involved, with a lack of familial history. Moreover, in FBCP patients in contrast to pemphigus vulgaris patients, there are no circulating antiepithelial antibodies.

Darier's disease lesions primarily occur in seborrhoic areas, such as the face, scalp, and upper trunk, rather than in intertriginous areas. Darier's disease lesions are persistent rather than cyclic, as in FBCP. The early lesions of Darier's disease are keratotic or crusted papules rather than vesicles, as in FBCP. When FBCP lesions are covered by crusts they may be distinguished from those of impetigo. The long duration of the disease with a tendency to recurrences, the sites involved, and the microscopic findings rule out impetigo. The mycotic lesions of the folds can be excluded by histology and with specific cultural and blood yeast tests.

Treatment. The systemic administration of steroids is effective in suppressing the manifestations of FBCP, but this therapy should be used only in severe cases. Topical applications of steroids are of limited value. The oral lesions can be treated successfully and without systemic side effects by iontophoresis with methylprednisolone [115]. Also interesting is the topical use of cyclosporine [116]. Generally, systemic therapy with antimicrobials (tetracycline, penicillin, and erythromycin) is quite effective because bacteria can produce and exacerbate the eruptions. In some instances, antimicrobial and antifungal ointment gives an improvement. Also, dapsone has been found to be effective in doses of 100/200 mg daily, and in maintenance doses of 50 mg daily [117]. Photochemotherapy with psoralen and a PUVA-22 chamber has been employed successfully and with long-term remission (19 months) [118]. The surgical procedures for excision of FBCP lesions followed by split-thickness grafting are interesting; however, there are sometimes recurrences [119]. Treatment with carbon dioxide laser vaporization has been performed successfully, with 40 % recurrences during 20-month follow-up [120]. Excellent treatment of FBCP was obtained with dermabrasion consisting of the removal of the entire epidermis. This treatment gives functional and cosmetic results and very few relapses, and it is the choice for FBCP unresponsive to conservative therapy [121].

6.6 Diseases of Connective Elastic Tissue

G. Hautmann, G.L. Campanile, and T.M. Lotti

6.6.1 Ehlers-Danlos Syndrome

Definition. Ehlers-Danlos syndrome is a group of hereditary connective tissue disorders which occur in various types. They are inherited as an autosomal dominant, autosomal recessive, or X-linked trait. On the basis of genetic, clinical, and biochemical criteria, at least 11 types of Ehlers-Danlos syndrome are now recognized. It has not been possible to identify the molecular defect in the dominant inherited Ehlers-Danlos syndrome types I, II, and III. However, the molecular defects of collagen biosynthesis of the other types are well known and can be used to establish the diagnosis.

Common to all types are cardinal symptoms such as overstretchability and vulnerability of the skin, with hyperextensibility of the joints. Slight stress and trauma tolerated by normal skin lead to rupture of vessels and to protracted, unsatisfactory wound healing. The frequent skin injuries bleed severely. Atrophic “fish jaw” scars and so-called molluscous pseudotumors are characteristic. Connective tissue hernias, spontaneous pneumothorax, perforated intestine, scoliosis, and muscular hypotonia are additional features. Eye involvement is also pathognomonic in many forms [122, 123].

Oral Manifestations. The oral mucosa is excessively fragile and subject to bruising. Wound healing may be delayed. Gingival bleeding and periodontitis are common. A hypermobility of the temporomandibular joint may occur. Approximately 50 % of patients have the ability to touch their nose with the tongue. Tooth mobility is not increased, but dental abnormalities, such as enamel, dentine, cementum defects, and an increased tendency to develop multiple pulp stones have been reported [124].

Diagnosis. Histopathologic and blood examinations are suggestive but not diagnostic.

Differential Diagnosis. Differential diagnosis includes cutis laxa, Marfan’s syndrome, and osteogenesis imperfecta.

Treatment. Only symptomatic treatment is possible. In severe types, genetic counseling is required.

6.6.2 Marfan’s Syndrome

Definition. Marfan’s syndrome is an inherited defect of connective tissue metabolism caused by an autosomal dominant gene, but the expressivity of the gene varies widely and about 5 % of cases are new mutations. The full syndrome is characterized by abnormally long extremities, arachnodactyly, ocular and cardiovascular defects, but partial forms are not uncommon and there are no absolute diagnostic criteria [125–130].

Oral Manifestations. The more common and characteristic oral manifestations of Marfan’s syndrome are represented by a narrow and high-arched palate; cleft palate, bifid uvula, and abnormalities in the shape of teeth are less common.

Associated Findings. The patient is often, but not invariably, exceptionally tall, with abnormal skeletal proportions: the extremities are long, the excess being greater distally, giving rise to arachnodactyly, and the length of the hallux is often particularly conspicuous. The skull is dolichocephalic and the paranasal sinuses are large. Lax capsules result in unstable or hyperextensible joints, kyphoscoliosis, pectus excavatus, and flat foot. Muscles may be underdeveloped and hypotonic.

Cutaneous defects are not constant or frequent, but serpiginous perforating elastosis may occur and the incidence and severity of atrophic striae may be increased.

Ocular abnormalities are common: they include ectopia lentis, trembling iris, myopia, and retinal detachment. Less frequent are blue sclerotics and heterochromia of the iris.

The cardiovascular system is affected: aneurysmal dilatation of the ascending aorta, aortic and mitral incompetence represent the most common abnormalities. Aortic dilatation may begin in childhood, whereas mitral valve prolapse occurs in about 80 % of cases. The prognosis is obviously related to the severity of the cardiovascular defects, the localization and progression of which are dependent on hemodynamic stresses.

Diagnosis. When the syndrome is fully expressed, it is unmistakable, but diagnostic certainty is impossible in the partial forms. It has been proposed to distinguish two types of Marfan's syndrome: major (mitral incompetence with a floppy valve, aortic incompetence, dilated aortic root, dissecting aneurysm of aorta, dislocation of lens, trembling iris) and minor (arachnodactyly, high-arched palate, funnel chest, asthenic build, instability of the joints, flat feet, scoliosis, spontaneous pneumothorax, floppy mitral valve without incompetence, severe myopia). Simple screening tests which may be helpful include the thumb sign (positive if the thumb, when completely opposed in the clenched hand, projects beyond the ulnar border), the wrist sign (positive if the thumb and little finger overlap when wrapped around the opposite wrist), and the ratio of the lower segment (pubic ramus to floor) to the upper segment (height minus lower segment), but this ratio varies with age and sex.

Differential Diagnosis. This includes Ehlers-Danlos syndrome, homocystinuria, marfanoid hypermobility syndrome, multiple endocrine neoplasia type IIb and mitral valve prolapse syndromes.

Treatment. Obviously, there is no specific treatment; patients should be seen by an ophthalmologist and an orthopedic surgeon; they should be reviewed regularly by a cardiologist. Beta-blockers may be used to retard the development of aortic dilatation. Pregnancy is inadvisable because of the 50 % risk of inheritance in the fetus and because of the risk of acceleration of aortic degeneration and vascular rupture.

6.7 Neurocutaneous Syndromes

G. Borroni and V. Brazzelli

6.7.1 Neurofibromatosis (Von Recklinghausen's Disease)

Definition. The term neurofibromatosis (NF) has been used to describe eight clinically and genetically distinct heritable disorders. NF_1 is the most frequent (85 % of patients) and it is characterized by tumors of the peripheral nervous system (neurofibromas), "café au lait" spots, axillary freckling and Lisch nodules. NF_2 is characterized by the occurrence of bilateral acoustic neuromas as well as meningiomas, ependymomas and schwannomas; cutaneous signs are less evident than in NF_1 [131–137].

Etiology. The prevalence of NF_1 is about 1 in 3000 individuals; the mutation rate is approximately 1 mutation per 10 000 gametes per generation and the genetic fitness is about 0.85. The genetic locus for NF_1 resides on chromosome 17q11.2. The gene responsible for NF_2 has been mapped to chromosome 22q12.

Oral Manifestations. Neurofibromas may affect any part of the body (Fig. 6.30) including the oral cavity, namely the tongue or palate. Oral neurofibromas may disturb phonation, respiration, and deglutition. Some facial plexiform neurofibromas tend to be be-

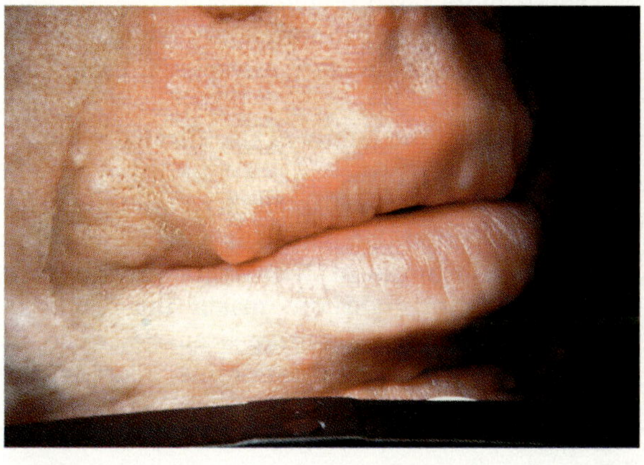

Fig. 6.30. Neurofibromas in the perioral area

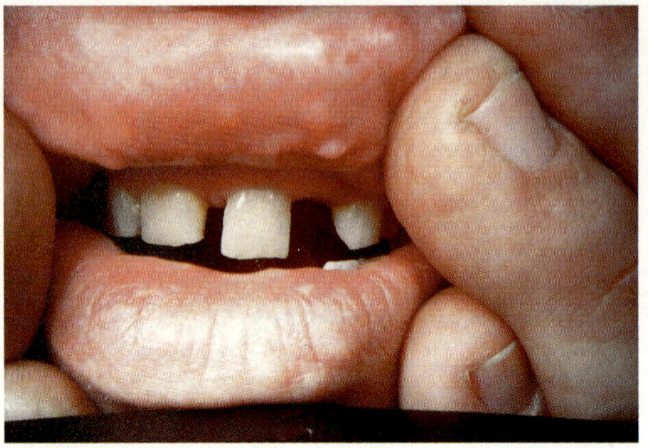

Fig. 6.31. Multiple neurofibromas involve the mucosa of the lips. In this patient hypodontia is also evident

low the zygomatic arch, with invasion to the buccal pad, gingivae and of lingual, pharyngeal, and laryngeal regions.

Associated Findings. Neurofibromas can occur in all parts of the body (Fig. 6.30); "cafè au lait" spots (Fig. 6.31) are characteristic of the NF_1 type, as well as the iris Lisch nodules; central nervous system tumors (commonly astrocytomas) are frequent in NF_2, as well as the acoustic neuromas and/or meningiomas. Pruritus associated with the presence of mast cells in the neurofibromas is characteristic of NF, especially during the growth of neurofibromas. Malignancy is a complication in 5% of NF_1 patients.

Diagnosis. The diagnosis of NF_1 includes the presence of two or more clinical signs:

1. Six or more "cafè au lait" spots
2. Two or more cutaneous neurofibromas or one plexiform neuroma
3. Axillary or perineal freckles
4. Optic gliomas
5. Two or more Lisch nodules
6. Presence of skeletal abnormalities (short stature, macrocephaly, craniofacial dysplasia, pseudoarthrosis)
7. NF patient in the family of the affected patient

Differential Diagnosis. Hereditary, multiple, and also circumscribed lipomatosis is a problem in the differential diagnosis of NF. Histologic study of an excised lesion, however, makes the diagnosis clear. Multiple lentigines have been described in some syndromes (leopard syndrome, Peutz-Jegher syndrome), but the number, size, distribution, and configuration of the individual lesions usually allow differential diagnosis.

Treatment. Pharmacological therapy includes ketotifen or other antihistamines for the pruritus. Surgery has to be considered to treat neurofibromas and some specific areas, such as orbital neurofibromas, and some plexiform, huge neurofibromas, including elephantiasiform variants. Bleeding is a common consequence of surgery, and should be carefully taken into account. NF patients should be monitored for central nervous and spinal neoplasm, and acoustic nerve involvement.

6.7.2 Down's Syndrome, Mongolism, Trisomy 21 Anomaly

Definition. Down's syndrome (DS) is a multisystem disorder featuring well established genotypic (trisomy 21) and phenotypic components, in most instances affecting children of elderly mothers. DS occurs approximately in 1:700 live births; there does not appear to be any racial or sexual bias [138–142].

Etiology. Over 95% of DS-affected individuals have 47 chromosomes including a trisomy 21. About 5% represent translocation at the 21-15 or 21-25 position with a normal component of 46 chromosomes. A small number of DS patients represent a mosaicism. Increasing maternal age is associated with an increased incidence of DS. A high risk of developing DS can occur in families in which a phenotypically normal mother has a translocation at the 21 chromosomal position, a defect which does not increase with maternal age. The mechanism by which this extra chromosome exerts its effect is unknown, but the somatic aberrations produced are remarkably constant.

Oral Manifestations. The mouth is small, round, and usually open. The dry mouth is a consequence of mouth-breathing because of nasal obstruction. Moreover, cheilitis and cracking of the lips are common (Fig. 6.32). The mandible is moderately hypoplastic, which gives the tongue an artificially large and protruding appearance; the tongue, moreover, is thick and fissured (Fig. 6.33). Palatal abnormalities, such as palatus ogivalis, are common. Teeth are delayed in eruption and are characterized by short roots; early loss of teeth is a feature (Fig. 6.34).

Associated Findings. The facies is the most recognizable feature of DS. Eyes present inner and outer epicanthal folds. The iris shows small white spots at the periphery (Brushfield spots). The ears are usually small and low set. Scalp hair is fine and somewhat sparse. Siringomas affect about 20% of DS patients. Short stature and brachycephaly

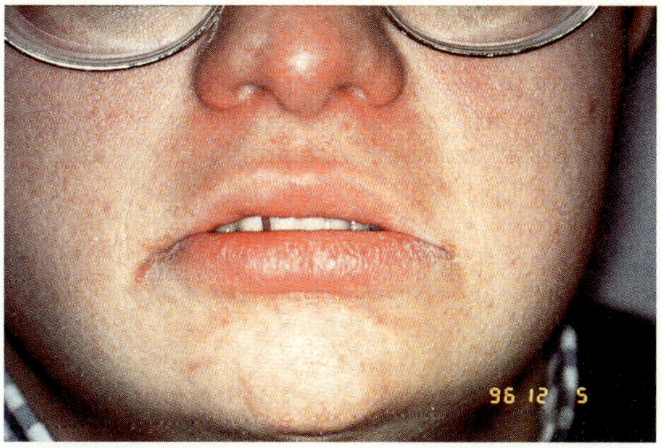

Fig. 6.32. Angular cheilitis and cracking of the lips, a common feature in DS patients due to mouth-breathing

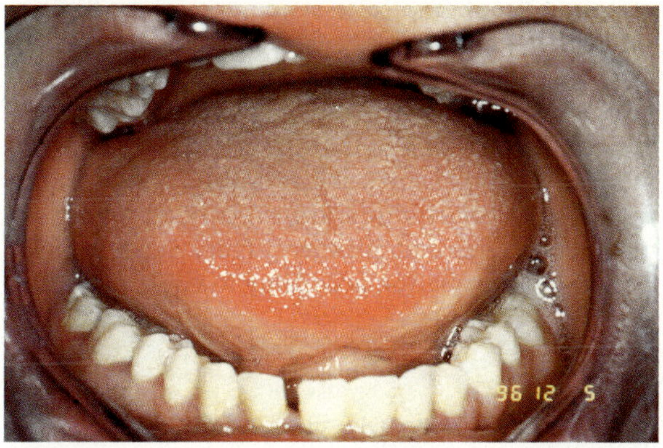

Fig. 6.33. Tongue is thick, broad (macroglossia) and slightly fissured

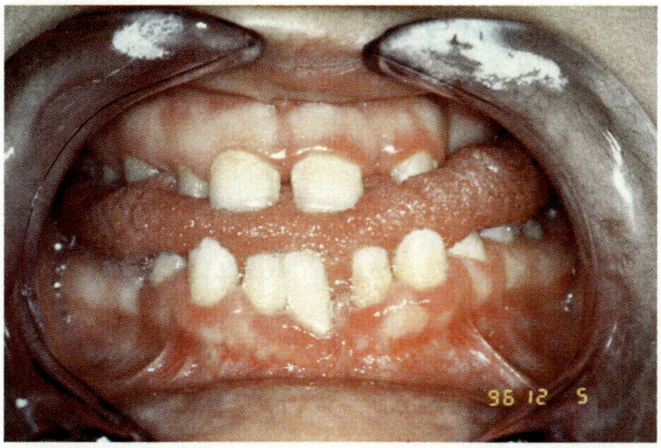

Fig. 6.34. Teeth are characterized by short roots with presence of periodontal disease. Both these conditions cause early loss of teeth

are characteristic features. Hands shown a single palmar crease (simian crease); clinodactyly of the fifth finger is common. Slow physical and mental development are evident (although variations may be seen). Congenital or acquired cardiac septal defects and pulmonary and aortic stenosis are common problems in DS. Moreover, patients with DS have multiple immune defects, with recurrent infections.

Diagnosis. The clinical diagnosis is based on the characteristic somatic features. Karyotyping is mandatory.

Differential Diagnosis. No single component of DS provides an absolute basis for the diagnosis, although the somatic features rarely need a differential diagnosis. Cretinism should be considered in the 1st month of life and it can easily be evaluated with thyroid functional tests.

Treatment. Some recurrent infections such as blepharitis, keratitis, and upper respiratory infections need antibiotic therapy. Congenital or acquired cardiac defects need surgical procedures.

6.7.3 Tuberous Sclerosis (Epiloia, Pringle-Bourneville's Disease)

Definition. Tuberous sclerosis (TS) is an autosomal dominant genetic condition with an incidence of 1 in 10 000, characterized by prominent cutaneous and brain involvement [143–149].

Etiology. Approximately 60 % of TS occurs as apparent sporadic cases. In families, it has autosomal dominant inheritance with high penetrance. Genetic linkage analysis indicates that about half of all TS families show linkage to chromosome 9q34 and about half to chromosome 16p13. There are no distinct features in the two groups of families showing linkage to the two genomic regions.

Oral Manifestations. Papilliferous oral mucosa lesions (Fig. 6.35) may be occasionally seen in 10 % of the patients; histologically, the lesions are characterized by an angiofibromatous pattern. Phenytoin-induced gingival hyperplasia (Fig. 6.35) has also been described in these patients. Congenital dental enamel pits are seen.

Associated Findings. Seizures are the most common presenting sign. The following findings are pathognomonic of TS: facial angiofibromas (Fig. 6.36), ungual fibromas (Koenen's tumors) (Fig. 6.37), retinal hamartomas, cortical tubers or subependymal nodules, multiple renal angiolipomas, cardiac rhabdomyoma, and pulmonary lymphangiomatosis.

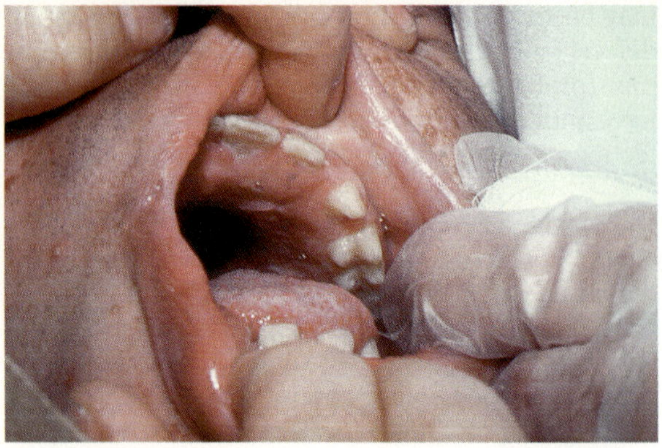

Fig. 6.35. Papilliferous oral mucosa lesions (angiofibromas of the oral mucosa) and phenytoin-induced gingival hyperplasia. Hypodontia is also present. This patient was both mentally handicapped and epileptic

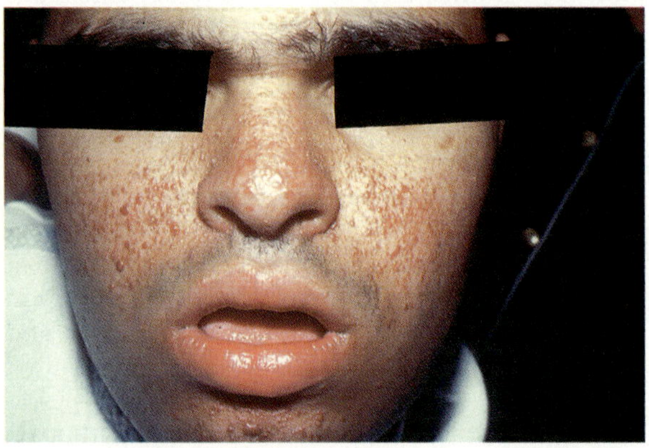

Fig. 6.36. Facial angiofibromas not only involving the nasolabial fold, but also nose, cheeks, and chin

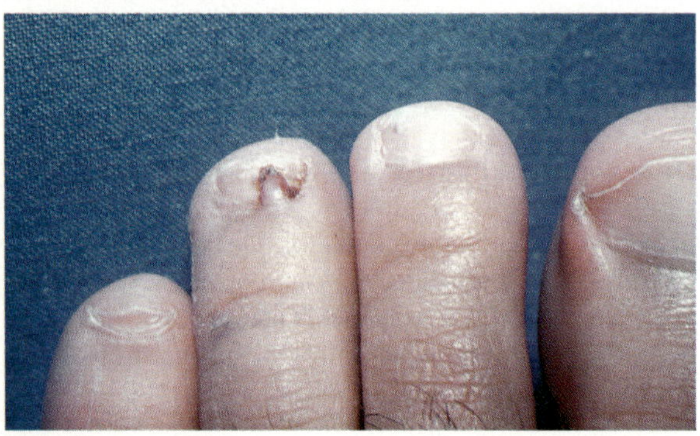

Fig. 6.37. Ungual fibroma (Koenen's tumors), another characteristic feature of TS

Microscopic Findings. Histologically, angiofibromas are characterized by dermal fibrosis and dilatation of capillaries. Large size and stellate fibroblasts are present giving the dermis a glial appearance. Occasionally, multinucleated giant cells are seen.

Diagnosis. Diagnosis includes major criteria and minor clinical features. These are summarized in Tables 6.3 and 6.4.

Differential Diagnosis. The diagnosis of TS is easy if adenoma sebaceum, epilepsy, and mental retardation coexist. If the diagnosis depends mostly on the presence of adenoma sebaceum, this must be differentiated from basal cell nevus syndrome, adenoid cystic basal cell epithelioma, cylindromas, syringomas, and Brooke-Spiegler syndrome. Thus, histologic studies need to be done.

Treatment. Treatment is largely dependent on the organ involvement and the severity of organ impairment. Anticonvulsants, barbiturates, antihypertensive drugs, antiarrythmic drugs, surgical tumor removal, dialysis, and plastic surgery may be used alone or in association according to clinical requirements.

Table 6.3. Criteria for definitive diagnosis of tuberous sclerosis. (From Rodriguez Gomez M. and Adams R. [144])

Facial angiofibromas
Ungual fibroma
Retinal hamartoma
Cortical tuber
Subependymal glial nodule
Renal angiomyolipomas

Table 6.4. Criteria for presumptive diagnosis of tuberous sclerosis. (From Rodriguez Gomez M. and Adams R. [144])

Hypomelanotic macules
Shagreen patches
Peripapillary retinal hamartoma
Gingival fibromas
Dental enamel pits
Single renal angiomyolipoma
Multicystic kidneys
Cardiac rhabdomyoma
Pulmonary lymphangiomyomatosis
Radiography "honeycomb" lungs
Infantile spasms
Myoclonic, tonic, or atonic seizures
Immediate relative with tuberous sclerosis

6.8 Hereditary Neoplasms

C. Feliciani and R. Jordan

6.8.1 Cowden Syndrome

Cowden syndrome (CD) (Figs. 6.38, 6.39), also known as *multiple hamartoma syndrome*, is a genodermatosis inherited as an autosomal dominant trait with variable expressivity. The gene for Cowden syndrome has been identified on chromosome 10q22-23. Cowden syndrome is a familial cancer syndrome with involvement of various organ systems such as skin, oral mucosa, thyroid, breast, female adnexa, and central nervous system. There is great variability in the clinical presentation. The syndrome typically presents in the 2nd decade and is characterized by multiple flesh-colored cutaneous papules, facial tricholemmonas, palmar and plantar keratoderma, and acral keratoses. Hamartomas, lipomas, fibromas, and angiomas are frequently present. Within the mouth, multiple papillomas, fibromas, and a fissured tongue represent the most common changes. Thyroid disease occurs in approximately two-thirds of patients and frequently consists of follicular adenoma or carcinoma. Gastrointestinal abnormalities occur in one-third of those afflicted and consist of multiple hamartomatous polyps and less commonly adenocarcinoma. Fibrocystic changes of the breast have been found in approximately two-thirds of women and are associated with a significant risk of breast cancer. A number of diseases of the central nervous system have also been described including meningiomas, medulloblastoma, and progressive macrocephaly with a mild to moderate delay in psychomotor development [150–153].

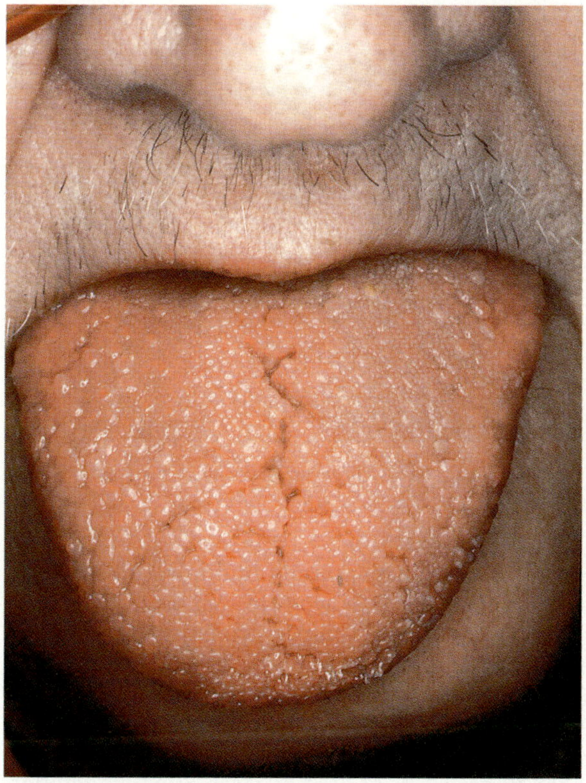

Fig. 6.38. Cowden syndrome (courtesy of M.D. FRCP, Benjamin K. Fisher, Dept. Dermatology, Women's college Hospital, Toronto, Ontario, Canada)

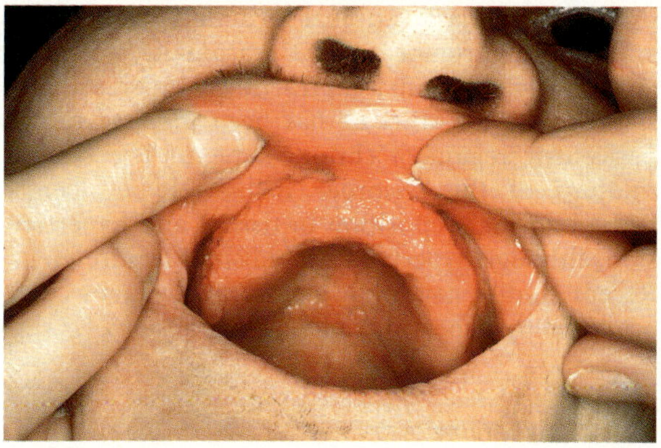

Fig. 6.39. Cowden syndrome. Papules on the upper gum (courtesy of M.D. FRCP, Benjamin K. Fisher, Dept. Dermatology, Women's college Hospital, Toronto, Ontario, Canada)

6.8.2 Multiple Endocrine Neoplasia Syndromes

These are a group of rare genetic conditions characterized by tumors or hyperplasias of neuroendocrine tissues. Three multiple endocrine neoplasia (MEN) syndromes are recognized and are associated with different patterns of organ involvement. The MEN 1 syndrome is characterized by tumors of the pituitary, parathyroid gland, and pancreas. The MEN 2A (Sipple) syndrome is characterized by the development of pheochromocytomas, medullary carcinoma of the thyroid, and parathyroid hyperplasia. Patients with MEN 2B (MEN 3) develop pheochromocytomas, medullary carcinoma of the thyroid gland, and mucosal neuromas.

6.8.2.1 *MEN 2A (Sipple Syndrome)*

Sipple syndrome (multiple endocrine neoplasia type 2 a) is an autosomal dominant disease included in ectodermal phakomatoses. It is characterized by hyperplasia and/or carcinoma of the parafollicular calcitonin-producing C cell of the thyroid, parathyroid hyperplasia, adrenal medullary hyperplasia, and/or pheochromocytoma. Occasionally, a cerebellar hemangioblastoma is present. By linkage analysis, the gene of MEN 2A has been mapped in the pericentric region of chromosome 10. The clinical findings of this disorder include hypocalcemia with abnormal deposition in tissues and hypertension, although hyperparathyroidism is less frequent. Recent studies have shown skin involvement characterized by lichen amyloidosis-like lesions [154].

6.8.2.2
MEN 2B Syndrome

The only MEN syndrome with oral manifestations is the MEN 2 B syndrome. Although it is inherited in an autosomal dominant fashion, up to 50 % of cases are believed to arise as new mutations. Patients typically have a marfanoid habitus with long, thin limbs, pectus excavatum, narrow face, thick lips, and occasionally everted eyelids. A characteristic feature is the development of bilateral mucosal neuromas at the commissures of the mouth. Approximately 50 % of affected individuals develop pheochromocytomas, with the prevalence increasing with age. Medullary carcinomas of the thyroid gland arise from the calcitonin-producing C cells and develop in 90 % of patients. Most of these tumors develop in the 2nd decade and are associated with metastatic disease.

6.8.3
Nevoid Basal Cell Carcinoma Syndrome
(Figs. 6.40–6.42)

The nevoid basal cell carcinoma syndrome, also known as Gorlin (Gorlin-Goltz) syndrome, is an autosomal dominant disorder that predisposes to multiple basal cell carcinomas of the skin, medulloblastoma, ovarian fibromas, and other neoplasms. Nevoid basal cell carcinoma was described in the late 19th century but was characterized in 1960 by Gorlin and Goltz. Although it is a genetic disease, the molecular basis of the disorder is not well understood. The clinical behavior of the associated neoplastic disease suggests that the underlying defect may be a mutation of a tumor-suppressor gene that plays a key role in normal embryonic development. An unusual and dominant mutation of a gene on chromosome 9q has been proposed recently. The characteristic clinical features of this syndrome include coarse face, strabismus, hypertelorism, and macrocephaly. Radiographic examination shows various skeletal and skull abnormalities such as spina bifida occulta, bifid ribs, dysgenesis of the corpus callosum, and calcification of the falx cerebri. Odontogenic keratocysts are a characteristic feature of the syndrome and are typically multiple and prone to recurrences. The cutaneous lesions appear between puberty and the mid-thirties, consisting of multiple basal cell carcinomas and palmar and plantar pits. Mental retardation and growth deficiency can also be present. Surgical removal of the cutaneous carcinomas is the only realistic therapy and, when extensive, these can be excised by laser. Supplementation with local injections of interferon-α may be helpful [155–161].

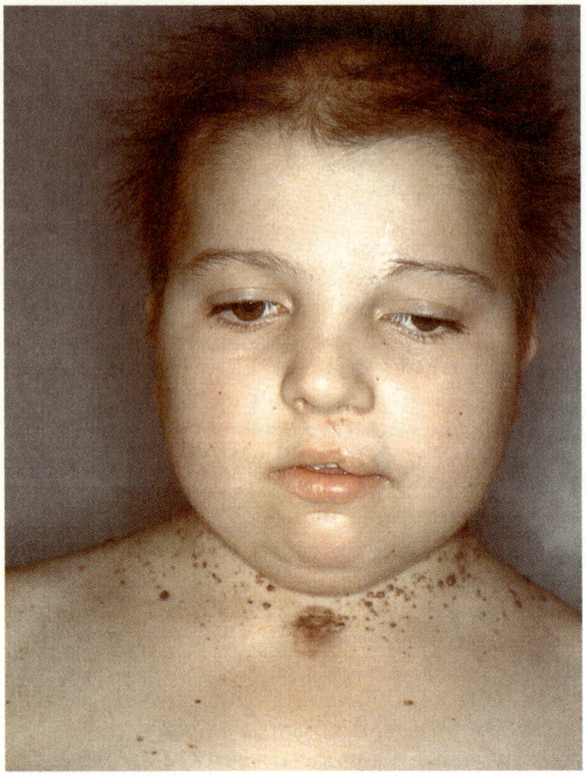

Fig. 6.40. Nevoid basal cell nevus syndrome, multiple epitheliomas on the neck in a patient with cleft lip

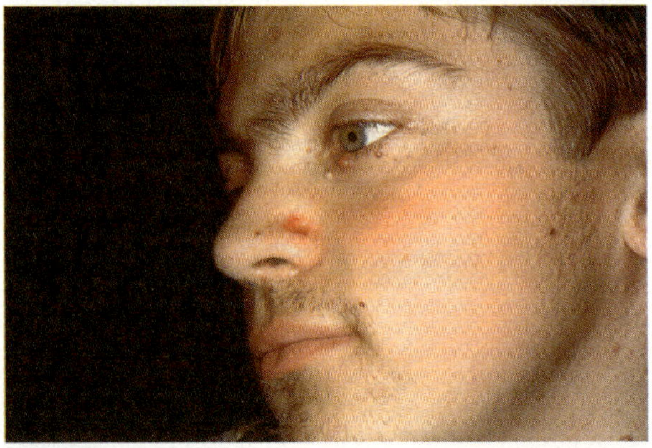

Fig. 6.41. Nevoid basal cell nevus syndrome, several epitheliomas on the face

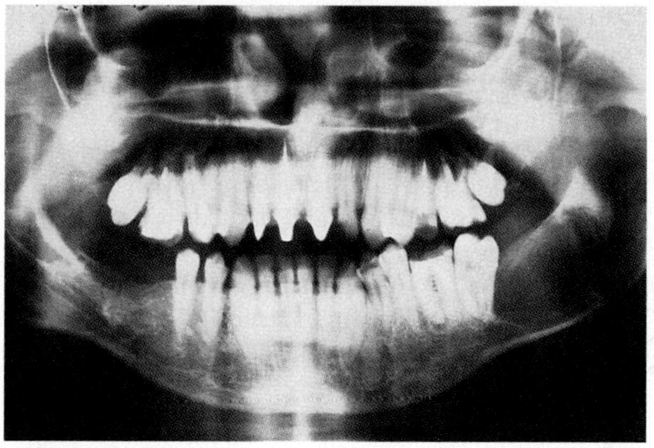

Fig. 6.42. Nevoid basal cell nevus syndrome, odontogenic cysts

6.8.4 Gardner's Syndrome

Gardner's syndrome is characterized by the presence of polyposis of the colon and rectum, associated with a wide range of extra-colon manifestations such as soft tissue tumors, bony abnormalities, retinal pigmentation, and dental abnormalities. Gardner's syndrome is caused by a mutation in the adenomatous polyposis coli (APC) gene located on chromosome 5q21. This disorder, inherited in an autosomal dominant pattern, has a marked propensity for multiple polyposis of the colon and rectum with a significant risk of malignant transformation. The polyps usually develop before the age of 10 years and are relatively asymptomatic. Melena, diarrhea, and vague abdominal pain usually appear around the age of 30 with 100 % of patients developing colorectal carcinoma in their mid-30s if colectomy is not performed. Extra-colon manifestations of Gardner's syndrome are common and include epidermal inclusion cysts of the skin and fibrous tumors, although a wide array of other tumors such as leiomyomas and lipomas have also been described. Fibromas and desmoid tumors frequently arise in surgical scars as well as de novo. Bone abnormalities are present in 50 % of patients and typically consist of osteomas of the mandible; however, any portion of the skeleton may be affected. Multiple bilateral retinal pigmented lesions, which are due to congenital hypertrophy of the retinal pigment epithelium, are often present at birth. Dental anomalies include supernumerary and unerupted teeth in both the mandible and the maxilla. Colorectal carcinoma is the most frequent tumor in all individuals. Periampullary carcinoma is the second most frequent, while intra-abdominal desmoids is the third. Other extracolonic tumors include papillary carcinoma of the thyroid (almost exclusively in women), gastric carcinoma (particularly in Japan), sarcomas, and brain tumors. Treatment is aimed at the polyposis consisting of colectomy with creation of an ileoanal reservoir. Management involves treatment of affected individuals, counseling of patients and their families, genetic screening of individuals at risk, and surveillance of affected patients for extra-colonic cancer [162–169].

6.9 Hereditary Diseases Caused by Disorders in Metabolism

G. Micali and A. Sapuppo

6.9.1 Amyloidoses

Definition. Amyloidoses are a group of disorders characterized by abnormal extracellular deposition of amyloid, a proteinaceous substance. Two distinct types of amyloidoses are known: systemic amyloidosis, in which several organs are involved, and localized amyloidosis, in which amyloid is restricted to a single organ.

Etiology. This is unknown in most cases. Rarely, both systemic and localized amyloidoses may be hereditary. Systemic amyloidosis may be primary or secondary to multiple myeloma or chronic inflammatory diseases (infections, rheumatoid arthritis, juvenile chronic arthritis, ankylosing spondylitis, Reiter's syndrome, Behçet's syndrome, Sjögren's syndrome, systemic lupus erythematosus, inflammatory bowel disease, various dermatoses). Localized amyloidosis primarily affects the skin, the lung, and the genitourinary tract.

The origin and chemical composition of amyloid varies according to the different forms of the disease: in primary and myeloma-related systemic amyloidosis and in localized amyloidosis, the intercellular deposits consist of immunoglobulin chain material (protein AL), while in systemic amyloidoses secondary to chronic inflammatory diseases amyloid is composed of an acute-phase reactant (protein AA). In the rare cases of hereditary amyloidosis it derives from prealbumin [170, 171].

Oral Manifestations. Involvement of oral mucosa is common in primary and myeloma-related systemic amyloidoses, with waxy translucent papules, nodules, plaques, bullae, and hemorrhagic spots on the tongue, gingiva, and inner surface of the lips and cheeks (Fig. 6.43). The tongue may be firm, enlarged, and protruding (macroglossia) (Fig. 6.44); its surface may be smooth, dry, or covered by fissures

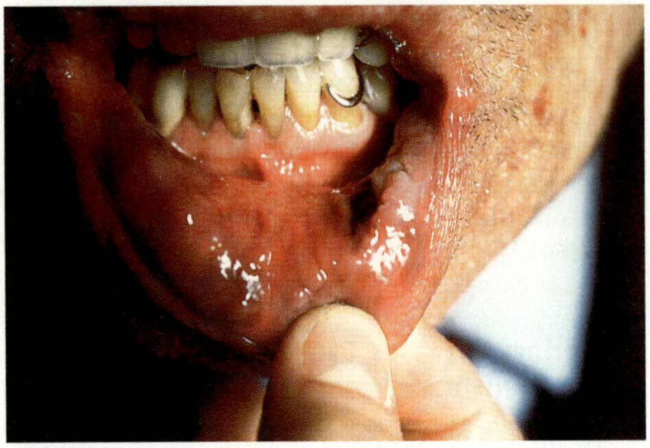

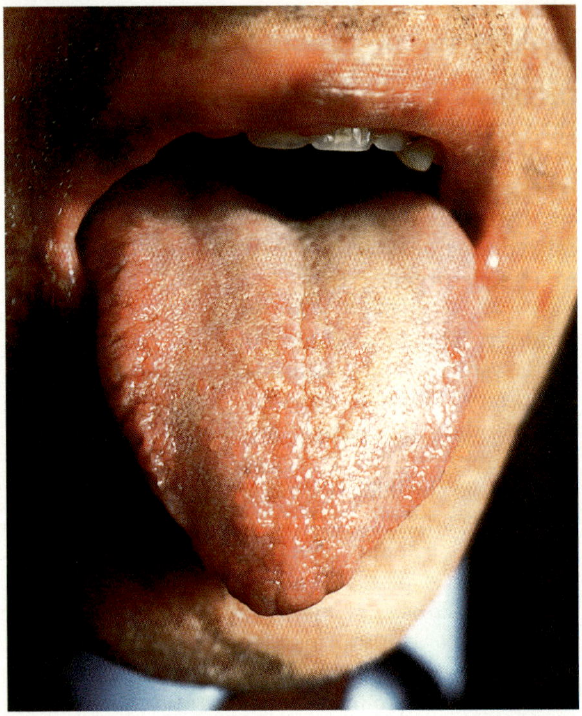

Fig. 6.43, 6.44. Clinical oral manifestations of amyloidosis. (Courtesy of Prof. M. Aricò, Department of Dermatology, University of Palermo, Palermo, Italy)

and ulcerations. Macroglossia may cause dysphagia, as well as tooth indentation along the lateral borders of the tongue. In all the other forms of amyloidosis, oral involvement is unusual [172, 173].

Clinical findings. In systemic amyloidosis, presenting symptoms include fatigue, weight loss, paresthesia, hoarseness, edema, and syncope. Further clinical features depend on visceral involvement and consist most frequently of nephrotic syndrome, congestive cardiac failure, hepatomegaly, ascites, protein-losing enteropathy, and malabsorption syndrome; the development of a "carpal tunnel syndrome" is also common. The skin may show hemorrhages, papules, nodules, diffuse infiltration, or bullae due to shearing within dermal amyloid deposits. Additional clinical findings may be observed according to the underlying disease.

In localized amyloidosis, skin involvement is characterized by macular and papular lesions. Amyloidosis of the lung shows nodular or diffuse infiltrations, while hematuria may be a symptom of amyloidosis of the genitourinary tract.

Microscopic Findings. Amyloid is a proteinaceous substance that has an extracellular localization and many characteristic tinctorial properties, like congophilia and green birefringence under polarized light. Under the electron microscope, amyloid has a fibrillar ultrastructure; the filaments have a diameter of 6–10 nm and a cross-B pattern on X-ray diffraction [174].

Diagnosis. The presence of macroglossia, carpal tunnel syndrome, and mucocutaneous lesions should lead to the diagnosis of systemic amyloidosis. However, histological examination of a sample obtained by fine-needle biopsy of the subcutaneous tissue from abdominal skin is necessary [171, 175]. In localized amyloidoses, diagnosis depends on histochemical, immunohistochemical, or ultrastructural demonstration of amyloid material in the biopsy specimen.

Treatment. There are no specific treatments for systemic amyloidosis; occasionally, results have been obtained with melphalan, colchicine, thymosin, and dimethyl sulfoxide. The prognosis of systemic amyloidosis is poor, especially in the primary and myeloma-related variants, and death usually takes place due to cardiac or renal failure. Therapy of localized amyloidoses may change according to the organ involved.

6.9.2 Lipoproteinosis

Synonyms. Hyalinosis cutis et mucosae, Urbach-Wiethe disease, lipoid proteinosis, lipoglycoproteinosis.

Definition. Lipoproteinosis is a rare metabolic disorder characterized by increased deposition of a hyaline material in the dermis of skin and mucosae; this deposition may also involve other organs [176, 177].

Etiology. The disease is inherited as an autosomal recessive trait. The hyaline deposits, produced by endothelial cells, pericytes, Schwann cells, and epithelial cells, arise from basal laminae. It has been suggested that lipoproteinosis may represent either a lysosomal storage disease due to single or multiple enzyme defects resulting in defective degradation, or a disorder in which cellular activity (fibroblasts, epithelial, and endothelial cells) is altered so that fibrous collagens are underproduced and basement membrane collagen overproduced [176].

Oral Manifestations. At onset, it frequently involves the oral mucosa; early in life the soft palate, tonsils, lips, and tongue show widespread papular lesions or firm yellow-white infiltrates. The tongue may be enlarged, stiffened, with short frenulum, and be difficult to protrude. Xerostomia, recurrent parotitis and dental anomalies may also be present [176, 179, 180].

Clinical Findings. Skin lesions usually appear during childhood as vesiculopustular lesions on the face and distal extremities which usually heal with residual depressed acneiform scars. With time, the deposition of hyaline material increases and gradually the involved skin and mucosa become irregularly filled with yellowish, pale hyaline deposits in plaques, and papules and nodules on the face and neck. Areas of increased friction (hands, elbows, and knees) are most affected and may be covered with hyperpigmented and hyperkeratotic patches. Papules on the eyelid margin are a typical finding. Other frequent manifestations are hoarseness secondary to the infiltration of the vocal cords, recurrent parotitis by obstruction of the Stensen duct, and epilepsy due to intracranial calcifications. Involvement of other organs is usually asymptomatic [176, 178, 179, 181].

Microscopic Findings. The hyaline material, acid-Schiff-positive, deposits in the dermis, surrounding blood vessels, and sweat glands; it is composed of a very fine network of procollagen filaments interlinked with amorphous granular material. In the affected dermis, excessive amounts of matrix glycoproteins and decreased quantities of collagen fibers are present [176, 177, 179].

Diagnosis. The presence in a child of hoarseness, enlargement and stiffening of the tongue, along with characteristic cutaneous lesions, may suggest the diagnosis, which, however, needs histological confirmation. Differential diagnosis includes erythropoietic protoporphyria, which involves exposed areas only, lichen myxoedematosus, which arises in adulthood, amyloidosis and xanthomatosis, which show different microscopic findings.

Treatment. There is no effective therapy although oral dimethylsulfoxide has been used successfully in one case. Carbon dioxide laser treatment of thickened vocal cords has proved to be effective for hoarseness. Anticonvulsants should be prescribed for those subjects who develop epilepsy. Tracheostomy is necessary in some cases due to laryngeal obstruction. In the majority of cases, the disease runs a chronic and benign course, with no shortening of life span [176].

6.9.3 Mucopolysaccharidoses

Definition. Mucopolysaccharidoses (MPS) are a hereditary group of diseases characterized by storage of mucopolysaccharides (or glycosaminoglycans), mainly dermatan sulfate, heparan sulfate, and keratan sulfate, secondary to different enzymatic defects in various tissues and organs. Based on the clinical findings and the type of enzymatic deficiency, 14 distinct types of MPS are known: I-H (Hurler syndrome), I-H/S, I-S (Scheie syndrome), II-A and II-B (Hunter syndrome), III-A, III-B, III-C and III-D (Sanfilippo syndrome), IV-A and IV-B (Morquio syndrome), VI-A and VI-B (Maroteaux-Lamy syndrome), and VII [182].

Etiology. Mucopolysaccharidoses are caused by deficiency of several lysosomal enzymes involved in the degradation of mucopolysaccharides; ten enzymatic defects have been identified (α-l-iduronidase, iduronate sulfatase, heparan *N*-sulfatase, arylsulfatase B, β-glucuronidase, etc.). All the MPS have autosomal recessive inheritance, except Hunter's syndroma, which is X-linked recessive [182–184].

Oral Manifestations. The oral mucosa involved may be different in each type; frequent findings are the enlargement of lips and tongue, which is protruded through the mouth, usually open (Fig. 6.45), and the delayed eruption of teeth, which are widely spaced and often exhibit severe attrition; localized areas of bone destruction, called "dentigerous cysts", and other dental abnormalities, like enamel hypoplasia, are frequently present. The mandible is often short and broad with wide bigonial distance and temporomandibular joint anomalies which may hamper mandibular movements; prognathism may also be present (Fig. 6.46) [184–187].

Clinical Findings. Somatic changes develop in the early months of life; there is clinical similarity between different enzymatic deficiencies and, conversely, wide phenotypic variety among every enzyme deficiency. Some findings occur most frequently:

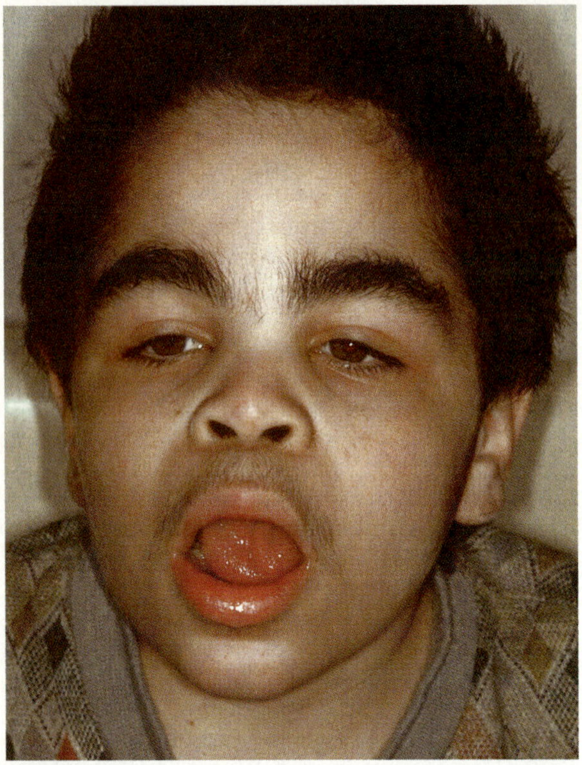

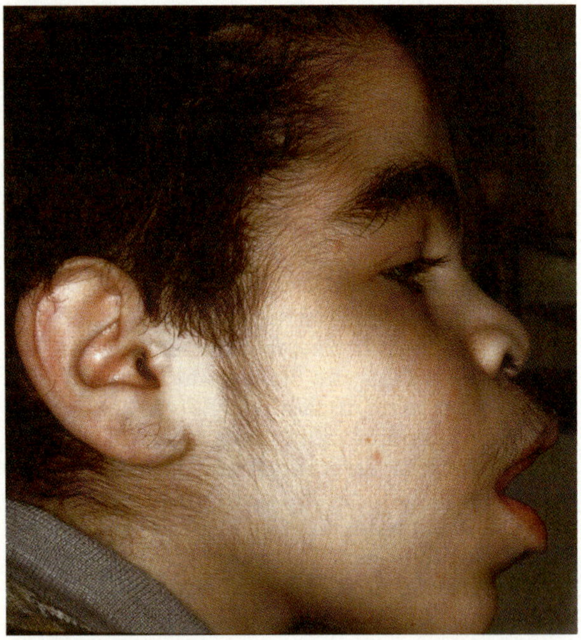

Fig. 6.45, 6.46. Clinical manifestations of mucopolysaccharidosis II-B. (Courtesy of Prof. L. Pavone, Department of Paediatrics, University of Catania, Catania, Italy)

coarsening of facial features, large head, low and depressed nasal bridge, hypertrichosis, hypertelorism, corneal opacities, deafness, short neck, bony changes (multiple dysostosis), short stature, joint abnormalities, umbilical and inguinal hernias, hepatosplenomegaly, skin thickening, and arteriosclerosis. In some syndromes (I-H, II.A, III-A, III-B, III-C, III-D), mental retardation is prominent. Cardiac failure and respiratory infections are the most common causes of death, which usually occurs in childhood. Patients with MPS I-S, II-A, IV-B, VI-A and VI-B may survive into adulthood [182, 183, 187, 188].

Microscopic Findings. Histologically, the presence of large cells with a pale distended cytoplasm, vacuolated for the presence of lysosomes stuffed with PAS-positive material, is characteristic. The nucleus is usually displaced to one side of the cytoplasm [183].

Diagnosis. Final diagnosis requires urinary assay of glycosaminoglycans, which are excessively excreted, by the toluidine blue test or by the gross albumin turbidity test. The enzymatic defect can be demonstrated in isolated leukocytes or cultured skin fibroblasts. X-rays of bones may be helpful. Prenatal diagnosis is possible at 8 weeks gestation through enzymatic assay in cultured chorionic villi cells.

Treatment. An effective causal treatment is not yet available. The treatment is only symptomatic and consists of physical therapy, surgical correction of joint anomalies and hernias, corneal transplantation and use of hearing devices. Bone marrow transplantation is under evaluation. Enzyme replacement therapies have shown no clinical benefits [182, 183].

6.9.4 Gaucher's Disease

Synonyms. Glucosylceramide lipidosis.

Definition. Gaucher's disease is the most common lipid storage disorder. It is characterized by lysosomal accumulation of glucocerebrosides in the histiocytes of various organs. According to the age of onset and neuronal involvement, three phenotypes have been described: an adult non-neuronopathic form (type I), the most frequent, an infantile neuronopathic form (type II), and a juvenile neuronopathic form (type III) [189, 190].

Etiology. Gaucher's disease, which has an autosomal recessive inheritance, is caused by deficient activity of a lysosomal enzyme, known as glucocerebrosidase (or glucosylceramidase), which is required for the hydrolysis of the β-glucosidic bond of glucocerebroside; the lack of the enzyme leads to the accumulation of insoluble glucocerebrosides in the histiocytes of various organs, including spleen, liver, bone marrow, and, in the more severe cases, central nervous system. About 40 mutations of the glucocerebrosidase gene have been identified for this disease; residual activity of mutant enzyme may explain phenotypic variability [189, 190].

Oral Manifestations. The oral mucosa is rarely involved and then only in the adult form, with dark brown patches or yellow pigmentation of the gingiva. Spontaneous gingival hemorrhages may also be present. Dental radiographs often reveal consistent bony changes, which result from encroachment of the bone marrow cavity; these changes may sometimes suggest the diagnosis of the disease [191, 192].

Clinical Findings. The adult type of Gaucher's disease can be diagnosed at any age. Its onset is often insidious, with weakness, growth retardation, anemia or bleeding diathesis; subsequently, abdominal enlargement from notable hepatosplenomegaly, and bone destruction (characterized by pain, pathologic fractures, aseptic necrosis) from expansion of medullary cavity, may develop. The skin may show brown or yellow hyperpigmentation of the face, neck, hands, or shins, while in about 25 % of cases yellow patches on the sclerae ("pingueculae") may occur. The age at onset in type II is approximately 3–6 months with hepatosplenomegaly and acute brainstem dysfunction, characterized by cranial nerve paralysis, trismus, strabismus, neck rigidity, laryngeal spasm; death usually takes place before 2 years of age due to aspiration pneumonia or apnea. A more prolonged survival with progressive neurologic deterioration usually occurs in type III or juvenile form of Gaucher's disease [189, 190].

Microscopic Findings. Histologically, "Gaucher's cells" are classically large lipid-laden histiocytic elements with a PAS-positive, wrinkled-appearing cytoplasm and an eccentric nucleus. They may be observed in the spleen, liver, lymph nodes, and bone marrow. These cells must be differentiated from those seen in leukemia, thalassemia, congenital dyserytropoietic anemia and multiple myeloma. Ultrastructurally, cytoplasmatic tubular inclusions are characteristic.

Diagnosis. The diagnosis, suspected by the clinical findings, is usually made by detecting Gaucher's cells in the bone marrow or spleen, and requires confirmation by the glucocerebrosidase assay in peripheral blood leukocytes or fibroblasts, and by DNA analysis [193]. Prenatal detection is possible, up to 8 weeks' gestation, through enzymatic determination in a chorionic villus sample.

Treatment. The most effective therapy for the treatment of type I Gaucher's disease is intravenous infusion of alglucerase or imiglucerase, a placentally derived form and a recombinant DNA-modified form, respectively, of glucocerebrosidase. Alglucerase, at a dose of 60 units/g every 2 weeks, improves quality of life, although the bone responds slowly. Splenectomy, bone marrow transplantation, and other symptomatic therapies give poor results. Gene therapy based on transfer of the therapeutic gene to hematopoietic stem cells was started in 1995 in the USA. The role of enzyme therapy in types II and III of Gaucher's disease is under evaluation [189, 193, 194].

6.9.5 Niemann-Pick Disease

Synonyms. Sphingomyelin lipidosis, sphingomyelinosis.

Definition. It is a rare lipid storage disease characterized by lysosomal deposition of sphingomyelin in proliferating macrophages of the reticulohistiocytic tissues (lymph nodes, spleen, bone marrow, thymus, Kupffer's cells, and neuroglia). Based on clinical, histological, and laboratory findings, six distinct types are known: A (acute neuronopathic form), B (chronic form without nervous system involvement), C (chronic neuronopathic form), D (Nova Scotia variant), E (adult non-neuronopathic form), F (a still undefined form) [195, 196].

Etiology. The disorder in all its variants is transmitted as an autosomal recessive trait. Types A and B are characterized by a defect of sphingomyelinase, a lysosomal enzyme. For the other types, the exact enzymatic defect is unknown: in most cases, an excessive deposition of cholesterol, which could be responsible for the inhibition of the sphingomyelin degradation, is present in various tissues [195, 196].

Oral Manifestations. Oral mucosa, as well as other mucous membranes, may be rarely involved in the advanced stage of the disease, with yellowish-brown hyperpigmentation or dark bluish spots. There may be retarded tooth eruption and precocious loosening of teeth.

Clinical Findings. The onset is generally during infancy for all types of Niemann-Pick disease, with weight loss, hepatosplenomegaly, generalized lymphadenopathy, and muscle weakness. Pulmonary infiltrations and severe involvement of the central nervous system (developmental delay, general functional deterioration, seizures, ataxia) may be the cause of death, which usually takes place in the early years of life; in types B and E, which are consistently free of neurological manifestations, the patients may survive into adulthood. In the late stages of the disease, yellowish papules of the skin and a cherry-red spot in the macula on ophthalmologic evaluation are seen in most cases. Finally, deafness and blindness may develop as common features [195, 197–199].

Microscopic Findings. Histologically, the typical finding is the "Niemann-Pick's cell", a mononucleate, large, pale, and foamy cell containing variably sized lipid cytosomes. PAS positivity is less marked than with Gaucher's cells.

Diagnosis. The diagnosis requires the identification of foamy cells in bone marrow, liver or spleen, and the demonstration of abnormal intracellular accumulation of spingomyelin. In types A and B, the diagnosis should be confirmed by the finding of low levels of leukocytic sphingomyelinase activity [195, 196, 200).

Treatment. No effective treatment is available. Supportive therapy includes the reduction of dietary cholesterol, the treatment of infective complications, the administration of anticonvulsants, transfusions, or splenectomy. For type B, bone marrow transplantation is under evaluation.

6.9.6 Acatalasia and Acatalasemia

Definition. Acatalasia is the deficiency of catalase in blood and tissues; the lack of this enzyme exclusively into the red cells is called acatalasemia. The clinical evidence of this defect is called "Takahara syndrome" [201, 202].

Etiology. The inheritance is probably autosomal recessive and many mutations may cause the biochemical anomaly with the production of a variant of the enzyme with very low specific activity or of an unstable variant. The lack of catalase hampers the degradation of hydrogen peroxide produced by the oral bacterial flora of the dental plaque deposits in the periodontal tissues; subsequently, hydrogen peroxide oxidizes hemoglobin, depriving the exposed tissues of oxygen and causing ulceration, necrosis, and decay [202–204].

Oral Manifestations. At its onset, the disease may appear with small painful ulcers of the gingival mucosa or of the tonsillar lacunae. Ulcerative and necrotic lesions may subsequently reach the dental alveoli with early tooth loss in childhood. In more severe cases, there may be widespread destruction, and gangrene of the maxilla or of the soft tissues of the mouth may occur [202, 203].

Clinical Findings. With the exception of oral lesions, physical examination of patients with Takahara syndrome is normal; occasionally, ulcerative lesions may be observed on the nasal mucosa. The life span is normal.

Diagnosis. Progressive gangrenous lesions of gingiva should suggest the correct diagnosis, which has to be confirmed by catalase activity assay [201]. Catalase is almost completely absent in the blood of homozygotes, while in heterozygotes it may vary between 35 % and 100 %. Adding a drop of blood to 2 ml of 2 % H_2O_2, if the sample contains less than about 5 % of the normal catalase concentration, the color changes to brown and then to white for the hemoglobin oxidation.

Treatment. This consists of excision of oral gangrenous lesions and extraction of affected teeth; systemic antibiotics and correct oral hygiene are necessary to control bacterial proliferation.

6.10 Hereditary Hematologic Diseases

R. S. Rogers, III

6.10.1 Cyclic Neutropenia

Definition. Cyclic neutropenia is a rare disease, usually presenting in childhood with oral ulcerations, fever, malaise, and recurrent infections associated with neutropenia. The severity of the infections usully parallels the severity of the neutropenia. The cyclicity of the neutropenia varies among patients from 12 to 30 days and lasts 3–4 days usually about every 3 weeks. The rhythmicity is constant for each patient [205].

Etiology. Recent studies have shown a T-lymphocyte defect with cyclic deficient production of GM-CSF, a growth factor for neutrophils.

Pathogenesis. With the neutropenia, particularly counts below 500/mm^3, residual or transient flora can proliferate, resulting in local sepsis (oral ulcerations) and systemic sepsis (chills, fever, and malaise).

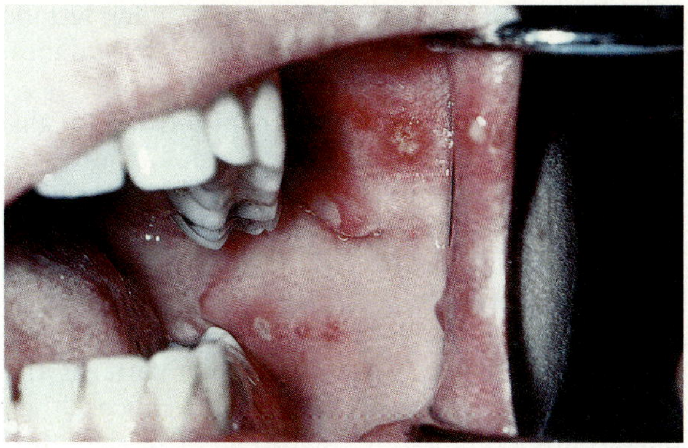

Fig. 6.47. Cyclic neutropenia. Note oral ulcers in various stages from red papules to confluent ulcers covered with a gray fibromembranous slough and surrounded by an erythematous halo. Note scar of left labial commissure from previous lesion

Oral Manifestations. Oral ulcerations develop on nonkeratinized and keratinized (masticatory) mucosal surfaces including alveolar gingivae and hard palate mucosa. The ulcerations are nonspecific in character, painful, and covered by a fibromembranous slough (Fig. 6.47). Breath may be fetid, the tongue coated, and the gingivae may bleed with dental hygiene measures.

Associated Findings. Neutropenia occurs as the early sign of an exacerbation and persists for 3–4 days. The neutrophil count may fall to less than $500/mm^3$.

Microscopic Findings. Nonspecific ulceration with a heavy round cell and a sparse polymorphonuclear leukocyte infiltrate.

Diagnosis. Characteristic cyclicity of the oral ulcerations and neutropenia.

Differential Diagnosis. Menstrually related aphthae may be confusing because of the rhythmicity, but aphthae tend to spare the masticatory mucosa, and patients with aphthosis do not usually suffer fever, malaise, and recurrent infections.

Treatment. Spontaneous improvement with decreasing severity can occur. Splenectomy may be helpful. Parenteral GM-CSF (experimental) is administered. Oral microflora are reduced with chlorhexidine astringent mouthwash in anticipation of a cyclic outbreak.

6.10.2 Hereditary Hemorrhagic Telangiectasia (Osler-Weber-Rendu Syndrome)

Definition. A hereditary disease characterized by multisystem vascular dysplasia presenting as cutaneous and mucosal telangiectasias which results in epistaxis and gastrointestinal hemorrhage. Pulmonary arteriovenous fistulas may be noted [206, 207].

Etiology. Autosomal dominant inheritance. Mutation of TGF-β binding protein, endoglin, which is critical to endothelial cell function. The genome resides on the 9q33-34 chromosome, named OWR1. Genetic heterogeneity is becoming apparent, leading to the concept that hereditary hemorrhagic telangiectasia is a family of disorders.

Pathogenesis. Vascular dysplasia can present as dilated vessels (telangiectasias), as ruptured vessels (hemorrhages), or as abnormal vessels (arteriovenous fistulas).

Oral Manifestations. Telangiectatic papules, mats, and nodules involving labial and glossal mucosa more commonly than other sites (Fig. 6.48). Spontaneous bleeding or bleeding after dental cleansing can occur.

Associated Findings. Nasal telangiectasias (epistaxis); cutaneous telangiectasia; pulmonary arteriovenous malformations (cyanosis, clubbing, embolic stroke, bruit); central nervous system arteriovenous malformations (headache, hemorrhage); gastrointestinal vascular dysplasia (bleeding).

Microscopic Findings. Dilated vessels in lamina propria; hemorrhage.

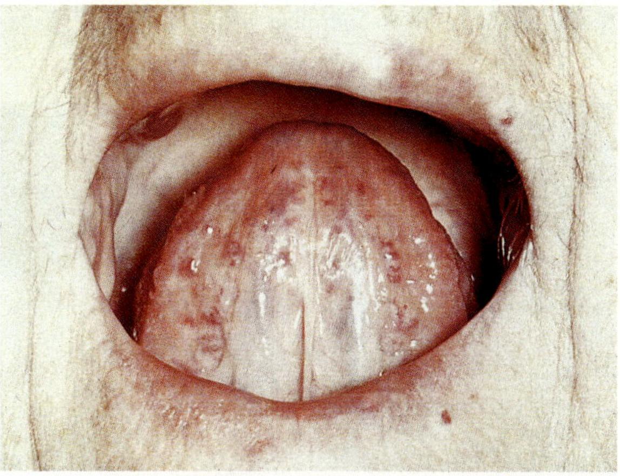

Fig. 6.48. Herditary hemorrhagic telangiectasia. Note telangiectatic macules (mats) and papules of perioral skin, lip vermilion, and undersurface of the tongue

Diagnosis. Characteristic telangiectasias and bleeding complications; family history.

Differential Diagnosis. CREST syndrome shows sclerodermoid cutaneous findings and esophageal dysmotility. Generalized essential telangiectasia is limited to the skin.

Treatment. Laser ablation of vessels which are the source of hemorrhage is recommended. Estrogen-progesterone therapy has been recommended for chronic gastrointestinal bleeding. Surgical approaches are used for major vascular abnormalities.

6.11 Hereditary Nevi

D. Ioannides

6.11.1 Fordyce Spots

Definition. Fordyce spots or the Fordyce condition are terms given to sebaceous glands which are observed on the vermilion border of the lips or on the oral mucosa. The incidence of Fordyce spots increases with age, so that they are found in about 80 % of the adult population.

Oral Manifestations. They appear as small, well-defined yellow or white macules or papules, which may present as single lesions or in a confluent way. They are noticed in the buccal mucosa over the alveolar process (Fig. 6.49) and the anterior pillar of the fauces. Large sebaceous glands are most often observed in the lower alveolobuccal sulcus. Fordyce spots are common on the upper lip, where they may be disturbing to the patient because of their appearance. They are asymptomatic and of no consequence, but seem to increase with rheumatic disorders, especially Reiter's syndrome. Similar lesions may occur on the glans penis and the labia minora.

Microscopic Findings. Microscopically, each globoid lesion consists of a group of small, mature lobules situated around a small sebaceous duct leading to the surface epithelium.

Diagnosis. Fordyce spots may be confused with lichen planus, but in the latter the mucous membrane lesions are white, arranged in reticular patterns and tend to be located more on the buccal mucosa than on the lips. Very rarely, involvement of the labial mucosa with pseudoxanthoma elasticum may simulate Fordyce spots.

Treatment. Treatment is not necessary.

6.11.2 White Sponge Nevus

Definition/Etiology. This condition has been reported under a variety of names, such as oral epithelial nevus or familial white folded gingivostomatosis. However, its original name, white sponge nevus, which was given by Cannon in the first report, is still the most widely used. It is inherited as an autosomal dominant disorder. It may be present at birth or have its onset in infancy, but its progression usually stops at puberty.

Oral Manifestations. The affected oral mucosa appears white or gray, thickened, folded, and spongy (Fig. 6.50). The degree of involvement varies even within a single family and sometimes the entire oral mucosa may be affected. Lesions are usually bilateral and symptomless. There are reports where the pharyngeal, esophageal, nasal, rectal, or vaginal mucosa are involved with lesions. Very rarely, iris coloboma has been observed.

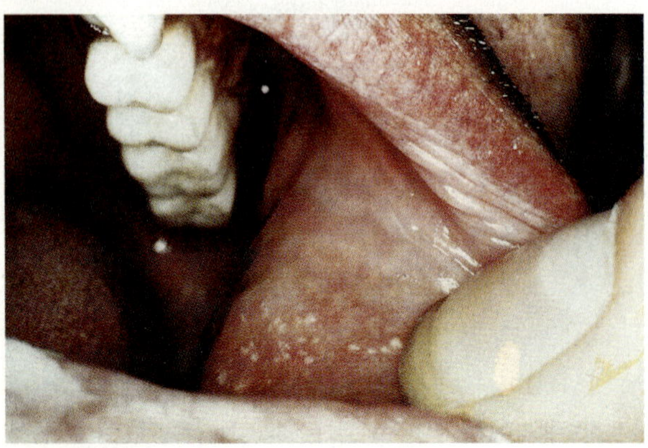

Fig. 6.49. Fordyce spots

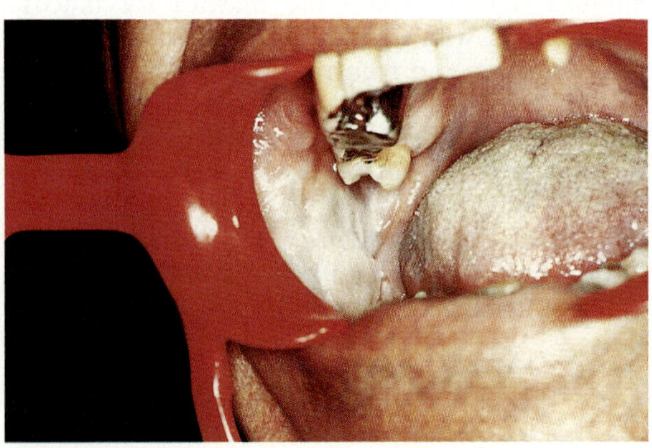

Fig. 6.50. White sponge nervus

Microscopic Findings. Microscopic evaluation of the mucosa reveals acanthosis and parakeratosis with vacuolated keratinocytes and focal cytoplasmic inclusions. Electron microscopic studies suggest abnormalities of tonofibril and keratohyaline granule formation.

Differential Diagnosis. White sponge nevus should be differentiated from pachyonychia congenita and leukoedema, because the histologic picture of these conditions is identical. In pachyonychia, the nails, palms, and soles are involved with lesions, whereas in leukoedema the lesions appear in adulthood and are no less white when stretched.

Treatment. White sponge nevus requires no treatment.

References

1. Peutz JL. A very remarkable of familial polyposis of mucous membrane of intestinal tract and masopharynx accompanied by peculiar pigmentation of skin and mucous membrane. Ned Maandschr Geneeskd 1921; 10: 134
2. Burdick D, Prior JT. Peutz-Jeghers Syndrome: A clinicopathologic study of a large family with a 27-year follow up. Cancer 1982; 50: 2139
3. Laskaris G. Color Atlas of Oral diseases. 2nd Ed. Stuttgart: Thieme Verlag, 1994; 28
4. Linos VA, Dozois RR, Dahlin DC et al. Does Peutz-Jeghers syndrome predispose to gastrointestinal malignancy? Arch Surg, 1981; 116: 1182–4
5. Spigelman AD, Murday V, Phillips RKS. Cancer and the Peutz-Jeghers syndrome. Cut 1989; 30: 1588–90
6. McAllister AJ et al. Seventeen patients with Peutz-Jeghers syndrome in four generations. Am J Surg 1967; 114: 839
7. Miller RL et al. Darier's disease of the oral mucosa: clinical case report with ultrastructural evaluation. J Oral Pathol 1982; 11: 79
8. Ferris T, Lamey PJ, Rennie JS. Darier's disease: oral features and genetic aspects. Br Dent J, 1990; 168: 71–3
9. Fenerly A, Laskaris G. Oral manifestation in Darier's disease. Hell Stomatol Rev 1984; 28: 40
10. Papillon MM, Lefevre P: Deux cas de keratodermie palmaire et plantaire symmetrique familiale (maladie de Meleda) chez le frere et la soeur. Coexistence dans les deux cas d'alterations dentaires graves. Bull Soc Fr Dermatol Syphilig 1924; 31: 82
11. Gorlin RJ et al. Syndromes of the head and neck. 2d Ed. New York: McGraw-Hill 1976
12. Vasilopoulou A, Laskaris G. Papillon-Lefevre syndrome: report of two brothers. J Dent Child 1989; Sept–Oct: 388
13. Laskaris G. Color Atlas of Oral diseases. 2nd Ed. Stuttgart: Thieme Verlag, 1994; 20
14. Gelmetti C, Nazzaro V, Cerri D et al. Long-term preservation of permanent teeth in a patient with Papillon-Lefevre syndrome treated with etretinate. Pediatr Dermatol, 1989; 6: 222–5
15. Nguyen TQ, Greer KE, Fisher GB et al. Papillon-Lefevre syndrome – report of two patients treated successfully with isotretinoin. J Am Dermatol 1985; 15: 46–9
16. Nazzaro V, Blanchet-Bardon C, Mimoz C. Papillon-Lefevre syndrome. Ultrastructural study and successful treatment with acitretin. Arch Dermatol 1988; 124: 533–9
17. Tchou PK, Kohn T. Dyskeratosis congenita: an autosomal dominant disorder. J Am Acad Dermatol, 1982; 6: 1034–9
18. Laskaris G: Color Atlas of Oral diseases. 2nd Ed. Stuttgart: Thieme Verlag, 1994; 16
19. Wormer R et al. Dyskeratosis congenita: two examples of this multisystem disorder. Pediatrics, 1983; 71: 603
20. Mills SE, Cooper PH, Beacham BE et al. Intracranial calcifications and dyskeratosis congenita. Arch Dermatol, 1979; 115: 1437–9
21. Koch HF. Effect of retinoids on precancerous lesions of oral mucosa. In: Orfanos CE, Braun-Falco O, Farber EM et al. (Eds.). Retinoids. Advances in Basic Research and Therapy. Berlin: Springer-Verlag, 1981; 307–12
22. Feinstein A, Friedman J, Schwach-Millet M. Pachyonychia congenita. J Am Acad Dermatol, 1988; 19: 705–11
23. Haber RM, Rose TH. Autosomal recessive pachyonychia congenita. J Am Acad Dermatol, 1986; 122: 919–23
24. Sharma VK, Sharma R, Kaus S. Pachyonychia congenita with tuberous sclerosis. Int J Dermatol 1989: 28: 332–33
25. Anneroth G et al. Pachyonychia congenita: a clinical, histological and microradiographic study with special reference to oral manifestations. Acta Derm Venereol (Stockh), 1975; 55: 387
26. Hunter J, Savin J, Dahen R. Clinical Dermatology, Oxford: Blackwell Sc, 1992; 42
27. Eastman JR, Goldblatt LJ. Psoriasis palatal manifestations and psychologic considerations. J Periodontol, 1983; 54: 736–9
28. Ulmasky M, Michelle R, Araj B. Oral psoriasis: report of six new cases. J Oral Pathol Med 1995; 24: 42–5
29. Sklavounou A, Laskaris G. Oral psoriasis. Report of a case and review of the literature. Dermatologica, 1990; 180: 157–159
30. Laskaris G. Color atlas of oral diseases, 2nd Ed. Stuttgart: Thieme Verlag 1994; 218
31. Moschella SL, Hurley HJ: Dermatology. Philadelphia: WB Saunders, 1992; 619–622
32. Laskaris G, Vareltzidis A Avgerinou G. Focal palmoplantar and oral mycosal hyperkeratosis syndrome. Oral Surg 1980; 50: 250
33. Young WG, Newcomb GM, Daley TJ. Focal palmoplanter and gingival hyperkeratosis syndrome: report of a family with cytologic, ultrastructural and histochemical findings. Oral Surg, 1982; 53: 473–482
34. Gerlin RJ. F.P. and marginal gingival hyperkeratosis syndrome. Birth Defects, 1976; 12: 239–242
35. Laskaris G. Color atlas of oral diseases. 2nd Ed. Stuttgart: Thieme Verlag, 1994; 18
36. Hassed SJ, Kincannon JM, Arnold GL. Clouston syndrome: an ectodermal dysplasia without significant dental findings. Am J Med Genet, 1996; 61: 274–6
37. Zirbel GM, Ruttum MS, Post AC, Esterly NB. Odonto-onychodermal dysplasia. Br J Dermatol, 1995; 133: 797–800
38. Ilyna HG, Amoashy DS, Grygory HA. "New" ectodermal dysplasia with mental retardation and syndactyly. Am J Med Genet, 1995; 58: 345–7
39. Tyler MT, Ficarra G, Silverman S Jr, Odom RB, Regezi JA. Malignant acanthosis nigricans with florid papillary oral lesions. Oral Surg Oral Med Oral Pathol Oral Radiol Endod, 1996; 81: 445–9
40. Kurzrock R, Cohen PR. Cutaneous paraneoplastic syndromes in solid tumors. Am J Med, 1995; 99: 662–71
41. Panidis D, Skiadopoulos S, Rousso D, Ioannides D, Panidou E. Association of acanthosis nigricans with insulin resistance in patients with polycystic ovary syndrome. Br J Dermatol 1995; 132: 936–41
42. Schwartz RA, Janniger CK. Childhood acanthosis nigricans. Cutis, 1995; 55: 337–41
43. Polymeropoulos MH, Ide SE, Wright M, Goodship J, Weissenbach J, Pyeritz RE, Da Silva EO, Ortiz De Luna RI, Francomano CA. The gene for the Ellis-van Creveld syndrome is located on chromosome 4p16. Genomics, 1996; 35: 1–5
44. Levi SE, Dansky R, Milner S, Benatar A, Govendrageloo K, du Plessis J. Atrioventricular septal defect and type A postaxial polydactyly without other major associated anomalies: a specific association. Pediatr Cardiol, 1995; 16: 242–6
45. Digilio MC, Marino B, Giannotti A, Dallapiccola B. Single atrium, atrioventricular canal/postaxial hexodactyly indicating Ellis-van Creveld syndrome. Hum Genet, 1995; 96: 251–2

46. Lukinmaa PL, Jensen BL, Thesleff I, Andreasen JO, Kreiborg S. Histological observations of teeth and peridental tissue in cleidocranial dysplasia imply increased activity of odontogenic epithelium and abnormal bone remodeling. J Craniofac Genet Dev Biol, 1995; 15: 212–21
47. Sharma A, Yadav R, Ahlawat K. Cleidocranial dysplasia. Indian Pediatr, 1995; 32: 588–92
48. Gelb BD, Cooper E, Shevell M, Desnick RJ. Genetic mapping of the cleidocranial dysplasia (CCD) locus on chromosome band 6p21 to include a microdeletion. Am J Med Genet 1995; 58: 200–5
49. Feldman GJ, Robin NH, Brueton LA, Robertson E, Thompson EM, Siegel Bartelt J, Gasser DL, Bailey LC, Zackai EH, Muenke M. A gene for cleidocranial dysplasia maps to the short arm of chromosome 6. Am J Hum Genet, 1995; 56: 938–43
50. Richardson A, Deussen FF: Facial and dental anomalies in cleidocranial dysplasia: a study of 17 cases. Int J Paediatr Dent, 1994; 4: 225–31
51. Jensen BL. Cleidocranial dysplasia: craniofacial morphology in adult patients. J Craniofac Genet Dev Biol, 1994; 14: 163–76
52. Jensen BL, Kreiborg S. Development of the skull in infants with cleidocranial dysplasia. J Craniofac Genet Dev Biol, 1993; 13: 89–97
53. Markovic MD: At the crossroads of oral facial genetics. Eur J Orthod, 1992; 14: 469–81
54. Gupta SK, Sharma OP, Malhotra S, Gupta S. Cleido-cranial dysostosis-skeletal abnormalities. Australas Radiol, 1992; 36: 238–42
55. Sule RR, Dhumawat DJ, Gharpuray MB. Focal dermal hypoplasia. Cutis, 1994; 53: 309–12
56. Arnold WP, Steijlen PM, Happle R. Focal dermal hypoplasia (Goltz-Gorlin syndrome). Br J Dermatol 1993; 129: 214–5
57. Kilmer SL, Grix AW Jr, Isseroff RR. Focal dermal hypoplasia: four cases with widely varying presentations. J Am Acad Dermatol, 1993; 28: 839–43
58. Anneren G, Arvidson B, Gustavson KH, et al. Orofacio-digital syndrome I and II: radiological methods for diagnosis and clinical variations. Clin Genet, 1984; 26: 178–186
59. Mohr OL. A hereditary lethal syndrome in man. Avh Norske Videnskad, 1994: 14: 1–18
60. Sugarman GI, Katakia M, Menkes JH. See-saw winking in a familial oro-facial digital syndrome. Clin Genet, 1971; 2: 248–54
61. Baraister M. The orofaciodigital syndromes. J Med Genet, 1986; 23: 116–119.
62. Cramer JA, Schmidt WJ. Incontinentia pigmenti. Arch Dermatol, 1955; 71: 699–702
63. Curth HO, Warburton D. The genetics of incontinentia pigmenti. Arch Dermatol, 1965; 92: 229–235
64. Nazzaro V, Brusasco A, Gelemtti C, et al. Hypochromic reticulated streaks in incontinentia pigmenti: an immunohistochemical and ultrastructural study. Pediatr Dermatol, 1990; 3: 174–178
65. Caputo R, Gianotti F, Innocenti M. Ultrastructural findings in incontinentia pigmenti. Int J Dermatol, 1975; 14: 46–55
66. Spallone A: Incontinentia pigmenti: seven case repots from one family: Br J Ophthalmol, 1987; 71: 629–634
67. Caputo R, Gelmetti C, Annessi G. Incontinentia Pigmenti. In: Pediatric dermatology and dermatopathology, vol III. Philadelphia: Williams and Wilkins, 1995, pp 35–40
68. Pye RJ. Bullous eruptions. In: Rook/Wilkinson/Ebling: Textbook of Dermatology 5th Ed. Oxford: Blackwell Scientific Publications, 1992
69. Gedde-Dahl T, Anton-Lamprect I. Epidermolysis bullosa: In Emory AEH, Rimoin DL (Eds). Principles and Practice in Medical Genetics New York: Livingstone, 1981
70. Coulombe PA, Hutton ME, Letai A et al. Point mutations in human keratin 14 genes of epidermolysis bullosa simplex patients: genetics and functional analyses. Cell, 1991; 64: 1301–1304
71. Ryynanen M, Knowlton RG, Uitto J: Mapping of epidermolysis bullosa simplex to mutations to chromosome 12. Am J Hum Genet 1991; 459: 978–983
72. Fine JD, Stenn J, Johnson L et al. Autosomal recessive epidermolysis bullosa simplex. Arch Dermatol, 1989; 125: 931–940
73. Salih MAM, Lake BD, Hag MA et al. Lethal epidermolythic epidermolysis bullosa: a new autosomal recessive type of epidermolysis bullosa. Br J Dermatol, 1985; 113: 135–140
74. Stepp MA, Spurr-Michaud S, Tisdale A et al. $\alpha 6 \beta 4$ integrin heterodimer is a component of hemidesmosomes. Proc Natl Acad Sci USA, 1990; 87: 8970–8979
75. Ryynanen J, Jaakkola S, Engvall E et al. Expression of B4 integrins in human skin: comparison of epidermal distribution with B1 integrin epitopes, and modulation by calcium and vitamin D3 in cultured keratinocytes. J Invest Dermatol 1991; 97: 562–569
76. Burgeson RE. Type VII collagen anchoring fibrils and epidermolysis bullosa. J Invest Dermatol, 1993; 101: 252–260
77. Ryynanen M, Knowlton RG, Parente MG et al. Human type VII collagen (COL7A1) on chromosome 3 to dominant dystrophic epidermolysis bullosa. Am J Hum Genet, 1991; 49: 797
78. Valle KJ, Bauer EA. Enhanced biosynthesis of human skin collagenase in fibroblasts cultures from recessive dystrophic epidermolysis bullosa. J Clin Invest, 1980; 66: 176–181
79. Winberg JO, Gedde-Dahl T, Bauer EA. Collagenase expression in skin fibroblasts from families with recessive dystrophic epidermolysis bullosa. J Invest Dermatol, 1989; 92: 82–90
80. Wright JT, Fine JD, Johnson LB. Oral soft tissues in hereditary epidermolysis bullosa. Oral Surg Oral Med Oral Pathol, 1991; 71: 440–446
81. Niemi KM, Sommer H, Kero M et al. Epidermolysis bullosa simplex associated with unusual dystrophy and recessive inheritance. Arch Dermatol, 1988, 124: 551–559
82. Haneke E, Anton-Lamprecht I. Ultrastructure of blister formation in epidermolysis bullosa hereditaria. V. Epidermolysis bullosa simplex localisata type Weber-Cockayne. J Invest Dermatol, 1982; 78: 219–224
83. Tidmann MJ, Eady RAJ. Hemidesmosome heterogeneity in junctional epidermolysis bullosa revealed by morphometric analysis. J Invest Dermatol, 1986; 86: 51–59
84. Tidman MJ, Eady RAJ: Evaluation of anchoring fibrils and other components of the dermal-epidermal junction in dystrophic epidermolysis bullosa by a quantitative ultrastructural technique. J Invest Dermatol, 1985; 84: 374–379
85. Bauer EA, Briggaman RA. Hereditary epidermolysis bullosa. In: Fitzpatrick TB, Eisen AZ, Wolff K et al (Eds). Dermatology in general medicine. 4th Ed. New York: McGraw-Hill, 1993
86. Carter DM, Lin AN, Varghese MC, Caldwell D, Pratt LA, Eisinger M. Treatment of junctional epidermolysis bullosa with epidermal autografts. J Am Acad Dermatol, 1987; 17: 246
87. Fine JD, Johnson L. Efficacy of systemic phenytoin in the treatment of junctional epidermolysis bullosa. Arch Dermatol, 1988; 124: 1402–1410
88. Gruskay DM. Nutritional management in the child with epidermolysis bullosa. Arch Dermatol, 1988; 124: 760
89. Grybosky JD, Toulokian R, Campanella RA. Gastrointestinal manifestations of epidermolysis bullosa in children. Arch Dermatol, 1988; 124: 746–751
90. Bauer EA, Cooper TW. Therapeutic considerations in recessive dystrophic epidermolysis bullosa. Arch Dermatol, 1981; 117: 529–532
91. Lin AN, Stern RS, Caldwell-Brown D. Phenytoin for recessive dystrophic epidermolysis bullosa. J Invest Dermatol, 1989; 92: 472–479
92. Bauer EA, Seltzer JL, Eisen AZ. Retinoic acid inhibition of collagenase and gelatinase expression in human skin fibroblast cultures: evidence for a dual mechanism. J Invest Dermatol, 1983; 81: 162–169
93. Griffin RP, Mayau BJ. The anaesthetic management of patients with dystrophic epidermolysis bullosa a review of 44 patients over 10 years period. Anaesthesia, 1993; 48: 810–815
94. Shenefelt PD, Castellano LM, Fensken A. Successful treatment of albopapuloid epidermolysis bullosa (Pasini variant) with pulse topical corticosteroid therapy. J Am Acad Dermatol, 1993; 29: 785–789
95. Evans GW, Johnson PE: Zinc binding factor in acrodermatitis enteropathica. Lancet, 1976; 2: 1310–1315

96. Van Wouwel JP, Uijlenbroek JJ. The role of the pancreas in the regulation of zinc status. Biol Trace Elem Res, 1994; 42: 143
97. Eckert CD, Sloan MV, Duncan JR et al. Zinc binding: difference between human and bovine milk. Science, 1977; 195: 789–799
98. Cousins RJ, Smith KT. Zinc binding properties of bovine and human milk in vitro: influence of change in zinc content. Am J Clin Nutr, 1980; 33: 1083–1089
99. Jensen RG, Clark RM, Ferris AM. Composition of the lipids in human milk: review. Lipids, 1980, 15: 345–351
100. Cunnane SC. Maternal essential fatty acid implementation increases zinc absorption in neonatal rats: relevant to the defect in zinc absorption in acrodermatitis enteropathica. Pediatr Res, 1982; 16: 599
101. Fukumuya KA, Sakamoto M, Olntani O, et al. Zinc binding proteins of newborn rats in the dermis. Curr Probl Dermatol, 1983; 11: 327–331
102. Fraker PJ, Jardieu P, Cook J. Zinc deficiency and immune function. Arch Dermatol, 1987; 123: 1699
103. Prasad AS. Clinical biochemistry and nutritional spectrum of zinc in human subjects: an update. Nutr Rev, 1983; 41: 197–200
104. Sandstrom B, Cederblad A, Lindblad BS, Lonnerdal B. Acrodermatitis enteropathica, zinc metabolism, copper status, and immune function. Arch Pediatr Adolesc Med, 1994; 148: 980
105. Sehgal WN, Jain S. Chronic familial benign pemphigus. J Dermatol, 1994; 21: 382–390
106. Abell E. Immunopathological investigation of glycocalyx material in Darier's and Hailey-Hailey disease. J Invest Dermatol, 1983; 80: 335–340
107. Cram DL, Muller SA, Winkelmann RA. Ultraviolet induced acantholysis in familial benign chronic pemphigus. Arch Dermatol, 1967; 96: 636–639
108. Burns RA, Reed WB, Swatek FE, Omieczinsky DT. Familial benign chronic pemphigus. Induction of lesions by Candida albicans. Arch Dermatol, 1967; 96: 254–258
109. Zaim MT, Bickers DR. Herpes simplex associated with Hailey-Hailey disease. J Am Acad Dermatol, 1987; 17: 701–708
110. Malchus R, Marsch WC, Ehlers G. HLA-B 16 in Hailey-Hailey disease. Acta Derm Venereol (Stockh), 1986; 66: 264–269
111. Ikeda S, Welsh EA Peluso AM, Leyden W, Duvic M, Woodley DT, Epstein EH Jr. Localization of the gene whose mutations underlie Hailey-Hailey disease to chromosome 3q. Hum Mol Genet, 1994; 3: 1147–1152
112. Bergman R, Levy R, Pam Z, Lichting C, Hazaz B, Friedman-Birnbaum R. A study of keratin expression in benign familial chronic pemphigus. Am J Dermatopathol, 1992; 14: 32
113. Wilgram GF et al. An electron microscopic study of acantholysis and dyskeratosis in Hailey and Hailey's disease. J Invest Dermatol, 1962; 39: 373–379
114. Haber H, Russell B. Sisters with familial benign chronic pemphigus (Gougerot, Hailey and Hailey). Br J Dermatol, 1950; 62: 458–461
115. Serpico R, Femiano F, Cozzolino F, Baeta GM. L'evoluzione della terapia in patologia orale: l'uso del cortisone per uso topico madiante inoforesi medicamentosa. XXII SIOCMF Congress. Bologna, Italy, 1992
116. Jutsukawa K, Ring J, Weyer U, Kimming W, Radloff H. Topical cyclosporine in chronic benign familial pemphigus (Hailey-Hailey disease). J Am Acad Dermatol, 1992; 27: 625–631
117. Sire DJ, Johnson BL. Benign familial chronic pemphigus treated with dapsone. Arch Dermatol, 1971; 103: 262–270
118. Il'in II, Molochov VA. The photochemotherapy of Hailey-Hailey disease. Vestn Dermatol Venerol, 1990; 7: 64–70
119. Aubert JP, Folchetti G, Berbis P, Magalon G. Surgical treatment of Hailey-Hailay disease or benign familial chronic pemphigus. A proposd case of submammary localization. Ann Chir Plast Esthet 1993; 38: 568–572
120. Kartamaa M, Reitamo S Familial benign chronic pemphigus (Hailey-Hailey disease). Treatment with carbon dioxide laser vaporisation. Arch Dermatol 1992; 128: 646–651
121. Hamm H, Metze D, Brocker EB. Hailey-Hailey disease. Eradication by dermabrasion. Arch Dermatol, 1994; 130: 1187
122. Sasaki T, Arai K, Ono M, et al. Ehlers-Danlos syndrome. A variant characterized by the deficiency of pro-a2 chain of type I procollagen. Arch Dermatol, 1987; 123: 76–79
123. Pope FM, Komorowska A, Lee KW et al. Ehlers-Danlos syndrome type I with novel dental features. J Oral Pathol, 1992; 21: 418–421
124. Barabas GM. The Ehlers-Danlos syndrome. Abnormalities of the enamel, dentine, cementum and the dental pulp: histological examination of 13 teeth from 6 patients. Br Dent J, 1969; 126: 509–512
125. Abraham PA, Peredja AJ, Carnes WH et al: Marfan syndrome: demonstration of abnormal elastin in aorta. J Clin Invest 1982; 70: 1245–1252
126. Pope FM. Clinical and genetic heterogeneity of the Marfan syndrome. Curr Prob Dermatol, 1987; 17: 218–225
127. Pyeritz RE, McKusick VA. Clinical variability in the Marfan syndrom Birth Defects Orig Artic Ser, 1979; 15(5B): 155–178
128. Loveman AB, Gordon AM, Fliegelmann MT. Marfan's syndrome. Arch Dermatol 1963; 87: 428
129. Pyeritz RE, McKusick VA. Basic defects in the Marfan syndrome. New Eng J Med, 1981; 305: 1011
130. Silver W, Kuskin L. Marfan's syndrome: cardiovascular manifestations. Angiology 1987; 29: 262–264
131. Scully C, Flint SR, Porter SR. Oral diseases. 2nd Ed. Martin Dunitz, London: 1996
132. Rodriguez Gomez M, Adams R. Neurocutaneous diseases. A practical approach. Boston: Butterworths, 1987
133. Zeller J, Hovnanian A. La maladie de Von Recklinghausen. Ann Dermatol Venereol, 1992; 119: 405–409
134. Viskochil D, Buchberg AM, Xu G et al. Deletions and a translocation interrupt a cloned gene at the neurofibromatosis type 1 locus. Cell, 1990; 62: 187–192
135. Cawthon RM, Weiss R, Xu Q et al. A major segment of the neurofibromatosis type 1 gene: cDNA sequence, genomic structure, and point mutations. Cell, 1990; 62: 193–201
136. Rouleau GA, Merel P, Lutchman M et al. Alteration in a new gene encoding a putative membrane-organizing protein causes neurofibromatosis type 2. Nature, 1993; 515–521
137. Geist JR, Gander DL, Stefanac SJ. Oral manifestations of neurofibromatosis types I and II. Oral Surg Med Oral Pathol, 1992; 73: 376–82
138. Scully C, Flint SR, Porter SR. Oral diseases. 2nd Ed., Martin Dunitz, London: 1996
139. Demis DJ, Dobson RL, McGuire J. Clinical Dermatology. Philadelphia: Harper & Row Publishers, Unit 12–33, 1983, Vol. 2
140. Reuland-Bosma W, van Dijk J. Periodontal disease in down's syndrome: a review. J Clin Periodontol, 1986; 13: 64–73
141. Scully C. Down's syndrome: aspect of dental care. J Dent, 1976; 4: 167–174
142. Kavanagh GM, Leeming JP, Marshman GM et al. Folliculitis in Down's syndrome. Br J Dermatol, 1993; 129: 696–99
143. Scully C, Flint SR, Porter SR. Oral diseases. London: Martin Dunitz, 2nd Ed., 1996
144. Rodriguez Gomez M, Adams R. Neurocutaneous diseases. A practical approach. Boston: Butterworths 1998
145. Kwiatkowski DJ, Short P. Tuberous sclerosis. Arch Dermatol, 1994; 130: 348–354
146. Caballero LR, Robles JLD, Caballero CR et al. Tooth pits: an early sign of tuberous sclerosis. Acta Derm Venereol (Stockh), 1987; 13: 457–9
147. Scully C. Oral mucosal lesions in association with epilepsy and cutaneous lesions: Pringle-Bourneville syndrome. Int J Oral Surg, 1981; 68–72
148. Monaghan HP, Krafchick BP, Mac Gregor DL et al. Tuberous sclerosis complex in children. Am J Dis Child, 1981; 135: 912–917
149. Berberian BJ, Sulica VI, Kao GF. Familia multiple eccrine spiroadenomas with cylindromatous features associated with epithelioma adenoides cysticum of Brooke. Cutis, 1990; 46: 46–50
150. Tucker MA, Mariman EC, Starink TM, Ponder BA, Ropers HH, Kremer H, Longy M, Eng C. Localization of the gene for Cowden disease to chromosome 10q22–23. Nat Genet, 1996; 13: 114–6

151. Mignogna MD, Lo Muzio L, Ruocco V, Bucci E. Early diagnosis of multiple harmatoma and neoplasia syndrome (Cowden disease). The role of the dentist. Oral Surg Oral Med Oral Pathol Oral Radiol Endod, 1995; 79(3): 295–9
152. Hanssen AM, Fryns JP. Cowden syndrome. J Med Genet, 1995; 32: 117–9
153. Mallory SB. Cowden syndrome (multiple hamartoma syndrome). Dermatol Clin 1995; 13: 27–31
154. Kousseff BG. Multiple endocrine neoplasia 2 (MEN 2)/ MEN 2A (Sipple syndrome). Dermatol Clin 1995; 13: 91–7
155. Shimkets R, Gailani MR, Siu VM, Yang Feng T, Pressman CL, Levanat S, Goldstein A, Dean M, Bale AE. Molecular analysis of chromosome 9q deletions in two Gorlin syndrome patients. Am J Hum Genet, 1996; 59(2): 417–22
156. Kanekura T, Kanzaki T, Kanekura S, Kawahara K, Nakashima T, Kitajima I, Maruyama I. p53 gene mutations in skin cancers with underlying disorders. J Dermatol Sci, 1995; 9: 209–14
157. Gorlin RJ. Nevoid basal cell carcinoma syndrome. Dermatol, Clin 1995; 13(1): 113–25
158. Rees J. Genetic alterations in non-melanoma skin cancer. J Invest Dermatol, 1994; 103(6): 747–50
159. Wicking C, Berkman J, Wainwright B, Chenevix Trench G. Fine genetic mapping of the gene for nevoid basal cell carcinoma syndrome. Genomics, 1994; 22(3): 505–11
160. Bale AE, Gailani MR, Leffell DJ. Nevoid basal cell carcinoma syndrome. J Invest Dermatol, 1994; 103: 126S–130S
161. Farndon PA, Del Mastro RG, Evans DG, Kilpatrick MW. Location of gene for Gorlin syndrome. Lancet 1992; 339: 581–2
162. Yuwono M, Rossi TM, Fisher JE, Tjota A. Oncogene expression in patients with familial polyposis coli/Gardner's syndrome. Int Arch Allergy Immunol, 1996; 111(1): 89–95
163. Ryan JC. Premalignant conditions of the small intestine. Semin Gastrointest Dis, 1996; 7(2): 88–93
164. Davies DR, Armstrong JG, Thakker N, Horner K, Guy SP, Clancy T, Sloan P, Blair V, Dodd C, Warnes TW. Severe Gardner syndrome in families with mutations restricted to a specific region of the APC gene. Am J Hum Genet, 1995; 57(5): 1151–8
165. Cohen MM Jr. Perspectives on craniofacial asymmetry. VI. The hamartoses. Int J Oral Maxillofac Surg, 1995; 24(3): 195–200
166. Narisawa Y, Kohda H. Cutaneous cysts of Gardner's syndrome are similar to follicular stem cells. J Cutan Pathol, 1995; 22(2): 115–21
167. Luk GD. Diagnosis and therapy of hereditary polyposis syndromes. Gastroenterologist 1995; 3(2): 153–67
168. Ko FY, Wu TC, Hwang B. Intestinal polyps in children and adolescents – a review of 103 cases. Acta Paediatr Sin, 1995; 36(3): 197–202
169. Perniciaro C. Gardner's syndrome. Dermatol Clin, 1995; 13(1): 51–6
170. Tan SY, Pepys MB. Amyloidosis. Histopathology, 1994; 25(5): 403–414
171. Adle-Biassette H, Vallat AB, Nochy D. Amyloidosis: definition and classification. Arch Anat Cytol Pathol, 1996; 44(2–3): 101–105
172. Kerner MM, Wang MB, Angier G, Calcaterra TC, Ward PH. Amyloidosis of the head and neck. A clinicopathologic study of the UCLA experience, 1955–1991. Arch Otolaryngol Head Neck Surg, 1995; 121(7): 778–782
173. Reinish EI, Raviv M, Srolovitz H, Gornitsky M. Tongue, primary amyloidosis, and multiple myeloma. Oral Surg Oral Med Oral Pathol, 1994; 77(2): 121–125
174. Bellotti V, Merlini G. Current concepts on the pathogenesis of systemic amyloidosis. Nephrol Dial Transplant, 1996; 11 (suppl. 9): 53–62
175. Dupond JL, de Wazières B, Saile R, Closs F, Viennet G, Kantelip E, Fest T, Vuitton DA. Systemic amyloidosis in the elderly: diagnostic value of the test of subcutaneous abdominal fat and the labial salivary glands. Prospective study in 100 aged patients. Rev Med Interne, 1995; 16(5): 314–317
176. Micali G. Lipoid proteinosis. In: Buyse ML (Ed). Birth defects encyclopedia. Oxford: Blackwell Scientific Publication, 1990; 1563–1564
177. Fabrizi G et al: Urbach-Wiethe disease: light and electron microscopic study. J Cutan Pathol, 1980; 7: 8–20
178. Chaudhary SJ, Dayal PK. Hyalinosis cutis et mucosae. Review with a case report. Oral Surg Oral Med Oral Pathol Oral Radiol Endod, 1995; 80(2): 168–171
179. Muda AO, Paradisi M, Angelo C, Mostaccioli S, Atzori F, Puddu P, Faraggiana T. Lipoid proteinosis: clinical, histologic, and ultrastructural investigations. Cutis, 1995; 56(4): 220–224
180. Disdier P, Harlé JR, Andrac L, Swiader L, Weiller PJ. Specific xerostomia during Urbach-Wiethe disease. Dermatology, 1994; 188(1): 50–51
181. Cinaz P, Guvenir T, Gonlusen G. Lipoid proteinosis: Urbach-Wiethe disease. Acta Paediatr, 1993; 82(10): 892–893
182. Fang-Kircher S. Mucopolysaccharidoses: current aspects of diagnosis and therapy. Wien Klin Wochenschr, 1995; 107(22): 698–701
183. Warzok R, Seidlitz G. Mucopolysaccharidoses. Genetics, clinical pathology, therapeutic regimes. Zentralbl Pathol, 1992; 138(3): 226–234
184. Roberts MW, Barton NW, Constantopoulos G, Butler DP, Donahue AH. Occurrence of multiple dentigerous cysts in a patient with the Maroteaux-Lamy syndrome (mucopolysaccharidois, type VI). Oral Surg Oral Med Oral Pathol, 1984; 58(2): 169–175
185. Downs AT, Crisp T, Ferretti G. Hunter's syndrome and oral manifestations: a review. Pediatr Dent, 1995; 17(2): 98–100
186. Gritli-Linde A, Linde A, Goldberg M Morphological alterations in dental and periodontal tissues in murine mucopolysaccharidosis type VII. Calcif Tissue Int, 1995; 57(3): 178–184
187. Sheridan O, Wortman J, Harvey C, Hayden J, Haskins M. Craniofacial abnormalities in animal models of mucopolysaccharidoses I, VI, and VII. J Craniofac Genet Dev Biol, 1994; 14(1): 7–15
188. Cleary MA, Wraith JE. The presenting features of mucopolysaccharidosis type IH (Hurler syndrome). Acta Paediatr, 1995; 84(3): 337–339
189. Morales LE. Gaucher's disease: a review. Ann Pharmacother, 1996; 30(4): 381–388
190. Kaminsky P, Belmatoug N, Billette de Villemeur T Maladie de Gaucher. Press Med, 1996; 25(3): 108–112
191. Regenye GR, Huberman BA, Itkin AB. Gaucher's disease: case report of mandibular trauma. Oral Surg Oral Med Oral Pathol, 1992; 73(1): 23–26
192. Bender IB, Bender AL. Dental observations in Gaucher's disease: review of the literature and two case reports with 13- and 60-year follow-ups. Oral Surg Oral Med Oral Pathol Oral Radiol Endod, 1996; 82(6): 650–659
193. Sidransky E, Tayebi N, Ginns EI. Diagnosing Gaucher disease. Early recognition, implications for treatment, and genetic counseling. Clin Pediatr, 1995; 34(7): 365–371
194. Ehlen C, Heintges T, Niederau C. Diagnose und Therapie des Morbus Gaucher. Med Klin, 1995; 90(5): 284–290
195. Elleder M: Niemann-Pick disease. Pathol Res Pract, 1989; 185(3): 293–328
196. Graber D, Salvayre R, Levade T. Accurate differentiation of neuronopathic and nonneuronopathic forms of Niemann-Pick disease by evaluation of the effective residual lysosomal sphingomyelinase activity in intact cells. J Neurochem, 1994; 63(3): 1060–1068
197. Gonzalez de Dios J, Fernandez Tejada E, Diaz Fernandez MC, Ortega Paez E, Hernandez Gonzalez J, de la Vega Bueno A, Hierro Llanillo L, Larrauri Martinez J, Jara Vega P. The current state of Niemann-Pick disease: evaluation of six cases. An Esp Pediatr, 1990; 32(2): 143–148
198. Touissaint M, Worret WI, Drosner M, Marquardt KH. Specific skin lesions in a patient with Niemann-Pick disease. Br J Dermatol, 1994; 131: 895–897
199. Van de Vlasakker CJ, Gabreaels FJ, Wijburg HC, Wevers RA. Clòinical features of Niemann-Pick disease type C. An example of the delayed onset, slowly progressive phenotype and an overview of recent literature. Clin Neurol Neurosurg, 1994; 96(2): 119–123

200. Levade T, Salvayre R, Douste-Blazy L. Sphingomyelinases and Niemann-Pick disease. J Clin Chem Clin Biochem, 1986; 24(4): 205–220
201. Crawford DR, Mirault ME, Moret R, Zbinden I, Cerutti PA. Molecular defect in human acatalasia fibroblasts. Biochem Biophys Res Commun, 1988; 153(1): 59–66
202. Hirono A, Sasaya-Hamada F, Kanno H, Fujii H, Yoshida T, Miwa S. A novel human catalase mutation (358 T del) causing Japanese-type acatalasemia. Blood Cells Mol Dis, 1995; 21(3): 232–234
203. Delgado W, Calderòn R. Acatalasis in two Peruvian siblings. J Oral Pathol, 1979; 8(6): 358–368
204. Ogata M. Acatalasemia. Hum Genet, 1991; 86(4): 331–340
205. Fink-Puches R, Kainz JT, Kahr A, Urban C, Smolle J, Kerl H. Granulocyte Colony-stimulating factor treatment of cyclic neutropenia with recurrent oral aphthae. Arch Dermatol, 1996; 132: 1399–1400
206. Guttmacher AE, Marchuk DA, White RI Jr. Hereditary hemorrhagic telangiectasia. N Eng J Med, 1995; 333: 918–924
207. McAllister KA, Grogg KM, Johnson DW, et al. Endoglin, a TGF-β binding protein of endothelial cells, is the gene for hereditary hemorrhagic telangiectasia type 1. Nature Genetics, 1994; 8: 345–351

CHAPTER 7

Infections of the Oral Cavity

M. La Placa and I. Ghersetich

7.1
Principles of Oral Microbiology

7.1.1
Introduction: The Oral Flora

Infections of the oral cavity are most commonly odontogenic in origin and include dental caries, periapical infections, gingivitis, periodontal infections and abscesses, and deep fascial space infections. Although rare, life-threatening complications, such as mediastinal or intracranial extension, retropharyngeal spread and airway obstruction, pleuropulmonary suppuration, and hematogenous dissemination to heart valves, prosthetic devices, and other metastatic foci are known, which indicate the potentially serious nature of these infections.

Nonodontogenic infections of the oral cavity include ulcerative and gangrenous stomatitis and infections of the major salivary glands. In addition, some systemic infections may involve the oral cavity with different lesions of variable severity.

The microbiology associated with odontogenic infections are complex and generally reflect the indigenous oral flora. Recent evidence, however, points to causative roles of specific microorganisms in different forms of odontogenic infections. This concept of specific microbial causes has created a considerable dilemma in the traditional approach to the diagnosis and management of such infections. The microflora associated with odontogenic infections are typically polymicrobial. It does not necessarily follow that each component of this complex microbiota has equal pathogenic potential, or that numerically predominant cultivable bacteria are the most important. Therefore, it may not be necessary to eradicate the entire microbial population for therapy to be effective.

The oral cavity cannot be regarded as a single, uniform environment. Although representative species of bacteria can be isolated from most areas of the mouth, unique ecologic niches are observed as certain sites, such as the tongue (*Streptococcus salivarius, Veillonella* spp.), tooth surface (*Streptococcus sanguis, S. mitis, S. mutans, Actinomyces viscosus*), and gingival crevice (*Fusobacterium, Bacteroides,* anaerobic spirochetes), tend to favor colonization by specific organisms. Factors that appear to control these localization patterns include selective adherence characteristics of certain bacteria for various types of cells, local environmental conditions such as oxygen tension, oxidation-reduction potential (Eh) and pH, interbacterial coaggregation, and reciprocal bacterial inhibition.

Apart from anatomic considerations, numerous other factors, such as age, diet and nutrition, eruption of deciduous dentition, oral hygiene, smoking habits, presence of dental caries or periodontal disease, antimicrobial therapy, hospitalization, pregnancy, and genetic and racial factors may influence composition of the oral bacterial population.

Quantitative studies indicate that obligate anaerobes constitute a large and important part of the resident oral microbial population. Overall, *Streptococcus, Veillonella, Lactobacillus, Corynebacterium,* and *Actinomyces* account for more than 70 % of the total cultivable oral bacterial population. Facultative gram-negative rods are uncommon in healthy adults but may be more prominent in seriously ill, hospitalized, and elderly patients. Few mycetes, usually represented by *Candida* spp. and protozoa (*Trichomonas tenax, Entamoeba gingivalis*) are occasionally present as resident oral microorganisms. Viruses are not a significant component of the normal oral microbiota. Members of the Herpesviridae family (Cytomegalovirus, Herpes simplex virus, Epstein-Barr virus, and human herpesvirus 6) can be present in the saliva of latently infected apparently healthy subjects.

7.1.2
Microbiology of Dental Caries

Dental caries are a slow decomposition of teeth resulting from the loss of hydroxyapatite crystals, with consequent mineralized matrix dissolution and reduced integrity of the teeth (Fig. 7.1). A large body of experimental evidence supports the belief that

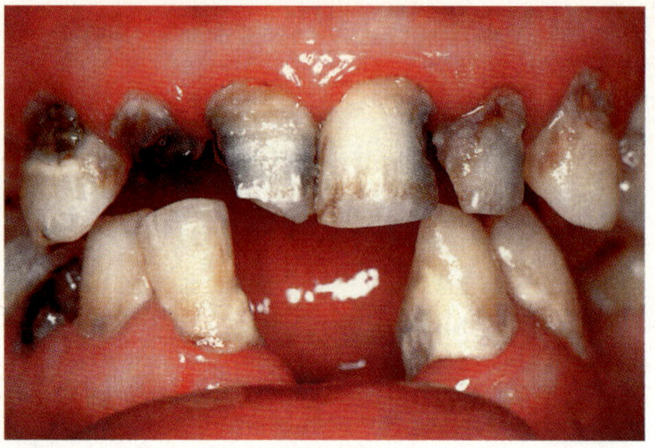

Fig. 7.1. Severe dental caries and reactive gingivitis in a partially edentulous subject

caries only occur in the presence of microorganisms [1]. In fact: (a) germ-free animals only develop caries in the presence of bacteria, (b) oral bacteria can cause demineralization of enamel in vitro, and (c) histological studies show bacteria within carious lesions of enamel and dentine. Current understanding supports the "plaque-host-substrate" theory of pathogenesis, according to which caries have a bacterial etiology interdependent with the host defense systems, dietary factors, and time (Fig. 7.2).

The bulk of available experimental evidence indicates that lowering the pH by bacterial acid production causes dissolution of the enamel. Enamel, which is 95 % calcified, is the most highly mineralized structure in the human body. The majority of the mineral is hydroxyapatite, a large family of calcium phosphate salts with the general formula: $Ca_{10}(PO_4)_6OH_2$. Hydroxyapatite has a finite solubility constant dependent upon the temperature, pH, and ionic strength

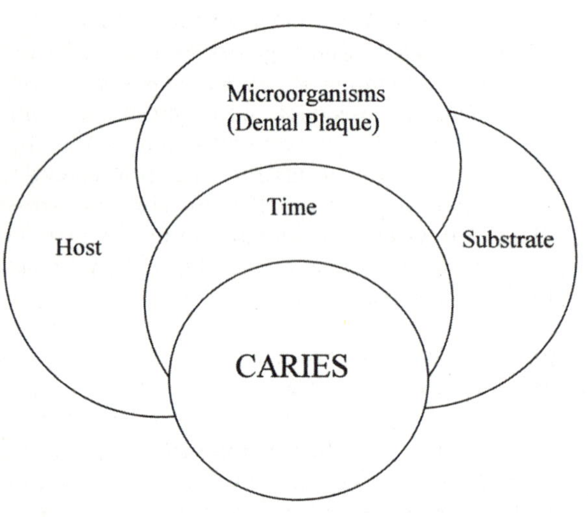

Fig. 7.2. Diagram illustrating the parameters involved in the development of human dental caries. All individual factors must be present before caries can occur

of the solvent surrounding the crystal. Alterations in these parameters and, in particular, lowering of pH, can result in solubilization of the crystals.

The production of acids from plaque bacteria and subsequent demineralization of enamel and formation of dental caries are the culmination of a highly selective process of bacterial adherence and colonization on the tooth surface.

After tooth eruption, several organic deposits may form on the surface of teeth. These deposits include dental plaque, materia alba, pellicle, and calculus. *Dental plaque* is defined as bacterial aggregations that are attached to the teeth or other solid oral structures. *Materia alba* describes bacterial aggregations, leukocytes, and desquamated oral epithelial cells accumulating at the surface of plaque and teeth, but lacking the regular internal structure observed in dental plaque (deposits removed by the mechanical action of a strong water spray are termed "materia alba," but if they withstand the water spray, they are called "dental plaque"). *Pellicle* is an organic film derived mainly from the saliva and deposited on the tooth surface. In its early stage, pellicle does not contain bacteria; however, it is soon colonized by bacteria and is then part of dental plaque. *Calculus* is calcified dental plaque, but it is always covered with a superficial layer of non-calcified plaque.

7.1.2.1 *Dental Plaque*

Dental plaque consists primarily of proliferating microorganisms, along with a scattering of epithelial cells, leukocytes, and macrophages, in an adherent intercellular matrix. The organic matrix is mainly a polysaccharide-protein complex produced by plaque microorganisms. Several oral streptococci synthesize levans (fructans) and glucans (mainly dextran) from dietary sucrose. The levans provide mainly energy, while the glucans not only provide energy, but also act as the organic skeleton of plaque, playing a fundamental role in bacterial adhesion and interbacterial coaggregation reactions.

The intermicrobial or extracellular matrix not only serves as a framework to bind the microorganisms into a coherent mass and as an extracellular storage of bacterial nutrients, but also contains numerous inflammation-inducing and other toxic substances, such as proteolytic enzymes, antigenic substances, endotoxin, and low-molecular-weight metabolites.

Dental plaque formation involves two major processes: (a) initial adherence and subsequent proliferation of salivary microorganisms to the acquired pellicle, and (b) further aggregation of bacteria to cells already attached. Initial adherence is mediated either by electrostatic forces (Ca^{2+}) or hydrophobic interactions (adhesion of bacterial cells to tooth surfaces through organic components: bacterial adhesins, glucans, etc.); subsequent accretion and "maturation" of dental plaque depends mainly on multiplication of attached bacteria, adhesion of new bacteria, and coaggregation of bacteria present in oral fluids to bacteria that are already attached. Plaque accretion is, in turn, influenced by bacterial (production of glucans), dietary (sucrose intake), and host-derived (oral cleansing mechanisms, leukocytes and antibodies in crevicular fluid, salivary glycoproteins, etc.) factors [2, 3].

7.1.2.1.1
Subgingival Plaque

Based on the relationship to the gingival margin, there are two categories: supragingival and subgingival plaque.

Supragingival plaque influences the establishment and relative proportions of subgingival microorganisms directly and indirectly. In association with supragingival plaque accumulation, there are inflammatory changes that modify the anatomic relationships of the gingival margin and the tooth surface. When these inflammatory changes occur, edema causes gingival enlargement, which increases the capacity of the subgingival area for bacterial colonization. This enlarged space protects bacteria from normal oral cleansing mechanisms. At the same time, there is a concomitant increase in the crevicular fluid flow and in pocket epithelial cell turnover. The end-result is a new ecologic environment protected from the supragingival milieu and bathed with gingival crevicular fluid, desquamated epithelial cells, and bacterial end-products, which subsequently influence the establishment and relative proportions of subgingival microorganisms. Many of these microorganisms lack the adherence ability to be first colonizers and have evolved mechanisms that can utilize supragingival bacteria as a means of colonization of the subgingival area. This environment has a low oxidation-reduction potential, which allows the most fastidious anaerobic bacteria to become established. Under these conditions, local environmental changes and local host defense reactions allow specific subgingival microorganisms to increase to a point where they can elicit pathology.

7.1.2.1.2
Plaque Bacteria Responsible for Acid Production

The bacteria which are the primary etiologic agents in various types of dental caries are not completely clear [4–6].

There are, in fact, three types of caries: enamel, dentine, and root surface caries. Enamel surface caries can be further divided into smooth surface and pit and fissure caries.

The smooth surface lesion has a well-defined microbiology characterized by the presence in the lesion of gram-positive facultative cocci, specifically *Streptococcus mutans* and *S. salivarius*. *S. mutans* is the primary etiologic agent in this type of caries, as (a) it ferments sugars to lactic acid, which is thought to be responsible for the dissolution of enamel matrix; (b) it is a prolific producer of insoluble extracellular dextrans, which allows bacteria to stick to the tooth surface; and (c) it is highly selective for pellicle-coated enamel surfaces.

Pit and fissure caries are the most common human lesions. Much less is known about their microbiology than about that of smooth surface caries, and of the several species of bacteria isolated from these lesions, *Streptococcus mutans* and lactobacilli are suspected as etiologic microorganisms.

Dentinal caries exhibit a somewhat different microbial ecology related to its location. Organisms growing here must be more anaerobic and derive most of their food from the tooth itself. The most commonly found pathogens in this region are lactobacilli. Other gram-positive anaerobic rods and filaments, such as *Bifidobacterium*, *Eubacterium*, and *Propionibacterium* have been identified. In addition, *Actinomyces* and *Bacillus* species have been noted at the invasive front of the deep dentinal lesion.

The root surface lesion is also initiated on pellicle-coated cementum by different flora than in the smooth surface lesions. Bacterial sampling of plaque from cemental caries reveals high numbers of *Actinomyces* spp., including *A. viscosus*, *A. naeslundii*,

Table 7.1. Bacteria associated with various types of caries

Caries type	Organisms isolated	Possible significance
Pit and fissure	*Streptococcus mutans*	High
	Lactobacillus spp.	High
	Streptococcus sanguis	Slight
	Actinomyces spp.	Possible
	Streptococcus mitis	None
Smooth surface	*Streptococcus mutans*	High
	Streptococcus salivarius	Little
Dentinal caries	*Lactobacillus* spp.	High
	Actinomyces naeslundii	High
	Actinomyces viscosus	Significant
	Streptococcus mutans	Possible
	Filamentous rod	Significant
Root caries	*Actinomyces viscosus*	High
	Actinomyces naeslundii	High
	Filamentous rod	High
	Streptococcus mutans	Some
	Streptococcus sanguis	Unclear
	Streptococcus salivarius	None clear

and *A. odontolyticus*. Other organisms including *Nocardia* and *Streptococcus mutans* have also been identified (Table 7.1).

7.1.2.2
Periapical Infections

Periapical infections result from pulpal trauma brought about by bacteria, temperature extremes, and physical forces. The most common cause is bacterial contamination of the pulp from carious lesions that have extended through the enamel and dentine. Bacteria and their products may also penetrate the pulp via accessory foramina which comunicate with periodontal pockets. Physical trauma, such a sudden blow to the face can compromise the pulpal blood supply, leading to pulpal death and subsequent bacterial colonization of the root canal. This phenomenon, called "anachoresis", comes about because of the attraction of bacteria into inflamed and/or necrotic tissue via the bloodstream.

Root canal infections are mixed bacterial infections with organisms from salivary contamination, carious lesions, and gingival/crevice pockets. These infections are predominantly by anaerobic bacteria, gram-negative anaerobic bacilli being the most common. These include species of *Actinomyces, Lactobacillus, Porphyromonas, Prevotella, Peptostreptococcus, Veillonella parvula, Enterocucus faecalis, Fusobacterium nucleatum,* and *Streptococcus mutans.*

7.1.3
Microbiology of Periodontal Disease

The main subgingival bacteria found in healthy subjects are *Streptococcus mitis, Streptococcus sanguis, Staphylococcus epidermidis, Rothia dentocariosa, Actinomyces viscosus, Actinomyces naeslundii* and small spirochetes.

The term "periodontal disease" describes a number of distinct clinical entities that affect the periodontium, including the gingiva, gingival attachment, periodontal ligament, cementum, and supporting alveolar bone. The classification of periodontal disease is based on clinical, bacterial, host, and environmental factors (Table 7.2).

The most common forms of gingivitis and periodontitis are caused primarily by bacteria, and the presence of subgingival dental plaque is necessary to initiate these diseases. The current paradigm for the pathogenesis of human periodontal diseases proposes that these afflictions occur as a result of subgingival plaque infection, frequently through familial transmission [7], with specific periodontal pathogenic bacteria (Fig. 7.3).

Table 7.2. Classification of periodontal diseases. Adapted from Current Procedural Terminology for Periodontics, 5th edn. Am. Acad. Periodontol. 1986

I. Gingival disease
  A. Gingivitis
    1. Nonspecific gingivitis
    2. Acute necrotizing ulcerative gingivitis (ANUG)
  B. Manifestions of systemic diseases and hormonal disturbances, e. g., desquamative gingivitis (associated with: cicatricial pemphigoid, pemphigus, Lichen planus, psoriasis), primary herpetic gingivostomatistis, "pregnancy stomatitis" and other hormonally mediated changes, diabetes, and other metabolic disases
  C. Drug-associated gingival inflammation, e. g., dilantin hyperplasia
II. Mucogingival conditions, e. g., gingival recession and aberrant frenun and/or muscle attachment
III. Periodontitis
  A. Adult periodontitis
    1. Slight
    2. Moderate
    3. Advanced
    4. Refractory and rapid progressive
  B. Juvenile periodontitis (JP)
    1. Prepubertal
    2. Generalized juvenile periodontitis (GJP)
    3. Localized juvenile periodontitis (LJP)
  C. Periodontal abscess
IV. Pathology associated with occlusion
V. Other conditions – miscellaneous (e. g., infection, trauma)

A small but varying amount of plaque can be controlled or tolerated without causing periodontal disease, probably as a result of host defense mechanisms. When specific periodontal pathogen bacteria within the plaque increase to significant numbers or produce virulence factors, or both, the "controlled environment" or balance shifts toward one favoring the development of disease. Disease also occurs when there is a reduction in the host's (local or systemic) defensive capacity.

7.1.3.1
Bacteria Associated with Periodontal Disease

Early theories on the role of dental plaque in periodontal disease suggested that there was only a quantitative change in the dental plaque bacterial population and that disease resulted from increased numbers of bacteria rather than the presence of specific pathogens. It was later discovered that bacterial plaque associated with gingival health differed from that seen in periodontal disease and most forms of periodontal disease had their own characteristic bacterial pathogens. In general, gram-negative, anaerobic microorganisms are the principal bacteria associated with most bacterially caused periodontal diseases. *Porphyromonas gingivalis, Prevotella intermedia, Bacteroides forsythus, Campylobacter rectus* (former *Wolinella recta*), and *Actinobacillus actinomycetemcomitans* are the most

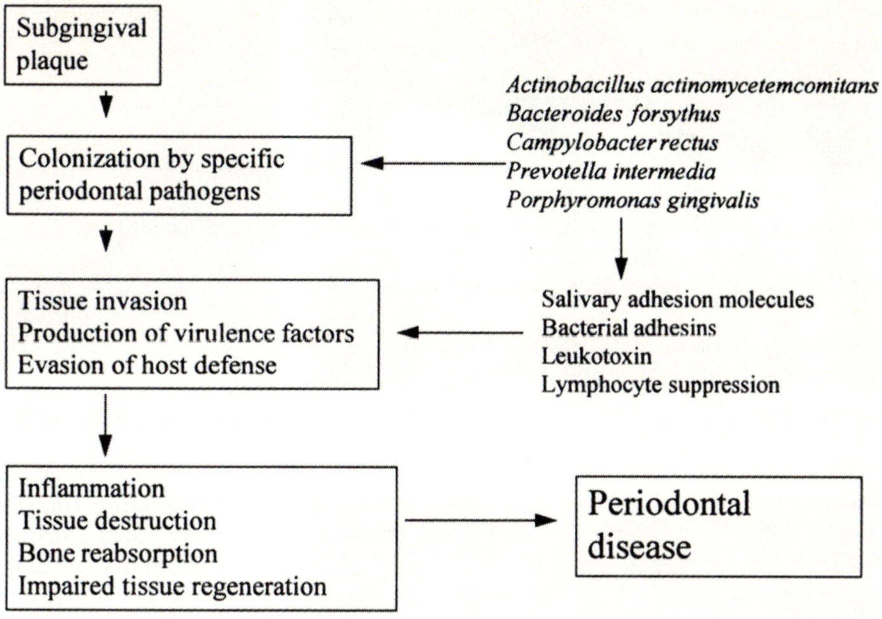

Fig. 7.3. Flow chart illustrating the sequence of events in the pathogenesis of periodontal disease

common bacteria significantly associated with periodontal disease (Table 7.3) [8, 9].

7.1.3.2 *Microbial Role in the Pathogenesis of Periodontal Disease*

The mechanisms by which subgingival bacteria can contribute to the pathogenesis of periodontal disease vary. These include factors influencing colonization (adhesion, coaggregation, multiplication, interbacterial relationships) and tissue damage. The pathogens involved in periodontal disease possess numerous factors that permit them to damage the periodontium directly, such as enzymes, endotoxins, and toxic low-molecular-weight metabolites, or to, compromise the host response by indirect means. Production of exotoxins in the true sense of the word by subgingival bacteria is rare. However, one type of exotoxin specifically directed toward human polymorphonuclear leukocytes is produced by *Actinobacillus actinomycetmcomitans.* This "leukotoxin" may enable *Actinobacillus actinomycetmcomitans* to destroy leukocytes in the gingival crevices, which assists the microorganism in its ability to colonize and invade the gingival tissue [10–12].

The disruption of collagen seen in periodontal disease, while mainly resulting from release of tissue collagenase, can also result from bacterial collagenase. *Porphyromonas gingivalis* and some strains of *Actinobacillus actinomycetmcomitans* produce collagenase and can degrade fibrinogen. Other bacterial enzymes of suspected periodontal pathogens that may cause periodontal destruction include gelatinase, aminopeptidase, phospholipase A, alkaline phosphatases, acid phosphatase, keratinase, arylsulfatase, neuraminidase, DNase, and RNase. Phospholipase A may initiate alveolar bone resorption as a precursor of prostaglandin. Alkaline and acid phosphatases may also cause alveolar bone loss [13].

Bacterial factors also aid in the evasion of host defenses. These factors influence both the cellular and the humoral immune response. Polymorphonuclear phagocytes may be influenced by leukotoxin and negative chemotactic factors, and bacteria can escape intracellular killing by the production of catalase and superoxide dismutase. Immunoglobulins and complement are inactivated or destroyed by bacteria such as *Porphyromonas gingivalis* and *Prevotella intermedia*, which have adverse effects on the bactericidal activity of serum.

Table 7.3. Principal microorganisms associated with periodontal diseases

Adult periodontitis	*Porphyromonas gingivalis, Prevotella intermedia, Bacteroides forsythus, Campylobacter rectus*
Refractory periodontitis	*Bacteroides forsythus, Prevotella gingivalis, Campylobacter rectus, Prevotella intermedia*
Localized juvenile periodontitis (LJP)	*Actinobacillus actinomycetemcomitans, Capnocytophaga*
Periodontitis in juvenile diabetics	*Capnocytophaga, Actinobacillus actinomycetem-comitans*
Pregnancy gingivitis	*Prevotella intermedia*
ANUG	*Prevotella intermedia*, intermediate-

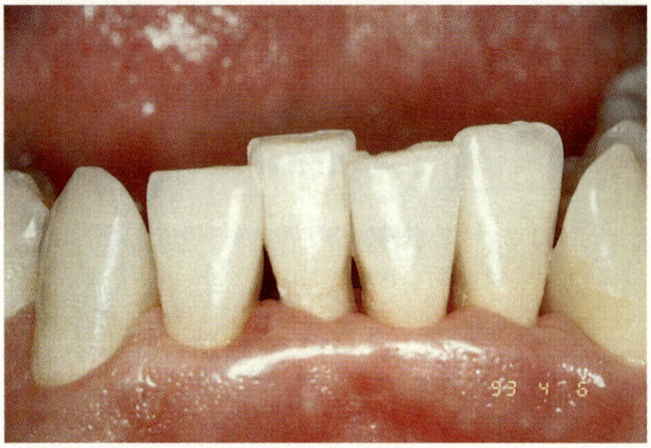

Fig. 7.4. Adult periodontitis

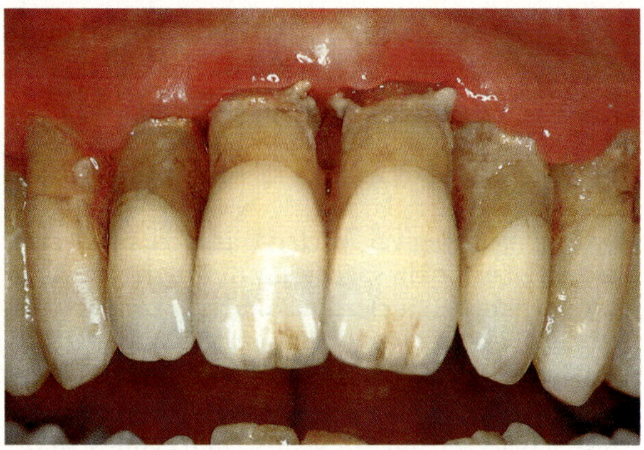

Fig. 7.5. Refractory and rapid progressive juvenile periodontitis

Subgingival bacteria may also affect the immune response by polyclonal B-cell activation [14], dysregulation of interleukin production, and induction of cytotoxic T-lymphocytes, and it is likely that some bacterial cell structural components may also act as superantigens. The combination of a direct effect of the bacteria on the periodontal tissues and indirect effects achieved by influences on host response represents the major pathogenetic element of periodontal disease (Figs. 7.4, 7.5).

7.1.3.3
Periodontal Abscesses

Periodontal abscesses occur with pre-existing periodontitis. This acute infection occurs in the walls of periodontal pockets as a result of the invasion of bacteria into the periodontal tissues (Fig. 7.6). While abscesses usually occur in patients with untreated periodontitis, it is more common in periodontitis patients with a systemic disease such as diabetes, in which the ability to combat infections is reduced. Early animal studies demonstrated

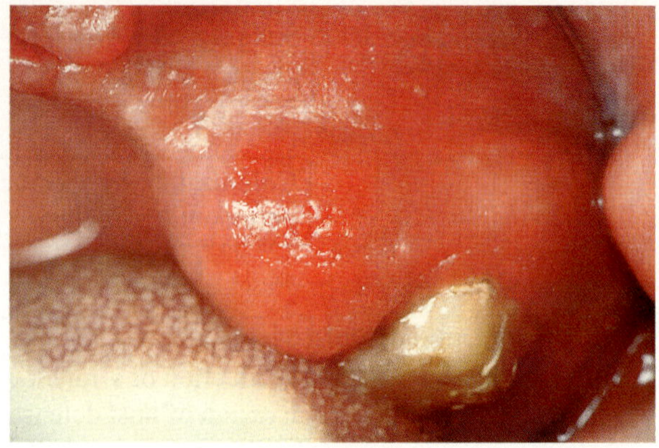

Fig. 7.6. Severe periodontal abscess

that fulminating, transferable abscesses could be induced by subcutaneous inoculation of plaque-derived materials (mixed anaerobic infections). Cultural examination of human abscesses reveals a microbiota with gram-negative anaerobic rods predominating. *Porphyromonas gingivalis, Fusobacterium* spp., *Capnocytophaga,* and *Vibrio* spp. are the most common gram-negative isolates, making up over 30 % of the total cultivable bacteria.

7.1.4
Microbiology of Soft Tissue Infections. Involvement of the Oral Cavity by Systemic Infections

The most important oral soft tissue infections are acute necrotizing ulcerative mucositis (ANUM) and actinomycosis of the mouth.

ANUM is a consequence of acute necrotizing ulcerative gingivitis (ANUG) spreading to adjacent sites. Formerly named "fusospirochetal disease" because of the large number of fusobacteria and different spirochetes present with the clinical picture of mucous membrane lesions, foul odor, and malaise, it is now considered to be caused by *Prevotella intermedia* and intermediate-sized spirochetes.

Actinomycosis is caused by the obligate anaerobe *Actinomyces israelii,* or, less commonly, *Actinomyes naeslundii,* or *Arachnia propionica. Actinomyces,* and presumably *Arachnia,* are present as normal flora in the mouth and from this source can cause infections of the periodontal tissues, oropharynx, tongue, neck, jaw, and lower respiratory tract. These infections are characterized by chronic induration, swelling, and sinus formation. Exudate from the sinuses contains typical "sulfur granules", which can be seen on gram staining to consist of aggregates of filamentous organisms.

Bacterial and viral infections can cause inflammation of the salivary glands. These agents may give

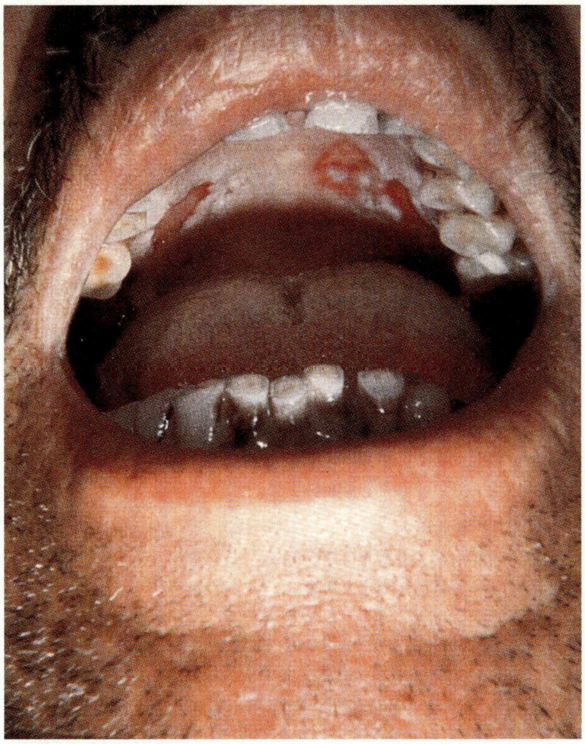

Fig. 7.7. Severe Herpes simplex (vesicles/ulcers) in the hard palatal area

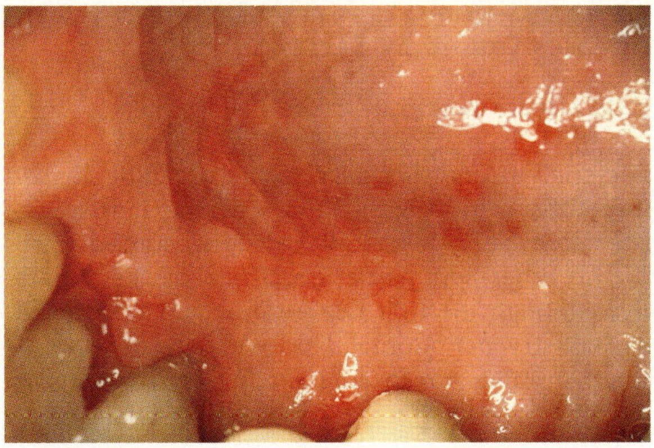

Fig. 7.8. Aphthous lesions of the hard palatal area

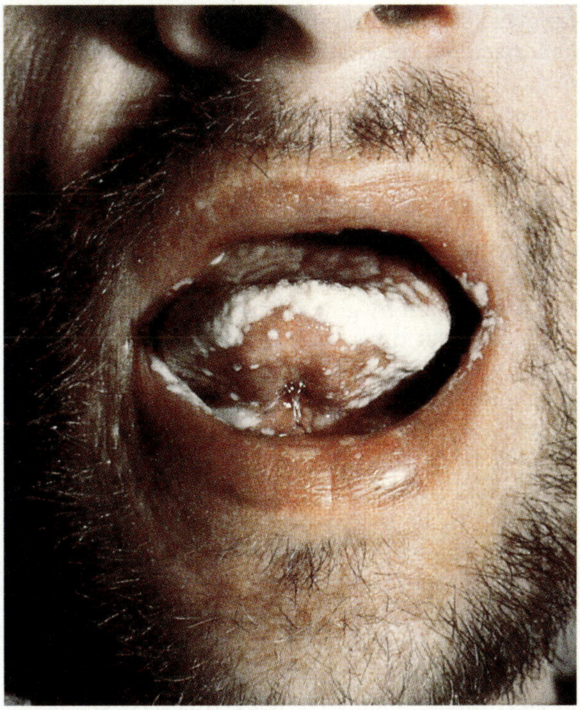

Fig. 7.9. Severe oral thrush (*Candida albicans* infection) in an HIV-1-infected (AIDS) patient

rise to acute and chronic sialadenitis and recurrent parotitis. Occasionally, the infectious process may spread to involve the submaxillary and sublingual spaces. The disease runs a violent and rapid course (Ludwig's angina) with marked swelling and little or no pus. The edema causes great difficulty in swallowing and a tracheotomy or intubation is frequently necessary. *Streptococcus* spp., *Staphylococcus* spp., and many anaerobic bacteria are frequently involved in these infections, which may occur after dental manipulation.

The oral cavity may also be involved during the course of various systemic infections, with different clinical manifestations. Vesicles/ulcers may be caused by herpes simplex virus (HSV) types 1 and 2, varicella-zoster virus (VZV), Coxsackievirus, mainly type A16 (hand, foot and mouth disease), tuberculosis, and syphilis (Figs. 7.7, 7.8).

Erythematous and macular lesions can be observed in the early stages of measles (Koplik's spots) and during scarlet fever and Epstein-Barr virus (EBV) infection (infectious mononucleosis).

Nodular and papular lesions (mucous patches) are frequent lesions of primary syphilis and during secondary syphilis, respectively.

Mucous plaques can arise as a consequence of papillomavirus infection (warts and condylomas) or may be caused by *Candida* spp. (white plaques: acute pseudomembranous candidiasis or thrush, acute atrophic candidiasis, chronic hyperplastic candidiasis, chronic localized mucocutaneous candidiasis with granuloma) (Fig. 7.9).

Acknowledgements. Prof. **Luigi Checchi**, Professor of Odontostomatologic Surgery in the Dentistry School of the Medical Faculty of the University of Bologna, Bologna, Italy, and Prof. **Elio Guido Rondanelli,** Professor of Infectious Diseases in the Medical Faculty of the University of Pavia, Pavia, Italy, provided the pictures illustrating the various clinical aspects of infectious oral pathology.

7.2 Diseases Caused by Bacteria

T. F. Mroczkowski

Bacterial infections of the oral cavity can be divided into three categories: diseases of the hard tissue (dental decay), periodontal disease, and diseases of the other soft tissue structures of the mouth. Even though the first two entities are the domain of dentistry, periodontal disease may be of some interest to other specialists including dermatologists.

7.2.1 Periodontal Disease

"Periodontal disease" is an umbrella term for a number of different pathologic processes which have bacterial etiology [15]. The disease is very common. It is likely that almost every adult has some degree of periodontal disease, and half of those who retain teeth to age 50 have gross and extensive periodontal tissue destruction. There are basically four types of periodontal disease [16] (Table 7.4).

a) Nonspecific gingivitis is an inflammatory process of the gingival tissue without bone loss [17]. It is characterized by gingival irritation, swelling, and bleeding, at times with formation of exudate in the gingival crevices. Since the process does not involve detachment of any of the periodontal structures or loss of alveolar bone, it is considered reversible: health can be restored by proper oral hygiene. Several bacterial species have been observed to be increased consistently and significantly in nonspecific gingivitis [17]; however, bacterial virulence factors have not been identified in this process. It seems that the pathology is due largely to host immune responses, which have a destructive effect on the gingival tissue.
b) Necrotizing ulcerative gingivitis (NUG) is an acute disease. It is seen most commonly in persons between adolescence and age 30. It appears that certain physiologic factors and stress may predispose to NUG. However, the disease is associated with specific microbial flora (Table 7.4). NUG is characterized by necrotic ulcerative lesions, with bleeding and pain that often result in destruction of the tips of the gingival papillae (Fig. 7.10). Successful treatment of the disease involves professional débridement of necrotic tissue, followed by carefully implemented personal and oral hygiene and plaque control. In some cases, when systemic symptoms occur (e.g., fever, malaise) administration of antibiotics is recommended.

Table 7.4. Bacterial agents implicated in periodontal disease.[a] (Based on [6])

Nonspecific gingivitis	*Actinomyces naeslundii* *Campylobacter concisus* *Streptococcus anginosus* *Streptococcus sanguis*
Necrotizing ulcerative gingivitis	*Prevotella intermedia* Spirochetes *Fusobacterium* spp.
Adult periodontitis	*Porphyromonas gingivalis* *Prevotella intermedia*
Localized early-onset periodontitis	*Antinobacillus actinomycetemcomitans*

[a] Other microorganisms may also be involved in initiation and/or progression of the disease.

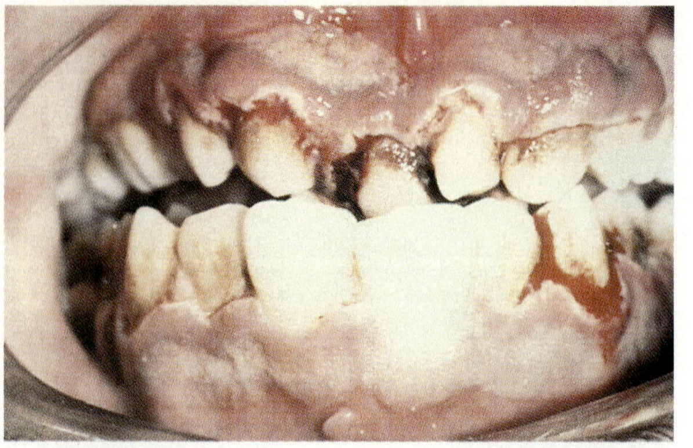

Fig. 7.10. Necrotizing ulcerative gingivitis. Necrotic ulcerative lesions resulting in necrosis of the gingival papillae. Courtesy of Dr. R.F. Carr and J. Tusa

c) Adult periodontitis is a chronic inflammatory disease characterized by gingival inflammation and the formation of periodontal pockets. This process is accompanied by alveolar bone loss, detachment of the periodontal ligament, and subsequent tooth mobility.
Both *Porphyromonas gingivalis* and *Prevotella intermedia* have been increasingly recognized in the etiology of this type of periodontitis [18, 19]. However, it appears that host factors play an important part in the disease process, by mounting inappropriate immune responses which have a destructive effect on the periodontium. The infiltration of plasma cells and B- and T-lymphocytes indicates local immune responses. Moreover, in the advanced phase, plasma cells make up most of the immune cells [18, 20].
d) Localized early-onset periodontitis (juvenile periodontitis) is characterized by periodontal pocket formation usually around incisors and first molars. The disease affects teenagers and young adults, and symptoms usually occur in the absence of pre-existing gingivitis and with lack of plaque. The process leads both to the loss of peri-

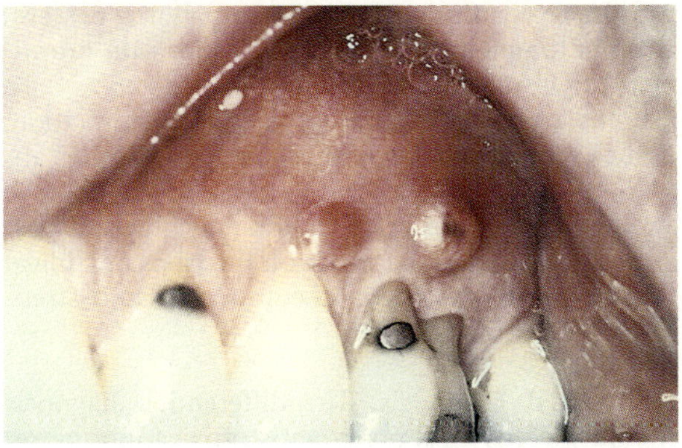

Fig. 7.11. Acute periodontal abscess results from obstruction to orifice of the periodontal pocket. This inhibits drainage of gingival fluid resulting in formation of abscess with signs of typical infection. Courtesy of Dr. R.F. Carr and J. Tusa

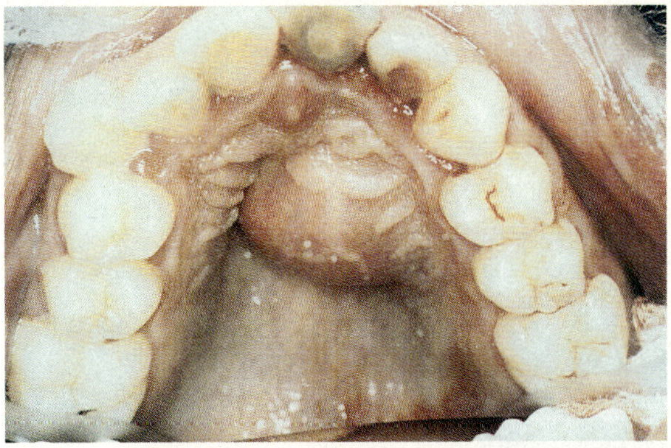

Fig. 7.12. Palatal abscess as frequently caused by aerobic and anaerobic flora. Courtesy of Dr. R.F. Carr and J. Tusa

odontal attachment structures and to alveolar bone loss. There seems to be a genetic predisposition based on familial occurrence of the disease, and there is mounting evidence to indicate that *Actinobacillus actinomycetemcomitans* is the principal etiologic agent [18, 19].

e) Acute periodontal abscess is an unusual consequence of ubiquitous chronic periodontal disease. It develops as a result of exacerbations of chronic periodontal disease, or as the result of a progressive destructive bacterial process involving the supporting structures that breaks through the pocket of epithelium. The abscess often develops secondary to the blockage of the alveolar pocket or may occur following trauma to the tooth or from a foreign body being lodged in the periodontal tissue. Oral examination reveals tender, edematous and erythematous gingiva, and a shiny elevation of the gingival margin. There is always tenderness with palpation over the affected area. The pain is unaffected by thermal changes (Fig. 7.11).

f) Cellulitis of the oral cavity usually results from a break in the integrity of the mucosal barrier, allowing oral pathogens to gain access to the underlying tissue. Trauma, microabrasions, or ulcerations are frequently the initiating injuries. At times, there may be contiguous spread from diseased skin or through hematogenous or lymphatic routes. The microorganisms multiply and initiate an inflammatory response with local and systemic signs. Fever and regional lymphadenopathy are frequent. Most infections are caused by both anaerobic and aerobic bacteria found in oral flora. If not recognized and treated, these infections may go to abscess formation, particularly those involving anaerobic flora (Fig. 7.12).

Periodontal disease should be distinguished from periodontal lesions seen in patients with uncontrolled diabetes or leukemia; gingival hypertrophy caused by drugs such as phenytoin or even contraceptive pills; viral and candidal stomatitis, Steven's Johnson syndrome, Behçet's disease, and various oral abnormalities frequently encountered in HIV infected patients.

Therapy includes administration of an antimicrobial agent effective against usual potential pathogens. If *Staphylococcus aureus* is present, appropriate coverage should be added. Frequently administered antimicrobials include: penicillin G or V, cephalexin, dicloxacillin, or clindamycin, and metronidazole. Tetracycline, doxycycline, and azithromycin are also effective. Treatment of periodontal disease may be ineffective if thorough débridement of necrotic tissue, local removal of bacteria with topical antiseptics (betadine) and mouthwashes (peridex), and long-term proper oral hygiene and plaque control is not maintained.

7.2.2 Bacterial Pharyngitis (Table 7.5)

Streptococcal pharyngitis (streptococcal sore throat – strep throat).

Table 7.5. Microorganisms causing bacterial pharyngitis

Streptococci group A
Streptococci non-group A
Neisseria gonorrhoeae
Anaerobes (Vincent's angina)
Corynebacterium haemolyticum
Corynebacterium diphtheriae
Mycoplasma pneumoniae

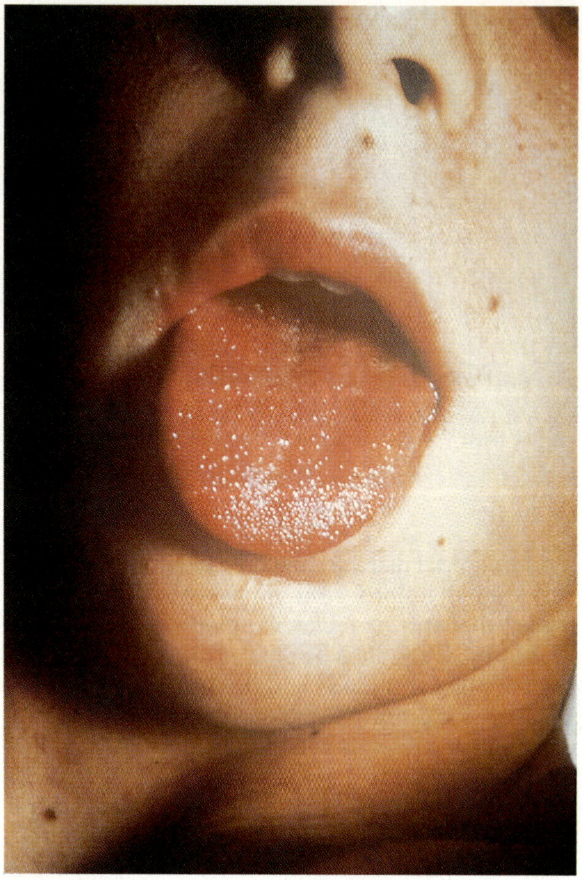

Fig. 7.13. "Strawberry tongue". A clinical feature seen in scarlet fever, Kawasaki syndrome and toxic shock syndrome. Courtesy of Dr. C.V. Sanders

This is caused by group A, β-hemolytic streptococci. The infection is primarily airborne but rare food-borne and milk-borne epidemics have been reported. The prevalence of streptococcal pharyngitis varies, but both the acute infection and the asymptomatic carrier state peak during the cold months of the year.

The signs and symptoms range from mild sore throat to severe disease with sudden onset of fever, severe pain on swallowing, malaise, headache, and nausea and/or vomiting. Physical findings vary from minimal erythema to severely edematous and erythematous pharynx, soft palate and tonsils with or without purulent exudate. Cervical nodes are enlarged and tender in a large proportion of patients. About 20 % of infections are asymptomatic. If the infecting streptococci produce erythrogenic toxin and the patient has no antitoxic immunity, scarlet fever (scarlatina) eruption occurs. The skin is diffusely erythematous with superimposed red papules which blanch on pressure. It fades in 2–5 days, leaving a fine desquamation. In scarlet fever, the face is flushed, circumolar pallor is present, and the tongue is usually coated white with prominent bright red papillae (strawberry tongue; 7.13). In rare instances, with the most intense inflammation, tissues may break down and form peritonsillar abscesses (quinsy) or Ludwig's angina where massive swelling of the floor of the mouth may block air passage. Diagnosis can be made on the basis of clinical findings, a positive bacterial culture, and anti-streptolysin O antibody test.

Differential Diagnosis. The differential diagnosis should include viral pharyngitis (this cannot be reliably distinguished on the clinical basis alone). Streptococcal pharyngitis is also commonly confused with infectious mononucleosis, which is characterized by generalized adenopathy, splenomegaly, abnormal lymphocytes, and positive serologic test. Diphtheria involves more confluent pseudomembranes. Candidiasis is distinguished by white patchy lesions on an erythematous base, and KOH tests shows yeasts. The petechial rash of scarlet fever should be distinguished from meningococcemia (positive culture for meningococci).

Treatment. Benzathine penicillin G intramuscularly or oral penicillin are the drug of choice. For patients allergic to penicillin, erythromycin for 10 days, or azithromycin for 5 days, are recommended. Untreated streptococcal infection is usually self-limiting. However, since rheumatic fever may follow (0.5 %–3 %) recurrent infection with group A streptococci early and effective treatment is advised.

7.2.2.1
Pharyngitis Caused by Corynebacterium diphtheriae

This disease occurs primarily in unvaccinated individuals. The organism gains entry through the respiratory tract and is spread mainly by respiratory secretions from patients with active disease or carriers. The microorganisms multiply on pharyngeal epithelial cells and secrete a potent toxin.

Characteristically, a tenacious gray membrane forms, which can spread over the entire pharynx and tonsils, and extend downward to the larynx or upward to the anterior nares (Fig. 7.14). The underlying mucosa bleeds easily when the membrane is touched. Early manifestations are mild sore throat, fever, and malaise, followed by signs of toxemia and prostration. Associated edema of the pharynx may cause swallowing and respiratory difficulties. Patients usually have enlarged tonsils and cervical lymphadenopathy. Irregularities of the cardiac rhythm may indicate damage to the heart (myocarditis), and later, there may be difficulties

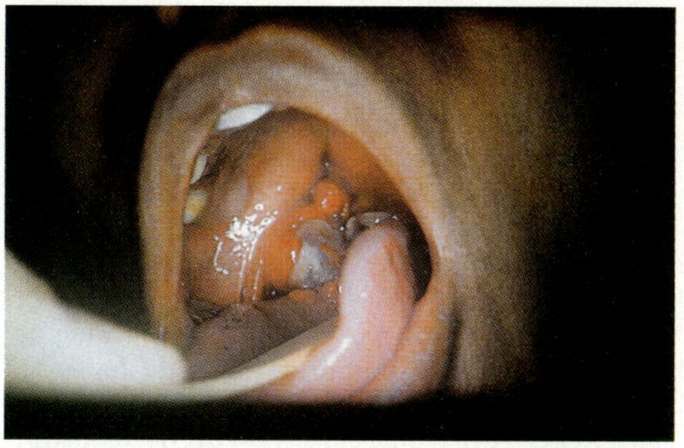

Fig. 7.14. Diphtheria. An adherent, thick, gray membrane, difficult to remove, develops on the tonsils and can spread over the entire pharynx

with vision, speech, or movements of the arms or legs. All of these manifestations tend to subside spontaneously.

Diagnosis. The condition is diagnosed on the basis of clinical features confirmed by demonstration of *C. diphtheriae* in gram-stained smear showing beaded rods in typical arrangement, and positive culture. Note: Specific treatment must never be delayed for laboratory reports if the clinical picture is strongly suggestive of diphtheria.

Differential Diagnosis. Differential diagnoses include: streptococcal pharyngitis, infectious mononucleosis, viral pharyngitis, Vincent's angina, and candidiasis.

Treatment. Diphtheria antitoxin must be given in all cases. Adjunctive therapy includes administration of penicillin G or erythromycin for at least 10 days.

7.2.2.2 *Pharyngitis Caused by Cornyebacterium hemolyticum*

This rare pharyngitis tends to occur in individuals in their second decade of life. Patients have low-grade fever, nonproductive cough, and lymphadenopathy. Most patients have enlarged tonsils with a purulent exudate. Some patients develop a scarlatiniform rash.

Diagnosis. Isolation of *C. hemolyticum* in culture allows the diagnosis. Gram-stained smear may reveal pleomorphic gram-positive rods associated with polymorphonucleosis.

Treatment. The infection responds readily to penicillin, azithromycin, or erythromycin.

7.2.3 Strawberry Tongue

Two clinical entities, toxic shock syndrome and Kawasaki disease, in addition to numerous skin and systemic symptoms, caused by enterotoxin producing *Staphylococcus aureus* are accompanied by so-called strawberry tongue [21, 22]. The same toxin may also be produced by group A streptococci which can cause *streptococcal* toxic shock syndrome, a recently recognized disorder that has the same clinical features as staphylococcal toxic shock syndrome, including strawberry tongue [22, 23] (Fig. 7.13).

7.2.3.1 *Toxic Shock Syndrome*

In most cases, this is caused by *Staphylococcus aureus* and in some, by group A streptococci. It occurs predominantly in menstruating women using tampons, though it may occur in men as well. The disease is characterized by acute onset with fever, vomiting, and diarrhea, followed by circulatory shock with hypotension. There is a widespread erythematous macular eruption and mucous membrane erythema, especially on the conjunctiva where there may also be hemorrhagic manifestations, in addition to those as on the tongue (strawberry tongue). Scattered petechiae, especially in the inguinal and antecubital areas, may be seen. The eruption is followed by desquamation of the affected skin, including hands and feet.

Diagnosis. Toxic shock syndrome can usually be diagnosed on clinical inspection. When necessary, cultures may confirm the diagnosis.

Differential Diagnosis. Other shock-type syndromes, Kawasaki disease, Reye's syndrome, scarlet fever, and Rocky Mountain spotted fever should be considered.

Treatment. Prompt and aggressive supportive therapy for shock is needed, and intravenous antistaphylococcal β-lactam-resistant antimicrobials are often given; the value of the latter, however, has been questioned by some authors.

7.2.3.2 *Kawasaki Disease (Mucocutaneous Lymph Node Syndrome)*

The manifestations of Kawasaki disease are similar in many ways to those of toxic shock syndrome. The disease was initially reported in Japan, where it predominantly affects young pre-school-age children.

The disease is rare in adults. Acute onset, fever of more than 5 days, bilateral conjunctival congestion, strawberry tongue, dry, red fissuring of the lips, an erythematous eruption more prominent on the trunk, palms and soles, followed by desquamation, are characteristic findings. Cervical adenopathy is present in the majority of patients and some patients may demonstrate arthritis, aseptic meningitis, and carditis. Cardiac involvement (coronary artery aneurysm) is the most serious late sequela.

Diagnosis. The diagnosis is based on clinical findings.

Treatment. Supportive treatment is given. Early administration of intravenous γ-globulin may reduce the cardiac complications.

7.2.4 Oral Lesions Caused by Sexually Transmitted Diseases

7.2.4.1 *Pharyngeal Gonorrhea*

Pharyngeal infection with *Neisseria gonorrhoeae* occurs predominantly in homosexual men (10 %–25 %) and in women practicing fellatio (10 %–20 %). In heterosexual men with gonorrhea, pharyngeal infection is encountered in 3 %–7 %. The pharynx as the sole site of infection is found in less than 5 % of patients regardless of gender and sexual orientation. The disease is asymptomatic in about 90 %, although acute exudative pharyngitis or tonsillitis with sore throat, pyrexia, and cervical adenopathy may occur. The clinical picture of gonococcal pharyngitis is nonspecific, and differentiation from viral or streptococcal pharyngitis is not possible on clinical grounds. Diagnosis of pharyngeal gonorrhea may create certain problems, since the gram-stained smear is useless and culture on selective media is insufficient. *N. gonorrhoeae* has to be differentiated from other *Neisseria* commonly present in the oropharynx, e.g., *N. meningitidis* and *N. lactamica.* The sugar fermentation test, immunofluorescence test, or DNA detection techniques including PCR and LCR are very helpful.

Treatment. Ceftriaxone 250 mg IM, in a single dose, or cefixime 400 mg orally or ciprofloxacin 500 mg orally as a single dose.

7.2.4.2 *Oral Lesions Caused by Chlamydia trachomatis*

Even though *Chlamydia trachomatis* can be detected in the pharynx after inoculation from oral-genital exposure, Chlamydia has not been established as a cause of pharyngitis [24, 25]; however, mucocutaneous lesions occur in Reiter's syndrome, the clinical entity in which chlamydial infection plays a significant role (80 % of cases). Reiter's syndrome occurs with increased frequency (ten-fold increased risk) in patients with the HLA-B27 haplotype. Typically, Reiter's syndrome consists of urethritis, arthritis, conjunctivitis, and stomatitits. The complete clinical picture is very rare. More often, one or two of these signs are present. Oral lesions occur in 10 %–25 % of patients with this condition, and are rather nonspecific. Stomatitis presents as painless, erythematous patches with superficial erosions on the tongue, soft palate, uvula, and buccal mucosa (Fig. 7.15). Occasionally, the tongue may show areas of erythema with loss of papillae.

Diagnosis. Clinical investigation will suggest the diagnosis, which is corroborated by detection of *C. trachomatis* in urethral exudate or antibodies to chlamydial antigens on microimmunofluorescent assay.

Differential Diagnosis. Aphthous stomatitis, candidiasis, Behçet's disease, Vincent's angina, and stomatitis caused by chemicals, drugs, alcohol, or tobacco must be considered.

Treatment. The treatment is symptomatic. Oral lesions in Reiter's syndrome are usually self-limiting. Chlamydial urethritis should be treated with doxycycline 100 mg orally twice a day for 7 days, or 1 g azithromycin as a single oral dose.

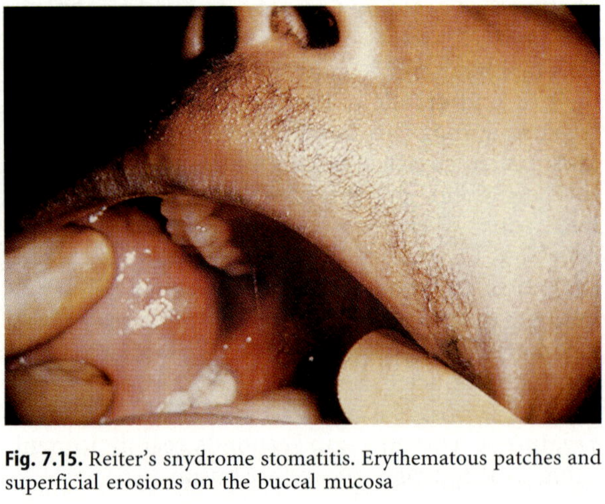

Fig. 7.15. Reiter's snydrome stomatitis. Erythematous patches and superficial erosions on the buccal mucosa

7.2.4.3
Syphilis

Syphilis (lues) is a chronic sexually transmitted disease cause by the spirochete *Treponema pallidum*. The disease can be acquired, or congenital if the offspring is infected transplacentally.

Both these entities are divided into early and late stages. Acquired syphilis is subdivided further into primary, secondary, and late or tertiary stages. The disease is characterized by a wide variety of manifestations including oral lesions which are encountered in all stages.

7.2.4.3.1
Primary Syphilis

After the incubation period (2–4 weeks) the primary lesion appears at the point of inoculation. Classically, a primary chancre is a painless, solitary lesion with a raised, well-defined border, located in the genital or anal areas. Extragenital primary chancres occur in less than 10 %, most commonly in the oral cavity (Fig. 7.16). The lips and tongue seem to be most frequently affected; however, primary chancres have been described on the tonsils, buccal mucosa, and soft palate. The primary chancre is usually associated with nontender regional adenopathy, which, in the case of oral location, is unilateral.

Diagnosis. The diagnosis is based on clinical manifestations and can be confirmed by demonstration of *T. pallidum* in dark-field examination and serologic testing. The latter can be non-reactive with the first 4–5 weeks of infection. The primary chancre in the mouth should be distinguished from herpes simplex (usually multiple, painful blisters/erosions); mucocutaneous histoplasmosis (painful ulceration with thick rolled edges); aphthosis (painful erosions on bright erythematous bases, with recurrences); and carcinoma (older age of patients, chronic indolent course).

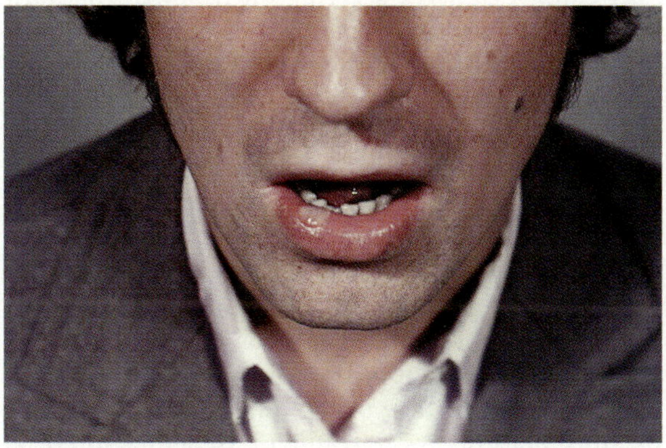

Fig. 7.16. Syphilis. Primary chancre on the lower lip

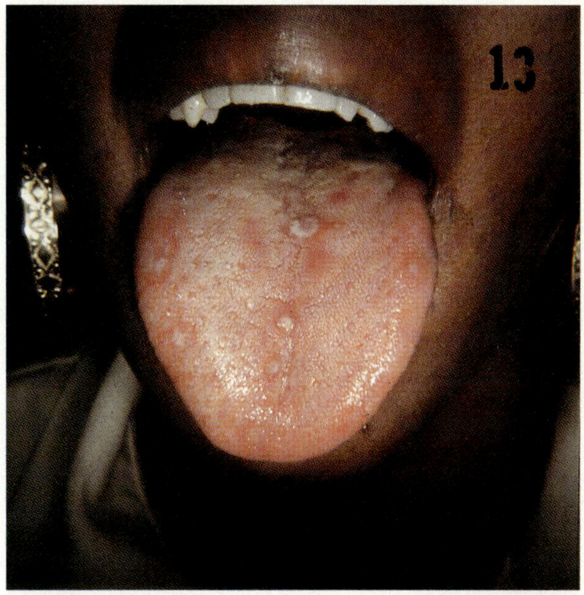

Fig. 7.17. Secondary syphilis. Mucous patches on the tongue

7.2.4.3.2
Secondary Syphilis

This stage begins 6–8 weeks after the appearance of the primary chancre. In contrast to the primary stage, patients with secondary syphilis may complain of flu-like symptoms and may demonstrate generalized lymphadenopathy. The most prominent feature of secondary syphilis is a skin eruption. About 80 % of patients have lesions of the skin or mucocutaneous junctions, and about 33 % have lesions in the mouth or throat. The most typical lesions are so-called mucous patches (Fig. 7.17), which appear in conjunction with the papular skin eruption. They can be found on the inner part of the lips, buccal mucosa, tongue, fauces, tonsils, and the pharynx and larynx. The typical mucous patch is sharply marginated, flat or slightly raised, faintly inflammatory, and covered with a whitish or grayish membrane (Fig. 7.18). On the soft palate and fauces, the lesions may be grouped into an elongated ulceration, the so-called small track ulcer. Lesions on the tongue usually lack papillae. In general, mucous membrane lesions, including oral changes, are painless unless secondarily infected. They are highly infectious and are more likely than skin lesions to recur during relapse.

Other common manifestations found in secondary syphilis include “moth-eaten” alopecia, syphili-

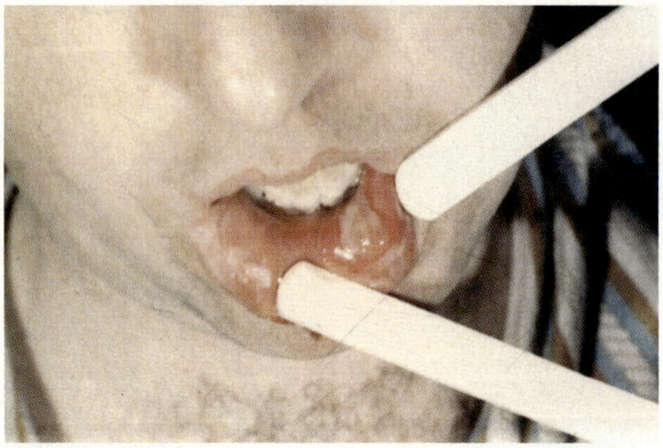

Fig. 7.18. Secondary syphilis. Typical mucous patch covered with a whitish membrane

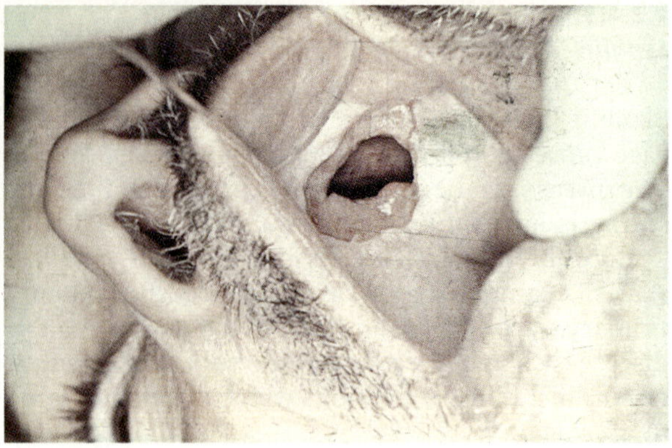

Fig. 7.20. Tertiary syphilis. Perforation of the hard palate

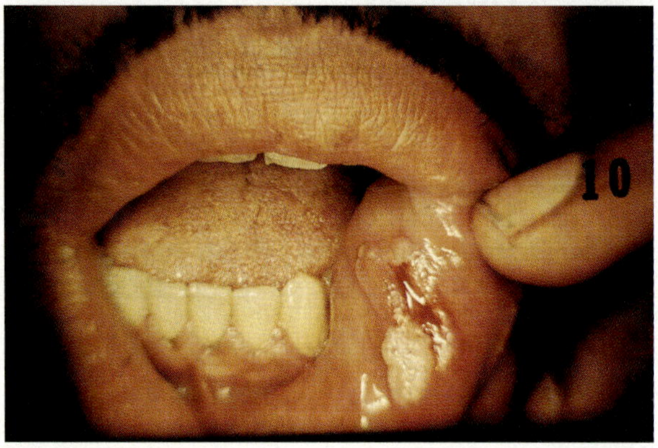

Fig. 7.19. Secondary syphilis. Condylomata lata on the inner site of the cheek. Courtesy of Dr. L.E. Millikan

tic leukoderma – patchy areas of hypopigmentation and condylomata lata – the hypertrophic broad-based, exuberant papules with flat moist tops (Fig. 7.19).

Differential diagnosis. Diagnosis of secondary syphilis is usually confirmed by serologic testing which, in this stage, demonstrates high titers. Moreover, *T. pallidum* can be demonstrated in moist lesions on dark-field examination. Mucous membrane lesions in the mouth or throat can be mistaken for aphthous ulcers, strep throat, viral exanthems, Vincent's angina, herpes labialis, Steven's Johnson syndrome, Behçet's disease, and pemphigus.

7.2.4.3.3
Tertiary Syphilis

The first manifestations of tertiary (late) syphilis may appear as early as 3 years and as late as 15 years after the primary stage. Although lesions of late syphilis can appear anywhere in the body, the most common forms are mucocutaneous, osseous, cardiovascular, neural and visceral. These forms can occur separately or in combination. Two major forms of mucocutaneous lesions of tertiary syphilis, nodular or nodulo-ulcerative and gummatous, may appear separately or may coexist. The nodular or nodulo-ulcerative lesions start as small painless nodules that develop gradually and regress even more slowly. They tend to be arranged in groups as rings, semicircles, or horseshoe shapes. Over the course of several months some nodules heal while new ones appear, usually at the periphery, resulting in a circular or serpiginous appearance that is pathognomonic for this stage of the disease.

The gumma usually occurs as a single lesion. It may be restricted to the skin or originate in the subcutaneous tissue, only secondarily involving the skin. Gummas have a predilection for the skin over the sternum, the sternoclavicular joints, the legs below the knees, the face, and the scalp. Gummas of the mucous membranes most often involve the mouth, tongue, and soft and hard palate. Involvement of the soft palate and uvula may lead to deformity and destruction of the tonsils that may cause extensive scarring on healing. The hard palate may perforate (Fig. 7.20) as a result of gummatous infiltrations of the roof of the mouth or the floor of the nose.

In late syphilis the tongue is a frequent target. Gummatous ulcerations may appear on the tongue, but interstitial glossitis is a more common sign. It results from diffuse gummatous perivascular infiltration of the blood vessels of the tongue. At the beginning of the process, there is painless enlargement of the tongue (macroglossia), but as healing occurs, interstitial fibrosis appears, which leads to irregular fissures of the surface of the tongue and atrophy of its musculature. As a result of ischemia, there is morbid loss of papillae. Chronic inflammation of the surface of the tongue is a common process which, in association with a decreased blood supply, creates an environment for development of leukoplakia, which is considered a precancerous lesion.

Diagnosis. The diagnosis of late mucocutaneous syphilis is basically dependent on the clinical features of lesions, aided by reactive serologic tests. They should to be distinguished from tuberculosis, sarcoidosis and malignancies and, in the early stages, from Vincent's angina and strep throat. Interstitial glossitis may resemble geographic tongue, scrotal tongue, and macroglossia resulting from acromegalism or hypothyroidism. Leukoplakia of the tongue should be distinguished from oral candidiasis, lichen planus and hairy leukoplakia, which occur in HIV-positive patients.

7.2.4.3.4
Congenital Syphilis

Clinical manifestations of congenital syphilis have traditionally been divided into early congenital syphilis, late congenital syphilis, and stigmata.

With the exception of bullous eruptions, the lesions of early congenital syphilis resemble in many ways those of secondary syphilis in adults, including lesions in the oral cavity. The mucous patches may be found in the nose and mouth, on the lips, and in the throat and larynx. Involvement of the pharynx combined with extension to the larynx may cause aphonia or a thin or hoarse cry or cough. The lesions around the mouth may become fissured, producing radiating scars (rhagades), which often persist for the rest of the patient's life (Fig. 7.21).

In late congenital syphilis, gummas located in the hard or soft palate, similar to those observed in acquired late syphilis, may result in palatal perforation, causing regurgitation of food and a nasal voice.

Stigmata, the third form of lesions seen in congenital syphilis, also include oral lesions. These are the residual effects of damage done to developing parts of the body in utero or during the early or late stages of syphilitic infection. Dental changes characteristic of late syphilis include Hutchinson's teeth (Fig. 7.22) and Moon's or "mullberry" molars (Fig. 7.23). Both abnormalities are found in the permanent teeth only. They are due to the effect of treponemal infection on the developing teeth buds shortly before and after birth. Hutchinson's teeth are changed, in that the sides are rounded (barrel shaped), while the cutting edge may be narrow (screwdriver-like) and may show a semilunar notch. Upper central incisors are most commonly affected. Moon molars are less common than Hutchinson's

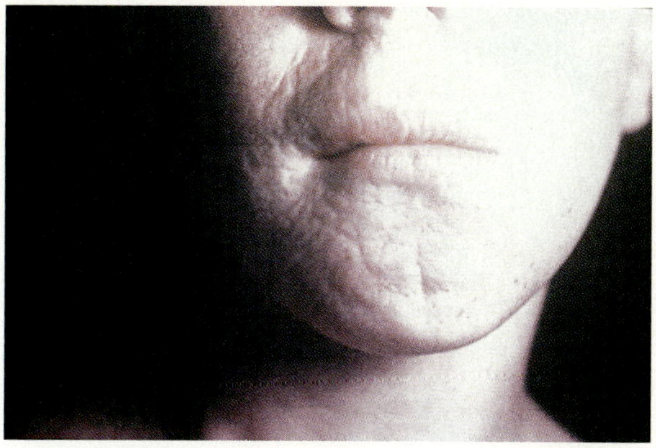

Fig. 7.21. Stigma of congenital syphilis: Rhagades – linear scars around the mouth, which persist for the rest of the patients life. Courtesy of Dr. L.E. Millikan

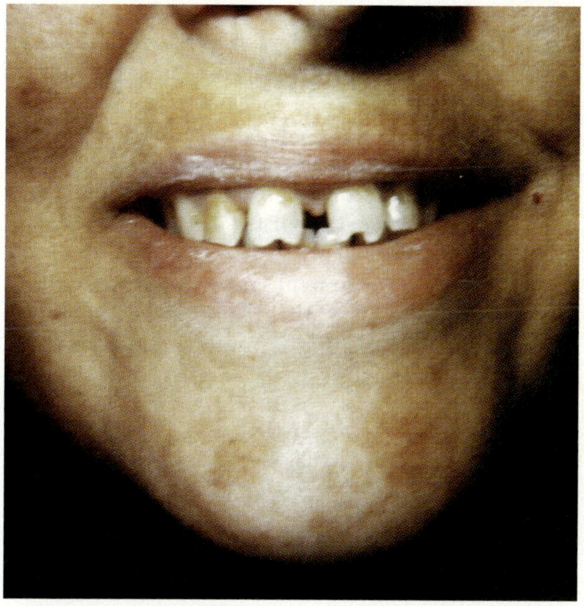

Fig. 7.22. Stigma of congenital syphilis. Hutchinson's teeth. Courtesy of Dr. L.E. Millikan

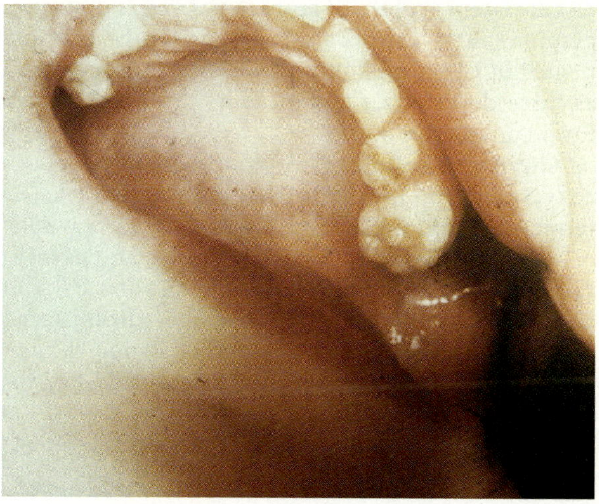

Fig. 7.23. Stigma of congenital syphilis. "Mulberry" molars. Courtesy of the Centers for Disease Control, Atlanta, GA

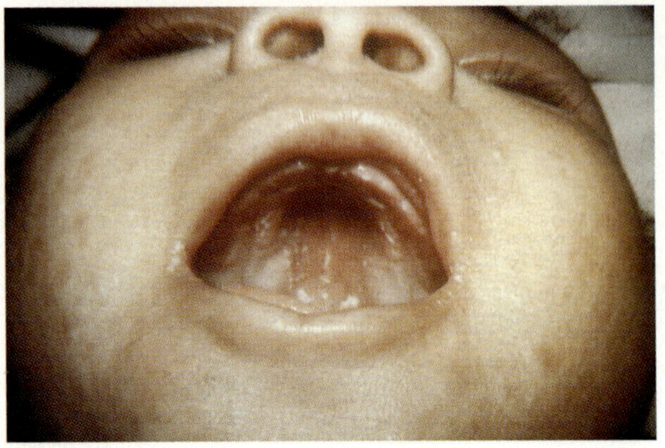

Fig. 7.24. Stigma of congenital syphilis: "Gothic palate". Courtesy of the Centers for Disease Control, Atlanta, GA

teeth. The first lower molars, which develop at the same time as the incisors, are the most frequently affected. Their biting surfaces are dome-shaped, with badly developed cusps, producing a mulberry-like surface. These teeth are poorly enamelized and are highly prone to decay. The other stigmata of the oral cavity are a high-arched palate called the "gothic palate" (Fig. 7.24) and the "bulldog jaw," a very prominent jaw owing to the failure of the maxilla to develop. Diagnosis of congenital syphilis is made on clinical grounds, and confirmed by positive serologic tests.

Treatment. Primary and secondary syphilis and early latent syphilis of less than 1 year's duration: benzathine penicillin G, 2.4 million units IM in one dose.

Alternative regimen for patients allergic to penicillin: doxycycline, 100 mg orally twice daily for 2 weeks or erythromycin, 500 mg orally four times daily for 2 weeks.

Late latent syphilis of more than 1 year's duration, gummas, and cardiovascular syphilis: benzathine penicillin G, 7.2 million units in total, administered as three doses of 2.4 million units IM, 1 week apart for 3 consecutive weeks.

Alternative regimens (for nonpregnant patients): coxycycline, 100 mg orally twice daily for 4 weeks, or tetracycline 500 mg PO four times daily for 4 weeks.

Congenital syphilis: for symptomatic and asymptomatic infants administer 100 000–150 000 U/kg of aqueous crystalline penicillin G daily (administered as 50 000 units/kg IV every 8–12 h) or 50 000 U/kg of procaine penicillin (administered once daily IM) for 10–14 days.

For detailed information, see the 1993 STD Treatment Guidelines [26].

7.2.4.4 *Chancroid, Granuloma Inguinale, and Lymphogranuloma Venereum*

7.2.4.4.1 *Chancroid*

Chancroid is an ulcerative sexually transmitted disease caused by *Haemophilus ducreyi.* It is clinically manifested by acute, painful ulcers on the genitalia, and inguinal lymphadenopathy with the possibility of bubo formation. Genital ulcers are sharply demarcated, have ragged undermined edges, and a sloughing base frequently covered with necrotic exudate. Upon removal of this exudate, an uneven, purulent granulation tissue is seen. The size varies from a few millimeters to 1–2 cm. Extragenital lesiôns are rare and have been described in the mouth and on the fingers, the breasts, and thighs. Lesions in the oropharynx have no particular characteristic features other than the concomitant presence of other, more classic, genital lesions.

Diagnosis. Diagnosis is often made on the basis of clinical presentation, confirmed by demonstration of *H. ducreyi* by culture and/or smear.

Differential Diagnosis. Chancroid should be distinguished from primary syphilis (*T. pallidum* in darkfield examination, positive syphilis serology tests); genital herpes (history of recurrences, positive Tzank tests, positive viral culture); LGV primary lesion is transient, often missed, positive test for *Chlamydia trachomatis;* granuloma inguinale – chronic disease, Donovan bodies in smears or in histology.

Treatment. The treatment of chancroid includes administration of antimicrobials such as azithromycin, 1 g PO once, ceftriaxone 250 mg IM in a single dose, or erythromycin base 500 mg PO four times a day for 7 days.

7.2.4.4.2 *Granuloma Inguinale (Donovanosis)*

This is a chronic, slowly progressive, and mildly contagious sexually transmitted disease caused by the gram-negative bacterium *Calymmatobacterium granulomatis.* It is characterized by granulomatous ulcerations usually affecting genitalia and neighboring sites. Oral lesions were first described by Donovan in 1905. They were described on the lips as extensive superficial ulcerations with well-defined, elevated granulomatous margins. Other cases involved oral and laryngeal lesions causing dysphagia and "bilateral ankylosis of the jaws" and also granuloma inguinale confined to the gingiva, causing "bleeding and a feeling of fullness of the lower gums" [27, 28]. In most instances, the oral lesions in granuloma inguinale are a result of self-inoculation from the genital or anal lesions.

Diagnosis. The diagnosis is made on clinical grounds confirmed by demonstration of Donovan bodies in a biopsy of the affected tissue.

Differential Diagnosis. Differential diagnoses include STD's causing genital ulcerations (see above section on chancroid).

Treatment. Tetracycline, 500 mg four times daily for 3 weeks or erythromycin, 500 mg four times daily for 3 weeks.

7.2.4.4.3
Lymphogranuloma Venereum

Lymphogranuloma venereum (LGV) is a sexually transmitted disease caused by one of three serovars of *Chlamydia trachomatis*, L_1, L_2, or L_3. It is characterized by a transitory primary lesion followed by suppurative regional lymphadenopathy, with fever and other constitutional symptoms. In the majority of cases, primary lesions occur on the external genitalia, followed by inguinal lymphadenitis and bubo formation. Oral lesions may result from orogenital contact or autoinoculation. A symptomatic triad consisting of iritis, aphthoid lesions of the mouth and the penis, and a positive Frei test, has been described [28]. The tongue appears to be a common site of oral involvement. The lesions on the tongue are usually small, slightly painful, superficial erosions with nonindurated borders. They are located usually at the tip of the tongue. In long-standing infection, there are zones of cicatricial retraction, dark red areas with loss of the superficial epithelium, or opaque lichenoid grayish papules. Erythematous soft palate and granulomatous lesions with regional lymphadenitis accompanied by dysphagia are commonly associated symptoms. Cervical lymphadenopathy follows primary lesions in the mouth. The skin covering the affected nodes is violaceous, swollen, and indurated. There may be one or more sinuses [28].

Diagnosis. LGV is usually diagnosed on the basis of positive serologic tests or isolation of chlamydia from infected tissue and secretions. However, the recovery rate is less than 30 %, so that the diagnosis is frequently based on clinical features and a positive complement fixation (CF) test.

Differential Diagnosis. In the cervical region, differential diagnoses should include actinomycosis, tuberculosis cutis, blastomycosis, and cat scratch disease. Lesions on the tongue should be distinguished from syphilis and tuberculosis. The presence of concomitant lesions in the anogenital area is very helpful.

Treatment. Doxycycline, 100 mg PO twice daily for 3 weeks or erythromycin, 500 mg PO four times daily for 3 weeks.

7.2.5
Actinomycosis

Actinomycosis is caused by the anaerobic gram-positive, filamentous bacterium *Actinomyces israelii*. Very occasionally, other species may be involved. Both *A. israeli* and other species of *Actinomycetes* occur in the normal flora of the mouth and tonsillar crypts; when introduced into traumatized tissue and associated with other anaerobic flora, these actinomycetes may become pathogens. Depending on the affected areas, there are three major types of actinomycosis: cervicofacial, thoracic, and abdominal.

Cervicofacial actinomycosis ("lumpy jaw") is the most common form (about two-thirds of cases) of infection, usually associated with odontogenic disease, e.g., tooth extraction, fracture, or other trauma to the mouth floor. The organism is introduced into traumatized tissue in an anaerobic environment. The infection then spreads to subcutaneous tissue and appears under the skin as a reddish or cyanotic induration. The disease develops slowly, forming woody-hard swellings, usually at the angle of the jaw in the parotid region or the neck (Fig. 7.25). A sinus tract usually extends externally to the skin, but may also extend internally to the tongue, larynx, bone, or other tissue. Cutaneous fistulas discharge

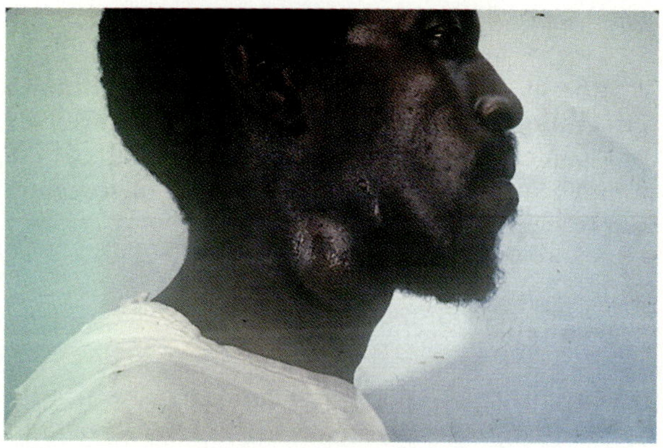

Fig. 7.25. Actinomycosis. Hard swelling at the angle of the jaw and draining sinuses. Courtesy of Dr. C.V. Sanders

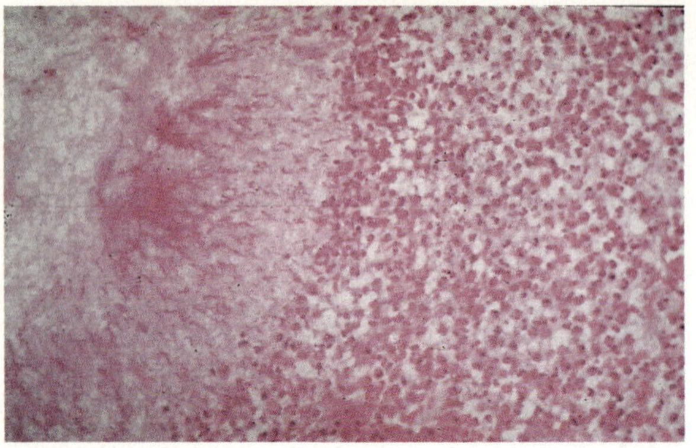

Fig. 7.26. Actinomycosis. "Sulfur granules" present in biopsy specimen. Courtesy of Dr. M. Kaminski

characteristic yellow pus. There is usually little pain unless there is marked secondary infection. Trismus indicates that the masticatory muscles are involved.

Diagnosis. The clinical picture is very suggestive. Diagnosis can to be confirmed by culture. When actinomycosis is suspected, exudate or tissue must to be cultured promptly under anaerobic conditions. Gram stain of pus or exudate will reveal filamentous, beaded, branching gram-positive rods that must be differentiated from nocardia. The hallmark of the infection is the presence of "sulfur granules" (masses of organisms appearing as yellow or white concentrations) in purulent material draining from the skin fistulas (Fig. 7.26).

Differential Diagnosis. Other diagnoses considered should include tuberculosis or staphylococcal, nocardial or deep fungal infections. Abscesses without a sinus tract should be distinguished from furuncles and carbuncles, lymphoma, and cyst. Chronic osteomyelitis tumors can mimic chronic actinomycosis. In osteomyelitis, pain is more severe, with greater destruction of bone and more rapidly developing suppuration. Radiological studies aid in the diagnosis.

Treatment. High doses of parenteral penicillin or a tetracycline should be given initially, followed by oral penicillin or tetracycline for a total of 3–6 months. Surgical excision and drainage of abscesses is very helpful.

7.2.6 Mycobacterial Infections

The mycobacteria comprise a large genus, which includes many species; *Mycobacterium tuberculosis* and *Mycobacterium leprae* are the most important human pathogens. Other mycobacteria, the so-called nontuberculous species, are also capable of infecting humans, but skin infections caused by them are rare. The mycobacteria responsible for most cutaneous diseases include *M. marinum, M. ulcerans, M. fortuitum, M. cheloneae,* and *M. avium intracellulare.*

7.2.6.1 *Tuberculosis*

Cutaneous manifestations of tuberculosis have been extremely rare in developed countries; however, in the era of AIDS, cutaneous tuberculosis is being seen again. Skin infections caused by *Mycobacterium tuberculosis* produce a variety of manifestations which are best classified on the basis of the route of inoculation (Table 7.6). Clinical findings depend a great deal on whether the host has been previously infected with *M. tuberculosis.*

7.2.6.1.1 *Exogenous Source*

Primary inoculation tuberculosis (tuberculous chancre) results from skin infection of an individual who has not been previously infected with *M. tuberculosis.* The mycobacterium presumably invades the skin through unnoticed minor abrasions or overt injuries. The organism multiplies locally and a lesion forms in about 2–4 weeks. The initial lesion is usually a papule or nodule located primarily on the exposed area of the skin at the site of trauma or an-

Table 7.6. Classification of cutaneous tuberculosis. (Adapted from [37, 38])

Source	Alternative nomenclature
A. *Exogenous source*	
1. Primary inoculation	Tuberculous chancre Tuberculosis primary complex
2. Post-primary inoculation	Tuberculosis verrucosa cutis Verruca necrogenica Prosector's warts
B. *Endogenous source*	
1. Contiguous spread	Scrofuloderma Tuberculosis colliquativa cutis
2. Autoinoculation	Orificial tuberculosis Tuberculosis cutis orificialis
C. *Hematogenous spread*	
1. Lupus vulgaris	Tuberculosis luposa cutis
2. Acute hematogeneous dissemination	Acute miliary tuberculosis of the skin Tuberculosis cutis miliaris disseminata Tuberculosis cutis acuta generalisata
3. Nodules or abscesses	Metastatic tuberculous abscess Tuberculous gumma

other skin abrasion. The initial lesion may develop into a shallow, ragged ulcer, usually painless, with undermined and indurated edges and a granular hemorrhagic base. Regional lymphadenopathy is common and may be the patient's presenting complaint.

The primary complex evolves slowly without systemic manifestations, and a healing process may take many months. Occasionally, tuberculous chancre proceeds to lupus vulgaris. The enlarged and draining lymph nodes subside slowly with subsequent calcification. At times, cold abscesses and sinuses may develop.

Mucosal Lesions. Uncommon oral and conjunctival lesions have been described. Oral lesions, often misdiagnosed, can form on the gums or in tooth sockets. They are usually painless.

Exogenous postprimary inoculation tuberculosis occurs in individuals who have been previously infected with *M. tuberculosis* and have developed some degree of immunity. Members of different occupational groups, such as pathologists, postmortem attendants, physicians, and butchers are traditionally at risk. Lesions occur on areas exposed to trauma, with the hands most commonly involved, producing a verrucous skin growth. Slow peripheral extension may result in the development of purplish or brown plaques that become fissured. Pus may sometimes be expressed. Regional lymphadenopathy, which is a prominent feature in primary inoculation, is rare and may be due to secondary bacterial infection.

7.2.6.1.2
Endogenous Source

Scrofuloderma results from contiguous spread of infection to the skin from adjacent foci such as lymph nodes, bones, or joints. The condition occurs most commonly after cervical lymphadenitis, less often with axillary or inguinal gland infection. The firm nodes frequently soften and liquefy and may drain serous or caseous material. Ulcerations often form along the chain of lymph nodes. The lesions heal with scarring, leaving characteristic marks at the site of the infection.

Orificial tuberculosis (tuberculosis cutis orificialis) occurs on mucous membranes or periorificial skin. The patients affected usually have advanced internal tuberculosis, primarily pulmonary, intestinal, or anogenital. They shed large numbers of organisms onto the mucous membranes and skin of the oral or anogenital regions. This form of cutaneous tuberculosis, which results from autoinoculation, manifests clinically as papules or small nodules, which break down to form irregular painful, and shallow ulcers. Traumatized areas are most susceptible, particularly the tip or lateral side of the tongue (Fig. 7.27). Occasionally the lips, the palate, or tooth sockets may be involved. The lesions are frequently tender and may be the cause of dysphagia. The lesions can be single or multiple. They rarely exceed 2 cm in diameter. They do not show a tendency to spontaneous healing.

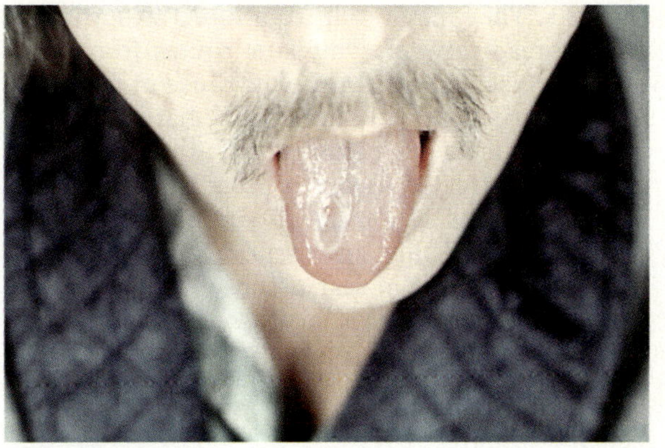

Fig. 7.27. Cutaneous tuberculosis. Shallow ulcer on the tongue in a patient with pulmonary tuberculosis

7.2.6.1.3
Cutaneous Tuberculosis from Hematogenous Spread

Lupus vulgaris, which is the most common type of cutaneous tuberculosis, may result from dissemination, usually from cervical adenitis, inoculation reexposure, or primary tuberculosis in nodes, lungs or elsewhere. In the case of pulmonary tuberculosis, organisms often disseminate by the hematogenous route, with resultant widely scattered, tiny tuberculomas. There can be numerous clinical manifestations, ranging from asymptomatic plaques, nodules and ulcerations with subsequent scars to hypertrophic lesions. The majority of these are located on the head and neck. Lesions usually begin as brown-to-red papules, solitary or multiple, that evolve into plaques with elevated borders. On diascopy, small yellow-brown "apple jelly" nodules may be visualized. Later, the center of the plaque becomes atrophic and may ulcerate. The lesions heal with scarring, contractures, and mottled pigmentation. Since healing and extension occur simultaneously, polycyclic and serpiginous plaques may develop. In the hypertrophic form, soft, tumorous, and hypersclerotic growth can be seen. In long-standing lesions, squamous cell carcinoma may develop.

In this form, mucous membranes are frequently affected. The oral, nasal and, to a lesser extent, conjunctival mucosa may be involved. Granulating, vegetating and ulcerating lesions can be seen on the buccal mucosa, the palate, the gingiva, or in the pharynx. They may result from direct extension or from spread through lymphatic routes from nasal lesions. Nasal lesions may be the cause of nasal cartilage destruction, and ulcers on the hard palate can be the cause of its perforation [29]. The natural course of untreated lesions is progressive; however, spontaneous resolution can also occur, leaving scarring, skin contracture, and tissue destruction. Active lupus may reoccur in scar tissue.

Miliary tuberculosis is mostly seen in infants and children with primary disease or, occasionally, in older patients, particularly if immunosuppressed. Skin lesions include disseminated papules, macules, vesicles, pustules, and hemorrhagic lesions. The last often occur when necrotizing vasculitis accompanies miliary tuberculosis. Erythematous nodules have also been described. The lesions are, in general, nontender. Pruritic lesions have also been described.

Other forms of hematogenous dissemination of cutaneous tuberculosis are multiple abscesses and/or nodules, which may form at the site of trauma.

Diagnosis. The diagnosis of cutaneous tuberculosis is made on the basis of a characteristic clinical picture confirmed by biopsy, smear, and culture. A PPD test should be positive except in cases of primary inoculation and, sometimes, miliary tuberculosis.

Differential Diagnosis. The form of the disease determines the differential diagnoses, which include numerous skin diseases. They can be excluded on the basis of histopathology, demonstration of acid-fast bacilli, and a positive PPD test.

Treatment. Standard antituberculous chemotherapy is effective for cutaneous tuberculosis. Prolonged treatment with at least two agents is indicated. The following drugs are recommended.

1. Isoniazid 300 mg daily for 6 months.
2. Rifampin 450–600 mg (depending on body weight) daily for 6 months.
3. Pyrazinamide 1.5–2.5 g daily (depending on body weight) for the first 2 months.
4. Ethambutol 15 mg/kg body weight daily for the first 2 months.

7.2.6.2
Cutaneous Lesions Caused by Nontuberculous Mycobacteria

Pathogenic nontuberculous mycobacteria are environmental saprophytes frequently found in soil, lakes, rivers, and swimming pools. They can be found in animal and human feces, human skin and sputum, and domestic water supplies and vegetation. They usually invade the skin by direct inoculation, but also by inhalation or ingestion. The exact mechanism that makes these bacteria pathogenic is unknown. The majority of infections are caused by *M. marinum* (swimming pool granuloma) in otherwise healthy persons. *M. chelonae* and *M. fortuitum* (*Mycobacterium fortuitum* complex) can cause both cutaneous and systemic infections, while other nontuberculous mycobacteria primarily cause infections in immunocompromised individuals, including patients with AIDS. In these last cases, *M. avium-intracellulare* and *M. haemophilum* are frequently isolated. The morphology of skin signs includes papular and pustular lesions, ulcerations, nodules, and scrofuloderma-like draining sinuses. Induration of the soft tissue or abscesses, as well as suppurative cervical lymphadenitis, have been described. Lesions in the oral cavity have also been reported. These included ulcerations of the buccal mucosa and indurations and nodules on the soft palate.

Diagnosis. Diagnostic procedures include biopsy, which should be submitted both for culture and histopathology with stain for acid-fast bacteria.

Differential Diagnosis. The differential diagnoses depend on the type of mycobacteria involved and include tuberculosis cutis, leprosy, mycoses, and bacterial infection. The differential diagnosis of lesions caused by *M. ulcerans* includes pyoderma gangrenosum, squamous cell carcinoma, foreign body granuloma, and deep fungal infections. Histopathology and culture aid diagnosis.

Treatment. The choice of antituberculous drugs should be guided by the sensitivity test. Minocycline or other tetracyclines are effective. Other antibiotics include rifampin or clarithromycin. In many instances (mainly after a poor response to treatment with antimicrobials) surgical excision is recommended.

7.2.6.3
Leprosy

Leprosy (Hansen's disease) is a chronic infectious disease caused by *Mycobacterium leprae.* The skin and peripheral nerves are primarily affected but other areas of the body, such as eyes, testes, nose and larynx, are also frequently involved. The disease is a rarity in Europe and North America, but is endemic to many geographical areas, such as south and southeast Asia (India, Indonesia, Burma), West and Central Africa, the Middle East, and Central and South America.

Although the exact mode of transmission has not been definitely established, the idea of respiratory transmission seems to be most convincing. The incubation period ranges from several months to over 20 years, with an average of 3–5 years. Though not hereditary, certain populations might be more susceptible to leprosy because of a genetically transmitted defect in their cell-mediated immune system specific for *M. leprae.* All races are susceptible and men are more likely to develop more serious forms of the disease than women; however, overall only 5 % are capable of contracting Hansen's disease.

The pathogenesis, and thus the clinical features, depend on the patient's ability to generate a cell-mediated immune response to *M. leprae.*

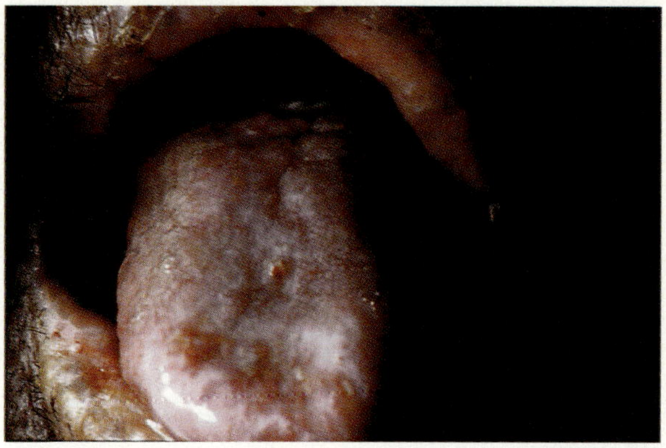

Fig. 7.28. Lepromatous leprosy (LL). Nodular infiltrating lesions on the tongue. Courtesy of Dr. D.M. Scollard and Ms. T. Thomassie of the GWL Hansen's Disease Center, Baton Rouge, LA

Clinical features. Disease manifestations lie along a spectrum that reflects the sometimes varying immune responsiveness of the host, but may be described as follows:

1. Indeterminate leprosy. This is the earliest form of the disease after exposure to *M. leprae,* and it is easily overlooked. It is characterized by the presence of (a) hypo- or hyperpigmented or erythematous macular lesion(s) located on the face, extremities, buttocks or trunk. The lesion is usually less than one to a few centimeters in diameter, with poorly defined margins. It causes no symptoms, but occasionally skin sensation may be diminished. The diagnosis can be supported by biopsy. Rarely, the presenting symptom is anesthesia caused by a peripheral nerve lesion, or blister or ulcer in an anesthetic hand or foot.
2. Tuberculoid leprosy. This form of leprosy, which is localized, occurs in individuals with intact immunity. The only tissues involved are skin and nerves. The lesions most often consist of a solitary, fairly large anesthetic plaque with loss of pigmentation, sweating, and tactile sensitivity inside the lesion. The surrounding skin may exhibit some reaction due to involvement of skin and peripheral nerves, which result in local tenderness and enlargement.
3. Lepromatous leprosy. This type of leprosy is encountered in patients with diminished or absent cellular immune response to the pathogen. This generalized form is characterized by numerous papules and plaques with shiny, flat-topped, erythematous or brownish surfaces. The lesions usually have poorly defined edges, and satellite lesions may develop outside the edge of the plaques. Often, the lesions are bilateral and symmetrical, and they may not be anesthetic. Another form with diffuse nonnodular infiltrative disease that lack discernible plaques or nodules is accompanied by loss of eyebrows and eyelashes, loss of body hair and the ability to sweat, or sensory loss in the distal extremities. Many years after onset, some patients with lepromatous leprosy may develop severe reactive episodes with sudden widespread tissue breakdown called the Lucio phenomenon. This reaction is due to infarction consequent upon deep cutaneous vasculitis, and causes the appearance of erythematous patches, bullae, and necrosis. It is systemic and can be fatal.
   In untreated cases, lepromatous leprosy is slowly progressive, coming to involve nearly the entire skin. On the face, the skin becomes thickened and corrugated ("leonine facies"); ear lobes are often thickened. The nose may become misshapen and may later collapse because of septal perforation and the loss of anterior nasal spine. Atrophic rhinitis (stuffy nose) is not uncommon. Lesions of the oral mucosa may take the form of papules on the lips. Granulomatous tissue may infiltrate the nose, ears, soft and hard palate, uvula, and larynx. Infiltration of the hard palate may cause its perforation. The tongue may show nodular infiltrations (Figs. 7.28, 7.29) that are also observed in the uvula and gums (Figs. 7.30, 7.31). The nasal mucosa may be hyperemic, causing epistaxis, or the mucous membrane may be covered with multiple ulcerations. In this form of leprosy, eye involvement is common (keratitis, iridocyclitis, or iris atrophy), as is testicular atrophy, which may cause gynecomastia, impotence, and sterility. Liver, kidney, and pulmonary involvement have all been recognized.
4. Borderline leprosy. This is an unstable form of the disease that may become either tuberculoid or lepromatous. It is manifested by few to numerous lesions, which also vary in size, shape and margin-

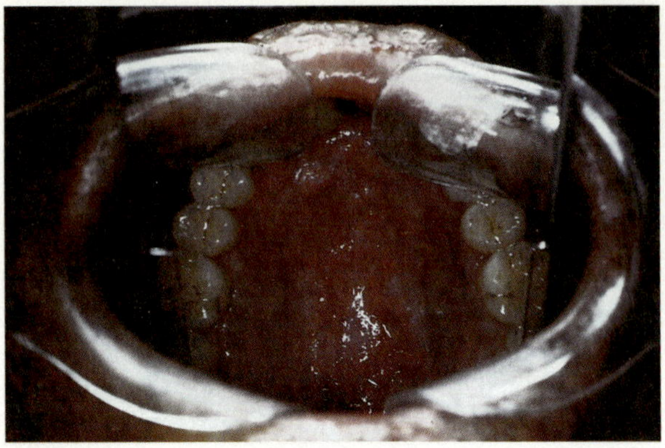

Fig. 7.29. Same patient as in Fig. 7.28. Nodular infiltrating lesions on the hard palate. Courtesy of Dr. D.M. Scollard and Ms. T. Thomassie of the GWL Hansen's Disease Center, Baton Rouge, LA

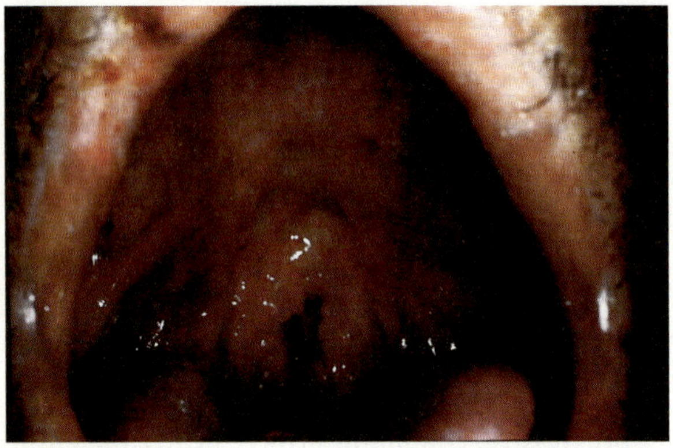

Fig. 7.30. LL, same patient as in Figs. 7.28, 7.29. Nodular infiltrating lesions of the oropharyngeal mucosa. Courtesy of Dr. D.M. Scollard and Ms. T. Thomassie of the GWL Hansen's Disease Center, Baton Rouge, LA

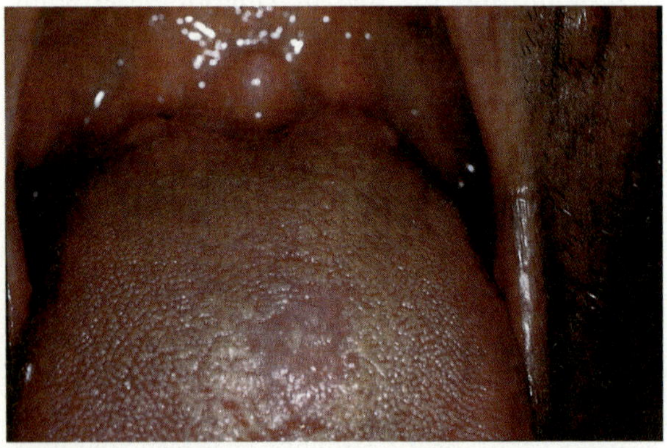

Fig. 7.31. LL: thickened plaque-like lesion on the tongue and anthropy of the uvula. Courtesy of Dr. D.M. Scollard and Ms. T. Thomassie of the GWL Hansen's Disease Center, Baton Rouge, LA

al definition. It can be divided into borderline tuberculoid (BT), borderline (BB), and borderline lepromatous (BL) disease. In BT disease, lesions are fewer, drier, and tend to be larger with diminished hair growth and sensation. There are fewer bacilli in smears and biopsies. In BB disease, the lesions are smaller and plaques with a "punched-out" center are common and characteristic. *M. leprae* may be found in tissue smears or biopsy. If the disease progresses toward lepromatous leprosy (LL), the lesions become extensive and numerous. They are usually smaller and symmetrical. Some of them may have punched-out centers. The lesions contain numerous bacilli. Reactive episodes before and after treatment occur in BB disease. Widespread and severe neuropathy is frequently observed, and permanent tissue destruction, especially in BL disease, is not rare (Fig. 7.32).

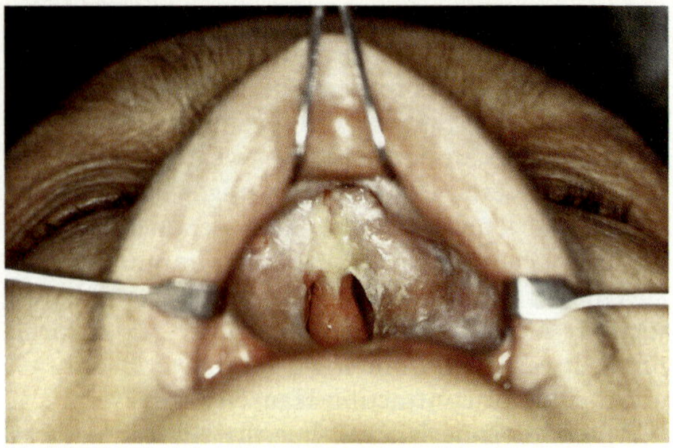

Fig. 7.32. Borderline leprosy (BL). Nasal septal perforation. Courtesy of Dr. D.M. Scollard and Ms. T. Thomassie of the GWL Hansen's Disease Center, Baton Rouge, LA

Diagnosis. Leprosy, in endemic countries, should be suspected in any patient with anesthetic skin lesions and signs of peripheral neuropathy. The diagnosis is corroborated by the presence of acid-fast bacilli in split-skin smears and biopsies. The histologic picture may be characteristic, showing histologic infiltration or obliteration of nerves. The lepromin test used in leprosy is not a diagnostic test. It is of value in determining patient ability to control *M. leprae* infection. It is strongly positive in TT, weakly positive in BT and BB, and negative in BL and LL.

Differential Diagnosis. Leprosy lesions can mimic many skin diseases, including lupus vulgaris, granuloma annulare, psoriasis, sarcoidosis, and syphilis or the treponematoses. Clues to diagnosis include residence in endemic countries, numbness, anesthesia, and enlarged nerves.

Treatment. The sulfones (dapsone) have been the treatment of choice until recently. However, owing to the rising incidence of sulfone-resistant disease, multidrug therapy is now recommended. The

WHO regimens for paucibacillary disease include dapsone 100 mg daily and rifampin 600 monthly, directly observed for 6 months. The multibacillary regimen is dapsone 100 mg daily plus clofazimine 500 mg daily and 300 mg monthly directly observed, plus rifampin 600 mg monthly directly observed for 2 years, preferably until the skin smear is negative.

The short-term therapy approach recommended in the United States consist of two regimens for paucibacillary cases; PB-1, which consists of dapsone 100 mg daily and rifampin 600 mg daily for 12 months, and PB-2, which consists of dapsone 100 mg daily and rifampin 600 mg monthly for 12 months. For multibacillary disease, there are three different regimens: MB-1, which is dapsone 100 mg daily and rifampin 600 mg daily for 2 years, with all treatment stopped if a mouse footpad study is successful; MB-2, which is dapsone 100 mg daily, rifampin 600 mg daily, and clofazimine 50 mg daily for 2 years, with all therapy stopped thereafter; and MB-3, which is dapsone 100 mg daily, rifampin 600 mg monthly directly observed, and clofazimine 50 mg daily with 300 mg monthly directly observed for 2 years, with therapy then discontinued.

7.2.7 Oral Lesions Caused by Bacteria in HIV-Positive Patients

Oral lesions are prominent features of AIDS and HIV infection. Some of them are reflections of reduced immune status manifested as opportunistic infections. Others represent the oral feature of HIV itself. Oral lesions caused by bacteria in association with HIV infection are listed in Table 7.7.

HIV-associated gingivitis is very common in HIV-infected persons and almost universal in AIDS. This form of gingivitis is severe and recurrent. The gingiva usually shows a fiery red marginal line, often with gum recession. Dental abscesses are common problems.

Periodontal disease is seen in about 30 %–50 % of AIDS clinic patients, but is much less common among HIV-positive patients who are asymptomatic (Fig. 7.33). The clinical picture resembles that of necrotizing ulcerative gingivitis or progressive periodontitis. The onset is usually rapid, with ulcerations and necrosis of the tips of interdental papillae. Many patients complain of severe, deep-seated pain that is not alleviated with the use of analgesics, and of spontaneous bleeding from the mouth. There may be progressive loss of gingival and periodontal tissues and massive destruction of supporting bones, causing loosening of the teeth. In severe cases, exposure and sequestration of bone may occur, producing necrotizing stomatitis [30], a condition resembling noma, which occurs in severely malnourished individuals. The etiology and pathology of periodontal lesions in patients with AIDS is not clear [31]. Standard therapy for periodontitis and gingivitis is ineffective. The therapeutic regimen involves thorough débridement and curettage, followed by application of topical antiseptics and short-course antibiotics such as Augmentin 250 mg t.i.d. for 4–6 days, metronidazole 250 mg q.i.d. for 7–10 days, or clindamycin 300 mg t.i.d. for 7 days. The effectiveness of treatment depends heavily on thorough removal of necrotic tissue and bacteria in the initial phase of therapy and on maintenance after this.

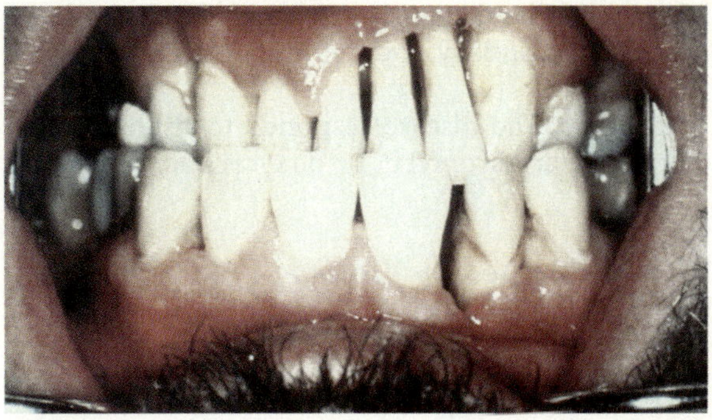

Fig. 7.33. Periodontitis in HIV patients. Courtesy of Dr. R.F. Carr and J. Tusa

Table 7.7. Oral lesions caused by bacteria in HIV-positive patients

Gingivitis
Periodontitis
Infection caused by *Mycobacterium avium-intracellulare*
Necrotizing stomatitis
Stomatitis caused by *Klebsiella*
Bacillary angiomatosis

There are reports of oral lesions caused by *Klebsiella pneumoniae* and *Enterobacter cloacae* in HIV-positive patients [32]. Both responded to antibiotic therapy based on sensitivity tests. Other oral ulcerations have been described in association with disseminated *Mycobacterium avium-intracellulare* infection in patients with AIDS [33].

Bacillary (epithelioid) angiomatosis, which is a vascular proliferation that mimics Kaposi's sarcoma, may produce oral lesions [34]. The condition, caused by *Rochalimaea quintana* and *Rochalimaea henselae*, most commonly occurs as a late manifestation of HIV infection, when CD4+ cell counts are below 100/mm^3 [35, 36]. Bacillary angiomatosis may affect many organs, including skin, lymph nodes, bone, bone marrow, brain, and gastrointestinal and respiratory tracts. The cutaneous lesions consist of papules or nodules that are violet to red in color, firm and nonblanching. The lesions are usually numerous.

Diagnosis. The diagnosis can be made on the basis of distinct histology and culture.

Treatment. The disease responds to three or four courses of erythromycin or doxycycline.

7.3
Diseases Caused by Viruses

7.3.1
Herpesvirus Group

S. R. Flint

7.3.1.1
Introduction

Members of the herpesviridae family of viruses (human herpesviruses, HHV) cause disease in man and most have a distinct oral component in the primary infection, expressed as an oral enanthem. The hallmark of infection is that it is lifelong and the viruses in this family possess the ability to remain latent in the tissues to which they are trophic following the primary infection. Latency of the viruses in this group has been described in neural, epithelial, endothelial, lymphoid, glandular, and connective tissues. Reactivation of the latent virus may result in specific disease, or there may be periodic asymptomatic shedding of free virus into body fluids. Asymptomatic viral shedding, particularly into saliva, is the main route of transmission, but virus may also be isolated periodically from other secretions, such as breast milk and genital fluids. Local reactivation episodes may occur in immunocompetent subjects, but may be particularly troublesome in the immunocompromised.

Eight different herpesviruses are described, six of which can exhibit specific oral manifestations. HHV-1, -2, and -3 (herpes simplex types 1 and 2 and varicella-zoster virus, respectively) together make up the alpha herpesvirinae subfamily. HHV-4 (Epstein-Barr virus) is designated a gamma herpesvirus and HHV5 (cytomegalovirus), a beta herpesvirus. HHV-6, 7, and 8 recently described members of this family. All are lipid covered, DNA viruses.

7.3.1.2
Primary Herpetic Gingivostomatitis (Gingivostomatitis Herpetica)

Etiology and pathogenesis. The causal agents of herpetic gingivostomatitis are the herpes simplex viruses (HSV). There are two closely related subtypes, HSV-1 and HSV-2, which can be distinguished

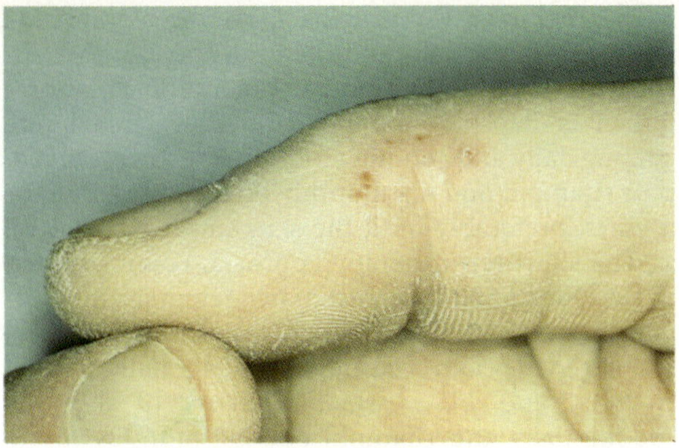

Fig. 7.34. Herpetic whithlow in a dentist, caused by a needlestick injury while treating an infected child

immunologically. Although HSV-1 generally causes herpetic gingivostomatitis and HSV-2 genital herpes, HSV-2 can also cause clinically indistinguishable oral lesions.

Approximately 5% of adults and children periodically shed HSV-1 asymptomatically into their saliva, and contact with infected saliva is probably the most important mode of transmission. Transmission of HSV-2 to nonimmune adults is usually by sexual contact. Both HSV-1 and HSV-2 can be transmitted by orogenital contact, and there is the potential for genital infection from primary oral contact. A particular occupational risk in nonimmune dentists and auxiliary personnel is infection of the fingers – the herpetic whitlow (Fig. 7.34).

Primary infection is seen mainly in children, although many infections are asymptomatic or are mild and may be attributed to "teething". Neonates may be protected by maternal passive immunity, and when the disease occurs in adults it is often more severe.

Oral and General Manifestations. The presentation is that of an acute febrile illness characterized by oropharnygeal ulceration and gingivitis [39]

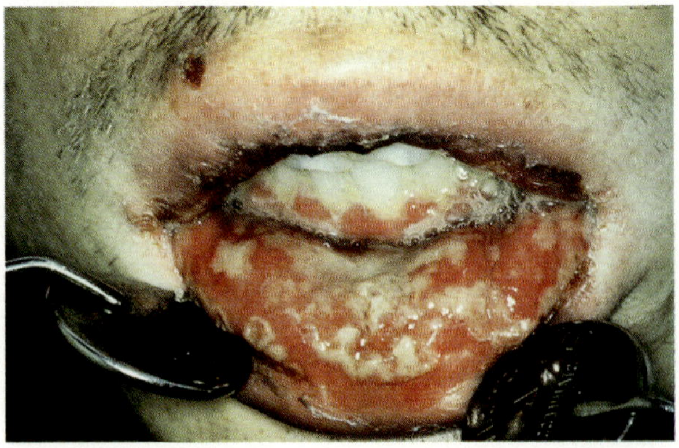

Fig. 7.35. Oral ulceration in primary herpetic gingivostomatitis

(Fig. 7.35). Herpes simplex may account for 2% of acute pharyngotonsillitis. There is malaise associated with lymphadenopathy and fever, which may precede the oral lesions by 1–3 days. The gingivitis is characteristic, with a rapid onset of florid, generalized swelling and erythema, particularly of the marginal gingiva, although the attached gingiva may also be affected (Fig. 7.36). Owing to the inability of patients to maintain their oral hygiene during this phase, and their debility, focal areas of acute necrotizing ulcerative gingivitis are often seen in association.

The disease is self-limiting, and complete healing of the ulceration occurs without scarring over a period of about 2 weeks, but infectious virus can be recovered from the saliva for up to 7 weeks following the primary infection. Dissemination of the virus may be seen in patients with perioral dermatoses, particularly dermatitis (eczema herpeticum, Kaposi's varicelliform eruption) or keratosis follicularis and in patients who use topical steroids. HSV-1 may also be a cause of meningoencephalitis.

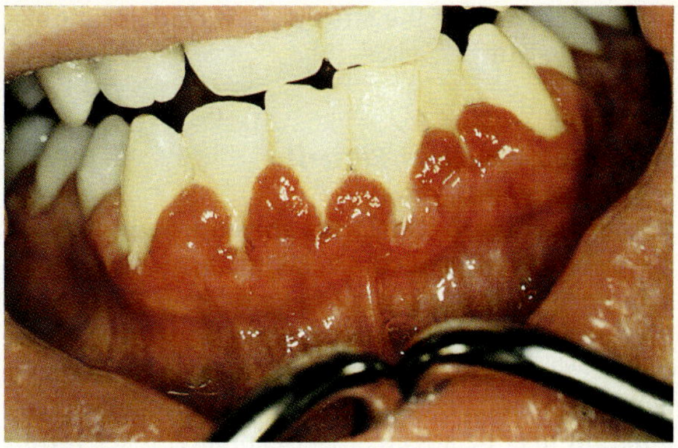

Fig. 7.36. Florid gingival swelling in primary herpetic gingivostomatitis

Diagnosis. The diagnosis is usually clinical but may be confirmed by viral culture or rising serial antibody titers. Acute serum IgM and IgG assays and convalescent IgG assay at 2 or 3 weeks are performed. A positive acute serum IgM and a more than four-fold rise in IgG antibodies in the convalescent serum confirms the diagnosis. HSV-1 and HSV-2 may be distinguished by both these techniques. The diagnosis is often retrospective, since recovery has usually occurred before the results are known. Exfoliative cytology with immunostaining may be useful for early diagnosis. Polymerase chain reaction techniques may become more widely available in the future for rapid diagnosis, but will not differentiate primary infection from reactivation or asymptomatic viral shedding.

Differential Diagnosis. The most important differential diagnoses are erythema multiforme (and other vesiculobullous dermatoses), the herpetiform variant of recurrent aphthous stomatitis, other herpesvirus group infections, and enterovirus infections. Although the diagnosis of these other conditions may be obvious from the history, or the presence of typical exanthemata, it may not be so obvious at the first presentation. Furthermore, a variant of erythema multiforme that is limited to the oropharyngeal mucous membranes has been described, although bloody extra-oral labial crusting is a fairly constant feature, which is rarely seen in herpetic gingivostomatitis. Although a degree of involvement of the gingivae is seen in erythema multiforme, it is much less florid than herpetic gingivostomatitis, and herpetiform aphthous stomatitis affects only the nonkeratinized mucosa. Paradoxically, erythema multiforme may occur 2 or 3 weeks after herpes simplex reactivation (herpes labialis), and HSV DNA has been demonstrated in lesional tissue in up to 80 % of cases of erythema multiforme. Hand, foot and mouth disease and herpangina may be distinguished by viral culture or serology, but clinically, the eruption of hand, foot and mouth disease and the fact that herpangina rarely affects the anterior oral mucous membranes are the diagnostic pointers.

Treatment. In mild cases, treatment is supportive and symptomatic. The importance of an adequate fluid intake should be stressed, particularly for children when they are pyrexial. Antipyretic analgesics, such as acetominophen, may be prescribed, but avoidance of salicylates is essential in children. Antimicrobial mouthwashes, such as chlorhexidine or benzymidine, are useful in the acute phase to assist oral hygiene and plaque control. In severe or complicated cases and in immunocompromised patients, antiviral agents can be prescribed. Acyclovir, a guanosine derivative activated by viral thymidine kinase (TK), inhibits herpes simplex replication. Clinical resistance is becoming a problem owing to herpes simplex strains which are TK-deficient [40, 41]. Since the disease is self-limiting and the drug may be life-saving in meningoencephalitis, prescription of the drug should be reserved for severe or complicated cases. The dosage is 200 mg five times daily for adults (100 mg five times daily for children), but in immunocompromised adults, the dose may be increased to 400 mg five times daily. The drug should be used with caution in the presence of renal impairment. An intravenous preparation is also available. Foscarnet, gancyclovir, and vidarabine are also effective, although less effective than acyclovir, but the efficacy of inosine pranobex is disappointing.

7.3.1.3
Herpes Labialis (Fever Blisters)

Etiology. Following primary infection with herpes simplex, the virus becomes latent in the trigeminal ganglion. Reactivation can occur from this site to produce blisters and crusting, typically at the mucocutaneous junction of the lip, the condition called herpes labialis (Fig. 7.37). Some 6%–12% of the population may be affected. Occasionally, reactivation occurs at other sites, such as the anterior nares, facial skin, or intraorally (recurrent intraoral herpes), when it simulated herpes zoster [42].

Oral Manifestations. The lesions of herpes labialis start as a macule, which rapidly becomes papular, vesicular, and pustular. Crusting occurs on rupture of the pustule (Fig. 7.38), and healing occurs over a period of 1 or 2 weeks, without scarring, unless bacterial superinfection occurs (Fig. 7.39). Often, in the prodromal phase, there is intense itching at the site of reactivation.

Triggers for reactivation include trauma, fever, intercurrent disease, ultraviolet light, immunosuppression, and, possibly, physiological hormonal changes. Recurrent intraoral herpes simplex is seen typically in the palate following administration of a greater palatine nerve block, but is extremely rare (Fig. 7.40). Why intraoral reactivation should not occur more commonly is not clear. Reactivation occurs in the presence of circulating antibodies, which are not elevated following the recurrence. There is evidence that the virus itself produces a herpes-specific immunodeficiency in some otherwise immunocompetent people with impairment of NK, macrophage, and neutrophil function. Susceptibility to herpes labialis is associated with the HLA-A1, HLA-B5 and HLA-DR1 histocompatibility antigens. In the immunocompromised, chronic intraoral ulcers can develop at any intraoral mucosal site. The lesions are often atypical, shallow, painful dendritic ulcers.

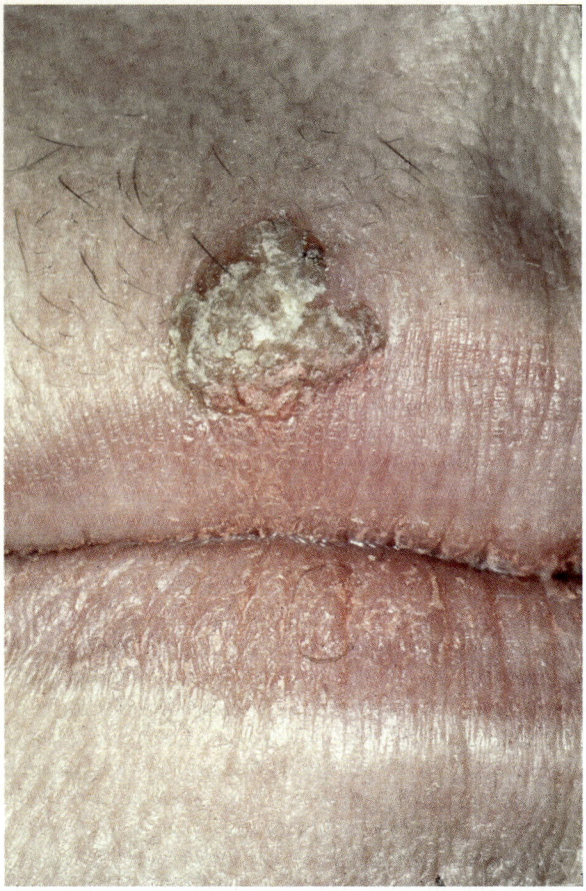

Fig. 7.38. Herpes labialis, late crusting stage

Diagnosis. The diagnosis of herpes labialis is clinical. When the presentation is atypical and when the

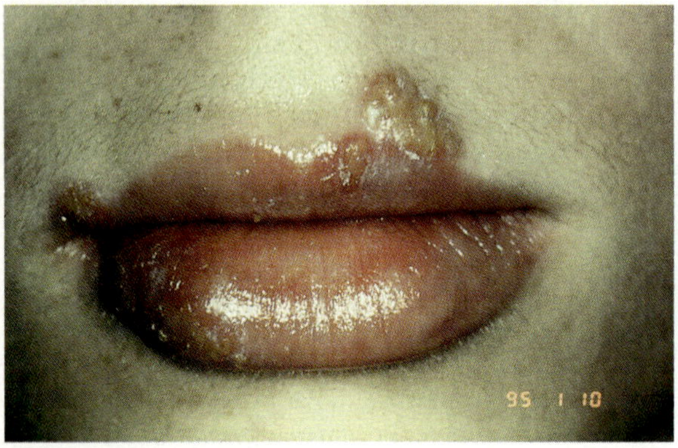

Fig. 7.37. Herpes labialis, late pustule stage

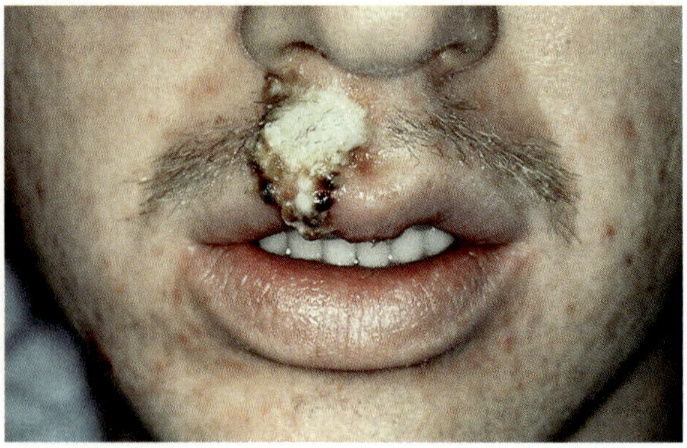

Fig. 7.39. Herpes labialis infected with *Staphylococcus aureus*

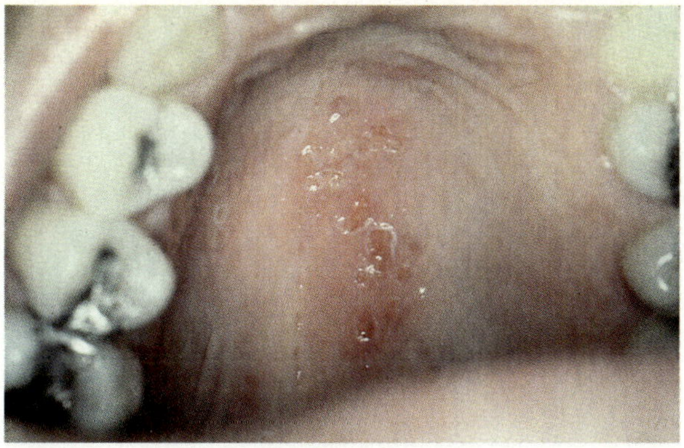

Fig. 7.40. Recurrent intraoral herpes simplex infection, following local anesthesia (a greater palatine nerve block)

patient is immunocompromised, viral culture and exfoliative cytology immunostaining may confirm the diagnosis.

Treatment. Herpes labialis can be treated by the application of topical acyclovir (5 % cream) or idoxuridine. If these are applied in the prodromal phase, the lesion may be aborted, but if treatment is not started early it is of dubious benefit. Once the lesion has reached the crusted stage, use of topical acyclovir has little therapeutic effect. Oral acyclovir has been shown to have little therapeutic advantage over topical application in herpes labialis. Prophylactic acyclovir may be used to suppress recrudescence in patients for whom the condition is very troublesome, particularly if they are immunocompromised, or in patients undergoing organ or bone marrow transplants [43]. In patients whose lesions are triggered by ultraviolet light, the use of sun-blocking lipsticks may prevent reactivation of the virus.

7.3.1.4
Varicella-zoster (Chickenpox)

Etiology and Pathogenesis. Varicella-zoster virus (VZV) causes varicella, or "chickenpox", in the primary infection. It remains dormant in latently infected dorsal root ganglia of sensory nerves and may later reactivate to produce herpes zoster, commonly known as "shingles" [44]. It is an alpha herpesvirus and genetically very similar to HSV-1 and HSV-2.

Varicella is an acute generalized disease characterized by sudden onset of low-grade fever, mild constitutional symptoms, and eruption. It occurs most commonly in winter and spring. After an incubation period of 2–3 weeks a variably dense rash appears, mostly on the trunk, head, and neck. It is extremely contagious, and by early adulthood 95 % of the population of metropolitan areas will have contracted the virus. Transmission is by direct contact, droplet, or airborne spread of secretions from the respiratory tract of infected cases. Asymptomatic and subclinical infection does occur, but in adults the fever and constitutional disturbance can be severe. It is very rarely fatal but may cause lethal primary viral pneumonia in adults, whereas in children, encephalomyelitis, Reye's syndrome, or septic complications are more often the cause of death. Following the acute infection, cellular and humoral responses usually confer lifelong immunity, but second attacks have been reported.

Oral and Associated Manifestations. The exathema begins as a maculopapular eruption lasting for only a few hours, becoming vesicular and pustular over a few days and eventually crusts. The lesions typically occur in crops over a 3- or 4-day period, so that lesions at different stages of maturity are seen in proximity to each other. The oral mucosa is commonly involved, although there may be only isolated lesions, which typically affect the soft palate (Fig. 7.41). Vesicles surrounded by an erythematous halo appear, which rupture to form ovoid ulcers.

Diagnosis. The diagnosis is clinical but may be confirmed by viral culture or rising antibody titers.

Treatment. Treatment is supportive and symptomatic unless complications ensue. Because of the close association of VZV infection with Reye's syndrome it is particularly important to avoid using salicylate in children, in whom attention should be paid to adequate fluid intake. A suitable antipyretic analgesic is acetominophen. The skin lesions should be bathed daily with an antiseptic solution such as chlorhexidine. The virus is sensitive to both vidarabine and acyclovir. Transmission can be prevented by giving VZIG (varicellazoster immune globulin) to susceptible contacts.

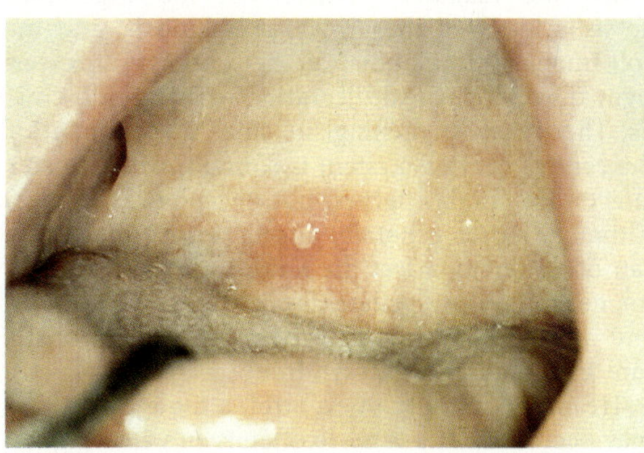

Fig. 7.41. Isolated palatal vesicle in varicella infection

7.3.1.5
Herpes Zoster (Shingles)

Etiology and Pathogenesis. Herpes zoster is a local manifestation of reactivation of latent VZV. It is seen mainly in the elderly, but there is a bimodal distribution. When seen in the young, it may be associated with immunosuppression and malignancies, such as acute leukemias. It has a particular association with Hodgkin's disease when this is treated with radiotherapy and chemotherapy [45]. In the elderly, herpes zoster may be a manifestation of an age-related decline in the cell-mediated immune response, but may also be a sign of the development of an internal malignancy, particularly chronic lymphatic leukemia.

Oral and Associated Manifestations. The initial symptoms of zoster are paresthesia and dysesthesia, usually confined to a single dermatome. After 2 or 3 days, lesions appear in crops along the affected dermatome, consisting of vesicles with an erythematous base which, as in varicella, become pustules and scab. Histologically, they are identical to the lesions of varicella, but clinically they are much more florid and closely aggregated. The eruption is usually unilateral and confined to one or two associated dermatomes. Occasionally, vesicles are seen outside the dermatome, and this is a particular feature of the condition in patients with internal malignancy or immunosuppression.

When zoster affects the trigeminal nerve, the presentation can be striking. Initially, the painful prodromal symptoms may be mistaken for pulpitis. There may be bone necrosis, tooth loss, and hypoplasia of developing teeth within a single quadrant. Occasionally, oral lesions may occur in the absence of a facial eruption. Multiple, fragile oral vesicles form in the skin and mucosa of the affected division, which break down rapidly to cause extensive, painful ulceration (Fig. 7.42). When the maxillary division of the trigeminal nerve is involved there may be chemosis, and involvement of the ophthalmic division may threaten sight through corneal ulceration or panophthalmitis. There may be meningism, since involvement of the central nervous system is common when zoster affects the cranial nerves, but encephalitis is rare. Although zoster generally affects sensory nerves, it can occasionally affect the facial nerve. Lower motor neuron palsy, ipsilateral pharyngeal ulceration, and a zosteric eruption in the external ear constitute the Ramsay-Hunt syndrome.

Healing is usually uneventful, although scarring may occur and this is more often seen when the cutaneous lesions become superinfected with bacteria, particularly *Staphylococcus aureus*. A particularly harrowing sequela to herpes zoster is postherpetic neuralgia. Tissue necrosis, disseminated infection, scarring, and postherpetic neuralgia are all the more common in the immunocompromised.

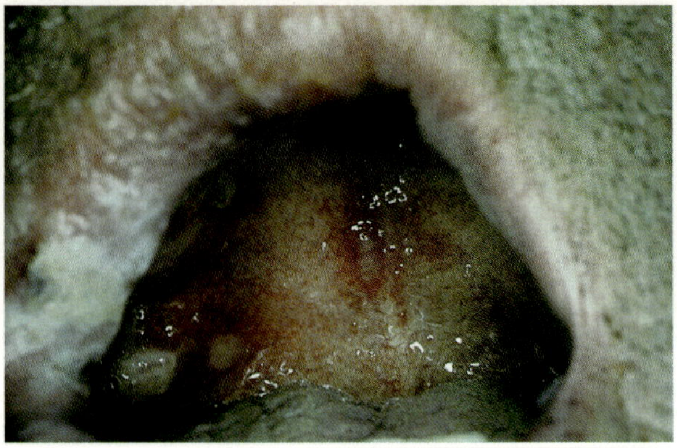

Fig. 7.42. Herpes zoster

Diagnosis. The diagnosis of zoster is clinical. The virus is very difficult to culture, and electron microscopy and the demonstration of multinucleate giant cells are nonspecific, although rising antibody titers may confirm the diagnosis in complicated cases.

Treatment. Treatment involves the use of acyclovir or vidarabine, antiseptic mouthwashes, and appropriate antimicrobials if superinfection of the rash occurs. The VZV is less sensitive to acyclovir than HSV, and larger doses are required for a therapeutic effect. In the normal host oral acyclovir, 800 mg five times daily for 7 days is the recommended dose. In the immunocompromised, for whom the disease may be life-threatening with dissemination causing pneumonitis, hepatitis, or meningoencephalitis, the drug should be administered IV. Early hopes that acyclovir therapy might prevent postherpetic neuralgia have not been substantiated. Postherpetic neuralgia responds poorly to drugs such as carbamazepine, but patients may respond to tricyclic antidepressant drugs such as amitryptiline.

7.3.1.6
Infectious Mononucleosis (Glandular Fever)

Etiology and Pathogenesis. Infectious mononucleosis (IM) is the clinical term used for the disease caused by primary infection with the Epstein-Barr virus (EBV). Although primary infection with this herpesvirus is often asymptomatic, particularly in childhood, about half of all infected young and older adults develop an acute, self-limiting, lymphoproliferative glandular fever syndrome [46].

EBV can be isolated from saliva in the majority of such cases and may continue to be shed for over a year. Some 20 % of normal individuals intermittently excrete EBV in the saliva at any one time, and this is thought to be due to asymptomatic reactivation episodes starting from the site of latency in the oropharyngeal epithelium and salivary glands. In immunocompromised patients and pregnancy, asymptomatic viral shedding is increased.

EBV seropositivity is virtually 100 % in underdeveloped countries, and in urban environments in developed countries seroconversion rates range from 60 % in towns to 94 % in densely populated areas, such as London, UK. Transmission occurs through infected saliva and during intimate contact, leading to the disease being described as the "kissing disease". There are occasional reports of EBV transmission from blood transfusions. Demonstration of EBV-infected epithelial cells in the uterine cervix raises the possibility of venereal transmission and the involvement of EBV in cervical pathology.

Oral and Associated Features. Clinical features of IM include: malaise, fever, tender lymphadenopathy with pharyngeal and tonsillar inflammation and edema, which may be severe. Occasionally, there may be ulceration of the tonsil or soft palate (Fig. 7.41). Often, during the prodrome, pintpoint petechial hemorrhages are seen at the junction of the hard and soft palate, and in more severe cases there may be hepatosplenomegaly, jaundice, periorbital edema, and respiratory embarrassment. Patients given synthetic penicillin therapy may develop a morbilliform eruption. The acute disease is self-limiting, but full recovery may take many weeks. In instances a protracted illness (chronic mononucleosis, chronic active EBV infection), nonspecific malaise, low-grade fever, weight loss, mild jaundice and persistent lymphadenopathy may ensue. Many such patients go on to develop clinical depression.

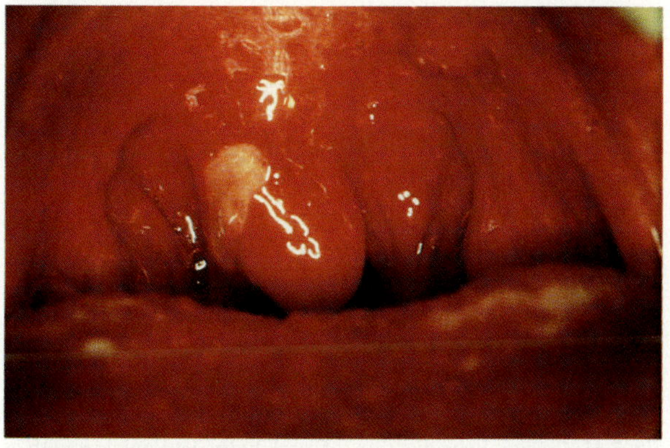

Fig. 7.43. Pharyngotonsillitis with ulceration of the uvula in infectious mononucleosis

Other rare complications include cranial nerve palsies, ruptured spleen, nephritis, thrombocytopenia and hemolytic anemia, pneumonitis, pericarditis, and meningoencephalitis. In the X-linked lymphoproliferative syndrome (Duncan's disease) persistent life-threatening infection is seen, and individual males with this disorder succumb either to overwhelming infection or to B-cell lymphoma in childhood or early adulthood.

Diagnosis. During the acute phase "monocytosis" is seen on a peripheral blood film, which gives rise to the term IM, but these cells are now known to be transformed T-lymphocytes. The diagnosis of IM is often clinical, but may be confirmed by demonstration of atypical lymphocytes in a peripheral blood film, heterophil antibodies (e.g., a positive "Monospot" test), or serum antibodies to a range of specific viral antigens such as early antigen (EA), EBV nuclear antigens (EBNAs), or the viral capsid antigen (VCA). False-positive Monospot tests may be seen in hepatitis B infection, lymphomas, leukemias, malaria, carcinoma of the pancreas, and systemic lupus erythematosus.

Differential Diagnosis. The glandular fever syndrome may be seen in other conditions, notably toxoplasmosis, brucellosis, diphtheria, cytomegalovirus and HIV infection, leukemias and lymphomas (which themselves may be EBV related). Infectious mononucleosis should be distinguished from bacterial and other viral causes of pharyngotonsillitis.

Treatment. Treatment of IM is supportive and symptomatic. In severe cases, antiviral agents, such as acyclovir, may be useful in conjunction with systemic steroids if there is respiratory embarrassment or jaundice.

Epstein-Barr virus was first isolated from Burkitt's lymphoma and is intimately related to the pathogenesis, not only of this tumor but also to nasopharyngeal carcinoma. Other disorders that may be EBV related include B-cell and T-cell lymphomas (particularly in patients with AIDS and in allograft recipients), Wegener's granulomatosis, thymic carcinoma, supraglottic and palatine tonsil carcinoma, histiocytic medullary reticulosis, recurrent parotitis, and periodic migrainous neuralgia. There is also a tenuous association with Sjøgren's syndrome.

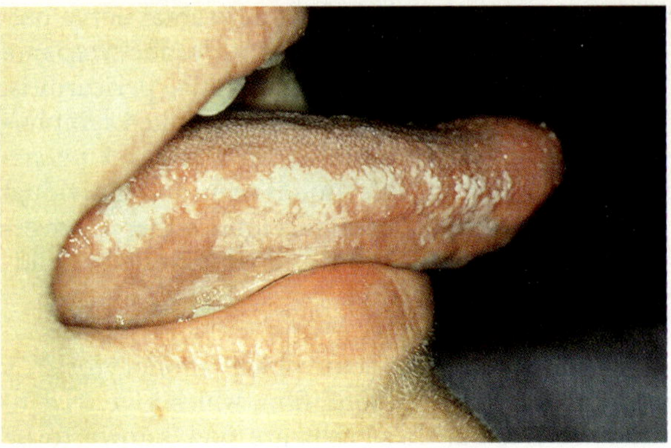

Fig. 7.44. Oral hairy leukoplakia at the typical site

7.3.1.7
Oral Hairy Leukoplakia

Etiology and pathogenesis. In patients infected with the human immunodeficiency virus (HIV), and rarely in patients who are immunosuppressed for other reasons, EBV is associated with an unique oral lesion – oral hairy leukoplakia (OHL) (Fig. 7.44).

Oral Manifestations. This lesion usually presents on the lateral and ventral surface of the tongue, and rarely at other mucosal sites. It has a characteristic appearance, with grayish-white ("hairy"), raised, vertical corrugations, and is sometimes seen early in HIV disease. When extensive, the leukoplakia may appear confluent. It has no reported malignant potential, but may be an important prognostic indicator for full-blown AIDS development [47].

Diagnosis. The diagnosis is by biopsy. The histopathological features of OHL are not pathognomonic and consist of hyperparakeratosis, vacuolation of the keratinocytes in the upper stratum spinosum (koilocyte-like cells), and absence of inflammatory infiltrate. Superinfection with *Candida* spp. may be seen. Since acanthosis and parakeratosis are normal features of the marginal tongue mucosa, and EBV-negative pseudo-OHL has been described, the definitive diagnosis can only be attained by the demonstration of EBV in the tissue by immunohistochemistry or in situ hybridization. Replicating virus can be demonstrated in the koilocyte-like cells, which are seen in the stratum spinosum (Fig. 7.43). A definitive diagnosis is important because of the prognostic implications of the lesion for HIV-seropositive patients and the medical and social implications for persons of unknown serostatus without any other cause for immunosuppression [48].

Differential Diagnosis. The differential diagnosis is extensive. Common causes of white lesions of the oral mucous membrane include: frictional keratosis and tobacco-related, candidal, and "idiopathic" leukoplakias. Syphilitic leukoplakia is seen in the tertiary form of the disease and is nowadays rare. The lateral border of the tongue is a site of predilection for oral lichen planus, but there will generally be evidence of the disease in other parts of the mouth. The oral lesions of discoid and systemic lupus erythematosus very rarely affect this site, being more common in the buccal mucous membrane and hard palate. Lesions of the rare genokeratoses (such as keratitis follicularis, white sponge nevus, pachyonychia congenita, and dyskeratosis congenita) are usually more widespread intraorally or associated with extraoral signs.

Treatment. Generally, the condition does not require treatment, but if it is symptomatic or very florid, or there is taste perturbation, it responds to oral acyclovir. Recurrence often occurs on cessation of therapy. The lesion has a relapsing natural history, but also may resolve if patients are started on antiviral agents such as azidothymidine (or other nucleoside analogues), presumably through immunomodulation.

7.3.1.8
Oral Manifestations of Other Herpesvirus Infections

Cytomegalovirus (CMV, HHV-4) can cause a primary infection that is indistinguishable from EBV, except that the patient is heterophil antibody-negative. The diagnosis can be confirmed by serology. Oral lesions caused by reactivation of the virus have been described only in immunocompromised patients [49], in whom there is an association with oral (along with pharyngeal and esophageal) ulceration (Fig. 7.46), and with submandibular sialadenitis

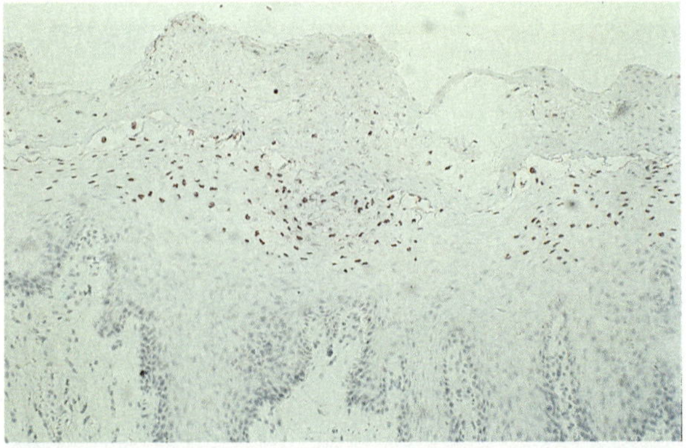

Fig. 7.45. In situ hybridization of oral hairy leukoplakia with a BamW DNA probe, demonstrating EBV (red coloration) in the koilocyte-like cells in the stratum spinosum

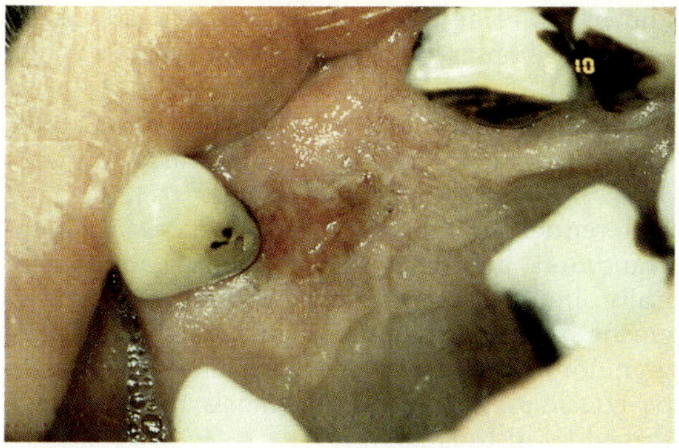

Fig. 7.46. Oral ulceration caused by cytomegalovirus in an immunocompromised patient

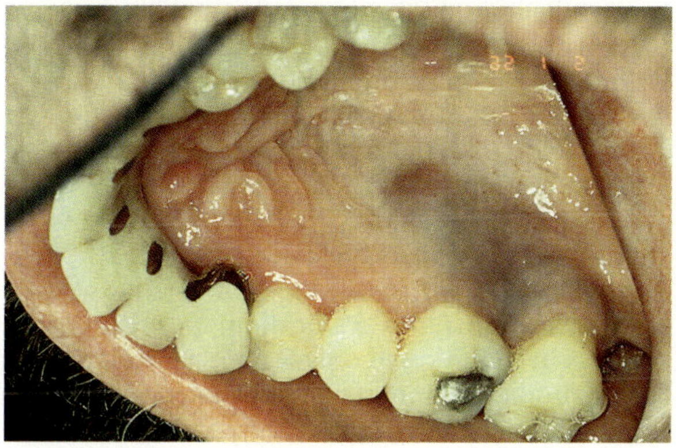

Fig. 7.47. Macular form of Kaposi's sarcoma in a patient with AIDS

in HIV disease and gingival hyperplasia in patients receiving cardiac transplants. Oral ulceration caused by CMV has also been reported in patients undergoing bone marrow transplantation and chemotherapy. Disease caused by CMV reactivation responds moderately to therapy with acyclovir, but the drug of choice is gancyclovir.

A relationship of CMV to Kaposi's sarcoma (KS) in AIDS has been suggested, but this is now thought to have a closer association with HHV-8, also called Kaposi's sarcoma-associated herpesvirus (KSHV). This virus is very similar to EBV and, while at the time of writing it had not yet been isolated in culture, it has been demonstrated by molecular techniques in AIDS-related, sporadic, and endemic KS [50]. Kaposi's sarcoma in AIDS is much more frequently associated with the homosexual risk group, which suggests a possible infectious etiology, and oral lesions are not uncommon, particularly where the disease is disseminated. The sites of predilection are the hard palate and gingivae (Fig. 7.45).

The remaining two herpesviruses (HHV-6 and HHV-7) are not known to cause intraoral disease. Human herpesvirus 6 causes exanthema subitum (roseola infantum), an acute specific fever of childhood, with a typical erythematous facial eruption (the "slapped cheek"), but without reported intraoral manifestations [51]. It is, however, trophic to the salivary glands and there is a speculative association with Sjøgren's syndrome. Both HHV-6 and HHV-7 can be isolated from saliva and have been demonstrated in salivary tissues [51, 52]. The clinical manifestations of HHV-7 remain unknown.

7.3.2 Poxviruses

M. Ramos-e-Silva

Poxviruses are the largest DNA viruses that affect animals. Humans can host three types: (1) orthopoxvirus, agents of variola or smallpox, and vaccinia; (2) parapoxvirus, which produce orf or ecthyma contagiosum, and milker's nodules; and (3) an unclassified group that includes molluscum contagiosum and tanapox, a virus only reported in Kenya and Zaire.

Smallpox, a highly contagious and fatal disease, disappeared after very intense worldwide vaccination campaigns coordinated by the World Health Organization. No cases are known to have occurred since October 1977, and WHO declared it eradicated in the early 1980s.

Oral manifestations of the other poxvirus diseases, although theoretically possible, are not very easily found. There are a few reports of oral vaccinia after immunization in humans, and of molluscum contagiosum in AIDS patients. Goats and sheep may present oral ecthyma contagiosum.

7.3.2.1 *Molluscum Contagiosum*

Definition. Molluscum contagiosum is a benign tumor-like viral disease seen in children. In adults, it is sexually transmitted and frequently associated with AIDS infection.

Etiology. The disease is caused by one of the largest poxviruses (200 by 300 nm), molluscum contagiosum virus, which has two subtypes: MCV-1 and MCV-2. Lesions caused by both subtypes are indistinguishable: MCV-1 is very frequent and has a worldwide distribution, while MCV-2 occurs mainly in male HIV patients. It does not grow in tissue cultures, and the disease is not experimentally reproducible in other species.

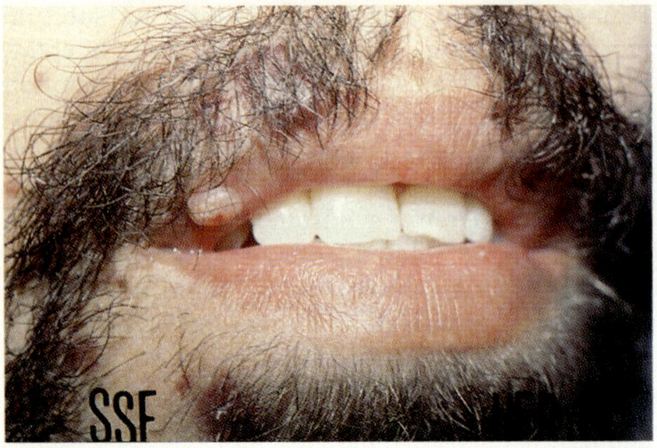

Fig. 7.48. Lip molluscum contagiosum in an HIV patient. Courtesy of Dr. Sonia Ferreira, Dr. Arley Silva Jr., and Dr. Sandra Torres, Brazil

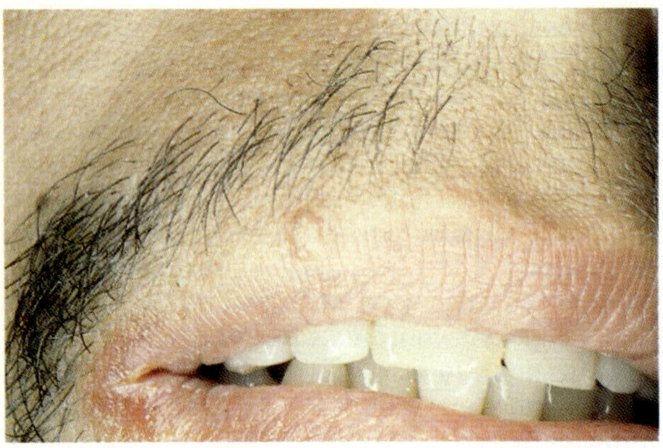

Fig. 7.49. Lip molluscum contagiosum in an HIV patient. Courtesy of Dr. Arley Silva Jr. and Dr. Sonia Ferreira, Brazil

Pathogenesis. Lesions are observed after an incubation period of 7–50 days and are transmitted directly or through fomes. Autoinoculation is very common.

Oral Manifestations. Oral lesions are rare and are reported in HIV patients (Figs. 7.48, 7.49). They are similar to cutaneous lesions and characterized by one to several persistent dome-shaped papules 1–3 mm across, with central umbilication. Giant elevations of more than 1 cm are exceptional. The predilection sites are the lips, but the tongue and buccal mucosa are occasionally affected.

Associated Findings. Mouth lesions are associated with HIV infection and with decreased number and impaired function of T-cells, but there are some reports of them in immunocompetent patients.

Microscopic Findings. Histopathology shows a cup-shaped papule in the epidermis with a central opening, forming a keratin crater. Intracytoplasmic eosinophilic viral inclusions, typical of poxvirus and known as Handerson-Patterson or molluscum bodies, are observed inside keratinocytes.

Diagnosis. Diagnosis of oral lesions is clinical, but a biopsy must be performed for confirmation.

Differential Diagnosis. Cryptococcosis, keratoacanthoma, and warts in HIV patients can be clinically indistinguishable from molluscum contagiosum. Lymphangioma, hemangioma, pyogenic granuloma and condyloma acuminatum must also be considered. The final diagnosis must be confirmed by histopathology.

Treatment. Curettage with or without diathermy is the method of choice for removal of the central viral core of the lesion. Cryosurgery is considered a good therapeutic option for widespread lesions, and large lesions may require surgical excision.

7.3.2.2
Vaccinia (Cowpox)

Definition. Vaccinia is the disease caused by a poxvirus (*Poxvirus officinalis*) used for smallpox vaccination. Since smallpox eradication, specific vaccination has been indicated only for special risk groups. The natural evolution of uncomplicated vaccination is limited by the host immune response and characterized by a local infection that heals with scarring.

Etiology. *Poxvirus officinalis* does not occur naturally and could be a mutant of smallpox or, more probably of cowpox virus. This last virus is the agent of a disease of cattle which begins as papules, changing into vesicles, and finally into pustules, providing immunity to smallpox virus in humans.

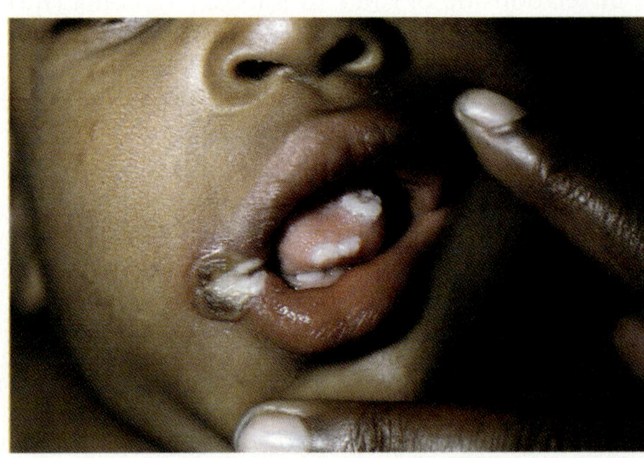

Fig. 7.50. Oral vaccinia. Courtesy of Dr. Kenneth Greer and Dr. Christopher Sheap, USA

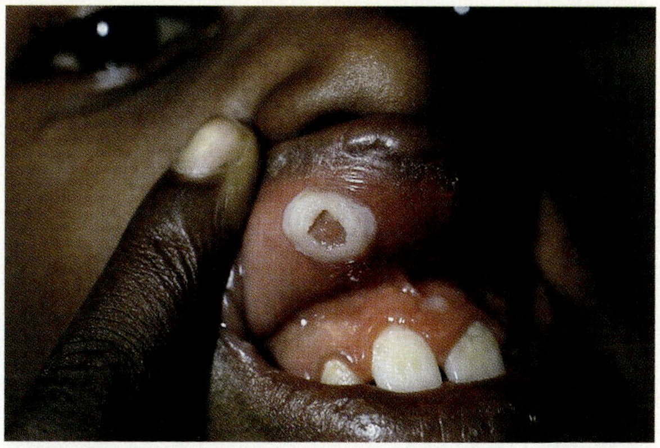

Fig. 7.51. Oral vaccinia. Courtesy of Dr. Kenneth Greer and Dr. Christopher Sheap, USA

Pathogenesis. Vaccinia is a complication of smallpox vaccination that may happen in the same person or in an individual who had close contact with a recently vaccinated person. It may appear through three basic mechanisms: secondary bacterial infection, exaggerated viral replication, and altered reactivity to the virus.

Oral Manifestations. Oral lesions are mostly due to accidental inoculation and are similar to those following a normal smallpox vaccination (Figs. 7.50, 7.51). The condition begins with an erythematous nodule, which turns into umbilicated vesicles and small pustules. It can also present as white plaques similar to diphtheric membrane. The only difference is that these do not tend to leave scars in the mouth.

Associated Findings. Other forms of this disease may be associated with mouth lesions, such as generalized vaccinia and eczema vaccinatum.

Microscopic Findings. Histopathology shows ballooning or reticular degeneration of keratinocytes, epidermal necrosis, and dermal inflammatory infiltrate.

Diagnosis. Recent history of vaccination or contact with a vaccinated person should suggest the possibility of vaccinia. Positive Tzanck test, serology, or viral culture are required for confirmation.

Differential Diagnosis. Accidental vaccinia must be differentiated from diseases that cause similar lesions, such as other viral infections, diphtheria, syphilis, herpes simplex, and aphthous stomatitis.

Treatment. Oral lesions after accidental inoculation are self-limiting and do not require treatment. They usually heal spontaneously without scarring in 7–10 days. Hyperimmune serum against vaccinia may be necessary for more severe cases.

7.3.3 Human Papillomaviruses

S. Jablonska

Human papillomaviruses (HPV) affect both skin and squamous epithelium of the genital and oral mucous membranes. Of the over 110 HPVs presently characterized, two, HPV13 and HPV32, are strictly specific for the oral mucosa, producing characteristic lesions of focal epithelial hyperplasia (FEH). The oral cavity can also be infected by other HPVs, mostly genital (HPV6, -11, -16), and rarely by cutaneous HPVs, specifically HPV2 and the closely related genital HPV57. These viruses are not consistently associated with defined clinical features, and have been found in benign, malignant, and premalignant conditions, and also in the normal mucosa. The results of various studies differ significantly, and this depends on the levels of sensitivity and specificity of the techniques used. In recent years, with the development of highly sensitive methods – PCR followed by dot blot hybridization with type-specific nucleotides – the detected prevalence of HPVs in oral tumors has steadily increased. The causative role of these viruses remains unclear, however.

The main HPV-associated oral conditions that are benign include: (1) squamous papilloma, (2) condylomata acuminata, and (3) common warts of the oral cavity. HPV-associated malignant tumors are squamous cell carcinomas and proliferative verrucous leukoplakia. The only disease associated with oral mucosa-specific HPVS is FEH.

7.3.3.1 *Focal Epithelial Hyperplasia (Heck's Disease)*

FEH is a disease of the oral mucosa, highly prevalent among native Americans and Eskimos in Alaska and Greenland, where, in some localities, it is present in over 30 % of the population, mainly children [53, 54]. It is extremely rare in Caucasians, but sporadic cases have been reported in many countries [55]. The geographic and racial distribution of the disease, which is very rare in Caucasian inhibitants of the same areas, suggests a role of genetic factors. Familial cases have been observed.

Etiology. The disease has been found to be associated with two specific HPVs: HPV13 [56] and HPV32 [57]. These HPVs have never been detected in any other cutaneous or mucosal lesions. Neither has it any oncogenic potential. Single reports on as-

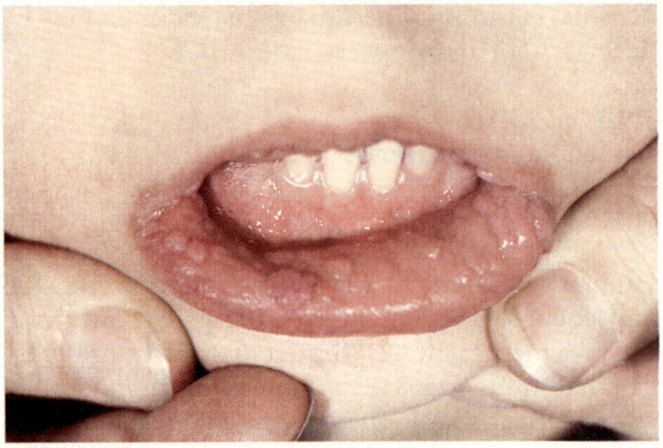

Fig. 7.52. Numerous soft, somewhat translucent nodules, with smooth surface and irregular margins, partly coalescent. The color does not differ from the surrounding mucosa. In this 11-year-old girl the lesions, found to be induced by HPV13, were widespread and also involved buccal mucosa and tongue

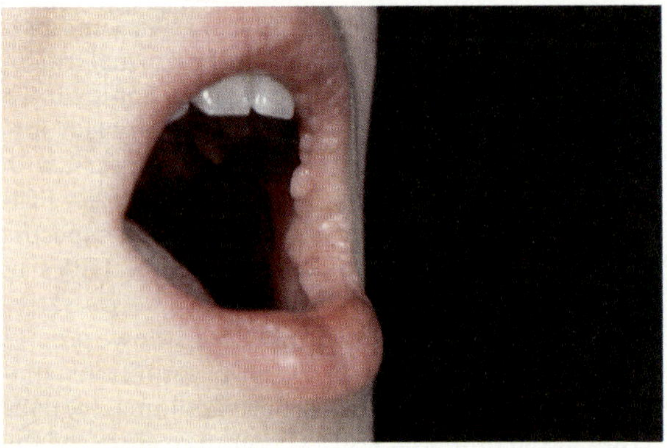

Fig. 7.53. Typical buccal lesions of FEH in a 7-year-old-girl, which lasted for several years and involved almost entire oral cavity

sociations of FEH with HPV1 [58] or HPV6 [59] might be due to the clinical similarity among all warty oral lesions.

Pathogenesis. Genetic factors are probably involved in the control of susceptibility to infection with FEH-specific HPVs. The immunogenetic associations are still unknown.

Oral manifestations. Multiple soft, not infrequently somewhat translucent, well-circumscribed nodules are roundish or have irregular margins, with a smooth surface, being whitish, grayish, or the color of adjoining normal mucosa. They are located on the oral mucosa of the lips, buccal mucosa, the tongue and hard palate, and never involve the peribuccal skin (Figs. 7.52, 7.53).

Associated Findings. There are no other HPV infections elsewhere on the skin and genital mucosa. The patients are not immunosuppressed.

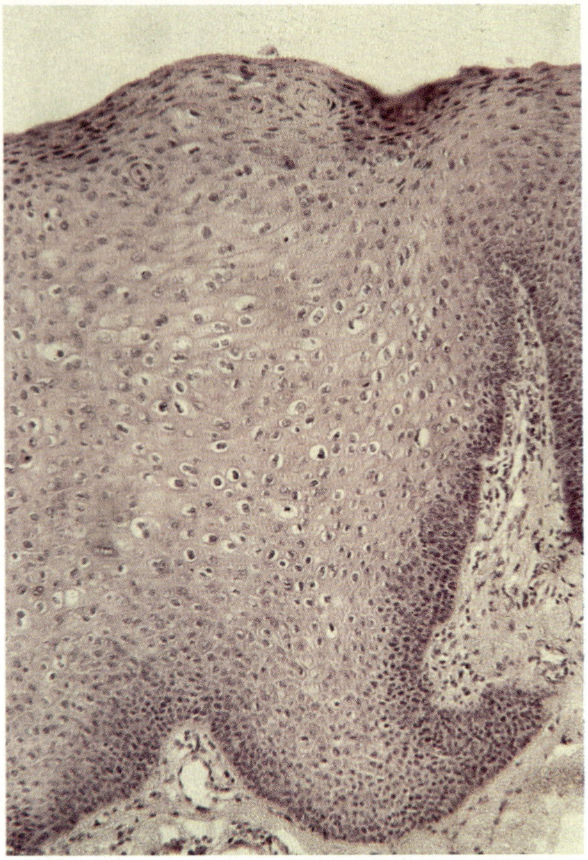

Fig. 7.54. Histology of FEH lesions. Hyperplasia of the epithelium with downward proliferating anastomosing rete ridges. Koilocyte-like vacuolization of keratinocytes

Microscopic Findings. There is pronounced acanthosis, with elongated rete ridges showing clubbing and horizontal anastomoses (Fig. 7.54). Spinous cells are present in some areas with koilocyte-like clarification. Electron microscopy rarely discloses viral particles, which are very scant.

Course of the Disease. The duration is variable, ranging from a few months to several years, with spontaneous regression of the lesions in most cases.

Diagnosis. This is based on characteristic clinical and histological manifestations and must be confirmed by detection of HPV13 or HPV32.

Differential Diagnosis. FEH should be differentiated from white sponge nevus, which differs in its more whitish surface and in the histological pattern (presence of large clarified cells replacing epithelium). Some condylomata acuminata may resemble FEH lesions [60], but are associated with HPV6. FEH should be also differentiated from oral common warts and squamous papillomas, which are less soft, usually not so abundant, and have a more keratotic and digitated surface.

Treatment. There is no specific therapy. The disease is self-limiting and painless, and does not cause any inconvenience to the patient. In our experience, removal of some nodules appears to accelerate the disappearance of all.

7.3.3.2
Papilloma or Squamous Papilloma

Definition. Squamous papilloma is the most frequent benign epithelial tumor in the oral cavity.

Etiology. In situ hybridization with the use of cutaneous and genital HPV probes disclosed HPV genome in 35 % of squamous papillomas, genital HPV6 or HPV11 in nearly all, and double infection with these HPVs and, in addition, with cutaneous HPV2 in 1 case [61]. More specific Southern blot hybridization of 6 of 7 oral papillomas revealed an association with HPV6 or its subtypes, and in 1 case with HPV16 [62]. With the use of PCR followed by dot blot hybridization, HPV DNA types 6 and 11 were identified in 68 % of papillomas [63].

Pathogenesis. The mode of infection is probably variable, but usually involves oral sex or contact with contaminated objects.

Oral Manifestations. These well-demarcated, usually single tumors, sometimes sessible (Fig. 7.55), not infrequently display similarity to other verrucous lesions in the oral mucosa.

Associated Findings. Other HPV-induced mucosal lesions (genital, anal, cervical) and skin warts might accompany or precede oral manifestations.

Microscopic Findings. There are typical features of papilloma formation with slight keratinization, acanthosis, papillomatosis, and clarification of the upper cell layers. The keratinization is less pronounced than in warts, and there is usually none of the koilocytosis characteristic of condylomata acuminata.

Diagnosis. The diagnosis is based on clinical and histological features and should be confirmed by virological findings, preferably by Southern blotting.

Differential Diagnosis. Differentiation from condyloma acuminatum might be difficult; however, condylomata are usually multiple and often confluent with a cauliflower-like surface, and display a more or less pronounced characteristic cytophatic effect (koilocytosis). Oral common warts differ in their appearance.
The most important differential diagnosis is that against Heck's disease, because of the different course and prognosis.

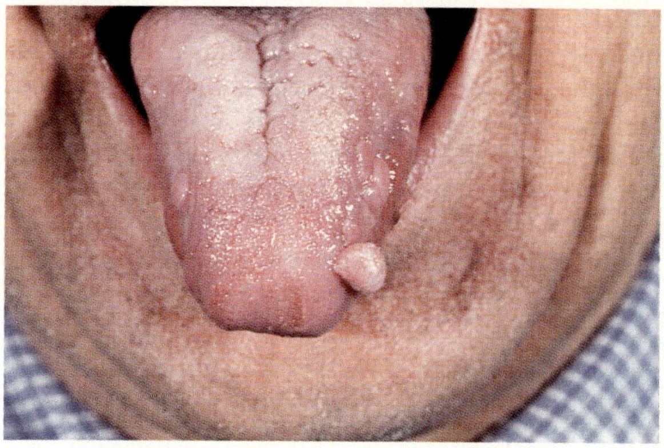

Fig. 7.55. Papilloma on the tongue. Sessile tumor with somewhat whitish keratotic surface

Treatment. Electrocautery, cryotherapy, and surgical removal are all effective.

7.3.3.3
Condylomata Acuminata

These oral warts (Fig. 7.56) are in essence a variety of oral squamous papillomas.

Etiology. Condylomata are nearly always induced by the same genital HPVs (6/11) as oral papillomas and genital condylomata acuminata.

Pathogenesis. Transmission takes place by oral contact with infected genitalia or through self-inoculation by contaminated hands in patients with anogenital infection.

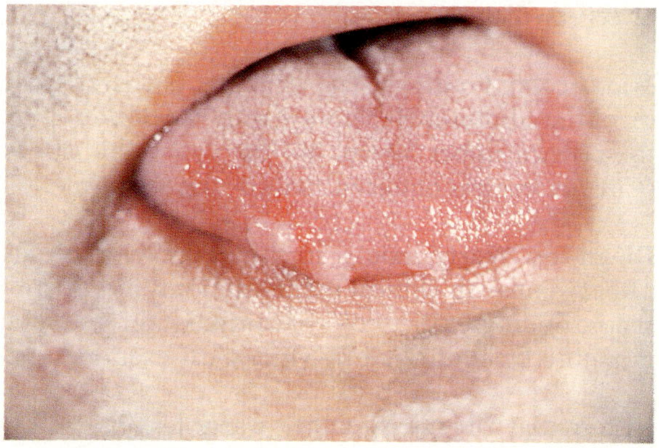

Fig. 7.56. Condylomata acuminata on the tongue, found to be induced by HPV 6. Multiple keratotic wart-like lesions

Manifestations. The lesions are usually multiple, frequently coalescent, forming cauliflower masses, although not so extensive as in the anogenital location.

Associated Findings. Genital warts are found in the patient and/or the sexual partner.

Microscopic Findings. Papillomas are seen with variously pronounced koilocytosis.

Diagnosis. The diagnosis must be confirmed by a virological study of the oral cavity and genital mucosa and, in femal patients, examination of the cervix.

7.3.3.4
Common Warts

Definition. Oral common warts have all the features of skin warts.

Etiology. Like cutaneous common warts, these oral lesions were found to be associated with HPV2 [64], which was detected in 20 % of the lesions [65]. More recent studies disclosed HPV DNA in 71 % of oral warts, 87 % of which contained HPV2 and closely related mucosal HPV57, which were not infrequently present in the same cells. Three of 22 patients had hand warts, suggesting possible autoinoculation [66]. The findings have been confirmed by an extremely sensitive PCR technique and direct DNA sequencing [67].

Manifestations. Papular, whitish, horny lesions with a digitated appearance are often localized on the lip vermillon, but can be present anywhere in the oral cavity: on the labial, buccal and gingival mucosa, and on the tongue.

Associated Findings. Not infrequently, warts are also present on the hands and face. The patients may be predisposed to HPV infection by a defect of cell-mediated immunity.

Microscopic Findings. The structure is characteristic of the common HPV2 wart with vacuolization of the cells in upper layers, but the cytopathic effect (CPE) is less pronounced than in the skin wart.

Diagnosis. Warty lesions in the oral cavity are all rather similar in clinical manifestations and microscopic findings; a diagnosis of common warts should therefore be confirmed by virological examination.

Differential Diagnosis. Other warty lesions (squamous papilloma, condylomata acuminata) are very similar.

Therapy. Electrocoagulation is the most effective treatment.

7.3.3.5
HPV-Associated Oral Cancers

Detectability of HPV in Oral Cancers. In early reports on oral tumors, HPVs had been detected in single cases [68–71], with a high prevalance of genital types: HPV11 and -16 [68], and HPV6 coexistent with HPV2 in tongue carcinoma [69] and with HPV16 [70, 71]. Of special interest is the coexistence of bowenoid papulosis of the genitalia with papules in the mouth and carcinoma of the tongue [71]. In recent studies with the use of more sensitive techniques (PCR and direct DNA sequencing), a strong association of oral tumors with HPVs, preferentially with HPV16, has repeatedly been reported. The prevalence varies from 20.8 % to 74 % [72–77].
Some cancers have also been associated with HPV6 and HPV11 [68, 69, 77] and/or with HPV2 [69, 78]. The cleavage pattern of the HPV2-positive tumors differed from that of the established HPV prototype, but it is not clear whether this is a primary event; however, HPV6/11 from the oral cancers did not differ from those detected in the benign genital warts.

The Etiological Role of HPVs in Oral Tumors. The impression that HPVs have an etiological role is supported by the presence of HPV16 in oral carcinoma and lymph node metastases [79]. A strong association of HPV with precancerous lesions, notably its presence in 89 % of proliferative verrucous leukoplakias [74], speaks in favor of its etiological role. HPV DNA was less frequent in cancers than in precancerous changes (33 %), which is consistent with the “hit-and-run” hypothesis, i. e., participation of HPVs only in the early stage of tumor development. According to Snijders et al. [75], viral oncogenesis may be accompanied by the loss of tumor suppressor genes that have still not been identified.
Although a high prevalence of HPVs in oral cancers favors their role in oncogenesis, it is not clear whether they are causative and indispensable factors, since they are not detectable in a proportion of tumors. In addition, various potentially oncogenic and nononcogenic HPVs are detected.

Latent HPV Infection. Most importantly, with the use of PCR, the same genital HPVs and in the same proportions were disclosed in normal oral mucosa [80, 81], and even more frequently in unaffected sites around carcinomas [72, 82]. Depending on the distance from the tumor, the detectability of HPV was found to be 3.8 %–26.9 % [76]. The rates for normal oral mucosa range from 1% [76] to 43% [82], which might depend on the techniques employed. Irrespective of how high the prevalence of HPVs is in normal mucosa, it is conceivable that HPS is present in a latent form, as it is in genital mucous membranes. However, the virus appears to be important in tumor development, but not the only cause. The best example illustrating the role of co-carcinogenes is that of the cancers in betel quid chewers, which are found to be HPV positive in 74% of cases [77].

Source of Infection. The source of HPVs is probably the genital mucosa. It has been reported that oral cancers in younger patients showed a higher prevalence of HPV (77.8%) than did similar lesions in patients above 60 years of age (29.4%) [75], which is probably due to more frequent genital infections in the younger sector of the population.
The presence of HPV oral cancers should be cautiously and critically interpreted, as its significance is not clear. All oral cancers should be studied for HPVs with the use of PCR and the more specific Southern blot technique, and the patients concerned should be investigated for the presence of genital HPV infections and skin warts.

Therapeutic Implications and Perspectives. The detection of HPVs in cancers has no therapeutic implications, except for the exclusion of X-ray irradiation, which is co-cancerigenic in all HPV infections.
It is conceivable that vaccination against HPV16 with the use of empty viral particles [83] will contribute to the prevention not only of genital HPV16 infection, but also of HPV16-associated oral cancers.

7.4 Diseases Caused by Fungi

E. M. Difonzo and G. L. Campanile

Fungi constitute a group of nonmotile eukaryotic organisms that have definite cell walls, are devoid of chlorophyll, and reproduce by means of spores. The spore can be produced either sexually ("fungi perfecti") or asexually ("fungi imperfecti") [84–86].

Fungi show two basic morphologic growth patterns. In the yeast form, cells multiply by budding, and the bud separates from the mother cells. Yeast fungi are round, oval, or elongated single cells (blastospores) and form smooth moist colonies in synthetic culture medium (Fig. 7.57). Examples of yeasts pathogenic in humans are *Candida* and *Cryptococcus* species. In contrast, in the mold form, fungi grow by forming branching filaments, with and without septa, named hyphae. A mass of such hyphae is called mycelium. The terms hypha and mycelium are usually used interchangeably. Mold fungi form colonies with a fuzzy surface on culture plates (Fig. 7.58). Examples of molds that are pathogenic in humans are dermatophytes and *Aspergillus* species. These two forms are not always mutually exclusive, and certain fungus species may assume one or both of these forms when growing in different surroundings and under different conditions. These dimorphic fungi often have the mold form in the environment and the yeast form in tissues. Examples of dimorphic pathogens include *Histoplasma capsulatum*, *Blastomyces dermatitis*, and *Sporothrix schenckii*.

In some yeasts, the bud may remain attached to the mother cell and bud continuously without separating, forming chains of elongated cells called pseudohyphae. The result is an end-to-end aggregation of elongated blastospores microscopically distinguishable from a true hypha only by constrictions of the pseudohypha at septal junctions. The species of the genus *Candida* produce pseudohyphae and true hyphae depending on the growth conditions.

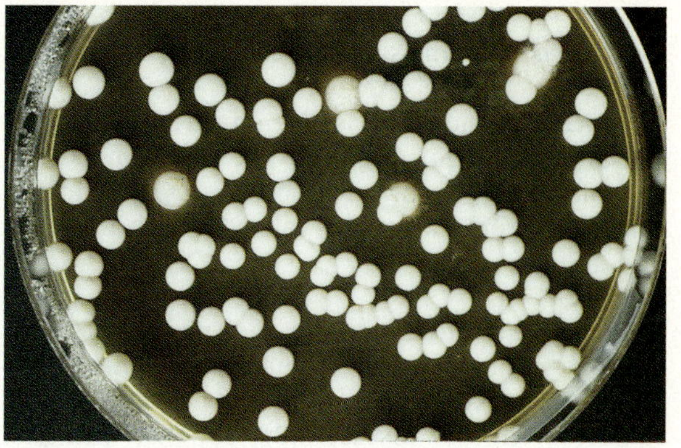

Fig. 7.57. Yeast colonies of *Candida albicans*, showing a smooth surface

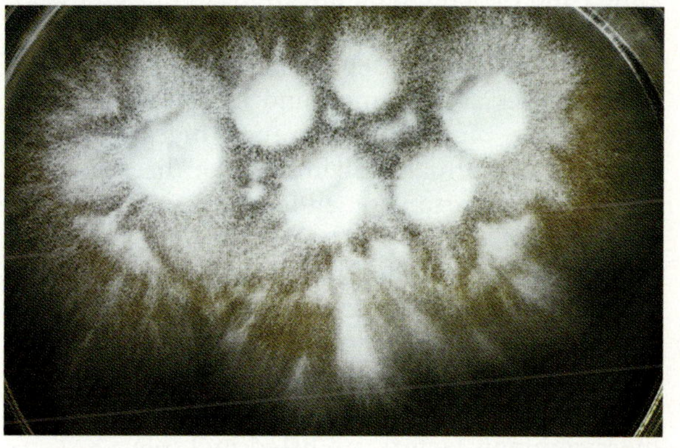

Fig. 7.58. Mold colony of *Microsporum canis*, showing a fuzzy surface

7.4.1 Candidosis: Candidiasis, Moniliasis, Thrush

Definition. Candidosis is the infection caused by yeasts of the genus *Candida*. The infection can involve any body tissue and produces manifestations that range from mild and localized lesions to severe and systemic ones.

Etiology. *Candida albicans* is the species most frequently responsible for human infections. Other species may occasionally cause infection, especially in certain clinical diseases [87, 88]. For example, *C. parapsilosis* is frequently found in cutaneous infections and endocarditis, *C. glabrata* produces vaginitis and disseminated infections in immunocompromised or debilitated patients, and *C. lusitaniae* is an important agent of septicemia. As *C. albicans* and other species are common and harmless commensales of the mucous membranes, digestive tracts, and skin in normal individuals, the disease is obviously an opportunistic endogenous infection.

Pathogenesis. Candidosis arises in subjects who are predisposed by illness or other debility to an overgrowth of their endogenous yeast flora. The severity and extent of the disease tend to increase with the number and severity of predisposing factors. The most common factors are listed in Table 7.8.
Candida infections are the results of an interplay between fungal virulence and host defenses. The most important *Candida* virulence attributes are: surface adhesion factors, surface hydrophobicity, lytic enzymes and propensity to switch phenotype. Hypha formation, which involves virulence attributes, increse in proteinase secretion and other metabolic transformations, is associated with the pathogenic behavior of the fungus [84, 89].

Table 7.8. Main factors predisposing to *Candida* infection

Impaired epithelial barrier Hydration/maceration Occlusion Wounds Burns	**Constitutional disorders** Diabetes mellitus Hypothyroidism Hypoadrenalism Deficiency of iron, zinc, or biotin deficiency
Neutrophil and macrophage disorders Neutropenia Leukopenia Agranulocytosis Myeloperoxidase deficiency	**Immune disorders** Thymic hypo-alymphoplasia Hyper-IgE syndrome Acquired immunodeficiency syndrome
Malignancy Leukemia Thymoma Lymphoma	**Drugs** Antimicrobials Cytotaxic agents Corticosteroids Immunosuppressive agents

Table 7.9. Most common *Candida* infections

Superficial cutaneous candidosis Intertrigo Paronychia Folliculitis	**Superficial mucosal candidosis** Vulvovaginitis Balanitis Oral candidosis
Chronic mucocutaneous candidosis **Deep candidosis** Esophagitis Gastrointestinal candidosis Respiratory tract candidosis Urinary tract candidosis	**Disseminated candidosis** Sepsis Endocarditis and pericarditis Arthritis Osteomyelitis Endophthalmitis Central nervous system candidosis

Host defenses against *Candida* are the barrier function of skin or mucous membranes and T-lymphocyte responses. The evidence for the importance of cellular immunity in defense against *Candida* infections is found in the predisposition to oropharyngeal candidosis in subjects with T-cell defects and patients with low CD4 counts resulting from HIV infection. The severity of the infectious process depends on the degree of immunological impairment of the host.

Clinical Manifestations. The clinical spectrum of candidosis is wide, although the most common manifestations are superficial lesions, especially infections of the mucous surfaces of the mouth or vagina (Table 7.9).
Superficial cutaneous and mucosal candidosis is a minor, often self-limiting, disease associated with one or more predisposing factors. Usually, the infection has a course with acute episodes. When the predisposing factors persist, chronic or relapsing infections may develop. Besides the oral candidosis dealt with in the present chapter, the most common superficial *Candida* infections are: vulvovaginitis, balanitis, intertrigo, paronychia and folliculitis.
Chronic mucocutaneous candidosis is a heterogeneous group of syndromes consisting of chronic infection of the skin, nails, and mucous membranes. The disease occurs in children who have defects of the thymus-derived immune system, leukocyte abnormalities, or polyendocrine diseases.
Deep and disseminated candidoses are major, life-threatening complications in debilitated immunocompromised subjects, in patients with burns, and in those with malignancies, predominantly lymphomas. Deep infection may involve esophagus, gastrointestinal tract (*Candida* peritonitis with intraabdominal abscess is also possible), respiratory and urinary tracts. Serious hematogenously disseminated infection can cause suppurative phlebitis, endocarditis and pericarditis, arthritis, osteomyeli-

tis, endophthalmitis, and central nervous system involvement.

Mycological Diagnosis. Because *Candida* is normally encountered as part of the flora of the mucous membranes, digestive tracts, and skin, its isolation in culture must be supported by direct demonstration of characteristic budding yeast, pseudohyphae and hyphae in the specimens of the lesions.

1. Direct demonstration. In the case of superficial infections, preparation of specimens (pus, smears, scrapings, etc.) with potassium hydroxide (10 % KOH) is the best diagnostic test for microscopic demonstration of *Candida.* Pseudohyphae or hyphae with yeast cells are evident in KOH mounts (Fig. 7.59). In deep infections, direct demonstration of the fungus in the tissue is obtained in stained slides (Giemsa or Wright's stain) of biopsy specimens.
   The presence of *Candida* in blood, urine, and other fluids (cerebrospinal, peritoneal, etc.) is detected in the sediment after their centrifugation.
2. Culture. The colonies of *Candida* species develop 24–48 h after inoculation of clinical specimens onto the culture media. They are small, creamy-white and smooth, with a fruit- or bread-like odor.
   On routine culture media, the various species of *Candida* produce only yeast cells, so that the identification of species is difficult. The two most rapid and reliable criteria for identifying *Candida albicans* are positive results of the germ-tube test (in fact only this species will form germ tubes in serum) and chamydospore formation on cornmeal agar medium (Fig. 7.60). Other species of *Candida* can be rapidly identified by the use of carbohydrate assimilation profiles [84–86].
   In addition to direct demonstration and culture, a variety of indirect methods have been proposed. These include detection of circulating antigens, detection of antibodies against these antigens, and detecting of fungal DNA by the polymerase chain reaction. These tests appear to be promising in the diagnosis of disseminated candidosis.
   For mycological findings to be interpreted correctly it must be remembered that *Candida* can be assumed to be the infecting fungus if it is repeatedly isolated from clinical specimens and if pseudohyphae are present in direct demonstration. *Candida* culture itself is not diagnostic.

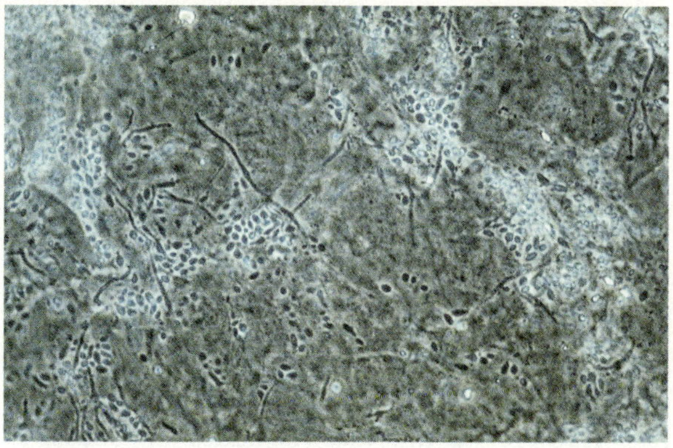

Fig. 7.59. Yeast cells, pseudohyphae and hyphae in specimen of superficial candidosis (KOH) mount

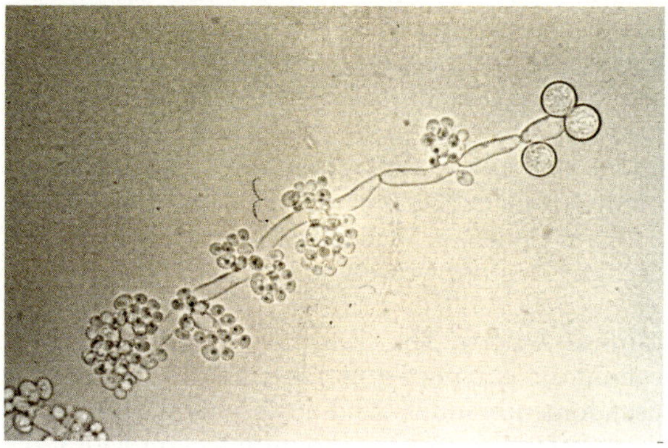

Fig. 7.60. Microscopic appearance of Candida albicans colony on cornmeal agar medium. Formation of chlamydospore

Treatment. Superficial candidoses usually respond to treatment with topical antifungal agents, such as azoles, amphotericin B, and nystatin. These products are available as creams and lotions for skin infection and as vaginal creams and suppositories for vulvovaginal candidosis. Spreading and recurrent infections may need oral therapy with fluconazole (50–100 mg daily), intraconazole (100 mg daily), or terbenifine (250 mg daily). Factors that promote *Candida* colonization of the terbenifine skin or mucosa should be eliminated whenever feasible.

Chronic mucocutaneous candidosis does not respond to topical therapy. Oral terbenifine and intraconazole are the drugs of choice, and the therapy may need to be continued for years.

Deep and severe life-threatening *Candida* infections are treated with intravenous amphotericin B, oral or intravenous fluconazole, oral intraconazole, or oral terbenifine.

7.4.2
Candidosis of the Oral Cavity

Definition. Oral candidosis (or oral thrush) is a common infection of the oropharynx, which is known to have a predilection for debilitated individuals and newborn infants. In recent times, with the advent of broad-spectrum antibiotics, immunosuppressants, and infection with HIV, this infection has become more prevalent and more severe.

Etiology. *C. albicans* is the most important agent. Other isolated species are *C. parapsilosis, C. tropicalis*, and *C. pseudotropicalis.*

Pathogenesis (see Sect. 7.4.1, Pathogenesis). According to Odds, the reported carriage rates of *C. albicans* in the mouths of healthy individuals range from 2 % to 69 % [87]. The infection begins with *Candida* adhesion to the oral mucosa. The adhesion appears to involve lectin-like interactions between mannoprotein of the yeast surface and glycoprotein receptors on the epithelial cells. *C. albicans* has also been shown to have an affinity to and bind to plastic surfaces, such as the acrylic resin of dentures [90]. The major host resistance mechanisms in oral candidosis are: barrier function of mucous membrane, high turnover rate of epithelial cells, salivary IgA, salivary lavage, and intact cellular immunity. The number of predisposing factors is elevated. In addition to those listed in Table 7.8, inadequate oral hygiene, smoking, and denture wearing are very important.

Clinical Aspects. The classification to types of oral candidosis is reported in Table 7.10 [87, 91]. Acute pseudomembranous candidosis (or oral thrush) is the best-known form of mouth infection with Candida. The infection is classically most prevalent among neonates, who acquire it during birth in the maternal birth canal, asthmatics treated with corticosteroid inhalation, and elderly subjects. In adults, it may be a harbinger of diabetes mellitus, malignancy, neutropenia, and HIV infection. The infection constitutes approximately 25 % of the oral candidosis seen in HIV-infected patients [92]. The disease is characterized by the presence of white patches on the mucosa of the cheeks, tongue, gingiva, palate, and pharynx. The lesions develop to become confluent pseudomembranes that resemble milk curds. The pseudomembranes can be scraped off with difficulty, to reveal an erythematous or erosive base. The infection is not normally painful.

Table 7.10. Oral candidosis

Acute pseudomembranous candidosis
Acute atrophic candidosis
Chronic atrophic candidosis
Angular cheilitis
Chronic hyperplastic candidosis

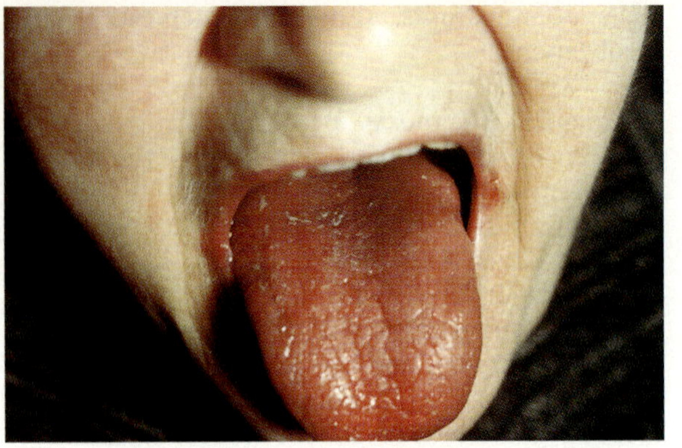

Fig. 7.61. Acute atrophic candidosis of the tongue

Acute atrophic candidosis (or erythematous candidosis or *Candida* glossitis) is commonly associated with the use of broad-spectrum antibiotics and topical or inhaled corticosteroid preparations. It is one of the most common forms in HIV-infected patients. The disease is characterized by painful, atrophic erythematous areas with shedding of the filiform papillae, located on any part of the oral mucosa, but most often affecting the dorsum of the tongue (median rhomboid glossitis) and the palate (Figs. 7.61, 7.62).

Chronic atrophic candidosis (or denture stomatitis) afflicts up to 60 % of denture wearers. Mechanical factors, inadequate denture hygiene, with consequent *Candida* colonization of the denture and uninterrupted denture wearing for long periods (longer than 24 h) facilitate the infection. The disease is characterized by chronic erythema and edema of the portion of the hard and soft upper palate that comes in contact with dentures. The lesions are commonly associated with angular cheilitis. The patient may experience slight soreness, but usually the lesions cause no symptoms.

Angular cheilitis (or perlèche) occurs most frequently in the elderly. In old subjects, the deep, occlusive folds of skin at the corners of the mouth, caused by loss of teeth or poorly fitting dentures, can result in saliva pooling and local maceration, with consequent *Candida* growth. HIV-infected subjects appear to be prone to develop this form of oral candidosis, which represents approximately 10 % of the oral infections seen in these patients. The disease is characterized by erythema, fissuring, maceration, and crusting at the oral commissures, with subjective symptoms of soreness, tenderness, burning, or pain (Fig. 7.63).

Chronic hyperplastic candidosis (or oral leukoplakia) is found in older adults who wear dentures, in children with underlyng immune defects, and in HIV-infected patients. The disease is character-

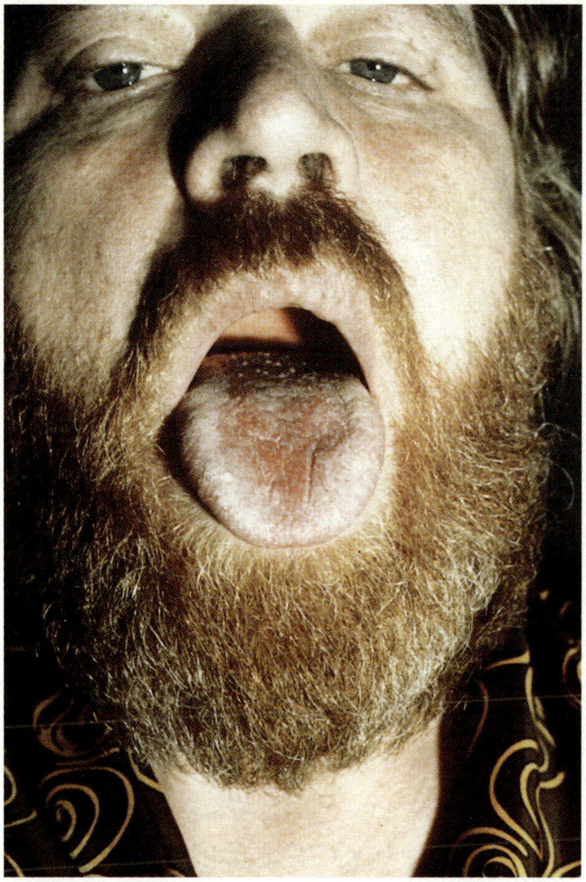

Fig. 7.62. Median rhomboid glossitis. Erythematous area on the dorsum of the tongue with papillary atrophy

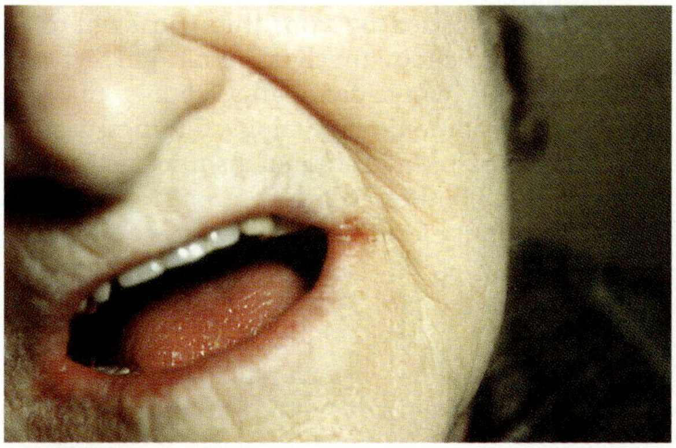

Fig. 7.63. Angular cheilitis. Erythema, fissuring and crusting at the oral commissures

ized by chronic, raised, whitish areas or plaques, which are hard and rough to the touch. The lesions are localized on the retrocommissural areas or, less commonly, on the buccal mucosa, palate, and tongue (Fig. 7.64). Malignant transformation has been reported [93].

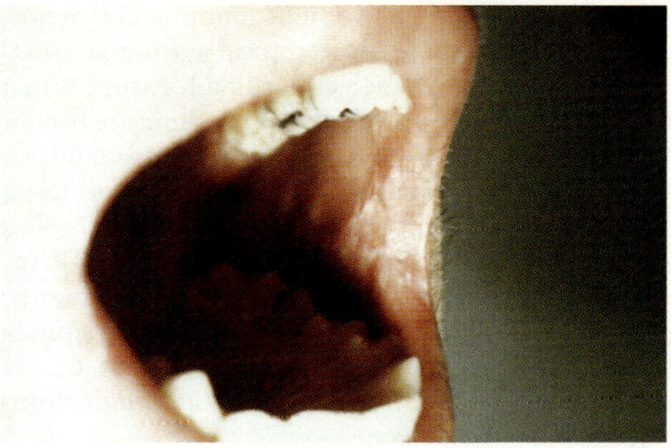

Fig. 7.64. Chronic hyperplastic candidosis. Raised, whitish plaque on the retrocommissural area

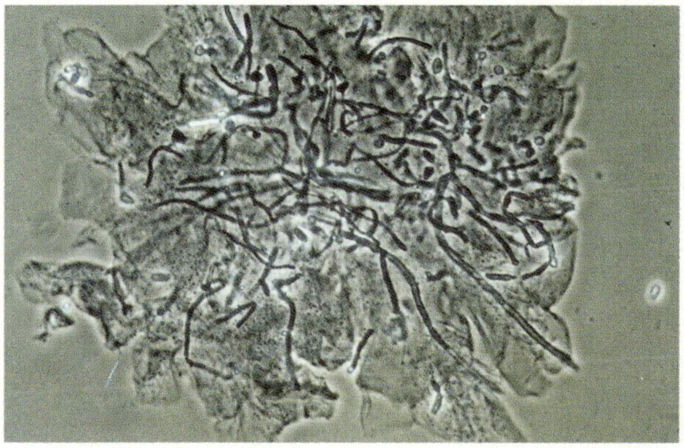

Fig. 7.65. Smear from angular cheilitis (KOH mount). It shows epithelial cells, yeast and hyphae

Diagnosis. The clinical picture in most forms of oral candidosis is characteristic, but diagnosis should be confirmed by the detection of yeasts and pseudohyphae in KOH mounts of scrapings from lesions (Fig. 7.65), and by the isolation of *Candida* in culture (see Sect. 7.4.2.1, Mycological Diagnosis).

Differential Diagnosis. Acute pseudomembranous candidosis should be distinguished from milk or food debris (which can be scraped off easily) and from lesions of lichen planus. The latter consist of white papules forming a lacework.
Chronic hyperplastic candidosis is often misdiagnosed as oral lichen planus or oral keratoses. The differential diagnosis can be particularly difficult when it is based on clinical symptoms alone.
Chronic hyperplastic candidosis in HIV-positive patients should be distinguish from the lesions of oral hairy leukoplakia. These are characterized by white patches with a hairy appearance along the lateral and dorsal aspects of the tongue.

Treatment. In patients without immune deficiency, it may be sufficient to give a topical antifungal treatment with nystatin or azoles in suitable forms. When topical therapy is unsuccessful, systemic treatment should be initiated. Fluconazole (100 mg daily for 10–14 days), itraconazole (200 mg daily for 10–14 days), and terbenifine (250 mg daily for 10–14 days) have all been shown to be efficacious. HIV-infected patients may also develop resistance to antifungal drugs. Treatment of oral candidosis requires careful oral hygiene. Antifungal treatment of the denture is essential, to remove the *Candida* colonization from its surface.

7.4.3 Deep Mycoses

G.L. Campanile, G. Hautmann, and T.M. Lotti

7.4.3.1 *Histoplasmosis*

Definition. Histoplasmosis is a chronic infectious disease acquired by the respiratory route, with a primary focus of infection in the lungs, with occasional hematogenous dissemination, and caused by a dimorphic fungus, *Histoplasma capsulatum.*
The disease is recognized most commonly in the eastern and central United States, where about 80 % of the adult population will have skin test evidence of prior infection. There is a marked preponderance of disease in patients above the age of 60 and in infants and children below the age of 10 years [94].
Histoplasma capsulatum can be recovered from soil naturally enriched with chicken or bird excreta. The causative fungus has been isolated from a large number of wild and domestic animals. However, animal-to-human and human-to-human spread do not occur. Three forms of histoplasmosis have been recognized: acute primary, chronic cavitary, and progressive disseminated [95].

Oral Manifestations. The oral lesions of histoplasmosis occur with sufficient frequency for it to be considered among the more common of the fungal infections involving this region. About 75 % of patients with the progressive disseminated form exhibit oral lesions [96].
Oral lesions can be single or multiple, nodular, ulcerative, or vegetative "sores" (Fig. 7.66), and are usually covered by a gray or pink membrane and show induration of the surrounding tissues. There seems to be no predilection for a particular oral site. Pain is the most common symptom [97].

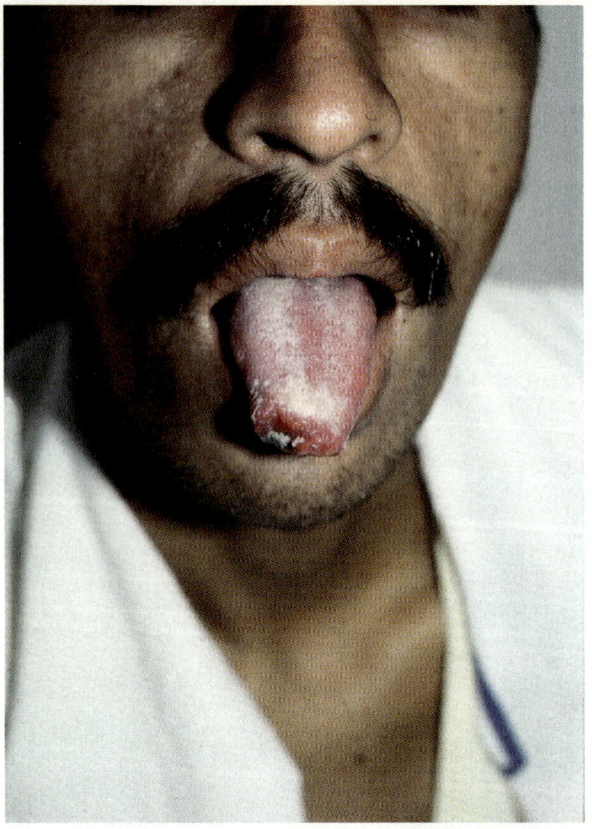

Fig. 7.66. Histoplasmosis in an HIV patient. Courtesy of Dr. Marcia Ramos-e-Silva, Brazil

Associated Findings. The *progressive disseminated form* is characterized by constitutional symptoms (fever, malaise, chills, myalgias, etc.) and hepatosplenomegaly, lymphadenopathy, bone marrow involvement, pulmonary radiologic findings, gastrointestinal disorders, and adrenal insufficiency, in addition to oral manifestations.
The *acute primary form*, which is more common and is self-limiting, is characterized by constitutional symptoms, pulmonary symptoms, and lymphadenopathy.
The *chronic cavitary form* is characterized exclusively by pulmonary signs and symptoms.

Diagnosis. The diagnosis is established by the isolation and identification of the causative fungus in culture from oral lesions, bone marrow, sputum, blood, urine, lymph node, or liver biopsy. Histopathologic examination shows a chronic granulomatous process, in which histiocytes may be present containing great numbers of organisms. The organisms, ranging in diameter from 1 to 5 μm, can usually be seen in routine H&E-stained sections. Special stains are usually advisable.

Differential diagnosis. Oral lesions may be mistaken for almost any inflammatory or neoplastic process.

Treatment. Amphotericin B is an effective agent, providing a systemic cure in most patients, although oral lesions have been successfully treated with ketoconazole alone [98].

7.4.3.2 *Lobomycosis*

Definition. Lobomycosis (or keloidal blastomycosis) is a rare fungal infection reported for the first time in 1931 by Lobo in Brazil. About 500 cases have been reported. The highest prevalence of lobomycosis is within the Brazialian Amazon region; however, this condition has also been reported in Mexico, Venezuela, Colombia, and Peru.
The disease most commonly occurs in otherwise healthy adult men. Farmers and other laborers who have close contact with areas rich in vegetation are most often affected. The disease is not transmitted among humans, and no plant or animal reservoir has been identified as yet. Interestingly, many cases of lobomycosis have also been reported in Atlantic bottle-nosed dolphins [99].
This disease is caused by the fungus *Paracoccidioides loboi.*

Clinical Manifestations. Lobomycosis presents clinically as solitary or multiple keloid-like plaques, nodules, or both. Areas of predilection include the distal extremities, lower back, and face. Lips are susceptible to this infection (Fig. 7.67). Most lesions of lobomycosis tend to be firm with a shining surface, whereas others may be verrucous or atrophic. The lesions are usually asymptomatic; however, pruritus and even anesthesia have occurred around the affected areas. Lymph node involvement has been reported.
The lesions of lobomycosis are chronic and may progress over decades, resulting in severe morbidity and cosmetic disfigurement. On occasion, squamous cell carcinomas have been identified within the scars of lesions that have previously been treated by surgery [100].

Diagnosis. Diagnosis of this infection is usually achieved histologically, as this organism is extremely difficult to culture [101]. Histologically, the epidermis may be normal or atrophic. Within the dermis, a granulomatous cellular infiltrate composed of giant cells and histiocytes is observed (Fig. 7.68). Additionally, the causative fungus is visualized with H&E stain as 10-μm-thick walled organisms with round, double contour membranes.

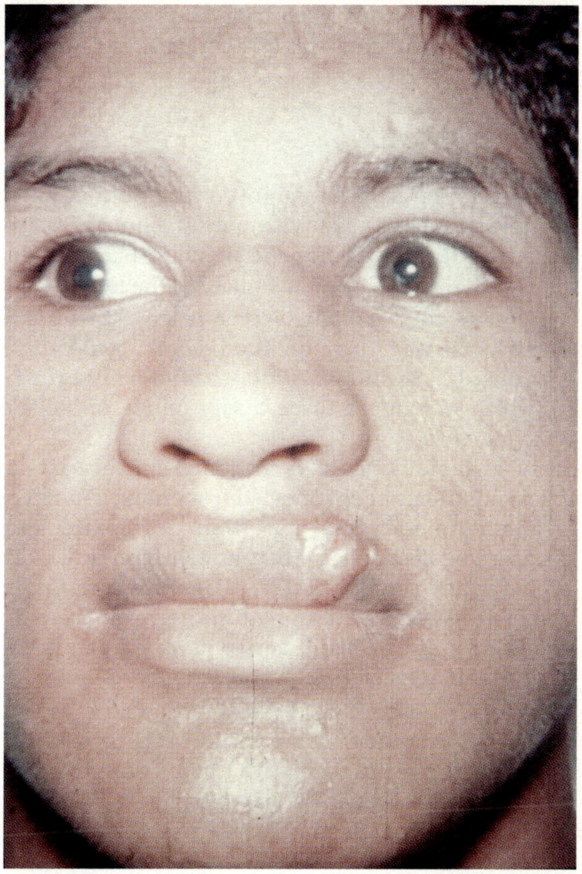

Fig. 7.67. Lobomycosis. Courtesy of Dr. Arival de Brito, Brazil

Differential Diagnosis. It is necessary to exclude sarcoidosis, chromomycosis, leishmaniasis, and true keloids.

Treatment. Many medications have been employed, including amphotericin B and ketoconazole; however, none have consistently provided a cure for lobomycosis. Clofazimine has afforded improvement

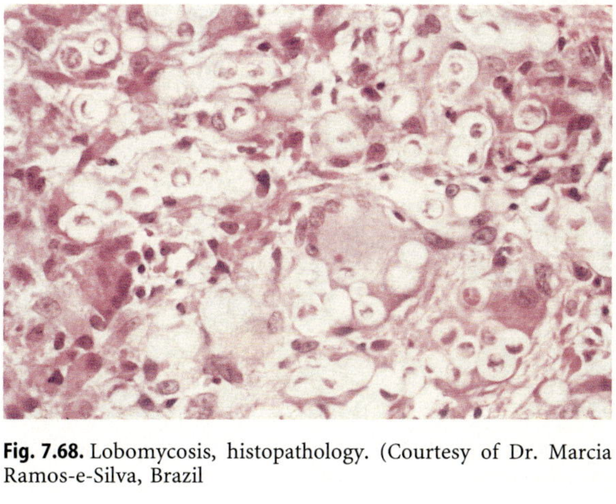

Fig. 7.68. Lobomycosis, histopathology. (Courtesy of Dr. Marcia Ramos-e-Silva, Brazil

in some early lesions [102]. Early surgical intervention remains the mainstay of therapy.

7.4.3.3
Paracoccidioidomycosis

Definition. Paracoccidioidomycosis (South American blastomycosis) is a chronic infectious disease characteristically affecting the skin or mucosa about the mouth or nose, or occasionally in the lungs, with subsequent involvement of regional lymph nodes, and occasionally dissemination hematogeneously. It is caused by the fungus *Paracoccidioides brasiliensis*, which is thought to be a saprophyte of soil or decaying vegetation.

Paracoccidioidomycosis is an important disease in Brazil, and it has been reported from most countries in South America and also from Costa Rica and Mexico. The disease is 5 times as common in whites as blacks, and about 10 times as common in males as in females. It is most frequent in the 20- to 30-year age group and it seems to occur more frequently in rural areas, especially in farmers [95].

Oral Manifestations. The vast majority of patients present with painful ulcerative lesions of the mouth with a granular surface. Perforation of hard palate associated with pain may be seen in severe cases. The soft and hard palate, tongue, and gingiva (Fig. 7.69) are frequently involved [103].

Assciated Findings. Ulcerative or verrucous lesions (Fig. 7.70) of the skin, most commonly seen about the lips and usually multiple, are characteristic of the disease. Less frequently, there is a solitary pustular lesion or subcutaneous abscess and draining sinus tract.

Involvement of the regional lymphatics is characteristic of the disease, and occasionally swelling or drainage of a lymph node, especially those of the cervical region, is the first sign noted by the patient. Occasionally, the disease begins with a cough, chest pain, and a pulmonary infiltrate seen on the chest roentgenogram.

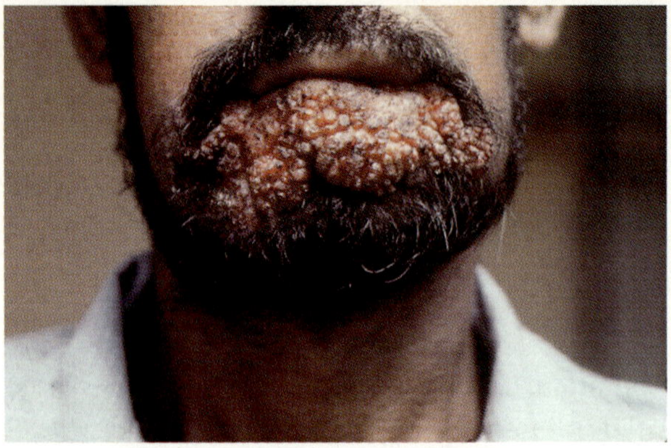

Fig. 7.70. Paracoccidioimycosis. Courtesy of Dr. Marcia Ramos-e-Silva, Brazil

From the above lesions, disease may disseminate to such organs as bone, adrenal glands, central nervous system, and spleen [104].

Diagnosis. The diagnosis is established by isolation and identification of the causative fungus in culture. By direct examination, the large (10–60 μm in diameter) spherical to oval cells are easily visualized (Fig. 7.71).

The histopathologic findings are characteristically both granulomatous (Fig. 7.72) and suppurative. In skin lesions, although the characteristic budding fungal cells stain with H&E, the special fungal stains, such as silver impregnation (Fig. 7.73), demonstrate them more strikingly.

Differential Diagnosis. This includes squamous cell carcinoma, tuberculosis, syphilis, leishmaniasis, and other systemic mycoses.

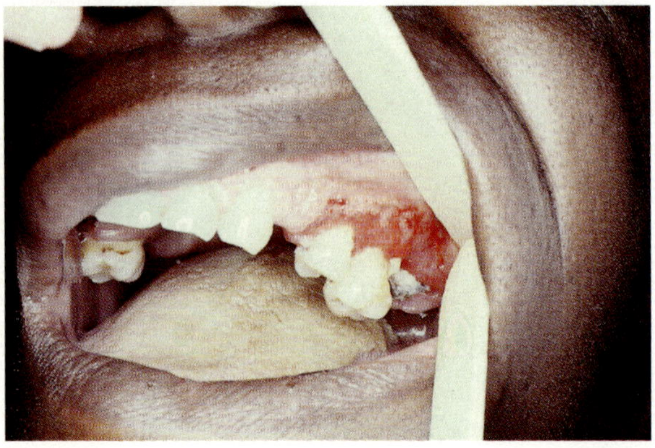

Fig. 7.69. Paracoccidioimycosis. Courtesy of Dr. Sandra Torres and Dr. Luis Carlos Moreira, Brazil

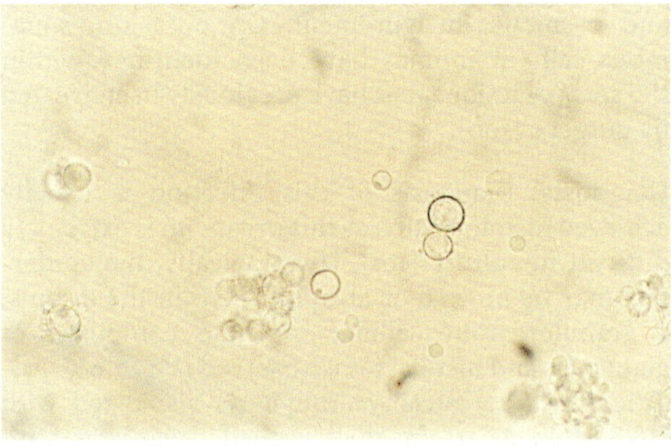

Fig. 7.71. Paracoccidioimycosis, direct examination. Courtesy of Dr. Marcia Ramos-e-Silva, Brazil

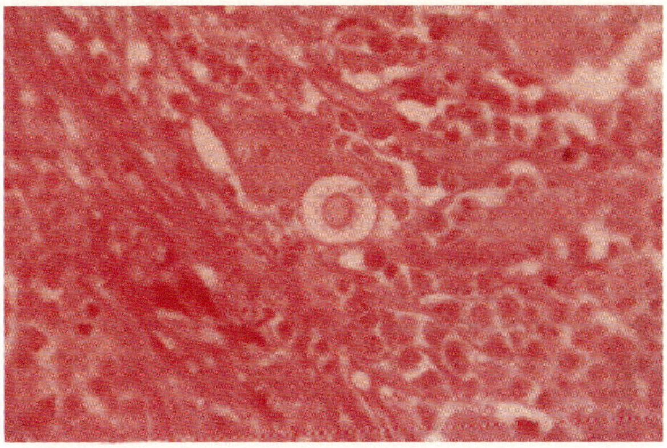

Fig. 7.72. Paracoccidioimycosis, pilot wheel aspect: lymph node. Courtesy of Dr. Marcia Ramos-e-Silva, Brazil

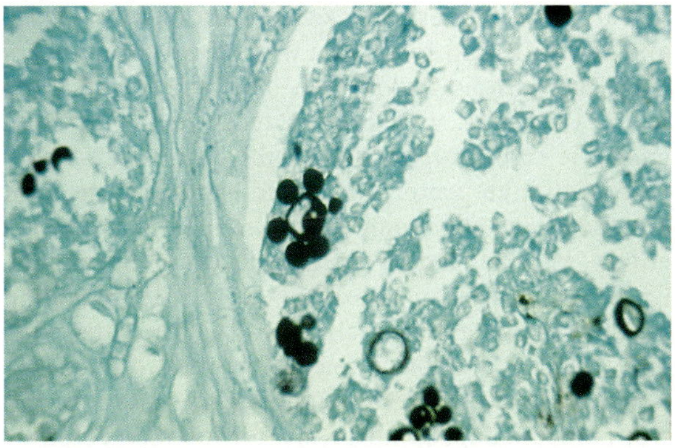

Fig. 7.73. Paracoccidioimycosis, skin, silver impregnation. Courtesy of Dr. Marcia Ramos-e-Silva, Brazil

Treatment. Intravenous amphotericin B, ketoconazole, and itraconazole are effective drugs.

7.4.3.4 *Blastomycosis*

Definition. Blastomycosis is a chronic infectious disease caused by a dimorphic fungus, *Blastomyces dermatitidis*, whose natural habitat has yet to be unequivocally demonstrated; meanwhile, wood has been implicated.
The disease occurs in the Americas and in Africa. It is common in males and in females and occurs more often in farmers and laborers aged 50 years and over. The disease occurs not infrequently in dogs, and has been reported once each in a horse and a sea lion.

Oral Manifestations. Approximately a quarter of the patients have oral or nasal mucous membrane lesions. Of this fraction, only one half are from a contiguous cutaneous lesion. Clinically, oral lesions at presentation are ulcers with a slightly verrucous surface and thin borders, or raised vegetating plaques [105].

Associated Findings. When infection disseminates from the lung, a number of cutaneous forms of the disease are seen. The most characteristic is an elevated, verrucous, crusted lesion, which has a serpiginous border and a tendency toward central healing. Another form of cutaneous disease is that of small superficial ulcerative lesions. A third form consists of a raised, firm, subcutaneous nodule, occasionally containing many small pustules over its surface.
Pulmonary involvement occurs in virtually all patients, but it is clinically important in only one-half of them.
Bone lesions in the form of osteomyelitis are seen most commonly in thoracic and lumbar vertebrae, pelvis, sacrum.
Disease of the genital tract occurs in approximately a third of the male patients. Rarely, the disease may be manifested by meningoencephalitis, cerebral abscess, endocarditis, or involvement of the liver, adrenals, spleen, or gastrointestinal tract [95].

Diagnosis. The diagnosis is established by isolation and identification of the causative fungus in culture from lesions. In the rare instances when material for culture is not available, the diagnosis rests on histopathologic examination.

Differential Diagnosis. It includes squamous cell carcinoma, tuberculosis, tertiary syphilis, and other systemic mycoses.

Treatment. Amphotericin B intravenously, ketoconazole, and itraconazole are effective drugs.

7.4.3.5 *Zygomycosis*

Definition. Zygomycosis (mucormycosis, phycomycosis) is an acute or fulminant infectious disease, which usually involves debilitated individuals. It is caused by fungi of the family Mucoraceae, mainly *Rhizopus* and *Rhizomucor*, and rarely other species. Zygomycosis is an opportunistic infection. The most common predisposing conditions are poorly controlled diabetes mellitus, hematologic malignancies, burns, malnutrition, uremia, liver cirrhosis, HIV disease, organ transplantation, cancer chemotherapy, and immunosuppressive therapy.
The fungus is acquired from the environment and erodes arteries, causing thrombosis, ischemia, and finally necrosis of the surrounding tissues.

Four clinical forms are recognized: rhinocerebral, pulmonary, gastrointestinal, and disseminated. The rhinocerebral form is the most common and presents with oral, cranial, and facial signs and symptoms.

Oral manifestations. Palatal ulceration and necrosis are the most characteristic oral lesions. The ulcer is shaply demarcated with a black necrotic eschar, while the bone is exposed. The mucosa surrounding the ulcer is usually thickened. Orbital and intracranial invasion is a common complication [106, 107].

Associated Findings. Clinically, the disease is characterized by low-grade fever, headache, malaise, sinus pain, bloody nasal discharge, periorbital or perinasal swelling and edema, ptosis of the eyelid, extraocular muscle paresis, and progressive lethargy [108].

Diagnosis. Laboratory tests useful for diagnosis are histopathologic examination and smear examination. Computerized axial tomography may be useful to demonstrate the extent of bone destruction.

Differential Diagnosis. It should include Wegener's granulomatosis, tertiary syphilis, tuberculosis, and other systemic mycoses.

Treatment. Intravenous amphotericin B and surgical débridement are indicated. Correction of underlying predisposing conditions is also important.

7.5 Diseases Caused by Protozoa

M. Ramos-e-Silva

Protozoa are unicellular organisms that range in size from submicroscopic to macroscopic. They are the simplest organisms of the animal kingdom; most are free-living, but some have a parasitic existence. Diseases caused by protozoa rarely produce oral lesions, except for the mucocutaneous form of leishmaniasis found in South and Central America, which is discussed in Chap. 8.
The medical literature includes very few case reports of amebiasis, American trypanosomiasis, toxoplasmosis, and trichomoniasis producing oral or perioral lesions.

7.5.1 Amebiasis

Definition. Amebiasis is an intestinal parasitic disease that can sometimes affect the skin, especially perianal and genital areas. Oral manifestations, although possible, are extremely rare.

Etiology. This disease is caused by a very common intestinal unicellular parasite present in all parts of the world, *Entamoeba histolytica*, the only human pathogenic species of this genus. The invasive form found in the tissues is a 20- to 40-μm elongated cell, with pseudopods on its surface.
Another species. *Entamoeba gingivalis*, morphologically very similar to *E. histolytica*, is often found in the mouth where it lives as a commensal. This species shows great proliferation when associated with inflammatory processes caused by other microorganisms

Pathogenesis. In humans, there are two pathogenically important distinct life cycle phases of *Entamoeba histolytica*: the trophozoite and the cyste. The trophozoite, or invasive form, produces the disease, penetrates the tissues, and sometimes blood vessels, and can be found inside the wall of the colon, especially the sigmoid and rectum. The cyst or infectious form is released with human feces to the outside, where it can survive for several days and is able to contaminate water, food, and fomites. Intestinal amebiasis, usually manifested as diarrhea or dysentery, is produced by the ingestion of these cysts, which turn into trophozoites in the ileum, being able to penetrate the intestinal wall again. Cutaneous and mucosal amebiasis may be provoked by direct inoculation from intestinal amebiasis, by continuity from amebic hepatic abscess, after infected colon or liver surgeries, hematogenous or lymphatic spread, and fecal-oral or genito-anal contact. Poor hygiene, promiscuity, poverty, and immunosuppression facilitate the disease, mainly in tropical areas.

Oral Manifestations. *Entamoeba gingivalis* oral infection may be suspected in the presence of generalized dental mobility, specially in young patients, enlarged tongue, fetid halitosis, vivid red color, frequent hemorrhages, and pruritus of gingiva, with no other causes. Cutaneous, genital, perianal or very rarely oral lesions provoked by Entamoeba histolytica, although extremely uncommon, are characterized when present by a single or few very painful unspecific serpiginous and destructive ulcers.

Associated Findings. Oral manifestations of *Entamoeba histolytica* infection may only be present in the advanced chronic form, which becomes manifest in various organs. Skin and mucosal lesions are almost always associated with intestinal amebiasis manifested by dysentery. There may be constitutional symptoms, ranging from mild, such as loss of appetite, fever, leukocytosis, and dehydration, to severe, such as massive intestinal hemorrhage, bowel perforation, and peritonitis. The most common extraintestinal manifestation is the hepatic abscess.

Microscopic Findings. In tissues the trophozoites, with a basophilic and elongated cytoplasm, single eccentric nucleus and central spherical cariosome, are very difficult to observe. In cutaneous and mucosal lesions they are more easily seen in biopsies of the borders rather than at the center of the ulcer.

Diagnosis. *Entamoeba gingivalis* can be recovered from dental plaques. The motile *Entamoeba histolytica* trophozoites may be found in lesion scrapings and the cysts on parasitologic examination of the feces. Other useful tests are hemagglutination, complement fixation, ELISA, immunoperoxidase, and especially indirect immunofluorescence.

Differential Diagnosis. All diseases that cause periodontal disease or large oral ulcerations, especially accompanied by pain, such as herpes simplex, donovanosis, tuberculosis, and squamous cell carcinoma, have to be included in the differential diagnosis. The main means of differentiation is histopathologic recognition of the occurrence of trophozoites.

Treatment. Complete cure can be rapidly achieved in 7–20 days with metroindazole, 20–40 mg/kg/per day, divided into three daily doses, for up to 8 days. Tinidazole, in a single daily dosage, 2 g for adults and 50–60 mg/kg for children, for 3–5 days, also shows good and fast results. Intravenous or intramuscular dehydroemetine hydrochloride, the drug of choice in the past, is cardiotoxic. Di-iodohydroxyquinoline, paramomycin, and diloxanide furoate can also be used. Severe dysentery associated with mucosal or cutaneous involvement requires supportive measures.

7.5.2 American Trypanosomiasis/Chagas' Disease

Definition. Trypanosomiasis is a tropical and mainly rural parasitic disease of blood and various organs. There are two different entities, the African, caused by trypanosomes of the *T. brucei* group (*T. gambiense* and *T. rhodesiense*) and transmitted by tsetse flies, also called sleeping sickness, and the American, known as Chagas' disease. Inoculation lesions on the lips can sometimes be observed in American trypanosomiasis.

Etiology. Chagas' disease is produced by a hemoflagellate protozoan, *Trypanosoma cruzi*, affecting humans and various domestic or wild mammals that act as reservoirs. It is transmitted by bloodsucking invertebrates of the order Hemiptera, genera *Triatoma*, *Panstrongylus*, and *Rhodnuis*, called reduviid, assassin or kissing bugs and "barbeiro" in Brazil. Transfusional and congenital infection are also possible, although very rare.

Pathogenesis. *Trypanosoma cruzi* goes through various stages in its life cycle. The trypomastigota or flagellated form is observed in the blood of the definitive vertebrate host, and amastigota in cells of various tissues. Other phases are only seen in the vector. The insect bites the definitive host and deposits infected stools on the skin or mucosa. Transmission occurs through the bite wound itself, small skin cuts and abrasions, or even through intact eye or lip mucosa.

Oral Manifestations. Mouth lesions are mainly seen on the lips and are similar to the skin chagoma. They are characterized by an erythematous nodule, swelling, or ulcer at the site of inoculation, which generally heals spontaneously in about 3 weeks.

Associated Findings. Inoculation occurs during the night, when the insect is active and needs to feed. Lesions appear on uncovered areas, usually the face. Romaña's sign (Fig. 7.74), a unilateral eyelid edema associated with dacryoadenitis (inflammation of the lacrimal gland), occurs in 80% of the cases, 5–10 days after transmission and is the most characteristic skin lesion. The acute phase, which is more prevalent in children, progresses with high fever, headache, morbilliform rash, regional lymphadenopathy, hepatosplenomegaly, and acute meningoencephalitis; death occurs frequently in this phase. The subacute form produces mild fever, malaise, and generalized lymphadenopathy.

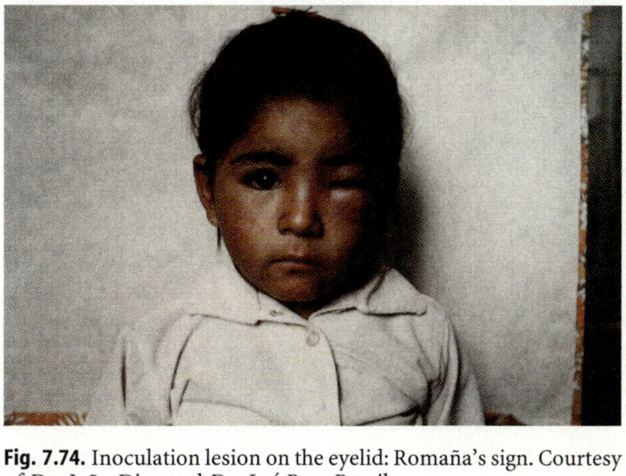

Fig. 7.74. Inoculation lesion on the eyelid: Romaña's sign. Courtesy of Dr. João Dias and Dr. Luí Rey, Brazil

Cardiac (chagasic myocarditis) and gastrointestinal (megaesophagus and megacolon) manifestations occur in the chronic phase.

Microscopic Findings. In blood smears, the trypomastigota form is a spindle-shaped, elongated and mobile protozoan, with an undulating membrane and an anterior flagellum, measuring 15–20 μm in length (Fig. 7.75). The form seen in the tissues, amastigota, measures 1.5–4.0 μm in diameter. It is a void and immobile obligatory intracellular parasite, found in groups, particularly inside muscle fibers.

Diagnosis. During the acute phase, direct examination of Giemsa - stained blood smears, imprints of skin, or lymph node biopsy can easily show the parasite. They can also be demonstrated by blood culture in NNN media, or animal inoculation.
Xenodiagnosis according to Brumpt is also helpful. For this, an uninfected reduviid bug (Fig. 7.76) is allowed to bite and feed on the patient's forearm: 30–60 days later the insect's feces are examined, searching for the infective form.
During the chronic phase, the Machado-Guerreiro complement fixation test using antigens of cultured *T. cruzi* is most useful. ELISA, hemagglutination, indirect immunofluorescence, and PCR can also be used to diagnose the disease.

Differential Diagnosis. Mucosal inoculation lesions have to be distinguished from other diseases that produce nodules, swellings, and ulceration, such as pyoderma, leishmaniasis, myiasis, angioedema, and especially primary syphilis chancre, which also heals spontaneously.

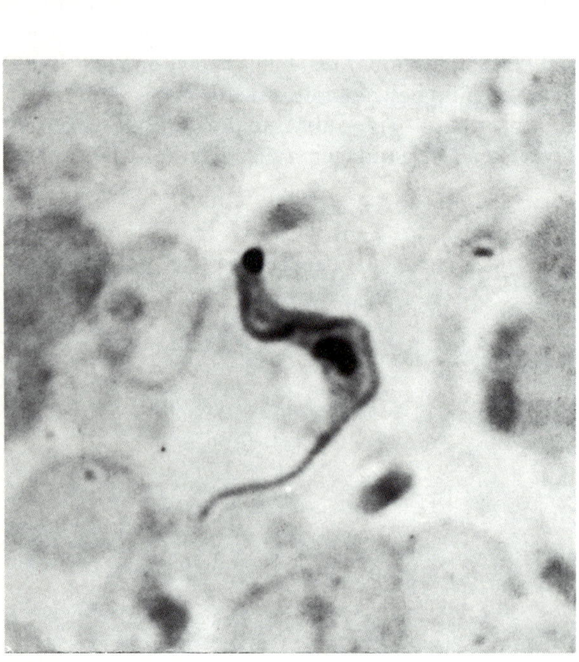

Fig. 7.75. Trypanosoma cruzi in blood. Courtesy of Dr. Luís Rey, Brazil

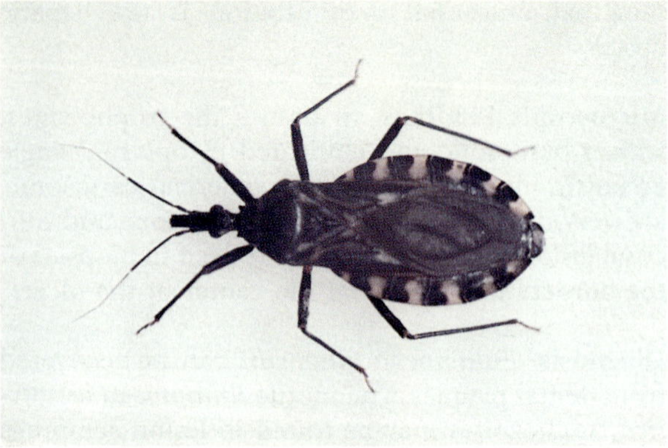

Fig. 7.76. Reduviid bug. Courtesy of Dr. Luís Rey, Brazil

Treatment. At present, oral trypanocidal medications such as benzonidazole, 5–7 mg/kg divided into two daily doses for 30–60 days, and nifurtimox 6–10 mg/kg, divided into three daily doses for 60–120 days, are the most effective, although both can cause serious side effects. Besides medication, improvement of rural housing conditions and control of vector proliferation are extremely important in this disease.

7.5.3 Toxoplasmosis

Definition. Toxoplasmosis is an acute or chronic, widespread and incidental disease of large mammals and humans. It is caused by a tiny sporozoon whose definitive hosts are cats.

Etiology. The obligate intracellular protozoan *Toxoplasma gondii* is transmitted by feces of the infected cat (definitive host) and is virtually capable of infecting all tissues except red blood cells.

Pathogenesis. *Toxoplasma gondii* is transmitted to humans in the form of oocysts present in the infected cat's feces, through contaminated soil, direct exposure to infected feces, tissue cysts in raw infected meat (specially pork), or tachyzoites (proliferating forms) in blood. The parasite invades the reticuloendothelial system and the endothelium of blood vessels, causing a necrotic granuloma.

Oral Manifestations. Cervical lymphadenopathy is the most common form of acquired toxoplasmosis, although other forms of oral and perioral manifestations are occasionally seen. Tongue, larynx, or pharynx myositis and parotid swelling may occur in the acquired form; enamel hypoplasia can be observed in congenital infection.

Associated Findings. Most human infections are asymptomatic. When symptoms occur, they range from a mild self-limiting disease, clinically resembling mononucleosis, to a fulminating disseminated condition that may cause extensive damage to the brain, eyes, skeletal and cardiac muscles, liver, and lungs, especially in AIDS patients. Severe manifestations causing intrauterine death, serious fetal damage, deafness or blindness can be seen in transplacental infection. Chorioretinitis may be associated with all forms, but is usually a late sequel of congenital toxoplasmosis.

Microscopic Findings. Histopathology is not diagnostic, but an enlarged lymph node, biopsy showing follicular hyperplasia, the characteristic 'immature sinus histiocytosis' and scattered foci of light pink histiocytes, very evident in a dense infiltrate of lymphocytes, with a lymphoma aspect, are highly suggestive of the disease.

Diagnosis. Confirmation can be achieved by demonstration of *Toxoplasma gondii* in lymph node, or any other infected organ or fluid. Serology by means of the Sabin-Feldman dye test, hemagglutination, complement fixation, indirect immunofluorescence, or ELISA are very useful. Specific IgM positivity indicates active disease.

Differential Diagnosis. Cervical lymphadenopathy of toxoplasmosis has to be distinguished clinically and histologically from lymph node enlargement from other causes, especially lymphomas, such as Hodgkin's disease.

Treatment. The drugs available for toxoplasmosis are pyrimethamine, 25 mg/day, and sulphonamides, 2–4 g/day. They act synergistically and are usually associated. Although very effective, this association has serious side effects, such as impairment of folic acid metabolism, that contraindicate its use in immunologically competent and asymptomatic patients.

7.5.4 Trichomoniasis/Trichomonosis

Definition. Trichomoniasis is a parasitic disease caused by flagellated protozoa of the genus *Trichomonas*, found mainly in the intestinal and genitourinary tracts of various invertebrates and vertebrates.

Etiology. There are three species of Trichomonas that can affect humans: *T. vaginalis*, a genitourinary parasite, *T. hominis*, a parasite of the intestinal tract, and *T. buccalis* or *tenax*, in general, a commensal of the mouth.

Pathogenesis. In the mouth, *T. tenax* is most often seen in the tartar formed around teeth, cavities of carious teeth, pockets associated with periodontal disease, and tonsillar crypts. Its presence is correlated with poor oral hygiene.

Oral Manifestations. This parasite has frequently been related to lesions of periodontium, the tissue that surrounds the tooth. Its abnormal proliferation is associated with the development of periodontal pockets, chronic inflammatory reaction, and ultimately destruction and loss of teeth in severe cases.

Microscopic Findings. *T. tenax* are found in scrapings from periodontal pockets and are characterized by four anterior flagella and an undulating membrane.

Treatment. All species of the genus *Trichomonas* can be easily treated with metronidazole, 250 mg, b. i. d. or t. i. d. for 7–10 days. Local hygiene improvement and appropriate treatment of periodontitis are more important for oral trichomoniasis than the administration of systemic drugs.

References

1. Asikanen S, Alaluusa S. Bacteriology and dental infections. Eur Heart J 1993; 14 [Suppl 1]:43–50
2. Gibbons RJ. Role of adhesion in microbial colonization of host tissues: a contribution of oral microbiology. J Dent Res 1996; 75:866–870
3. Marsh PD. Microbial ecology of dental plaque and its significance in health and disease. Adv Dent Res 1994; 8:263–271
4. Marsh PD. The role of microbiology in models of dental caries. Adv. Dent Res 1995; 9:244–269
5. Watanabe K, Frommel TO. Porphyromonas gingivalis, Actinobacillus actinomycetemcomitans, and Treponema denticola detection in oral plaque samples using the polymerase chain reaction. J Clin Periodont 1996; 23:212–219
6. Bjarnason S, Kohler B, Wagner KA. A longitudinal study of dental caries and cariogenic microflora in a group of young adults from Goteborg. Swed Dent J 1993; 17:191–199
7. Tutte-McDonnell M, Griffen AL, Moescherberger ML, Dalton RY, Fuerst PA, Leys EJ. Concordance of Porhyromonas gingivalis colonization in families. J Clin Microbiol 1997; 35:455–461
8. Zambon JJ. Microbiology of periodontal disease. In: Genco RJ et al. (Eds) Contemporary periodontics. St Louis: Mosby, 1990; pp 147–160
9. Hamada S, Holt C, McGhee JR (Eds). Periodontal disease: pathogens and host immune response. Tokyo: Quintessence Publishing 1991
10. Zambon JJ, Haraszthy VI, Hariharan G, Lally ET, Demuth DR. The microbiology of early onset periodontitis: association of highly toxic Actinobacillus actinomycetemcomitans strains with localized juvenile periodontitis. J Periodont 1986; 67:282–290

11. Brogan JM, Lally ET, Demuth DR. Regulation of Actinobacillus actinomycetemcomitans leukotoxin: analysis of the promoter region of leukotoxic and minimal leukotoxic strains. Infect Immun 1994; 62:501–508
12. Socransky SS, Haffajee AD. The bacterial etiology and destructive periodontal disease: current concepts. J Periodontol 1992; 63 [Suppl]:322–331
13. Loomer PM, Ellen RP, Tenebaum HC. Characterization of inhibitory effects of suspected periodontopathogens on osteogenesis in vitro. Infect Immun 1995; 63:3287–3996
14. Tew J, Engel D, Mangan D. Polyclonal B-cell activation in periodontitis. J Periodontal Res 1989; 24:225–241
15. Zambon J. Microbiology of periodontal disease. In: Contemporary periodontics. In: RJ Genco, HH Goldman, DW Cohen (Eds) St Louis: Mosby 1990; pp 147–160
16. Macrina FL. Bacterial diseases of the oral tissues. Adv Exp Med Biol 1992; 327:25–34
17. Genco RJ. Classification and clinical and radiographic features of periodontal disease. In: R Genco, HM Goldman, DW Cohen (Eds) Contemporary periodontics. St. Louis: Mosby, 1990; pp 63–81
18. Hamada S, Holt SC, McGhee (Eds). Periodontal disease: pathogens and host immune responses. Tokyo: Quintessence, 1991; pp 2–29
19. Slots J. Listgarten, Bacteroides gingivalis, Bachteroides intermedius and Actinobacillus actinomycetemcomitans in human periodontal disease. J Clin Periodontal 1988; 15:85
20. Page RC, Schroeder HE. Periodontitis in man and other animals. Basel: Karger, 1982
21. Leung DY, Meissner HC, Fulton DR, et al. Toxic shock syndrome toxin-secreting Staphylococcus aureus in Kawasaki syndrome. Lancet 1993; 342: 1385–1388
22. Stevens DL, Tanner MH, Winship J, et al. Severe group A streptococcal infections associated with a toxic shock-like syndrome and scarlet fever. N Eng J Med 1989; 321:1–7
23. Hoge CW, Schwartz B, Talkington DF, et al. The changing epidemiology of invasive group A streptococcal infection and the emergence of streptococcal toxic shock-like syndrome. JAMA 1993; 269:384–389
24. Schachter J, Atwood G. Chlamydial pharyngitis? J Am Vener Dis Assoc 1975; 2:12
25. Neistein LS, Inderlied F, Inderlied C. Low prevalence of Chlamydia trachomatis in the oropharynx of adolescents. Pediatr Infect Dis 1986; 5:660–662
26. Centers for Disease Control. STD Treatment Guidelines. MMWR 1993; 42, RR-14:27–46
27. Ferro ER, Richter JW. Oral lesions of granuloma inguinale: Report of three cases. J Oral Surg 1946; 4:121–124
28. Brightman VR. Sexually transmitted diseases. In: MA Lynch, (Ed.). Burket's oral medicine. J.B. Philadelphia: Lippincott 1984; p 865
29. Brooks BJ Jr, Marier R, Sanders CV. Ulcer of the hard palate. JAMA 1982; 247:819–820
30. Williams CA, Winkler JR, Grassi M, Murray PA. HIV-associated periodontitis complicated by necrotizing stomatitis. Oral Surg Oral Med Oral Pathol 1990; 69:351–355
31. Zambon JJ, Reynolds HS, Genco RJ. Studies of the subgingival microflora in patients with acquired immunodeficiency syndrome. J Periodontal 1990; 61:699–704
32. Schmidt-Westhausen A, Fahrenbach FL, Reichart PA. Oral Enterobacteriaceae in patients with HIV infection. J Oral Pathol 1990; 19:229–231
33. Volpe F, Schimmer A, Barr C. Oral manifestations of disseminated Mycobacterium avium-intracellulare in a patient with AIDS. Oral Surg 1985; 60:567
34. Speight PM. Epithelioid angiomatosis affecting the oral cavity as a first sign of HIV infection. Br Dent J 1991; 171:367–370
35. Koehler JE, Tappero JW. AIDS Commentary: Bacillary angiomatosis and bacillary peliosis in patients infected with human immunodeficiency virus. Clin Infect Dis 1993; 17:612–624
36. Koehler JE, Quinn FD, Berger TG et al. Isolation of Rochalimaea species from cutaneous and osseous lesions of bacillary angiomatosis. N Engl J Med 1992; 372:1625–1631
37. Beyt BE. Cutaneous mycobacteriosis. Medicine 1981; 60:95–111
38. Feingold DS. Cutaneous tuberculosis. In: Sanders CV, Nesbit LT (Eds) The skin and infection. Baltimore: Williams & Wilkins 1995: 130
39. Vestey JP, Norval M. Mucocutaneous infection with herpes simplex viruses and their management. Clin Exp Dermatol 1992; 17:221–237
40. Crumpacker CS. Significance of resistance of herpes simplex virus to acyclovir. J Am Acad Dermatol 1988; 18:169–172
41. Whitley J, Gnann JW. (1992) Acyclovir: a decade later. N Engl J Med 1992; 327: 782–789
42. Miller CS, Redding SW. Diagnosis and management of orofacial herpes simplex virus infections. Dent Clin N Amer 1992; 36(4):879–893
43. Mandell A. Is it meaningful to treat patients with recurrent herpetic infections? Scand J Infect Dis 1991; suppl 78:27–32
44. Straus SE, Ostrove JM, Inchuaspe G, et al. Varicella-zoster virus infection. Ann Intern Med 1988; 108:221–237
45. Mandel BK. Herpes zoster and the immunocompromised. J Infect Dis 1987; 14: 1–5
46. Schuster V, Kreth HW. Epstein-Barr virus and associated diseases in children. Eur J Paediatr 1992; 151(10):718–725
47. Greenspan D, Greenspan JS, Hearst NG. Relation of oral hairy leukoplakia with human immunodeficiency virus infection and risk of developing AIDS. J Infect Dis 1987; 155:475–481
48. EC-Clearinghouse. On oral problems relating to HIV infection and WHO Collaborating Centre on oral manifestations of the human immunodeficiency virus. Classification and diagnostic criteria for oral lesions in HIV infection. J Oral Pathol Med 1993; 22:289–291
49. Schubert MM, Epstein JB, Lloid ME, et al. Oral manifestations of cytomegalovirus in immunocompromised patients. J Oral Pathol Med 1993; 22(6):268–273
50. Levy J. A new human herpesvirus: KSHV or HHV8? Lancet 1995; 34:786
51. Bagg J. Human herpesvirus 6: the latest human herpesvirus. J Oral Pathol Med 1991; 20:465–468
52. Black JD, Inoue N, Kite-Powell K, et al. Frequent isolation of human herpesvirus 7 from saliva. Virus Res 1993; 29(1):91–98
53. Praetorius-Clausen F, Mögeltoft M, Roed-Petersen B, et al. Focal epithelial hyperplasia of the oral mucosa in a south-west Greenlandic population. Scand J Dent Res 1970; 78:287–294
54. Preatorius-Clausen F, Emmertsen M. Occurrence of focal epithelial hyperplasia among Amerindians in Ecuador. Int J Oral Sur 1973; 2:45–53
55. Obalek S, Janninger C, Jablonska S, et al. Sporadic cases of Heck disease in two Polish girls: Association with human papillomavirus type 13. Pediatr Dermatol 1993; 10:240–244
56. Pfister H, Hettich J, Runne U, et al. Characterization of human papillomavirus type 13 from focal epithelial hyperplasia Heck lesions. J Virol 1983; 47:363–366
57. Beaudenon S, Praetorius F, Kremsdorf D, et al. A new type of human papillomavirus associated with oral focal epithelial hyperplasia. J Invest Dermatol 1987; 88:130–135
58. Petzoldt D, Pfister H. HPV1 DNA in lesions of focal epithelial hyperplasia Heck. Arch Dermatol Res 1980; 268:313–314
59. De Villiers EM, Weidauer H, Le JY, et al. Papillomviren in benignen und malignen Tumoren des Mundes und des oberen Respirationstraktes. Laryngol Rhinol Otol 1986; 65:177–179
60. Paradisi M, Mostaccioli S, Celeno G, et al. Infantile condylomata of the oral cavity. Pediatric Dermatol 1992; 9:107–111
61. Eversole LR, Laipis PJ. Oral squamous papillomas: detection of HPV DNA by in situ hybridization. Oral Surg Oral Med Oral Pathol 1988; 65:545–550
62. Naghashfar Z, Sawada E, Kutcher E, et al. Identification of genital tract papillomaviruses HPV6 and HPV16 in warts of the oral cavity. J Med Virol 1985; 17:313–324
63. Ward KA, Napier SS, Winter PC, et al. Detection of human papilloma virus DNA sequences in oral squamous cell papillomas by the polymerase chain reaction. Oral Surg Oral Med Oral Pathol Radiol Endod 1995; 80:63–66

64. Lutzner M, Kuffer R, Blanchet-Bardon C, et al. Different papillomaviruses as the causes of oral warts. Arch Dermatol 1982; 118:393–399
65. Eversole LR, Laipis PJ, Merrell P, et al. Demonstration of human papillomavirus DNA in oral condyloma acuminatum. J Oral Pathol 1987; 16:266–272
66. Padayachee A, Van Wyk CW. Human papillomavirus /HPV/ in oral squamous cell papillomas. J Oral Pathol 1987; 16:353–355
67. Padayachee A, Sanders CM, Maitland N. A polymerase chain reaction investigation of oral verrucae which contain HPV types 2 and 57 by in situ hybridization. J Oral Pathol Med 1995; 24:329–334
68. Löning T, Ikenberg H, Becker J, et al. Analysis of oral papillomas, leukoplasias, and invasive carcinomas for human papillomavirus type related DNA. J Invest Dermatol 1985; 84:417–420
69. De Villiers EM, Weidauer H, Otto H, et al. Papillomavirus DNA in human tongue carcinomas. Int J Cancer 1985; 36:575–578
70. Ostrow RS, Manias DA, Fong WJ, et al. A survey of human cancers for human papillomavirus DNA by filter hybridization, Cancer 1987; 59:429–438
71. Lookingbill DP, Kreider JW, Howett MK, et al. Human papillomavirus type 16 in bowenoid papulosis, intraoral papillomas, and squamous cell carcinoma of the tongue. Arch Dermatol 1987; 123:363–368
72. Mao EJ. Prevalence of human papillomavirus 16 and nucleolar organizer region counts in oral exfoliated cells from normal and malignent epithelia. Surg Oral Med Oral Pathol Oral Radiol Endod 1995; 80:320–329
73. Brandwein M, Zeitlin J, Nuovo GJ, et al. HPV detection using "hot start" polymerase chain reaction in patients with oral cancer: a clinicoopathological study of 64 patients. Mod Pathol 1994; 7:720–727
74. Polefsky JM, Silverman S, Abdel-Salaam M, et al. Association between proliferative verrucous leukoplakia and infection with human papillomavirus type 16. J Oral Pathol Med 1995; 24:193–197
75. Snijders P, Cruz I, Steenbergen R, et al. Human papillomavirus involvement in carcinomas of the oral cavity, Quebec. International Papillomavirus Workshop Abstract Book 1995; p. 12
76. Ostwald C, Muller P, Barten M, et al. Human papillomavirus DNA in oral squamous cell carcinomas and normal mucosa. J Oral Pathol Med 1994; 23:220–225
77. Balaram P, Nalinakumari KR, Abraham E, et al. Human papillomarivuses in 91 oral cancers from Indian betel quid chewers: high prevalence and multiplicity of infections. Int J Cancer 1995; 61:450–454
78. Adler-Storthz K, Newland JR, Tessin BA, et al. Identification of human papillomavirus types in oral verruca vulgaris. J Oral pathol 1986; 15:230–233
79. Howell RE, Gallant L. Human papillomvirus type 16 in an oral squamous carcinoma and its metastasis. Oral Surg Oral Med Oral Pathol 1992; 74:620–626
80. Scully C, Cox MF, Prime SS, et al. Papillomaviruses: the current status in relation to oral disease. Oral Surg Oral Med Oral Pathol 1988; 65:526–532
81. Kellokoski JK, Syrjanen SM, Chang F, et al. Southern blot hybridization and PCR in detection of oral human papillomavirus infections in women with genital HPV infections. J Oral Pathol Med 1992; 21:459–464
82. Jalal H, Sanders CM, Prime SS, et al. Detection of human papilloma virus type DNA in oral squames from normal young adults. J Oral Pathol Med 1992; 21:465–470
83. Dillner J. Immunobiology of papillomavirus. Prospect for vaccination. Cancer 1992; 5:181–187
84. Kwon-Chung KJ, Bennett JE. Medical Mycology. Philadelphia: Lea and Febiger, 1992; 20–44
85. Rippon JW. Medical mycology: the pathogenic fungi and the pathogenic actinomycetes. 3rd ed. Philadelphia: Saunders, 1988
86. Crissey T, Lany H, Parish LC. Manual of medical mycology. Cambridge: Blackwell Science, 1995
87. Rindum JL, Stenderup A, Holmstrup P. Identification of Candida albicans types related to healthy and pathological oral mucosa. J Oral Path Med 1994; 23:406–412
88. Odds FC. Candida and candidosis 2nd ed. London: Bailliere Tindall, 1988; 11–19
89. Senet J-M, Robert R. Physiopathologie des candidoses. J Mycol Mèd 1995; 5:145–166
90. Ruechel R. Virulence factors of Candida species. In: Samaranayake LP, MacFarlane TW (Eds) Oral candidosis. London: Wright, 1990; pp 47–65
91. Mooney MA, Thomas I, Sirois D. Oral candidosis. J Int Dermatol 1995; 34:759–765
92. Samaranayake LP. Oral mycoses in HIV infection. Oral Surg Oral Med Oral Pathol 1992; 73:171–180
93. Walker DM, Arendorf TM. Candidal leucoplakia, chronic multifocal candidosis and median rhomboid glossitis. In: Samaranayake LP, MacFarlane TW (Eds) Oral candidosis. London: Wright, 1990; pp 184–199
94. Wheat Lj, et al. A large urban outbreak of histoplasmosis: clinical features. Ann Intern Med 1982; 94: 331–335
95. Utz JP, Shadomy HJ. Deep fungal infections. In: Fitzpatrick TB, Eisen AZ, Wolff K, Freedberg IM, Austen KF (Eds) Dermatology in General Medicine, 3rd ed. New York: McGraw-Hill, 1987; 2248–2275
96. Miller RL, et al. Localized oral histoplasmosis. Oral Surg 1982; 53:367–70
97. Young LL, et al. Oral manifestations of histoplasmosis. Oral Surg 1972; 33:191–194
98. Toth BB, Frame RR. Oral histoplasmosis: diagnostic complication and treatment. Oral Surg 1983; 55:597–601
99. Migaki G, Valerio MG, Irvine B, Garner FM. Lobo's disease in an Atlantic bottle-nosed dolphin. J Am Vet Med Assoc 1971; 159:578–582
100. Gross ML, Millikan LE. Deep fungal infections in the tropics. Dermatologic Clinics 1994; 12:695–700
101. Sampaio MM. A note on the cultivation of the aetiological agent of Jorge Lobo's disease in 199 TC medium containing phytohaemagglutinin. Rev Inst Med Trop Sao Paulo 1974; 16:121–122
102. Silva D. Traitement de la maladie de Jorge Lobo par la clofazimine (B663). Bull Soc Pathol Exot 1978; 71:409–412
103. Almeida O, Jorge J, Scully C, Bozzo L. Oral manifestations of paracoccidioidomycosis (South American blastomycosis). Oral Surg 1991; 72:430–433
104. Franco M, Mendes RP, Moscardi-Bacchi M, et al. Paracoccidioidomycosis. Clin Trop Med Commun Dis 1989; 4:185–189
105. Page LR, Drummond JR, Daniels HT, et al. Blastomycosis with oral lesions. Oral Surg 1979; 47:157–161
106. Hauman CHJ, Raubenheimer EJ. Orofacial mucormycosis. Oral Surg, 1989; 68:624–627
107. Jones AC, Bentsen TY, Freedman PD. Mucormycosis of the oral cavity. Oral Surg 1993; 75:445–449
108. Laskaris G. Fungal infections. In: Laskaris G (ed) Color atlas of oral diseases, 2nd ed. New York: Thieme Medical, 1994; pp 164–173

Suggested Further Reading

Alyssa Kim Y, Schwartz R. The United States of America. In: Parish LC, Millikan LE (Eds). Global dermatology - diagnosis and management according to geography, climate, and culture. New York: Springer-Verlag, 1994; pp 45–50

Appel BN, Mendelow H, Pasqual HN. Acquired toxoplasma lymphadenitis. Oral Surg Oral Med Oral Pathol 1979; 47:529–32

Arenas R. Dermatologia. Atlas, diagnostico y tratamiento. 2nd ed. Mexico: McGraw-Hill Interamericana, 1996; pp 375–376, 548–549

Azulay RD, Azulay DR. Dermatologia. 2nd ed. Rio de Janeiro: Guanabara Koogan, 1997; pp 161, 232

Barsh LI. Molluscum contagiosum of the oral mucosa. Oral Surg Oral Med Oral Pathol 1996; 22:42–6

Bryceson ADM, Hay RJ. Parasitic worms and protozoa. In: Champion RH, Burton JL, Ebling FJG (Eds) Rock Wilkinson, Ebling Textbook of Dermatology. 5th ed. London: Blackwell Scientific 1994; pp 1217–64.

Caumes E. Dermatoses virales generalités. In: Piérard GE, Caumes E, Franchimont C, Arrese Estrada JA (Eds) Dermatologie tropicale. Brussels: Éditions de l'Université de Bruxelles, 1993; pp 81–3

Caumes E. Pox viruses. In: Piérard GE, Caumes E, Franchimont C, Arrese Estrada JA. (Eds) Dermatologie tropicale. Brussels: Éditions de l'Université de Bruxelles, 1993; pp 103–7

Caumes E, Danis M. Trypanosomiases. In: Piérard GE, Caumes E, Franchimont C, Arrese Estrada JA (Eds) Dermatologie tropicale. Brussels: Éditions de l'Université de Bruxelles, 1993; pp 335–40

Cawson RA, Binnie WH, Eveson JW. Color atlas of oral disease. Clinical and pathologic correlations. 2nd ed. Hong Kong: Wolfe, 1993; pp 13.4, 18.20–21

Farah FS, Klaus SN, Frankenburg S, Klion AD, Nutman TB. Protozoan and helminth infection. In: Fitzpatrick TB, Eisen AZ, Wolff K, Freedberg JM, Austen KF (Eds) Dermatology in general medicine. 4th ed. New York: McGraw-Hill, 1993; pp 2769–87

Fujita WH, Barr RJ, Gottschalk HR. Cutaneous amebiasis. Arch Dermatol 117(5):309–10

Fulginiti VA. Smallpox and complications of smallpox vaccination. In: Fitzpatrick TB, Eisen AZ, Wolff K, Freedberg JM, Austen KF. Dermatology in general medicine. 4th ed. New York: MacGraw-Hill, 1993; pp 2596–602

Grassi L Jr, Gatti R, Carneri I. Protozoosi orali rilevate nel 1984 all'ospedale Niguarda-Ca' Granda, Milano. Ann Ist Super Sanita, 22(1):249–52

Greer KE, Sheap CN. A family outbreak of oral accidental vaccinia. Arch Dermatol 1974: 110(1):107–8

Grossetê G. Amibiase cutanéee. In: Piérard GE, Caumes E, Franchimont C, Arrese Estrada JA (Eds). Dermatologie tropicale. Brussels: Éditions de l'Université de Bruxelles, 1993; pp 341–2

Gundersen SG, Bjorvatn B. Vaccinia and topical steroids: a case report. Acta Derm Venereol (Stockh) 1980; 60(5):445–7

Harman R. Toxoplasmosis. In: Canizares O, Harman R. Clinical tropical dermatology. 2nd ed. Boston: Blackwell Scientific, 1992; pp 322–3

Highet AS, Kurtz J. Viral infections. In: Champion RH, Burton JL, Ebling FJG (Eds) Rock Wilkinson, Ebling textbook of dermatology. 5th ed. London: Blackwell Scientific, 1992; pp 867–951

Kerdel-Vegas F. American trypanosomiasis. In: Champion RH, Burton JL, Ebling FJG (Eds) Rock Wilkinson, Ebling textbook of dermatology. 5th ed. London: Blackwell Scientific, 1992; pp 1250–1

Knobler R. Human immunodeficiency virus infection. Dermatol Clin 1989; 7:369–85

Laskaris G. Color atlas of oral diseases. Stuttgart: Thieme, 1988; pp 100–16

Lowy DR. Milker's nodules and molluscum contagiosum. In: Fitzpatrick TB, Eisen AZ, Wolff K, Freedberg JM, Austen KF (Eds) Dermatology in general medicine. 4th ed. New York: McGraw-Hill 1993; pp 2606–10

Lyons T, Scholten T, Palmer JC, Stanfield E. Oral amoebiasis: alternatives in oral disease. Ont Dent 1982; 59(2):16–20

Magaña Lozano M, Magañana-Garcia M. Cutaneous amebiasis. In: Canizares O, Harman R (Eds) Clinical tropical dermatology. 2nd ed. Boston: Blackwell Scientific, 1992; pp 278–82

Nocodemo EL, Nicodemo AC, Amato Neto V, Sampaio S. American trypanosomiasis (Chagas' disease). In: Canizares O, Harman R (Eds) Clinical tropical dermatology. 2nd ed. Boston: Blackwell Scientific, 1992; pp 286–92

Paul M, Abeyaratne M. Cutaneous amebiasis. Br J Surg, 1961; 49: 288–91

Praetorius-Clausen F. Rare oral viral disorders (molluscum contagiosum, localized keratoacanthoma, verrucae condyloma acuminatum, and focal epithelial hyperplasia). Oral Surg Oral Med Oral Pathol, 1972; 34:2606–10

Richman TB, Kerdel FA. Amebiasis and trypanosomiasis. Dermatol Clin, 1989; 7:301–11

Schaller KF (Ed). Color atlas of tropical dermatology and venereology. Berlin: Springer-Verlag, 1994; pp 103–14

Scully C, Flint SR, Porter SR. Oral diseases. 2 ed. Singapore: Martin Dunitz, 1996; p 99

Whitaker SB, Wiegand SE, Budnick SD. Intraoral molluscum contagiosum. Oral Surg Oral Med Oral Pathol 1991; 72:334–6

CHAPTER 8

Tropical Pathology of the Oral Mucosa

C. Zaitz and M. Ramos-e-Silva

8.1 Paracoccidioidomycosis (South American Blastomycosis, Brazilian Blastomycosis, or Lutz's Mycosis)

Definition. Paracoccidioidomycosis is a rural endemic condition that mainly affects male manual workers (15:1) between the ages of 29 and 40 years, being rare in children. The sites involved are the lungs, oral, nasal, and gastrointestinal mucous membranes and the lymphatic system [1, 2].

Etiology. *Paracoccidioides brasiliensis* is a saprophytic dimorphic fungus. It is a eukariotic cell with a chitin wall, that likes humid places with land rich in proteic material and minimal temperature variation. It has been isolated from sand in endemic areas. Man is its only natural host, and it is found in Central America and in South America, with the exception of Chile.

Pathogenesis. Invasion is mainly pulmonary by spore inhalation, but there are reports of cutaneous, oral, and anogenital mucosal inoculation. Man-to-man transmission is unknown, and familial cases are rare. Dissemination occurs by either the lymphatic or the hematogenous route or by contiguity.

The immunological state of the patient will determine the degree of severity of the disease. Depending on this immunological response, the patient will have the infection without disease; benign, localized disease that can be cured spontaneously; or severe, chronic, generalized disease, which is the most common form [3–6].

Oral Manifestations. In the mucous membranes, especially the mouth, the characteristic lesion is an erythematous ulcer with hemorrhagic and granular dots (Figs. 8.1, 8.2). Macrocheilitis, infiltrations, and vegetations can also be present (Figs. 8.3, 8.4) Sialorrhea is frequent.

Associated Findings. Cutaneous inoculation is very rare. Most skin lesions occur by either hematogenous or lymphatic dissemination, and they take the form of papules, tubercles, vegetations, or ulcers. At the base of the ulcer, hemorrhagic dots like those on oral ulcers can be seen. Regional or generalized adenopathy is usually present and the lymph nodes develop fistulas. Pulmonary paracoccidioidomycosis occurs in 90 % of cases, affecting both lower half of the lungs, and in 12 % of cases there is an association with tuberculosis. Besides the skin, other organs commonly involved are: gastrointestinal system, liver, spleen, central nervous system, and adrenals.

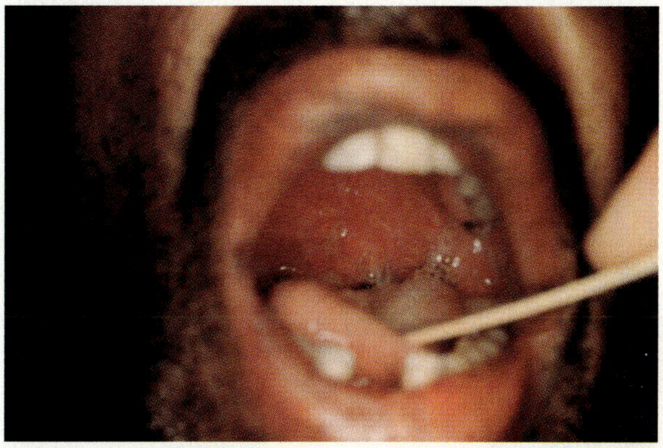

Fig. 8.1. Paracoccidioidomycosis. Erythematous ulcer with hemorrhagic dots on the palate

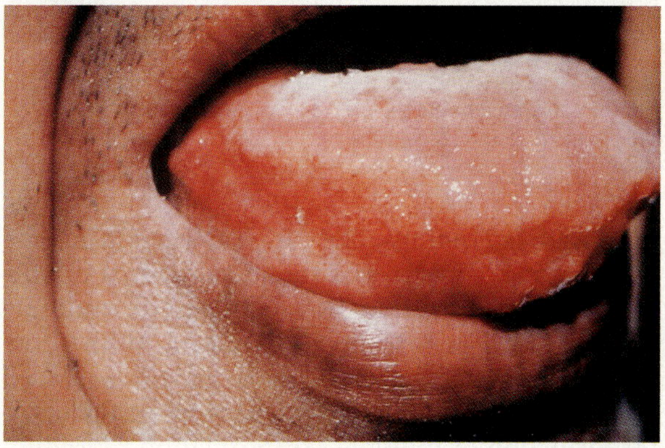

Fig. 8.2. Paracoccidioidomycosis: erythematous ulcer with hemorrhagic dots on the tongue

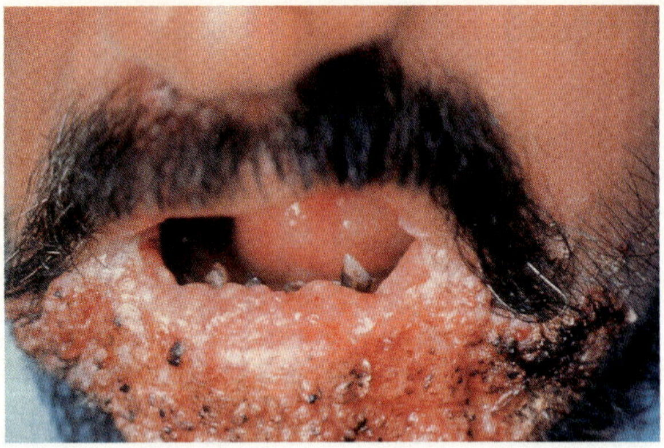

Fig. 8.3. Paracoccidioidomycosis macrocheilitis, infiltration, and vegetation on the lip

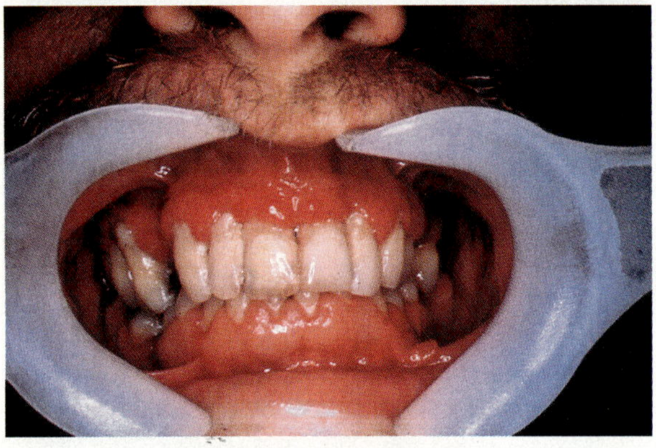

Fig. 8.4. Paracoccidioidomycosis gingivitis and erythema of the oral mucous membrane

Microscopic Findings. The parasite, when inside the lymph node, appears as a round cell with a double refringent wall, with or without single or multiple budding, and is 5–25 µm in diameter. With some stains other than hematoxylin-eosin, the so-called pilot wheel aspect can be seen because of the cryptosporulation or multiple exosporulation reproduction of the fungus.

The histopathological structure, a uniform pattern in all affected organs, is similar to that in other inflammatory chronic diseases, differing in the finding of the fungus better seen with silver methenamine or PAS stains. This paracoccidioidic granuloma is an immunospecific tissue response type IV or cellular hypersensitivity reaction against the fungal antigens that destroy or block it; it has a tuberculoid pattern, showing foreign body- and Langhans-type giant multinucleated cells, sometimes very numerous, of variable sizes. The fungus inside giant cells can be degenerated, latent, or in active reproduction by way of simple or multiple budding.

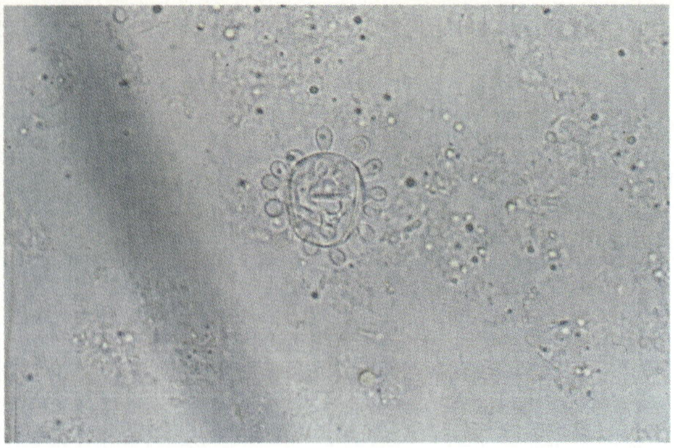

Fig. 8.5. Paracoccidioidomycosis: round forms with a double contour membrane. "Pilot wheel" appearance. Direct examination

Diagnosis. A clinical diagnosis can be confirmed by mycological examination (both direct and culture) and histopatholgy. The paracoccidioidin test can be of some aid.

Direct examing of materials from the lesions reveals round forms, with a double contour membrane, single or multiple budding) and sometimes a pilot wheel appearance (Fig. 8.5). In agar-Sabouraud and agar-blood at room temperature, growth of a white colony adherent to the medium is slow (20–30 days). The microscopy of these colonies shows thin septated mycelial filaments with terminal or intercalated spores. At 37 °C, mainly in enriched media, the colony acquires a cerebriform or leveduriform surface and microscopic examination reveals round cells similar to those found in tissues.

Histopathology shows the granuloma, and with Grocott and PAS stains, the fungi can be easily visualized. The paracoccidioidin test can be useful, but it is also positive in silent infection [7–13].

Differential Diagnosis. Sometimes it is difficult to differentiate paracoccidioidomycosis from leishmaniasis, cutaneous tuberculosis, and lethal midline granuloma on clinical examination, but laboratory studies usually confirm the diagnosis.

Treatment. Among sulfonamides, sulfamethoxipyridazine, 500–1000 mg per day, can be used for 2 years. Intravenous amphotericin B, which is reserved for severe cases, is given daily or on alternate days in glucose, as a slow infusion over several hours. The total dose is 2–4 g.

Oral and daily administration of ketoconazole, 200–400 mg, fluconazole, 150–300 mg, or itraconazole, 200–400 mg, is also effective.

8.2 Myiasis

Definition. Myiasis is an infestation of any part of the skin and mucous membrane by the larvae of Diptera, especially flies. It is mainly a disease of domestic animals, but it can accidentally infest man [14–19].

Etiology. There are two types of cutaneous myiasis: the cavitary form, caused mostly by the genera *Chrysomyia, Calliphora, Lucilia, Musca, Phormia, Sarcophaga*, and *Wohlfahrtia*, and the furunculoid form, produced by the genera *Hypoderma, Gasterophilus, Dermatobia, Callitroga, Chrysomyia*, and *Cordylobia*.

Pathogenesis. In cavitary myiasis, the larvae infest decaying flesh. Furunculoid myiasis affects living flesh. The parasite is an obligatory myiasis producer, because its larvae need to parasitize skin for its biological cycle to be completed. In Central and South America, the species most frequently responsible for furunculoid myiasis is *Dermatobia hominis*.

Oral Manifestations. Cavitary myiasis shows many larvae in suppurating tissues that show marked destruction. Sometimes, it also affects the upper respiratory tract. There are mild to severe constitutional symptoms and eosinophilia.

In furunculoid myiasis there are one or more papules or nodules. Each of them has at least one larva inside (Figs. 8.6, 8.7). There is discrete discomfort, pruritus, and slight movement of the larva at the opening of the lesion can be observed.

Associated Findings. If there is infestation in other areas, the findings observed are analogous to those observed in the case of oral infestation (Fig. 8.8).

Diagnosis. Cavitary myiasis is diagnosed by the finding of multiple larvae in ulcers. Furunculoid myiasis is diagnosed by observation of the movement of the single larva at the opening of the lesion.

Differential Diagnosis. Both cavitary and furunculoid myiasis are easily diagnosed by the finding of the larva or observation of its movement. When there are a few larvae in cavitary myiasis and they are not found promptly, the lesion looks like an ulcer, sometimes very extensive.

Treatment. Removal of all larvae is the most important objective of treatment. In the case of cavitary myiasis, they can be removed by the application of ether, which makes the larva come out, and extraction with a fine forceps. Furunculoid myiasis can be extracted either by pressure with the fingers or by the application of a thick layer of solid vaseline: the larva comes out and into the vaseline, leaving the skin. In rural areas, people apply a piece of pork fat on top of the lesion, for the same effect. In more difficult cases, it can be removed by surgery.

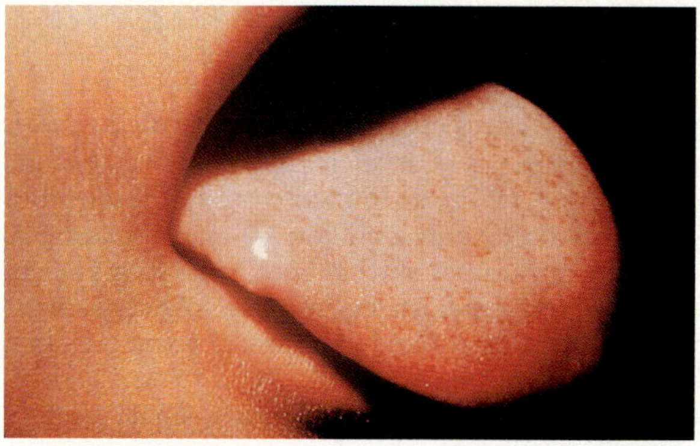

Fig. 8.6. Furunculoid myiasis. Nodule with larva inside on the tongue. Courtesy of Dr. Alberto Eduardo Cox Cardoso, Maceió, Brazil

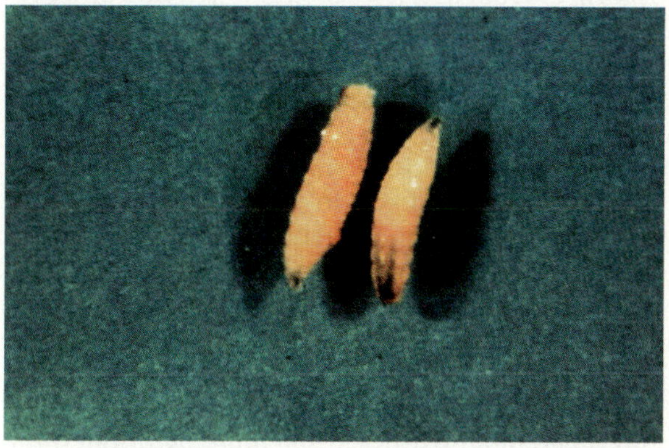

Fig. 8.7. Furunculoid myiasis: two larvae

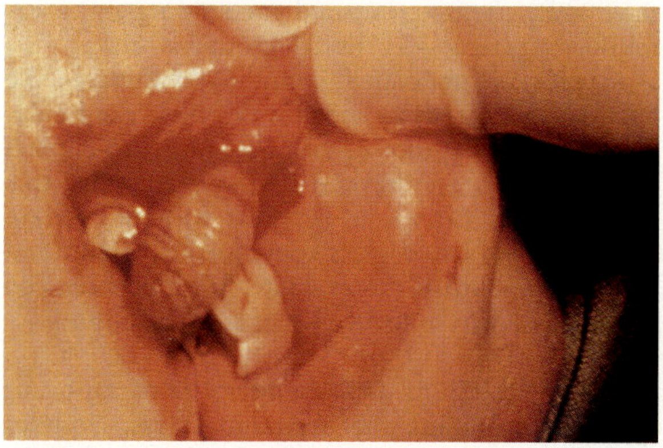

Fig. 8.8. Furunculoid myiasis: nodule with larvae on the cheek. Courtesy of Dr. Ivo Bussoloti Filho, São Paulo, Brazil

8.3 Leprosy (Hansen's Disease)

Definition. Leprosy is a chronic curable disease with a good prognosis with reference to survival, but incapacitating. Of the 20 million cases in the world, it is estimated that only 2 million are under treatment. Over the centuries, there has been wide geographical variation in its incidences, but it is now considered endemic in tropical and subtropical areas [20–27].

Etiology. *Mycobacterium leprae* is a small, slightly curved rod that turns red on Gram and acid-fast Ziehl-Neelsen staining. It is an intracytoplasmic parasite of macrophages, in which it can be isolated or form globoid masses, called globi, in skin and peripheral nerves, sparing the central nervous system. It only affects humans, although it has been found and reproduced in the armadillo, monkey, and mouse.

Pathogenesis. The incubation period is long, 2–7 years. Bacilli are spread in through nasal droplets or from open lesions of bacilliferous patients, passing into the nasal mucosa or into open lesions on the skin of healthy individuals. In 1966, Ridley and Jopling classified leprosy, based on the notion of polar forms first described by Rabello (1953), into lepromatous leprosy at one end of the spectrum and tuberculoid leprosy at the other, with the three types of borderline leprosy in between: one tending to the immune-depressed end, the BL group, one in the middle, the BB group and one tending to the immunocompetent side, the BT group.

Specific cell-mediated immunity eliminates the bacilli in most people, and this response can be detected by the lepromine test. Because the clinical form depends on the late immune reaction, this can cause the disease to progress without restrain to limit itself or to regress spontaneously. Humoral immunity is difficult to evaluate, but it is enhanced in forms that have low cell-mediated response.

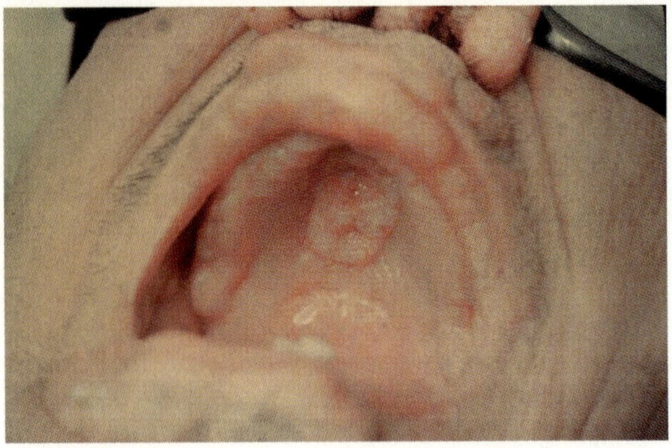

Fig. 8.9. Leproma on the hard palate. Courtesy of Dr. Sinésio Talhari, Manaus, Brazil

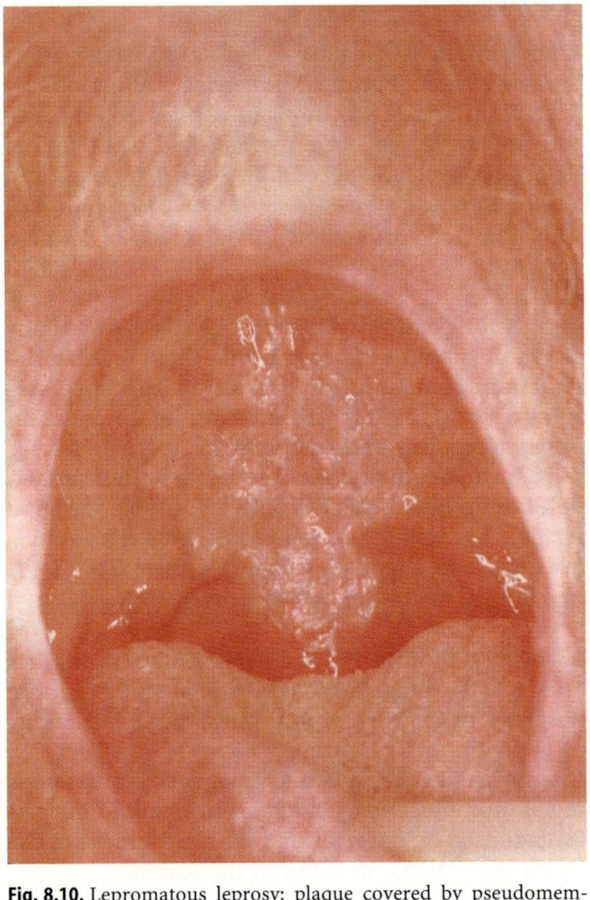

Fig. 8.10. Lepromatous leprosy: plaque covered by pseudomembranous material on the palate. Courtesy of Dr. Ivo Bussoloti Filho, São Paulo, Brazil

Oral Manifestations. Oral manifestations can occur in the lepromatous and borderline form. Nodules (lepromas), plaques, papules, and ulcers can be present. The main sites are the hard and soft palate, the dorsal aspect of the tongue, the lips, and the gingiva (Figs. 8.9, 8.10) [21].

Associated Findings. All forms affect skin and present thickened nerves, alterations in sensitivity to pain, temperature and touch, and motor, trophic, vasomotor, and secretory disturbances.

Lepromatous leprosy, which is the most contagious form, is characterized by multiple erythematous macules, papules, nodules, and plaques. There are ill-defined borders, usually bilateral with a tendency to symmetry. Patients sometimes have bilateral infiltration of the earlobes, madarosis, and desquamation of the legs.

The tuberculoid form shows few lesions and can be only neural. Lesions are papular or plaque-like, with well-defined borders and depressed centers.

They are usually hypopigmented in black skin, and erythematous in white skin. Lesions are usually hairless, and unilateral bone reabsorption may be present.

The borderline form has features in between the lepromatous and tuberculoid forms. It is asymmetrical. Unilateral earlobe infiltration may occur. The severity of skin and nerve alterations (Fig. 8.11) depends which end of the spectrum the patient's disease is (BL, BB, or BT). Hair also does not grow on the lesion.

Microscopic Findings. There are three basic histopathological structures: the lepromatous, the tuberculoid, and the borderline structure. Lepromatous structure shows an infiltrate in the dermis, hypodermis, and internal organs, with Virchow cells which are macrophages with many bacilli and lipid drops in their cytoplasm. On hematoxylin-eosin staining, these cells have a foamy appearance. Bacilli, isolated or in globi, can be detected by Ziehl-Neelsen or Wade staining (Fig. 8.12). Sudan III and Scarlet R can show the fat inside the Virchow cells. A normal aspect band, called the Unna band, separates the epidermis from the infiltrate composed of lymphocytes and plasmocytes.

The tuberculoid structure has a dermal infiltrate that can touch the epidermis, showing an aspect of nodules of epithelioid cells. There are lymphocytes at the edges and Langhans giant cells at the center of the granuloma.

The borderline structure shows features of Virchow cell infiltrate (LL) and of tuberculoid granuloma (TT). The predominance of one or the other of these depends if it is the BL, BB, or BT. There can be three histopathological situations in this form: in the first, the patient has some lesions with lepromatous structure and others with tuberculoid structure; in the second, there are Virchow and tuberculoid areas in the same biopsy, and the third has a mixed structure of foamy and epithelioid cells.

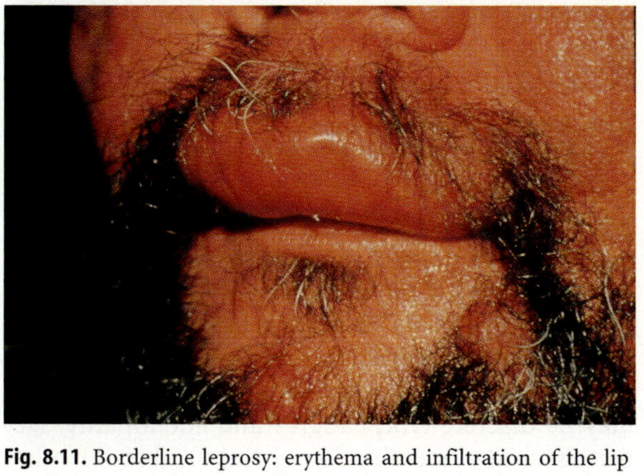

Fig. 8.11. Borderline leprosy: erythema and infiltration of the lip

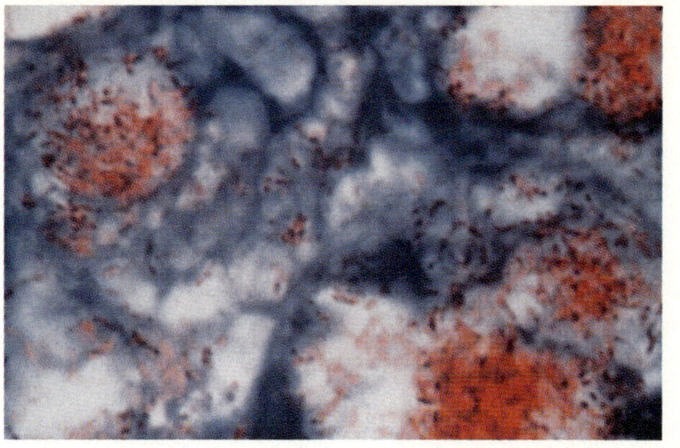

Fig. 8.12. Wade staining shows many mycobacteria leprae

All three forms of leprosy show alteration in the nervous structures in the skin.

Diagnosis. The diagnosis of the disease and its forms is made by the finding of the bacilli in cutaneous lymph and nasal secretion. Ziehl-Neelsen stain is used and only the presence of globi is diagnostic. They are found in 100 % of lepromatous leprosy, in 75 % of borderline, and in only 5 % of tuberculoid cases.

Other tests used are evaluation of sensitivity to heat, pain, and touch, the histamine, pilocarpine and Mitsuda test, which is all intradermal reaction read 21–28 days after the injection, and which can also be positive in 80 % of the general population older than 19 years in endemic areas.

In addition, a skin and sometimes a nerve biopsy are performed for diagnosis, and there are other tests that can be used.

Differential Diagnosis. Oral manifestations of leprosy can be diagnosed as lymphoma, tertiary syphilis, and lethal midline granuloma. Features on other sites and the biopsy are usually diagnostic.

Treatment. Multidrug therapy is used, as recommended by the World Health Organization. Bacilloscopy is performed in three to five different sites on the skin. The patient is considered paucibacillary if no bacillus is found, and is then treated with rifampicin (600 mg/month) and dapsone (100 mg/day) for 6 months. If there are one or more bacilli, the patient takes rifampicin (600 mg/month), dapsone (100 mg/day), and clofazimine (300 mg/month plus 50 mg/day) for 2 years. Some new drugs in different combinations such as pefloxacin (800 mg/day), ofloxacin (400 mg/day), claritromycin (500 mg/day), and minocycline (100 mg/day), are still in the research stage.

8.4 Mucocutaneous Leishmaniasis

Definition. Leishmaniasis is an infectious disease that affects mainly skin, mucous membranes, and lymph node. Usually, it does not affect the internal organs or the central nervous system [28–35].

Etiology. The condition is caused by a protozoa of the genus *Leishmania*. Transmission occurs through the bite of an infected female mosquito, mainly of the genera *Phlebotomus* and *Lutzomya*. The species classification of the genus *Leishmania* is still controversial. Some have suggested than one species causes different clinical forms, while others classify this genus into various species, each one causing a particular form of the disease: cutaneous, muco-cutaneous, visceral (Kala-azar), and anergic.

Pathogenesis. The clinical classification is made with reference to the type of lesion and the species of *Leishmania* and *mosquito* involved. The immunological state of the patient, the evolution, and the prognosis of leishmaniasis also depend basically on the cell-mediated response which, depending on its state, may lead to a clinical and even biological cure or to more severe forms.

There are two types of transmission: the sylvestral, in which the reservoirs are wild animals and humans become infected when they enter the forests and are bitten by mosquitos, and the urban type, where the biological cycle occurs in the domiciliary or peridomiciliary area and the reservoir is the sick person or a domestic animal.

The promastigote, the flagellated or leptomonad form, is transmitted to animals or healthy humans by the female mosquito which needs warm blood to mature its ovarian follicles. In the affected person or animal, it develops into the amastigote or ovoid aflagellated form, called the leishmania, which can again be transmitted to a female mosquito. This is the form found in the tissues.

Oral Manifestations. Mucous membranes can also be affected after hematogenous dissemination. The mouth, nose, larynx, and pharynx are mostly involved (Figs. 8.13–8.16). There are infiltrative, ulcerous, vegetating, and atrophic-crusted lesions. Infiltration of the upper lip and nasal region give a tapiroid appearance. Parrot beak-like nose is caused by partial destruction of the subseptum. A gangosiform aspect is present when oral and nasal cavities combine into a single cavity. Deforming osteoarthritis occurs with severe ulcero-cicatricial involvement [30, 31].

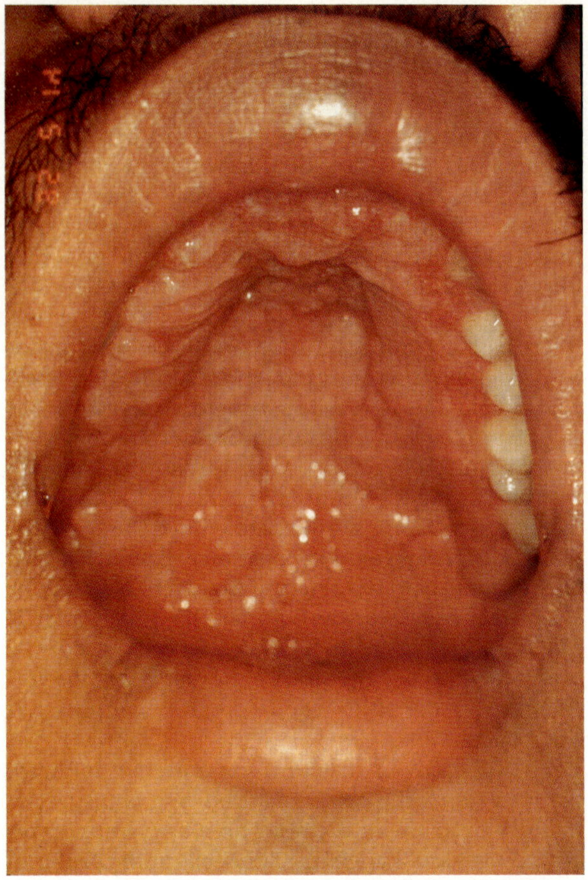

Fig. 8.13. Mucocutaneous leishmaniasis: infiltration of the palate

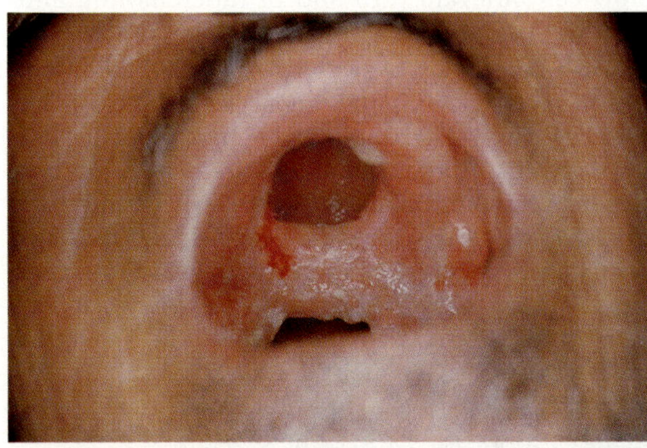

Fig. 8.14. Mucocutaneous leishmaniasis: destruction of the palate. Oral and nasal cavities have become combined into a single cavity

Associated Findings. There is an incubation period, ranging from 3 weeks to many months, before a lesion appears at the site of inoculation. The predilection site is the leg. There can be an erythematous area, edema, papule, tubercle, or ulcer, ranging from millimeters to centimeters in size, and there may be discrete lymphangitis and adenopathy. Hematogenous dissemination is responsible for other

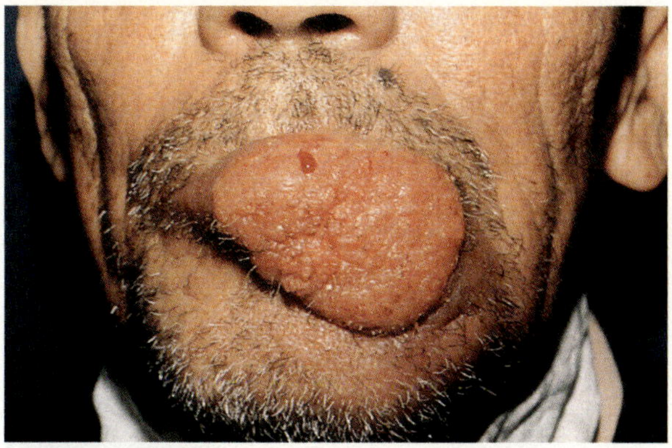

Fig. 8.15. Mucocutaneous leishmaniasis: tongue with infiltrative and vegetating aspect

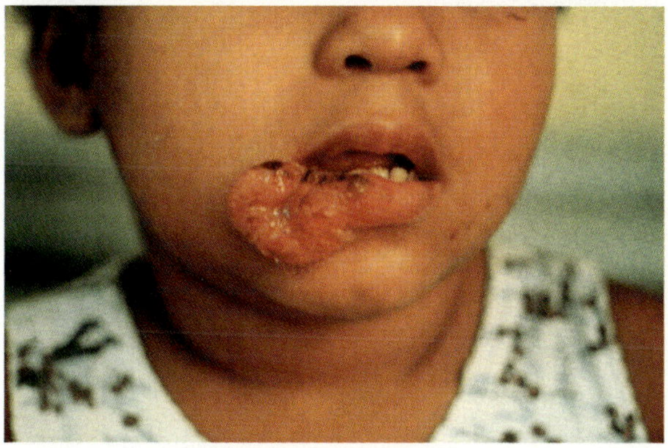

Fig. 8.16. Mucocutaneous leishmaniasis: vegetating and infiltrative lesion on the lip

skin lesions, called leishmanids, variable in number and size, which are papulo-crusted, ulcero-crusted, papulo-follicular, tuberous, or vegetating.

Microscopic Findings. The characteristic finding is a granulomatous structure with leishmania in macrophages.

Diagnosis. Laboratory examinations should be performed when the clinical aspect of the lesion and the patient's origin suggest this diagnosis. Direct examination using Giemsa stain will show amastigota formed inside macrophages in 100 % of smears taken from recent lesions. Culture is performed in NNN medium in which promastigota or leptomonas, the flagellated form, grow. Histopathology can be diagnostic if very small oval structures are observed inside the macrophages: amastigotes or the ovoid form of the parasite (Fig. 8.17).

The Montenegro test, an intradermal reaction of a suspension of leptomonas or antigenic fractions of leishmania and read after 48–72 h will be positive forever after inoculation. Indirect immunofluorescence reveals anti-*Leishmania* and anti-*Trypanosoma cruiz* antibodies as a cross reaction.

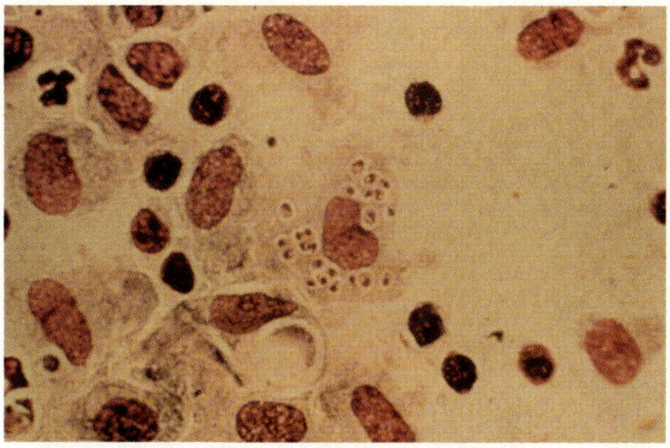

Fig. 8.17. Mucocutaneous leishmaniasis: amastigota or ovoid forms of the parasite inside the macrophages

Differential Diagnosis. Paracoccidioidomycosis, squamous cell carcinoma, lethal midline granuloma, and Wegener's granuloma can be differentiated by biopsy and the finding of leishmania.

Treatment. Glucantime, an antimonial, in a dosage of 0.1 g/kg per day IM or IV in two cycles of 30 days 2 weeks apart, is still the medication used for leishmaniasis. For more severe cases, amphotericin B, 1 mg/kg per day in dextrose as a very slow IV injection, with a maximum total dose of 2 g , is used. More recently two newer drugs: intramuscular pentamidine, an aromatic diamine, 2.5 mg/kg used in ten daily or alternate-day doses, and oral itraconazole, in a dosage of 400 mg/day, have been used with very good results. Another one, paromycin, is still in trials for topical and systemic use.

8.5 Donovanosis (Granuloma Venereum, Granuloma Inguinale)

Definition. Donovanosis is a sexually transmitted disease that is found in tropical and subtropical regions and affects mostly the anal and genital areas (Fig. 8.18) [36–41].

Etiology. The causative agent is a gram-negative intestinal saprophyte, *Calymmatobacterium (Donovania) granulomatis.*

Pathogenesis. In general, but not exclusively, this is regarded as a sexually transmitted disease mainly of homosexual men with low socio-economic level of 20–45 years of age. Hematogenous dissemination is rare.

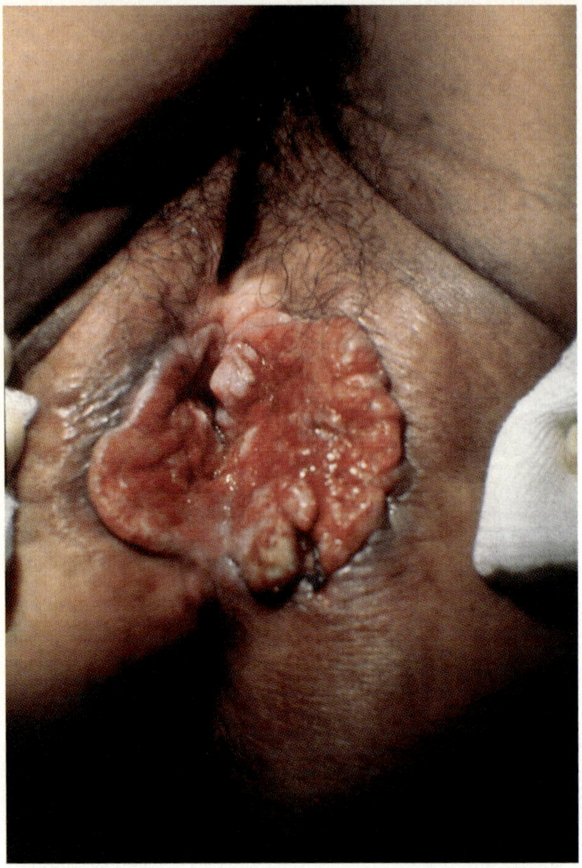

Fig. 8.18. Donovanosis: ulcerated and vegetating lesion in the anal region. Courtesy of Dr. Cleide Ishida, Rio de Janeiro, Brazil

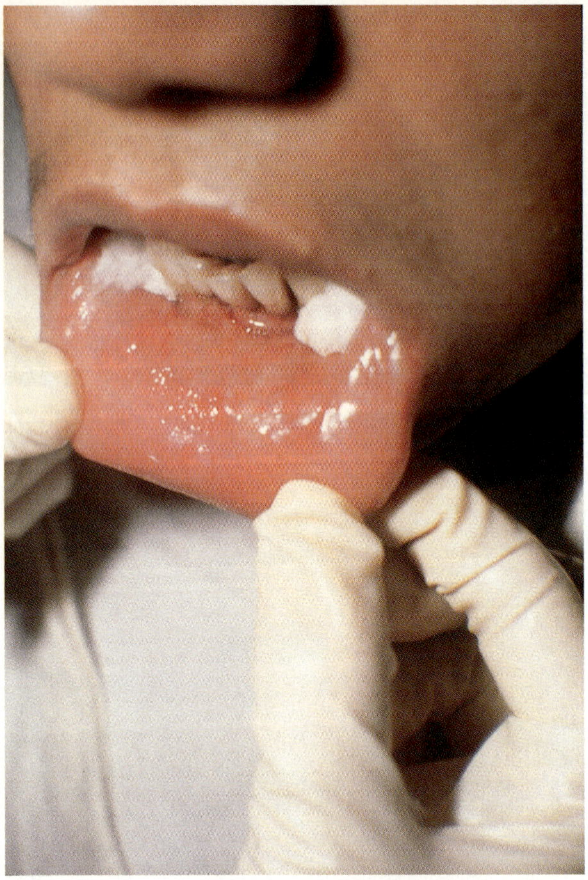

Fig. 8.20. Donovanosis: Irregular ulcer on the oral mucous membrane of the lip. Courtesy of Dr- Cleide Ishida, Rio de Janeiro, Brazil

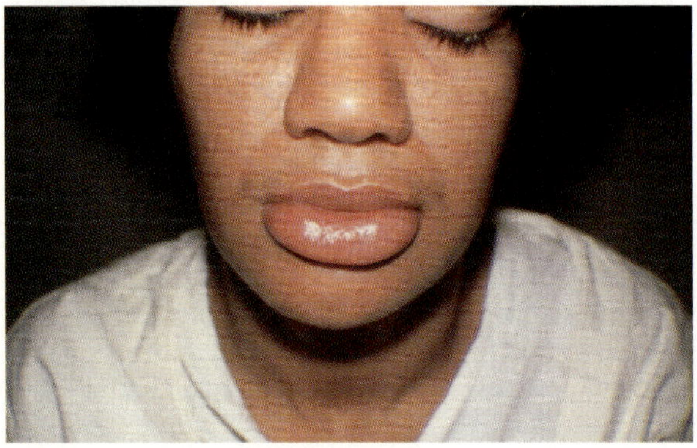

Fig. 8.19. Donovanosis: infiltration of the lip. Courtesy of Dr. Cleide Ishida, Rio de Janeiro, Brazil

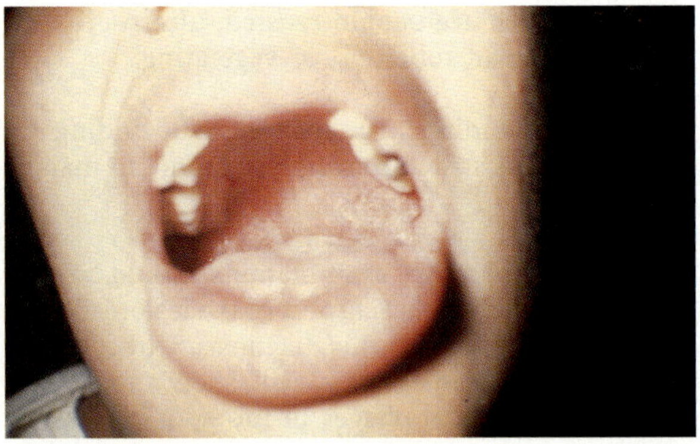

Fig. 8.21. Donovanosis: irregular ulcers on the palate. Courtesy of Dr. Cleide Ishida, Rio de Janeiro, Brazil

Oral Manifestations. Oral manifestations are very rare. Unilateral, chronic, progressive, and indolent ulcers with satellite lesions caused by autoinoculation are the characteristic findings. The initial lesion is a small indurated nodule that soon ulcerates and becomes a painless shallow ulcer, with some vegetation, that easily bleeds. There is a serous exudate and destructive lesions can achieve a size of many centimeters (Figs. 8.19–8.22) [37].

Associated Findings. In men, it generally affects the prepuce, glans or anal area, and in women, the labia

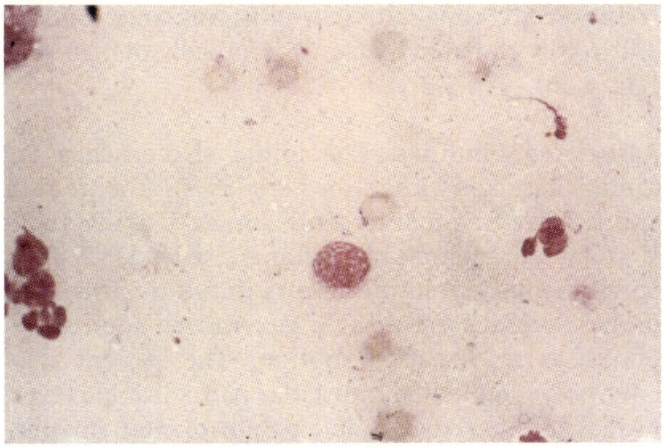

Fig. 8.22. Calymmatobacteria (Donovania) granulomatis

minora or majora and, less frequently, the inguinal and anal regions. There is no adenopathy and sometimes elephantiasis of the scrotum or esthiomene occurs, resulting from the cicatricial process.

Microscopic Findings. In histopathology, small rods can be found inside the macrophages.

Diagnosis. The diagnosis is confirmed by the finding of the agent on direct examination with either Giemsa or Wright staining. Inoculation of the material in the vitellin sac of chicken embryo can be performed.

Differential Diagnosis. Oral syphilitic chancre, ulcerous tuberculosis, and squamous cell carcinoma are easily excluded when the agent is found.

Treatment. Streptomycin, 1–2 g/day for 10–20 days, tetracycline, 2 g/day for 15–20 days or sulfamethoxazol, 800 mg, and trimethoprim, 160 mg, twice a day for 15–30 days are used. Erythromycin, gentamicin, minocycline, ampicillin, and other drugs can also be employed in the case of allergy.

8.6 Syphilis

Definition. Syphilis is an exclusively human treponemal venereal disease that leads to both cutaneous and internal lesions [24–48].

Etiology. The agent is a flagellated and very mobile spirochete, *Treponema pallidum*, which is morphologically and serologically identical to other treponemas.

Pathogenesis. Transmission can be sexual, congenital, or by other contacts. There is no predilection for either sex, and it is universal, with a higher incidence in the tropical areas because of the low socio-economic level. Its incidence depends on human sexual behavior. Penetration occurs through mucous and semimucous membranes. There are two forms, each with various phases: sexually transmitted, with recent (primary and secondary), latent, and late (tertiary) phases, and congenital, with recent and late phases.

The initial lesions are caused by cellular and vascular responses to the agent. These lesions disappear, and usually 2–3 months or more later there is an immunocomplex deposition, which causes a generalized eruption. The late phase is characterized by an intense hypersensitivity reaction.

Oral Manifestations. Oral lesions can appear in all phases. In the recent part of the primary phase, if the inoculation site was the oral mucosa, a typical chancre appears 3–4 weeks after penetration, as a round, painless, superficial ulcer with a raised and indurated border (Figs. 8.23, 8.24). During the secondary period of the recent phase, mucous patches may be present (Fig. 8.25). Gummatous ulcers, the

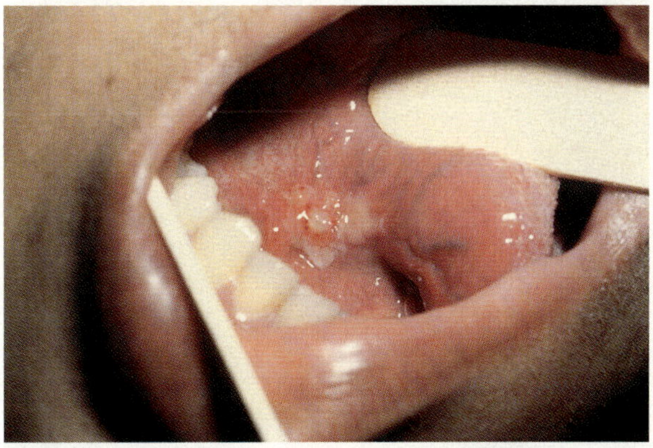

Fig. 8.23. Recent syphilis, primary period: chancre, a round ulcer with an indurated border on the oral mucosa

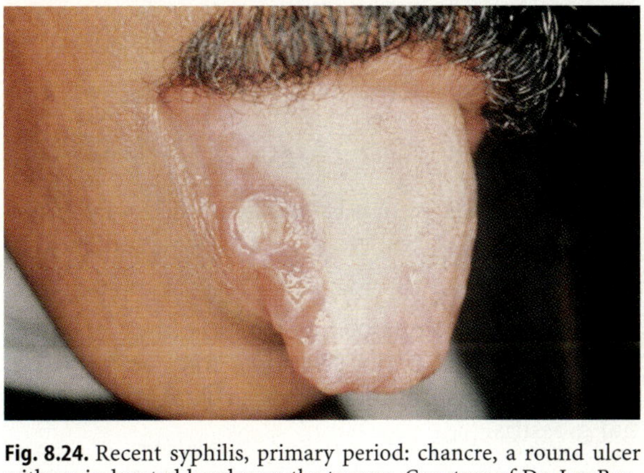

Fig. 8.24. Recent syphilis, primary period: chancre, a round ulcer with an indurated border on the tongue. Courtesy of Dr. Ivo Bussoloti Filho, São Paulo, Brazil

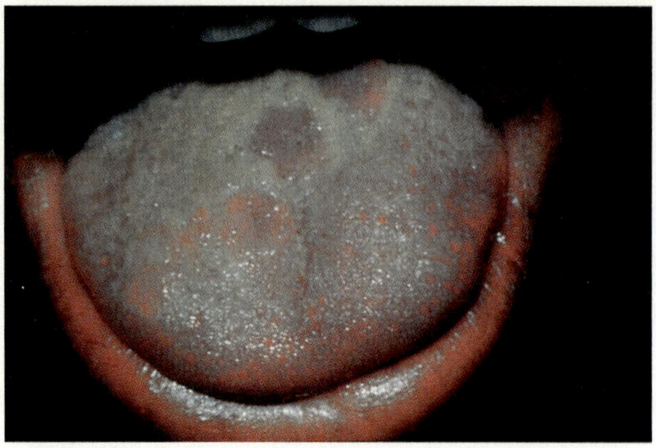

Fig. 8.25. Recent syphilis, secondary period: mucous patches on the tongue. Courtesy of Dr. Iphis Campbell, Brasilia, Brazil

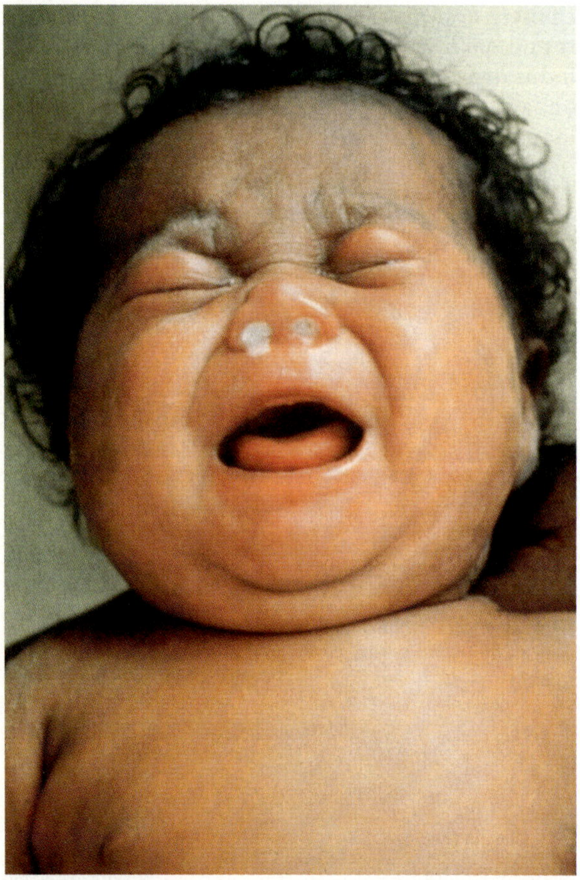

Fig. 8.26. Recent congential syphilis: mucous patches and oral radiated fissures

characteristic lesions of late syphilis, may occur in the mouth during this phase, as may leukoplakia, hard palate perforation, and superficial and interstitial glossitis.

In recent congenital syphilis, mucous patches and oral radiated fissures can all be present (Fig. 8.26) [45].

Associated Findings. The initial chancre has the same characteristics elsewhere as in the mouth and is more frequent in genital areas. Usually, there is bilateral, painless, regional polyadenopathy. Spontaneous involution occurs in 1–4 months. Secondary syphilis arises as a generalized monomorphous asymptomatic eruption. The patient may have polyadenopathy, muscular pain, discrete fever, headache, pharyngitis, and palmo-plantar involvement. This generalized eruption, called syphilides, can be erythematous (roseola), papular, papulodesquamative (psoriasiform), or follicular (lichenoid). In this phase, patchy alopecia, anal and genital lesions (condylomata lata), madarosis, and paronychia may occur. The late phase is characterized by nodular and/or gummatous lesions on the skin and skeletal, eye, cardiovascular, and nervous system involvement.

Congenital syphilis, when transmitted early in pregnancy, causes abortion of the fetus or its death at birth. If transmission occurs later in pregnancy, the affected children are underweight and pale. A bullous eruption, particularly of the palmoplantar regions, may be followed by a generalized maculopapular or papulopustular eruption. In its late phase, there are gummatous and nodular lesions, painful bone involvement, keratitis, deafness, and articular alterations. Severe active congenital syphilis may lead to characteristic signs: saddle nose, Hutchinson teeth, high-arched palate, atrophy of upper maxilla, mulberry molars, and others.

Microscopic Findings. Histopathology in early syphilis may reveal some treponema around walls and an intense vasculitis with a dense infiltrate of lymphocytes and plasmocytes. Usually, during the secondary period, treponema are present, as is an infiltrate of hystiocytes, lymphocytes, and numerous plasmocytes. In late syphilis, a granuloma with no treponema is found, and sometimes caseous necrosis.

Diagnosis. A finding of treponema in an early phase confirms the diagnosis. Dark-field observation (Fig. 8.27), silver impregnation (Levaditi and Warthin-Starry stains), and direct immunofluorescence may help in this search. VDRL (venereal disease research laboratory) and FTA-abs (fluorescent treponema antibody absorption) are the serological tests most widely used. When nervous system involvement is suspected, a neurologic examination must be performed.

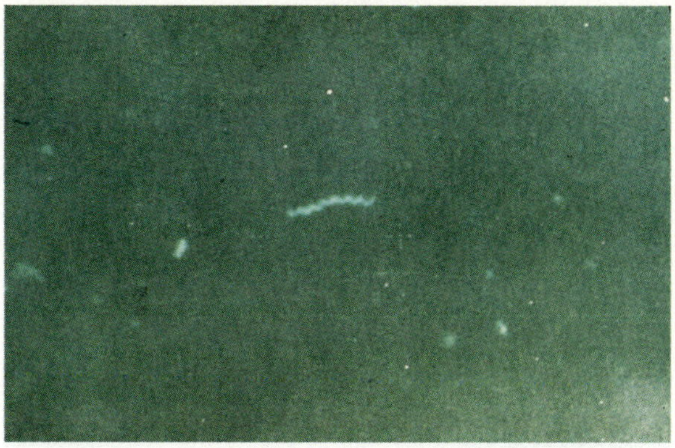

Fig. 8.27. Recent syphilis: treponema in dark-field observation

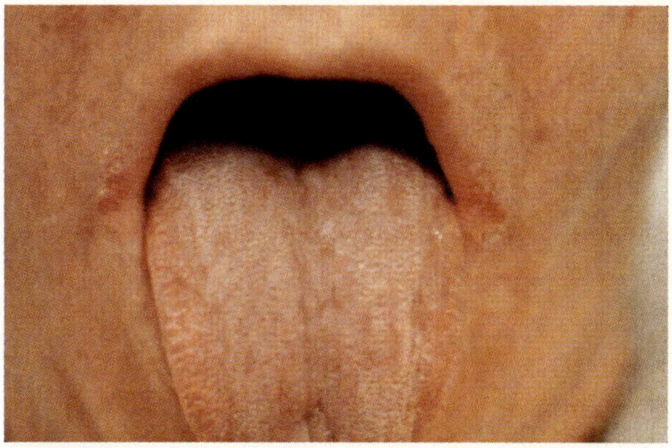

Fig. 8.28. Oral candidosis: creamy white pseudomembrane plaques on the tongue

Differential Diagnosis. Depending on the phase, oral lesions may be confused with a variety of other diseases. Syphilitic chancre may resemble aphtha, leishmaniasis, and ulcerous tuberculosis; mucous patches may mimic candidosis, lichen planus, lupus erythematosus; gummatous lesions can be confused with squamous cell carcinoma, paracoccidioidomycosis, and other types of ulcers. Serological tests confirm the diagnosis. Late syphilis is the phase most difficult to diagnose.

Treatment. The treatment of choice is benzathine penicillin in an IM total dose of 2.4 million units for primary syphilis, 4.8 million units for secondary syphilis, and 12 million units for tertiary syphilis, divided over 10 days. For neurosyphilis, procaine or aqueous penicillin must be used, since benzathine penetrates the blood-brain barrier. Congenital syphilis is treated with 50000 U/kg per IM or IV for 10 days with aqueous or procaine penicillin. For patients with penicillin allergy, erythromycin or tetracycline, 2 g/day for 30 days, can be administered.

8.7 Oral Candidosis (Moniliasis)

Definition. Candidosis is a primary or secondary infection involving yeasts of the genus *Candida,* which are normal inhabitants of the alimentary tract and the mucocutaneous regions [49–59].

Etiology. *Candida albicans* is the predominant yeast of the genus *Candida* and is found in most cases of oral candidoses. Other species that belong to the normal flora of the mucocutaneous areas can also be pathogenic (*C. tropicalis, C. krusei,* and others).

Pathogenesis. There are various predisposing factors and general conditions in which the normal equilibrium between *Candida* and host is sufficiently disturbed to lead to a pathologic state: (a) extreme youth; (b) pregnancy; (c) administration of steroids; (d) endocrine dysfunctions; (c) diabetes; (f) prolonged administration of antimicrobials; (g) immunosuppressive agents; (h) drug abuse; (i) accidents destroying barriers such as trauma, burns; and (j) general debility (genetic, iatrogenic, and acquired).

Oral Manifestations. A creamy white to gray pseudomembrane covers the tongue, soft palate, buccal mucosa, and the oral surfaces (Figs. 8.28, 8.29). Erythematous candidosis (Fig. 8.30) is usual in AIDS patients and also in old people, who may also present chronic cheilitis (Fig. 8.31) [50, 54].

Associated Findings. Patients with general debility may develop systemic disease.

Microscopic Findings. Direct examination reveals necrotic material, leukocytes, loose epithelial cells, bacteria, and food material along with intertwined pseudohyphae and hyphae of yeast cells (Fig. 8.32).

Diagnosis. Diagnosis is made through clinical signs and symptoms, mycological examination, and histopathologic appearance, and depends on demonstration of the organism.

Differential Diagnosis. In some patients, leukoplakia, lichen planus, tertiary syphilis, and other lesions resemble cutaneous candidosis.

Treatment. As candidosis is primarily an opportunistic infection, the prognosis depends almost entirely on the type and severity of the predisposing conditions or diseases.

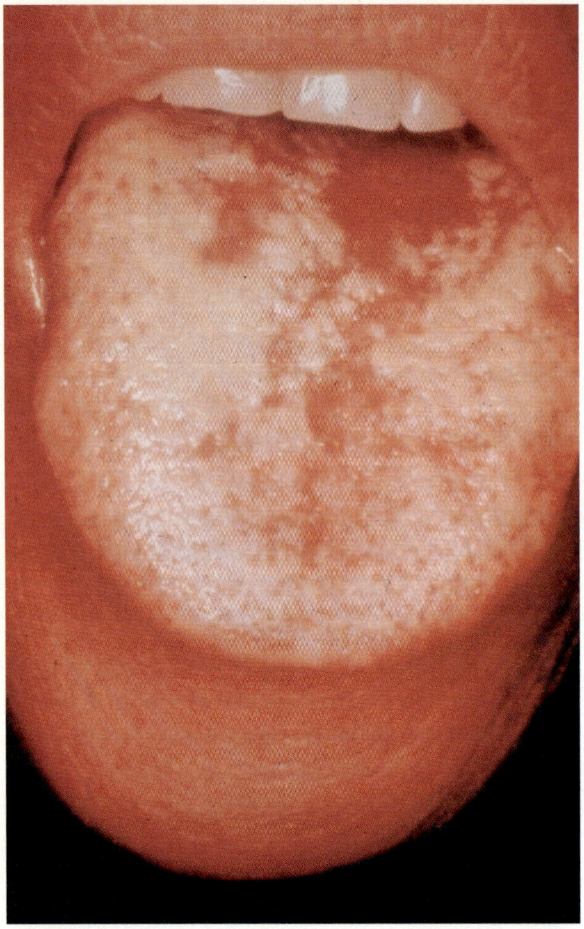

Fig. 8.29. Oral candidosis: creamy white pseudomembrane plaques covering the tongue

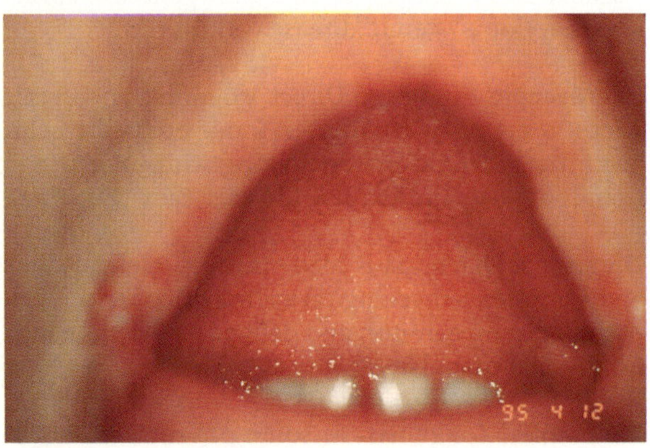

Fig. 8.30. Oral candidosis: erythematous candidiasis on the palate and chronic cheilitis

Topical treatment has been considered the therapy of choice, with the use of 1 % crystal violet, 1 % nystatin, amphotericin B suspensions, clotrimazole, ketoconazole, or econazole cream.

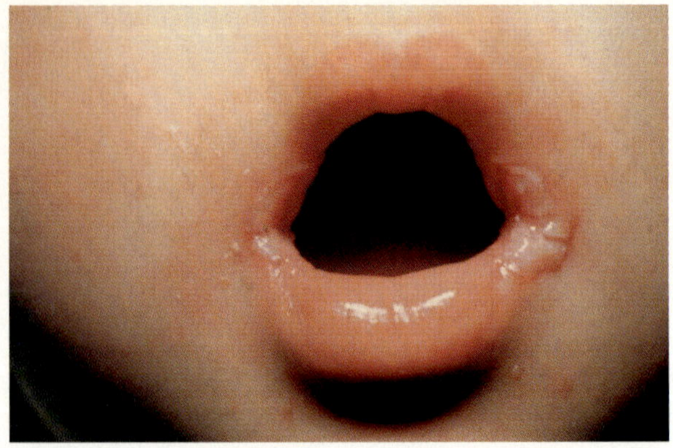

Fig. 8.31. Oral candidosis: chronic cheilitis

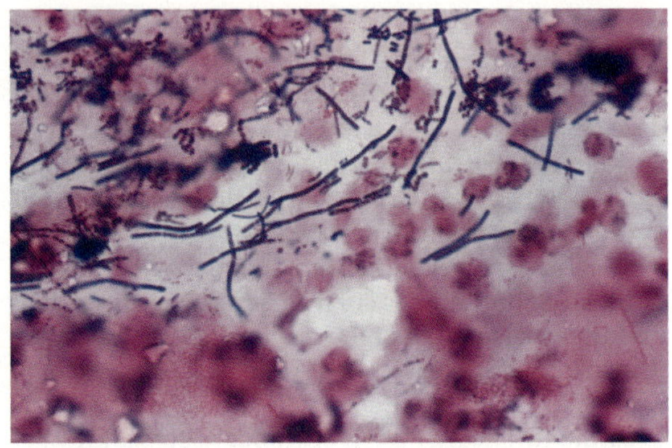

Fig. 8.32. Oral candidosis: pseudohyphae and hyphae of yeast cells. Direct examination. Gram staining

New oral agents in single doses, such as ketoconazole (200–400 mg), itraconazole (200–400 mg), and fluconazole (150–300 mg) can be prescribed. For more severe and extensive infections, amphotericin B (1 mg/kg per day IV in dextrose with a maximum total dose of 2 g) can be administered very slowly.

8.8 Entomophthoromycosis Conidiobolae (Chronic Rhinofacial Zygomycosis, Rhinoentomophthoromycosis)

Definition. This is a chronic and rare infection of the nose and adjacent areas, involving fungi that are members of the phylum Zygomycota and order Entomophthorales. Most cases have occurred in Central and West Africa, Brazil, Colombia and Caribbean, mainly in formerly healthy adults [60–68].

Etiology. *Conidiobolus coronatus* is the etiologic agent.

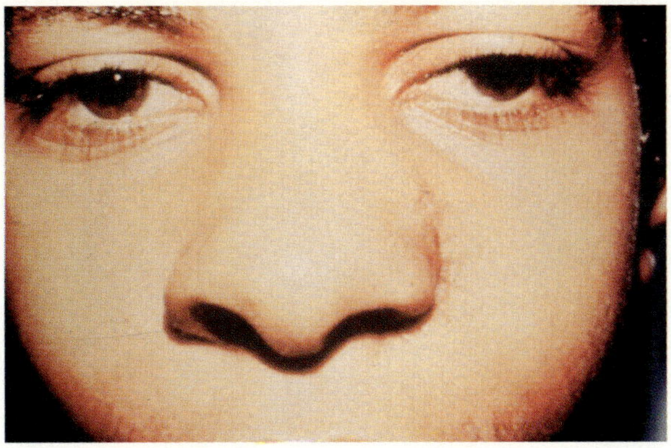

Fig. 8.33. Entomophthoromycosis. Bilateral distortion of the nasal region. Courtesy of Dr. Valdir Bandeira, Recife, Brazil

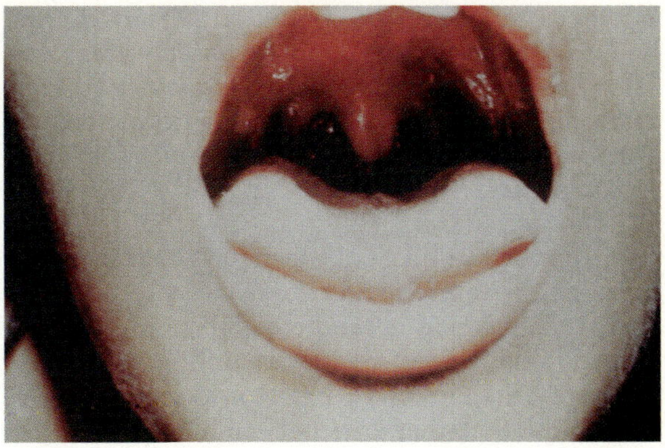

Fig. 8.35. Erythematous infiltrated plaque on the palate

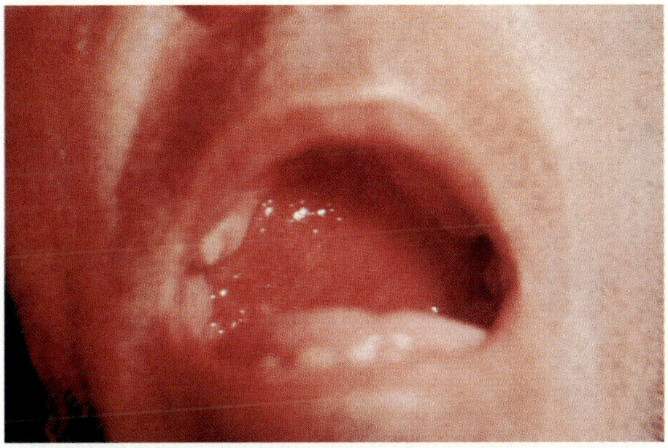

Fig. 8.34. Entomophthoromycosis. Erythematous infiltrated plaque on the palate. Courtesy of Dr. Valdir Bandeira, Recife, Brazil

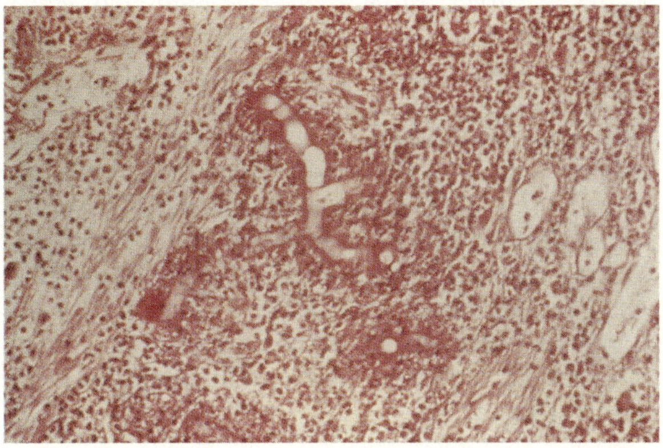

Fig. 8.36. Inflammatory reaction with sparsely septate hyphae

Pathogenesis. Infection by *C. coronatus* results from direct implantation of spores on nasal mucosa. Local trauma can facilitate the implantation that probably starts in the turbinates inferior and extends, slowly or sometimes rapidly, to ostia, foramina, paranasal sinuses, oropharynx, and palate.

Oral Manifestation. Large erythematous infiltrated and progressive plaques occur mainly on the palate [61, 64].

Associated Findings. There is usually bilateral, or less frequently unilateral, distortion of the subcutaneous tissue of the nasal region, associated with a mucoid discharge and nasal obstruction (Fig. 8.33). There can also be erythematous infiltrated plaque on the palate (Figs. 8.34, 8.35).

Microscopic Findings. Histopathology shows pyogranulomatous inflammatory reaction in the tissue with sparsely septate hyphae with an eosinophilic halo (Splendore-Hoeppli phenomenon) surrounding them (Fig. 8.36).

Diagnosis. The diagnosis is made from the clinical signs, histopathologic appearance and laboratory identification of the fungus.

Differential Diagnosis. The main conditions that need to be excluded are lymphatic edema and subcutaneous malignant lymphoma.

Treatment. Some lesions clear spontaneously after surgery. Lesions usually respond to oral treatment with potassium iodide (40–60 drops of saturated potassium iodide three times a day for 3–4 months). Amphotericin B (1 mg/kg per day), clotrimoxazole, ketoconazole, and itraconazole can also be used [65].

8.9 Larva Migrans (Creeping Eruption)

Definition. Larva migrans is characterized by itchy serpiginous tracks that primarily affect the feet, hands or buttocks and, rarely, the mouth. It is common in tropical countries) [69–75].

Etiology. Larva migrans is caused by larvae from hookworms of various animals, mainly dogs and cats. The nematode *Ancilostoma braziliense* is the main etiologic agent. Other larvae can cause the disease, such as *A. caninum, A. ceylonicum, Uncinaria stenocephala.*

Pathogenesis. Adult hookworms live mainly in the intestines of animals and release ova into the feces. Ova are thus found in sand or soil contaminated by animals and, under favorable conditions of temperature and humidity, hatch into noninfectious rhabdoid larvae that later become filariform infective larvae. They are found in the upper half-inch of the sand or soil.

The mouth infection, like the skin one, probably occurs by direct contact with contaminated sands, but the ingestion of contaminated food may also be responsible.

Oral Manifestations. Larva migrans is rare in the mouth, but when it happens it can involve the tongue, lips, cheeks, floor of the mouth, palate, and oropharynx. The symptoms are itching and burning. Clinical examination shows erythematous areas and tortuous whitish lines (Figs. 8.37, 8.38). Many larvae may be active, producing bizarre patterns. Larvae move a few millimeters to a few centimeters each day.

Associated Findings. Oral infestation may be associated with cutaneous larva migrans.

Microscopic Findings. Circular or ovoid structures, compatible with nematode larva can be found inside cavities of subepithelial regions of the mouth.

Diagnosis. The diagnosis is made mainly from clinical examination.

Treatment. Broad-spectrum antihelminthics such as thiabendazole: 5–50 mg/kg for 2–4 days and occasionally longer, and albendazole: 400 mg daily for 1–3 days can be used with success; topical thiabendazole as a 15 % cream is also effective in cutaneous larva migrans.

8.10 Cervicofacial Actinomycosis

Definition. Chronic suppurative and granulomatous disease is characterized by peripheral spread and formation of multiple framing sinus tracts. These sinuses drain from suppurative pyogenic lesions and the exudate contains firm, lobulated grains or microcolonies of the etiologic agent [76–85].

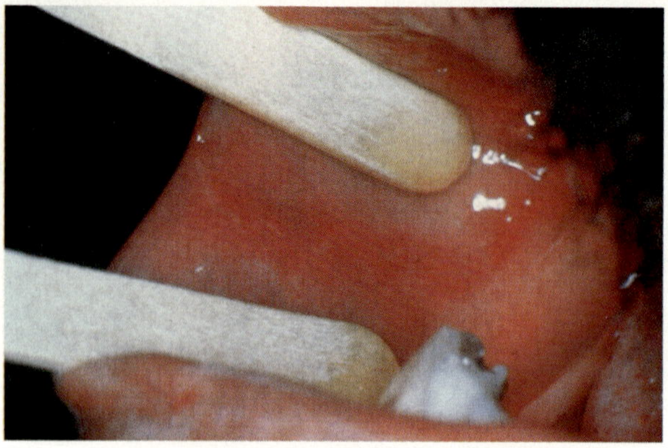

Fig. 8.37. Larva migrans: erythematous areas and tortuous whitish lines on the cheek. Courtesy of Dr. Oslei Paes de Almeida, Piracicaba, Brazil

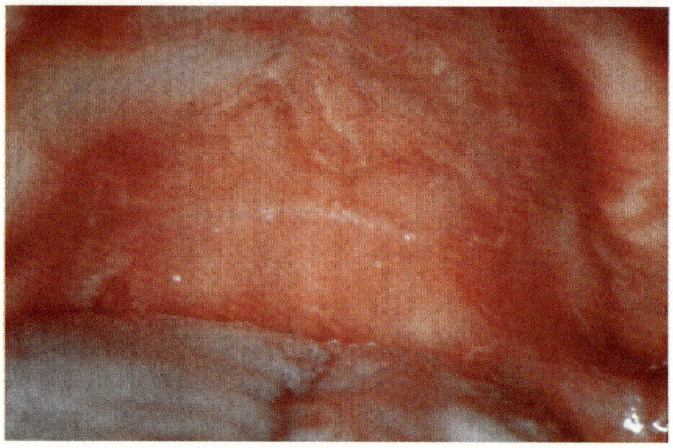

Fig. 8.38. Larva migrans: erythematous areas and tortuous whitish lines on the palate. Courtesy of Dr. Oslei Paes de Almeida, Piracicaba, Brazil

Etiology. Members of the family Actinomycetaceae, called higher bacteria, a group that consist of commensals, is found in oral-cavity and other mucosal areas. *Actinomyces israelli* is the predominant organism in human infections.

Pathogenesis. The organism penetrates through trauma in mucous membrane of the mouth, by way of carious teeth. Salivary glands are sometimes involved.

Oral Manifestations. The most common initial symptoms are pain and swelling. Primary lesion is usually in the mandible or maxilla and probably arises as a direct extension from a periodontal abscess formed in turn as the result of carious teeth, dental extraction, or trauma to the jaw.

Associated Findings. Dull red indurated nodule on the cheek or submaxillary region (Fig. 8.39) may be associated, and multiple sinuses, discharging puru-

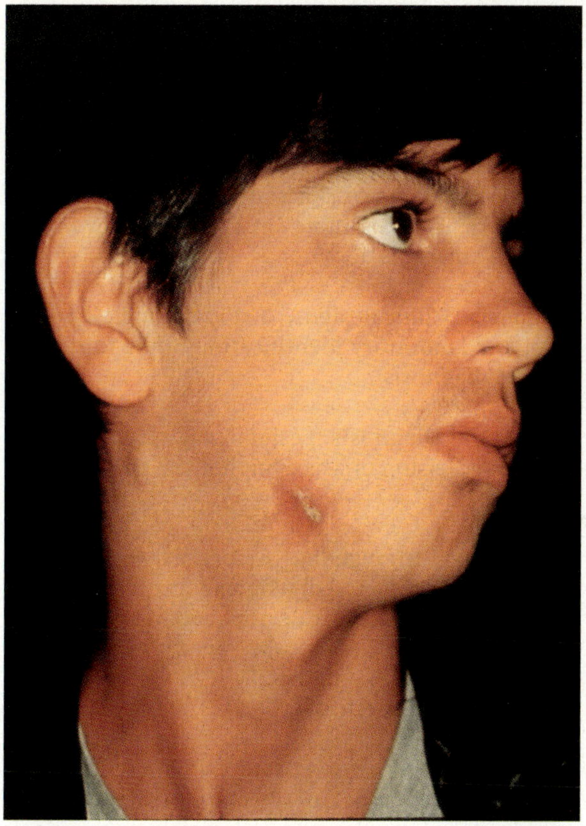

Fig. 8.39. Cervicofacial actinomycosis: red indurated nodule in the submaxillary region. Courtesy of Dr. Ivo Bussoloti Filho, São Paulo, Brazil

lent material containing sulfur granules, may close temporarily and reopen later.

Microscopic Findings. Microscopy reveals an acute pyogenic response, which evolves into a chronic granulomatous lesion, suppuration, and abscess formation (Fig. 8.40). Granules have an adherent mass

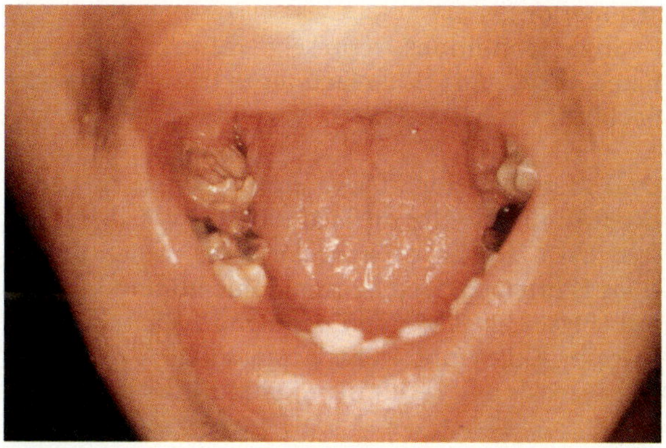

Fig. 8.40. Cervicofacial actinomycosis. Chronic granulomatous lesion. Courtesy of Dr. Ivo Bussoloti Filho, São Paulo, Brazil

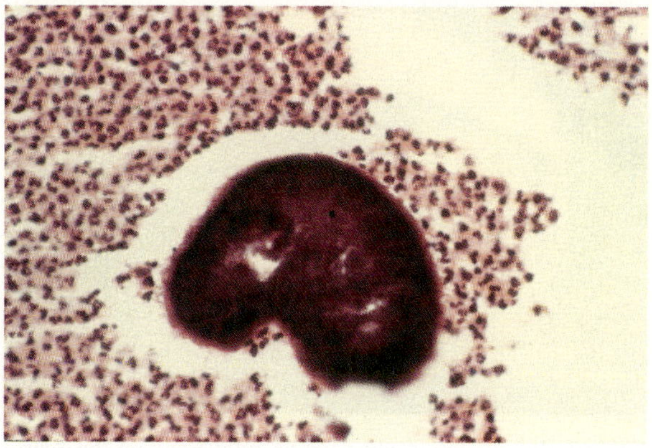

Fig. 8.41. Cervicofacial actinomycosis. A typical granule

of polymorphonuclear neutrophils that are attached to radially arranged eosinophilic "clubs" (Fig. 8.41).

Diagnosis. The diagnosis is made from the clinical signs and symptoms, laboratory examination, direct and culture methods, and histopathologic appearance, depending on the demonstration of organisms.

Differential Diagnosis. Cervicofacial actinomycosis must be differentiated from a number of chronic infections and neoplastic diseases.

Treatment. Penicillin is considered the treatment of choice. Regimens vary from 1–6 million units to 10–20 million units of penicillin G IV per day, depending on the severity of disease. Therapy is administered for 30–45 days before surgical incision, drainage, or excision, or the lesions are allowed to heal by secondary intention.

8.11 Histoplasmosis (*Histoplasmosis Capsulatum*)

Definition. Histoplasmosis is a deep fungal infection with worldwide distribution [86–96].

Etiology. Histoplasmosis is caused by *Histoplasma capsulatum* var. capsulatum, a dimorphic fungus found in soil or in excrement of chickens, starlings, blackbirds, pigeons, and bats.

Pathogenesis. Infection is initiated after inhalation of spores and results in a variety of clinical manifestations. Approximately 95 % of cases are subclinical. The remaining patients may have a chronic progressive lung disease, a chronic cutaneous or systemic disease, or an acute fatal systemic infection.

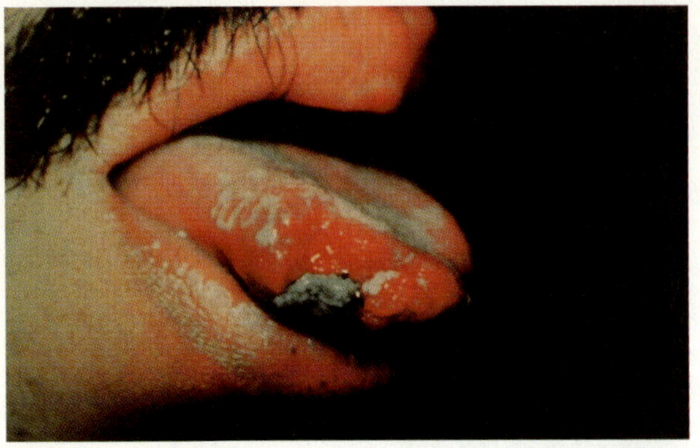

Fig. 8.42. Histoplasmosis: ulcer and necrotic lesion on the tongue before treatment

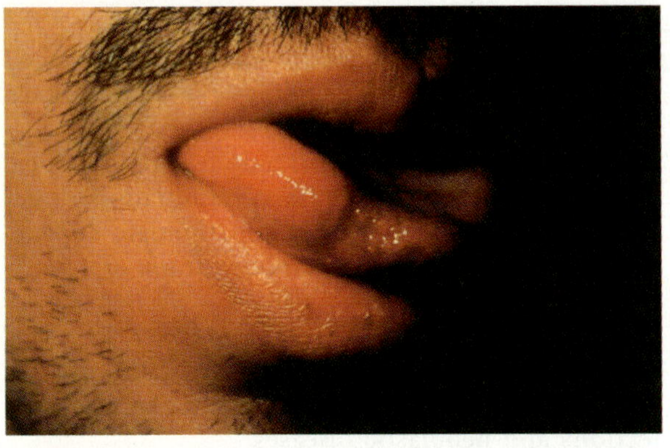

Fig. 8.43. Histoplasmosis: same patient as in Fig. 8.42 after treatment

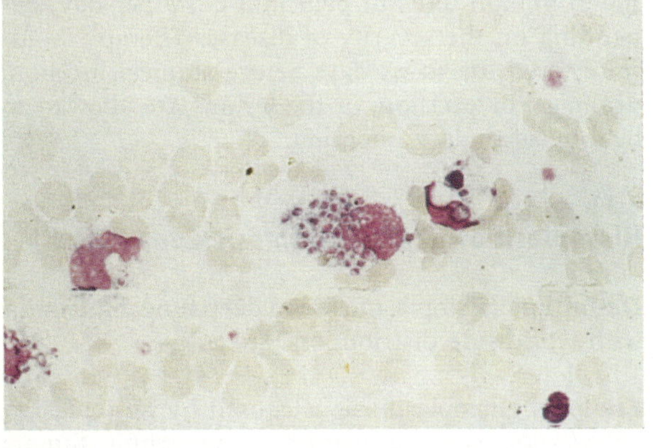

Fig. 8.44. Histoplasmosis: yeast cells within histiocytes. Hematoxylin and eosin

Oral Manifestations. Histoplasmosis can occur mainly in the mouth of patients infected with HIV. Mucous lesion includes painful ulcers, nodules, vegetating and necrotic lesions (Figs. 8.42, 8.43).

Associated Findings. Skin lesions resemble molluscum contagiosum, erythematous macules, necrotic papules and nodules.

Microscopic Findings. Yeast cells within histiocytes have a uniform size and are visible in Gram, Giemsa, Wright's, or hematoxylin and eosin-stained smears (Fig. 8.44). They resemble *Leishmania donovani* but lack the kinetoplast.

Diagnosis. Clinical signs, histopathologic appearance, and laboratory identification of the fungus allow the diagnosis.

Differential Diagnosis. Lesions may resemble cryptococcosis, leishmaniasis, lymphomas, and even sarcoidosis.

Treatment. Intravenous amphotericin B, 0.5–0.6 mg/kg, is given daily during the acute stage, and then oral itraconazole 200–400 mg weekly.

8.12 Cutaneous Tuberculosis

Definition. Tuberculosis of the skin is a spectrum of skin conditions due to infection with obligatory mycobacterial pathogens. Orificial tuberculosis and papulonecrotic tuberculid can occur in the mouth [97–105].

Etiology. Etiologic agents are *Mycobacterium tuberculosis, M. bovis*, and, under certain conditions, bacillus Calmette-Guérin (BCG), an attenuated strain of *M. bovis.*

Pathogenesis. Infection may be exogenous (from an outside source), it may occur after autoinoculation (orificial tuberculosis), or it may be endogenous (continuous extension of a tuberculosis process by way of the lymphatics or by hematogenous dissemination).

Some conditions represent recurrent disseminated or systemic skin reactions to toxins of tubercle bacilli: the tuberculids.

Oral Manifestation. There are two types that may occur in the mouth; orificial tuberculosis characterized by a circular or irregular ulcer, which on the floor is often covered by pseudomembranous material (Figs. 8.45, 8.46), and papulonecrotic tuberculid showing red, symptomless papules that develop central necrosis and result in red pitted scars (Fig. 8.47).

Associated Findings. Cavitary pulmonar tuberculosis, ulcerative tuberculosis of the pharynx and larynx

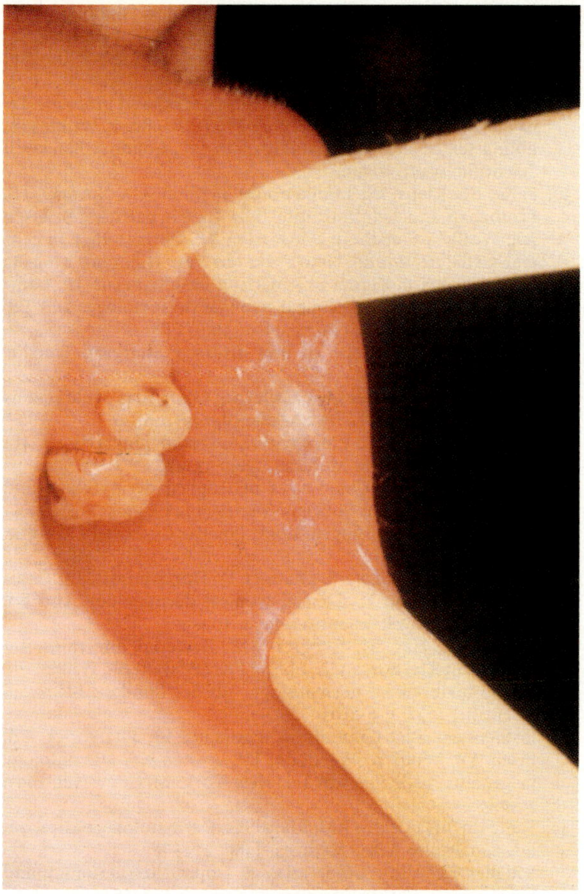

Fig. 8.45. Orificial tuberculosis: irregular ulcer covered by pseudomembranous material on the cheek. Courtesy of Dr. Ivo Bussoloti Filho, São Paulo, Brazil

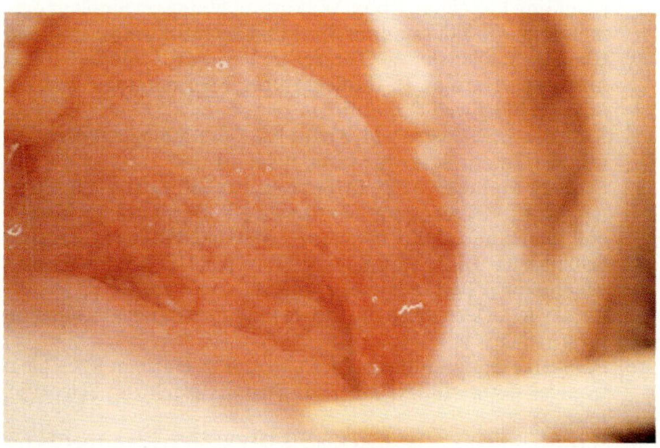

Fig. 8.46. Orificial tuberculosis: irregular ulcer covered by pseudomembranous material on the palate. Courtesy of Dr. Ivo Bussoloti Filho, São Paulo, Brazil

are frequently associated with oral lesions. Papulonecrotic tuberculids, characterized by papules and pitted scars on the knees, elbows, buttocks, and lower trunk, are also associated.

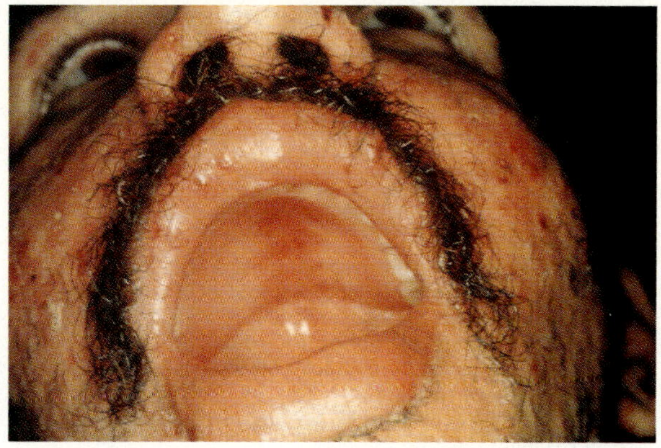

Fig. 8.47. Papulonecrotic tuberculid: red papules with central necrosis and red pitted scars. Courtesy of Dr. Iphis Campbell, Brasília, Brazil

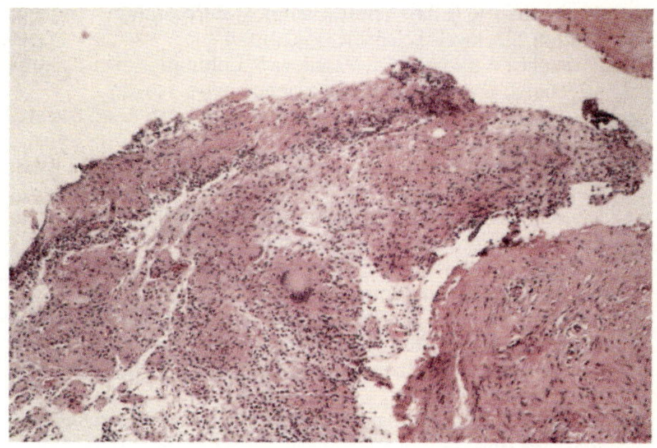

Fig. 8.48. Orificial tuberculosis: tubercles with caseation in deep dermis

Microscopic Findings. In the presence of orificial tuberculosis, tubercles with caseation may be found deep in the dermis (Fig. 8.48) and papulonecrotic tuberculid, necrosis of the upper dermis, and inflammatory tuberculoid infiltrate surrounding the necrotic area are also seen. Obliterative or granulomatous vasculitis of blood vessels may also be present.

Diagnosis. The diagnosis of orificial tuberculosis is made from the finding of painful ulcers inside the mouth in patients with pulmonary tuberculosis, the presence of acid-fast organisms and positive culture. Papulonecrotic tuberculid is diagnosed from the clinical picture and histopathology.

Differential Diagnosis. Orificial tuberculosis must be differentiated from syphilitic lesions, aphthous ulcers and carcinomas, and papulonecrotic tuberculid from pityriasis lichenoides et varioliformis acuta.

Treatment. Triple chemotherapy is used with isoniazid (5–10 mg/kg per day up to 300 mg per day), rifampicin (10–20 mg per day up to 600 mg) and ethambutol (15–25 mg/kg per day) for 6 months.

References

1. Azulay RD. Dermatologia. Rio de Janeiro: Guanabara Koogan, 1985: 153–155
2. Franco M, Lacaz CS, Restrepo-Moreno A, Del Negro G (Eds). Paracoccidioidomycosis. Boca Raton: CRC Press 1994: 20–62
3. Hay RJ, Roberts SOB, MacKenzie DWR. Mycology. In: Champion RH, Burton JL, Ebling FJG (Eds). Rook, Wilkinson, Ebling Textbook of Dermatology, 5th Edn. London: Blackwell Scientific 1992: 1127–216
4. Kwon-Chung KJ, Bennett JE. Medical mycology. Malvern: Lea and Febiger 1992: pp 594–619
5. Lacaz CS, Porto C, Martins JEC. Micologia médica, 8th edn. São Paulo: Sarvier 1991: pp 248–92
6. Negroni R. Paracoccidioidomycosis (South American blastomycosis, Lutz's Mycosis). Int J Dermatol 1993: 32:847–59
7. Padilha-Gonçalves A. Paracoccidioidomycosis. In: Canizares O, Harman R (Eds). Clinical tropical dermatology. 2nd Ed. Boston: Blackwell Scientific, 1992: 61–9
8. Parish LC, Witkowski JA, Vassileva S. Color atlas of cutaneous infections. Oxford: Blackwell Science, 1995: 139–40
9. Restrep A. Treatment of tropical mycoses. J Am Acad Dermatol 1994: 31 (3 Pt 2): Suppl. 91–102
10. Rippon JW. Medical mycology. 3rd Ed. Philadelphia: W.B. Saunders, 1988; 506–31.
11. Sampaio SAP, Castro RM, Rivitti EA. Dermatologia basica. 4th Ed. São Paulo: Artes Médicas, 1989: 343–58
12. Schaller KF (Ed). Color atlas of tropical dermatology and venereology. Berlin: Springer-Verlag, 1994: 97–8
13. Shadomy HJ, Utz JP. Deep fungal infections. In: Fitzpatrick TB, Eisen AZ, Wolff K, Freedberg JM, Austen KF. Dermatology in general medicine. 4th Ed. New York: McGraw-Hill, 1993: 2468–97
14. Azulay RD. Dermatologia. Rio de Janeiro: Guanabara Koogan, 1985: 168–169
15. Burns DA. Diseases caused by arthropods and other noxious animals. In: Champion RH, Burton JL, Ebling FJG (Eds). Rook, Wilkinson, Ebling textbook of dermatology. 5th Ed. London: Blackwell Scientific, 1992: 1265–324
16. Canizares O. Myiasis. In: Canizares O, Harman R. Clinical tropical dermatology. 2nd Ed. Boston: Blackwell Scientific, 1992: 404–11
17. Sampaio SAP, Castro RM, Rivitti EA. Dermatologia básica, 4th Ed. São Paulo: Artes Médicas, 1989: 373–88
18. Schaller KF (Ed). Color atlas of tropical dermatology and venereology. Berlin: Springer-Verlag, 1994:140–1
19. Wilson DC, Leyva WH, King Jr LE. Arthropods bites and stings. In: Fitzpatrick TB, Eisen AZ, Wolff K, Freedberg JM, Austen KF. Dermatology in general medicine. 4th Ed. New York: McGraw-Hill, 1993: 2810–26
20. Azulay RD. Dermatologia. Rio de Janeiro: Guanabara Koogan, 1985: 124–32
21. Bryceson ADM, Leprosy. In: Champion RH, Burton JL, Ebling FJG (Eds). Rook, Wilkinson, Ebling textbook of dermatology 5th Ed. London: Blackwell Scientific, 1992: 1065–83.
22. Canizares O, Harman R, Adriaans B. Leprosy. In: Canizares O, Harman R. Clinical tropical dermatology. 2nd Ed. Boston: Blackwell Scientific, 1992: 165–200
23. Grosset JH, Progress in the chemotherapy of leprosy. Int J Lepr 1980; 62: 268–76
24. Laskaris G. Color atlas of oral diseases. Stuttgart: Thieme, 1988: 134–5
25. McDougall AC, Ulrick MI. Mycobacterial disease: leprosy. In: Fitzpatrick TB, Eisen AZ, Wolff K, Freedberg IM, Austen KF. Dermatology in general medicine. 4th Ed. New York: McGraw-Hill, 1993: 2365–410
26. Sampaio SAP, Castro RM, Rivitti EA. Dermatologia básica. 4th Ed. São Paulo: Artes Médicas, 1989: 287–310
27. Schaller KF (Ed). Color atlas of tropical dermatology and venereology. Berlin: Springer-Verlag, 1994: 1994: 22–36
28. Azulay RD. Dermatologia. Rio de Janeiro: Guanabara Koogan, 1985: 159–65
29. Bryceson ADM and Hay RJ. Parasitic worms and protozoa. In: Champion RH, Burton JL, Ebling FJG (Eds). Rook, Wilkinson, Ebling textbook of dermatology. 5th Ed., London: Blackwell Scientific, 1992: 1217–64
30. Farad SF, Klaus SN, Frankenburg S, Klion AD, Nutman TB. Protozoan and helminth infection. In: Fitzpatrick TB, Eisen AZ, Wolff K, Freedberg JM, Austen KF. Dermatology in general medicine. 4th Ed. New York: McGraw-Hill, 1993: 2769–87
31. Kerdel-Vegas F, Kerdel F. American leishmaniasis. In: Canizares O, Harman R. Clinical tropical dermatology. 2nd Ed. Boston: Blackwell Scientific, 1992: 301–12
32. Laskaris G. Color atlas of oral diseases. Stuttgart: Thieme, 1988: 146–7
33. Parish LC, Witkowski JA, Vassileva S. Color atlas of cutaneous infections. Turin: Blackwell Science, 1995: 163–6
34. Sampaio SAP, Castro RM, Rivitti EA. Dermatologia básica. 4th Ed. São Paulo: Artes Médicas, 1989: 373–88
35. Schaller KF (Ed). Color atlas of tropical dermatology and venereology. Berlin: Springer-Verlag, 1994: 110–3
36. Azulay RD. Dermatologia. Rio de Janeiro: Guanabara Koogan, 1985: 196–7
37. Canizares O, Olansky S, Olansky D. Donovanosis. In: Canizares O, Harman R. Clinical tropical dermatology. 2nd Ed. Boston: Blackwell Scientific, 1992: 504–9
38. Highet AS, Hay RJ, Roberts SOB. Bacterial infections. In: Champion RH, Burton JL, Ebling FJG (Eds). Rook, Wilkinson, Ebling textbook of dermatology. 5th Ed. London: Blackwell Scientific, 1992: 953–1031
39. Rothenberg RB. Granuloma inguinale. In: Fitzpatrick TB, Eisen AZ, Wolff K, Freedberg JM, Austen KF. Dermatology in general medicine, 4th Ed. New York: McGraw-Hill, 1993: 2757–9
40. Sampaio SAP, Castro RM, Rivitti EA. Dermatologia básica. 4th Ed. São Paulo: Artes Médicas, 1989: 279–86
41. Schaller KG (Ed). Color atlas of tropical dermatology and venereology. Berlin: Springer-Verlag, 1994: 77–8
42. Azulay RD. Dermatologia. Rio de Janeiro: Guanabara Koogan, 1985: 137–43
43. Laskaris G. Color atlas of oral diseases. Stuttgart: Thieme, 1988: 124–30
44. Morton RS. The treponematoses. In: Champion RH, Burton JL, Ebling FJG (Eds). Rook, Wilkinson, Ebling textbook of dermatology. 5th Ed. London: Blackwell Scientific, 1992: 1085–126
45. Olansky S, Olansky A, Olansky D. Venereal Syphilis. In: Canizares O, Harman R. Clinical tropical dermatology. 2nd Ed. Boston: Blackwell Scientific, 1992: 509–24
46. Sampaio SAP, Castro RM, Rivitti EA. Dermatologia Básica. 4th Ed. São Paulo: Artes Médicas, 1989: 311–26
47. Sanchez M, Luger AFH. In: Syphilis. In: Fitzpatrick TB, Eisen AZ, Wolff K, Freedberg JM, Austen KF. Dermatology in general medicine. 4th Ed. New York: McGraw-Hill, 1993: 2703–43
48. Schaller KF (Ed). Color atlas of tropical dermatology and venereology. Berlin: Springer-Verlag, 1994: 70–3
49. Azulay RD. Dermatologia. Rio de Janeiro: Guanabara Koogan, 1985: 150–2
50. Canizares O. Candidiasis. In: Canizares O, Harman R. Clinical tropical dermatology. 2nd Ed. Boston: Blackwell Scientific, 1992: 34–7
51. Hay RJ, Roberts SOB, MacKenzie DWR. Mycology. In: Champion RH, Burton JL, Ebling FJG (Eds). Rook, Wilkinson, Ebling textbook of dermatology. 5th Ed. London: Blackwell Scientific, 1992: 1127–216
52. Kwon-Chung KJ, Bennett JE. Medical mycology. Malvern: Lea and Febiger, 1992: 280–336
53. Lacaz CS, Porto C, Martins JEC. Micologia médica. 8th Ed. São Paulo: Sarvier, 1991: 216–224.
54. Laskaris G. Color atlas of oral diseases. Stuttgart: Thieme, 1988: 138–43
55. Martin AG, Kobayashi GS. Yeast infections: candidiasis, pytiriasis (tinea) versicolor. In: Fitzpatrick TB, Eisen AZ, Wolff K,

Freedberg JM, Austen KF. Dermatology in general medicine. 4th Ed. New York: McGraw-Hill, 1993: 2452–67
56. Parish LC, Witkowski JA, Vassileva S. Color atlas of cutaneous infections. Oxford: Blackwell Science, 1995: 121–25
57. Rippon JW, Medical mycology. 3rd Ed. Philadelphia: W.B. Saunders, 1988: 532–81
58. Sampaio SAP, Castro RM, Rivitti EA. Dermatologia básica. 4th Ed. São Paulo: Artes Médicas, 1989: 327–42
59. Schaller KF (Ed). Color atlas of tropical dermatology and venereology. Berlin: Springer-Verlag, 1986
60. Azulay RD. Dermatologia. Rio de Janeiro: Guanabara Koogan, 1985: 159
61. Harman R. Subcutaneous zygomycosis. In: Canizares O, Harman R. Clinical tropical dermatology. 2nd Ed. Boston: Blackwell Scientific, 1992: 85–7
62. Hay RJ, Roberts SOB, MacKenzie DWR. Mycology. In: Champion RH, Burton JL, Ebling FJG (Eds). Rook, Wilkinson, Ebling textbook of dermatology. 5th Ed. London: Blackwell Scientific, 1992: 1127–216
63. Kwon-Chung KJ, Bennett JE. Medical Mycology. Malvern: Lea and Febiger, 1992: 447–63
64. Lacaz CS, Porto C, Martins JEC. Micologia médica. 8th Ed. São Paulo: Sarvier, 1991: 355–70
65. Restrepo A. Treatment of tropical mycoses. J Am Acad Dermatol 1994; 31: Suppl. 91–102
66. Rippon JW. Medical Mycology. 3rd Ed. Philadelphia: W.B. Saunders, 1988: 681–713
67. Sampaio SAP, Castro RM, Rivitti EA. Dermatologia básica. 4th Ed. São Paulo: Artes Médicas, 1989: 343–58
68. Schaller KF (Ed). Color atlas of tropical dermatology and venereology. Berlin: Springer-Verlag, 1994: 102
69. Azulay RD. Dermatologia. Rio de Janeiro: Guanabara Koogan, 1985: 169–70
70. Burns DA. Diseases caused by arthropods and other noxious animals. In: Champion RH, Burton JL, Ebling FJG (Eds). Rook, Wilkinson, Ebling textbook of dermatology. 5th Ed. London: Blackwell Scientific, 1992: 1265–324
71. Canizares O. Larva migrans. In: Canizares O, Harman R. Clinical tropical dermatology. 2nd Ed. Boston: Blackwell Scientific, 1992: 332–4
72. Farah FS, Klaus SN, Frankenberg S, Klion AD, Nutman TB. Protozoan and helminth infections. In: Fitzpatrick TB, Eisen AZ, Wolff K, Freedberg JM, Austen KF. Dermatology in general medicine. 4th Ed. New York: McGraw-Hill, 1993: 2769–87
73. Lopes MA, Zaia AA, de Almeida, OP, Scully C. Larva migrans that affect the mouth. Oral Surg oral Med oral Pathol 1994; 77: 362–7
74. Sampaio SAP, Castro RM, Rivitti EA. Dermatology básica. 4th Ed. São Paulo: Artes Médicas, 1989: 373–88
75. Schaller KF (Ed). Color atlas of tropical dermatology and venereology. Berlin: Springer-Verlag, 1994: 115–6
76. Azulay RD. Dermatologia. Rio de Janeiro: Guanabara Koogan, 1985: 157–9
77. Hay RJ, Roberts SOB, MacKenzie DWR. Mycology. In: Champion RH, Burton JL, Ebling FJG (Eds). Rook, Wilkinson, Ebling textbook of dermatology. 5th Ed. London: Blackwell Scientific, 1992: 1127–216
78. Kwon-Chung KJ, Bennett JE. Medical mycology. Malvern: Lea and Febiger, 1992: 560–93
79. Lacaz CS, Porto C, Martins JEC. Micologia medica. 8th Ed. São Paulo: Sarvier, 1991: 59–84
80. Padilha-Gonçalves A, Canizares O, Hay R, Harman R. Actinomycosis. In: Canizares O, Harman R (Eds). Clinical tropical dermatology. 2nd Ed. Boston: Blackwell Scientific, 1992: 99–101
81. Parish LC, Witkowski JA, Vassileva S. Color atlas of cutaneous infections. Oxford: Blackwell Science, 1995: 145–6
82. Rippon JW. Medical mycology. 3rd Ed. Philadelphia: W.B. Saunders, 1988: 30–52
83. Sampaio SAP, Castro RM, Rivitti FA. Dermatologia básica. 4th Ed. São Paulo: Artes Médicas, 1989: 343–58
84. Schaller KF (Ed). Color atlas of tropical dermatology and venereology. Berlin: Springer-Verlag, 1994: 92–3
85. Shadomy HJ, Utz JP. Deep fungal infections. In: Fitzpatrick TB, Eisen AZ, Wolff K, Freedberg JM, Austen KF (Eds). Dermatology in general medicine. 4th Ed. New York: McGraw-Hill, 1993: 2468–97
86. Azulay RD. Dermatologia. Rio de Janeiro: Guanabara Koogan, 1979: 92–98
87. Dobleman TJ, Scher N, Goldman M. Invasive histoplasmosis of the mandible. Head Neck 1989; 11:81–84
88. Hay RJ, Roberts SOB, MacKenzie DWR. Mycology. In: Champion RH, Burton JL, Ebling FJG (Eds). Rook, Wilkinson, Ebling textbook of dermatology. 5th Ed. London: Blackwell Scientific, 1992: 1127–216
89. Kwon-Chung KJ, Bennett JE. Medical mycology. Malvern: Lea & Febiger, 1992: 464–513
90. Lacaz CS, Porto B, Martins JEC. Micologia médica. 8th Ed. São Paulo: Sarvier, 1991: 327–39
91. Laskaris G. Color atlas of oral diseases. Stuttgart: Thieme, 1988: 144–5
92. Parish LC, Witkowski JA, Vassileva S. Color atlas of cutaneous infections. Oxford: Blackwell Science, 1995: 140–1
93. Rippon JW. Medical Mycology. 3ed. Philadelphia: W.B. Saunders, 1988: 381–423
94. Sampaio SAP, Castro RM, Rivitti EA. Dermatologia básica. 4th Ed. São Paulo: Artes Médicas, 1989: 343–58
95. Shadomy HJ, Utz JP. Deep fungal infections. In: Fitzpatrick TB, Eisen AZ, Wolff K, Freedberg JM, Austen KF. Dermatology in general medicine. 4th Ed. New York: McGraw-Hill, 1993: 2468–97
96. Swindells S, Dureham T, Johansson SL et al. Oral histoplasmosis in a patient infected with HIV. A case report. Oral Surg oral Med oral Pathol 1994; 77: 126–30
97. Adriaans B, Dominguez-Soto L, Canizares O, Harman R. Tuberculosis of the skin. In: Canizares O, Harman R (Eds). Clinical tropical dermatology. 2nd Ed. Boston: Blackwell Scientific, 1992: 201–15
98. Azulay RD. Dermatologia. Rio de Janeiro: Guanabara Koogan, 1985: 132–5
99. Laskaris G. Color atlas of oral diseases. Stuttgart: Thieme, 1988: 132–4
100. Parish LC, Witkowski JA, Vassileva S. Color atlas of Cutaneous Infections. Oxford: Blackwell Science, 1995: 43–6
101. Sampaio SAP, Castro RM, Rivitti EA. Dermatologia básica. 4th Ed. São Paulo: Artes Médicas 1989: 287–310
102. Savin JA. Mycobacterial infections. In: Champion RH, Burton JL, Ebling FJG (Eds). Rook, Wilkinson, Ebling textbook of dermatology. 5th Ed. London: Blackwell Scientific, 1992: 1033–63
103. Schaller KF (Ed). Color atlas of tropical dermatology and venereology. Berlin: Springer-Verlag, 1994: 37–8
104. Sehgal VN, Bhattacharya SN, Jain S, Loganik K. Cutaneous tuberculosis. The evolving scenario. Int J Dermatol 1994; 33: 97–104
105. Tappeiner G, Wolff K Tuberculosis and other mycobacterial infections. In: Fitzpatrick TB, Eisen AZ, Wolff K, Freedberg JM, Austen KF. Dermatology in general medicine. 4th Ed. New York: McGraw-Hill, 1993: 2370–95

CHAPTER 9

Oral Lesions in Acquired Immunodeficiency Syndrome (AIDS)

M. Ramos-e-Silva and B. Moritz Trope

9.1 Introduction

In the early days of the HIV epidemic, the oral mucosa was regarded as a frequent site for HIV virus-related lesions but, as with many other features of this disease, opinion has changed, and most of these infections, neoplasms, drug reactions, and other groups of diseases are now considered "unusual" in HIV-infected patients. Classic or atypical forms of many diseases may develop inside the mouth in association with HIV infection. Some are regarded as markers of immune status, especially related to circulating CD_4^+ T-lymphocytes, while others are seen as indicators of HIV infection on apparently healthy individuals, thus leading to its diagnosis. Early adequate diagnosis of these oral lesions is relevant for early treatment and, to a certain extent, for a better prognosis.

Hairy leukoplakia and pseudomembranous candidosis have the strongest predictive value for progression into full-blown AIDS, and although there is a clear association between the severity of immunosuppression and the severity and extent of periodontal breakdown and its rate of progression, periodontal status does not seem to be particularly helpful in predicting the progression of AIDS.

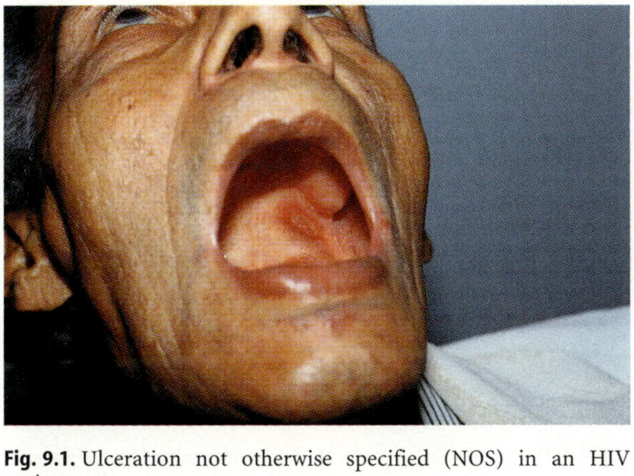

Fig. 9.1. Ulceration not otherwise specified (NOS) in an HIV patient

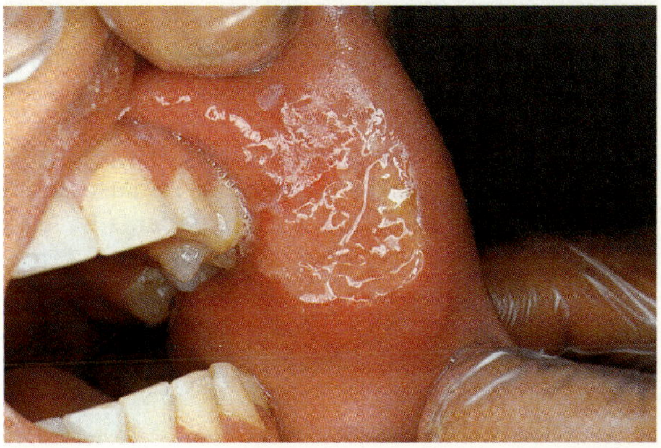

Fig. 9.2. Ulceration NOS in an HIV patient. Courtesy of Dr. Sandra Torres, Brazil

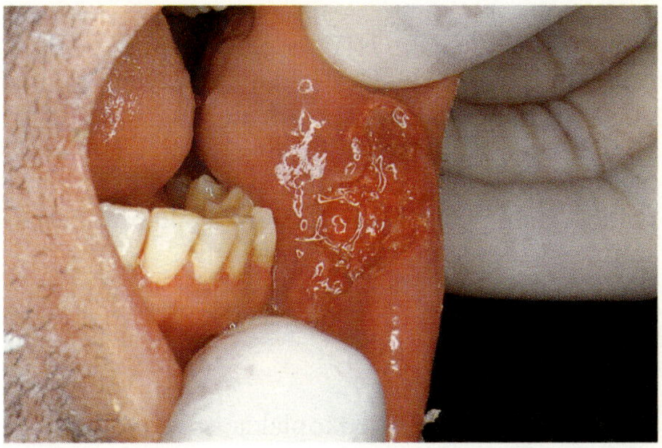

Fig. 9.3. Ulceration NOS in an HIV patient. Courtesy of Dr. Sandra Torres, Brazil

A recent classification [1] attempts to group HIV-associated oral lesions into the three following categories: (1) strongly associated with; (2) less commonly associated with; and (3) seen in HIV infection. Group 1 includes candidosis, hairy leukoplakia, Kaposi's sarcoma, non-Hodgkin's lymphoma, and periodontal disease. Group 2 and group 3 include a wide variety of manifestations, some of which still have controversial positions in this classification. Among those not presented in depth in this chapter, ulceration NOS (not otherwise specified) (Figs. 9.1–9.3) recurrent aphthous ulcers, bacterial infections,

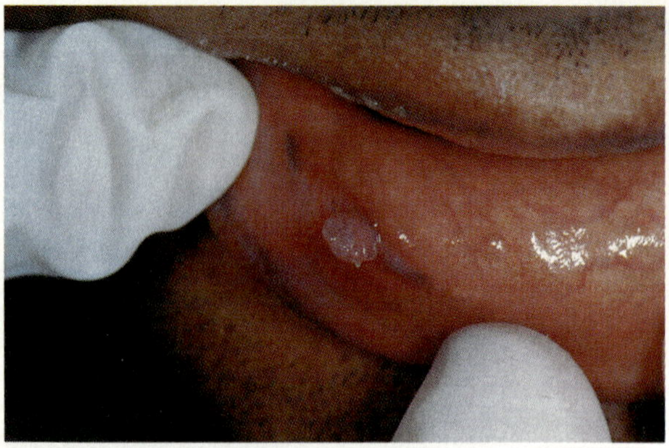

Fig. 9.4. Human papillomavirus lesion in an HIV patient

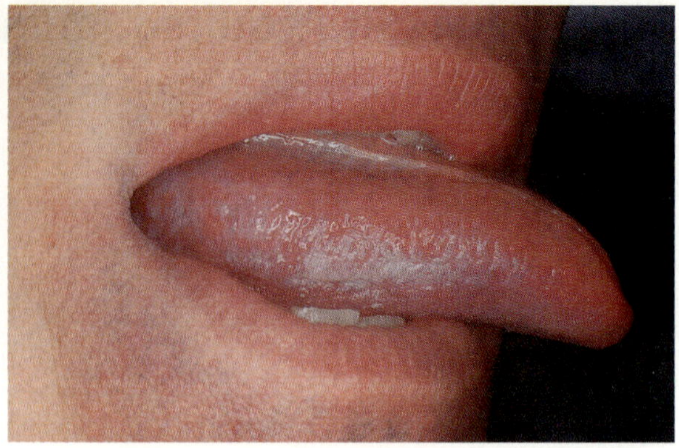

Fig. 9.5. Hairy leukoplakia in an HIV patient. Courtesy of Dr. Sandra Torres, Brazil

human papillomavirus infections (Fig. 9.4), salivary gland enlargement and rug reactions, because of the large quantity of medication AIDS patients have to take, must at least be cited for their relative frequency in the presence of HIV infection.

In this chapter, all oral manifestations included in group 1 of the EC Clearinghouse classification and some belonging to groups 2 and 3 will be presented.

9.2 Viral Infections

The most important HIV-associated oral diseases caused by virus are hairy leukoplakia, herpes simplex infection, molluscum contagiosum, and human papillomavirus infection. Of these, hairy leukoplakia, even though not specific, is considered almost pathognomonic of HIV infection, while oral herpes simplex is observed quite frequently.

9.2.1 Hairy Leukoplakia

Definition. Oral hairy leukoplakia is a characteristic white lesion usually on the sides of the tongue, which is considered an important marker of HIV infection (Fig. 9.5). It is included in group 1, (lesions strongly associated with HIV infection) of the EC Clearinghouse classification [1].

Etiology. This lesion is the most common Epstein-Barr virus (EBV)-related manifestation in AIDS.

Pathogenesis. This type of lesion is regarded as a specific result of replicating EBV in mucosal keratinocytes.

Oral Manifestations. The clinical features are rather typical, although not a pathognomonic characteristic or diagnostic: white or grayish, nonremovable patches, usually occurring on the lateral margins of the tongue (Fig. 9.6). They are often corrugated and shaggy with a 'hairy' appearance, can be uni- or bilateral, and rarely occur on the ventral surface of the tongue.

Associated Findings. Lesions are symptomless, although in a few cases a burning sensation may occur, especially if a *Candida* coinfection is present. Unlike HIV infection, it is rarely observed in other immunosuppressed patients, such as organ-transplant recipients, or in immunocompetent individuals. It is frequently associated with a low CD_4^+ T-lymphocyte count, in general less than $300/mm^3$.

Microscopic Findings. Histological features are not specific. Keratin projections, parakeratosis and acanthosis, ballooning of cells in the prickle cell layer, mild inflammation, and mild epithelial atypia in some cases may be present. Basophilic nuclear inclusion bodies of epithelial cells in the prickle cell layer are an indication of viral infection.

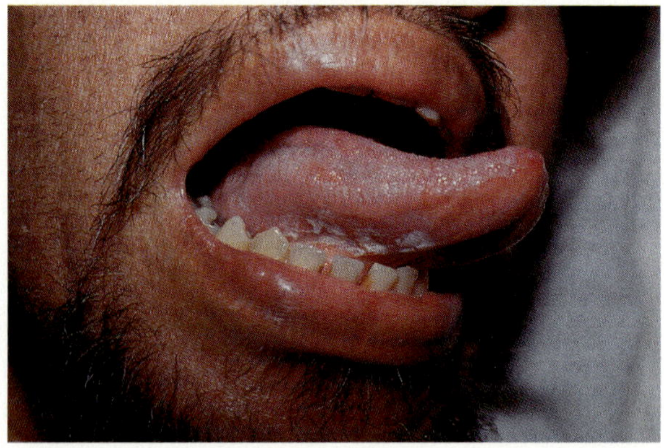

Fig. 9.6. Hairy leukoplakia on the side and pseudomembranous candidosis on the ventral surface of the tongue in an HIV patient

Diagnosis. In questionable cases, the presence of EBV is required for diagnosis and can be documented by exfoliative cytology for electron microscopy and in situ hybridization or PCR.

Differential Diagnosis. A number of oral white lesions can mimic hairy leukoplakia, such as candidal infection, with which it is associated in many cases. Lesions caused by restorative material, oral lichen planus, white sponge nevus, tongue biting, and classic leukoplakia may also be similar. A squamous cell carcinoma in an initial phase can mimic hairy leukoplakia and, because of its relatively poor prognosis, this differential diagnosis must be well established.

Treatment. In most cases, treatment is not required, although several modalities of therapy, including topical caustics and antiviral drugs, have been tried with varying results.

9.2.2 Herpes Simplex Infection

Definition. Herpes simplex infection is caused by herpesviruses mainly affecting mucosa (Fig. 9.7). Recurrence at the same site is one of its main characteristics. It is classified in group 2 (lesions less commonly associated with HIV infection) of the EC Clearinghouse classification [1]. However, an ulcerated herpes simplex lesion lasting for more than 1 month is one of the AIDS-defining factors used for its diagnosis.

Etiology. As a rule, herpes simplex virus type 1 causes extragenital lesions, although type 2 can also be responsible for lesions in the mouth, especially in HIV patients.

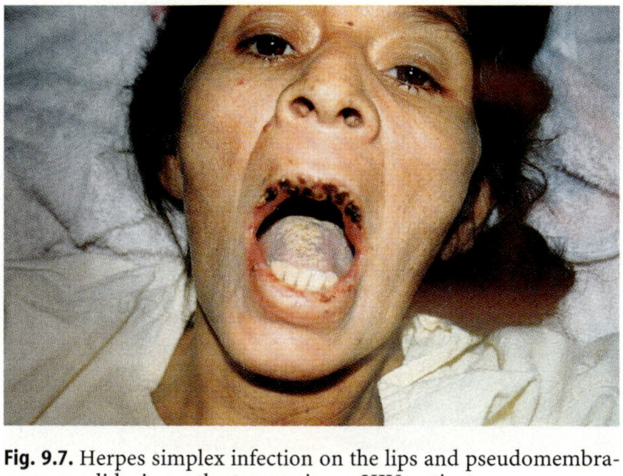

Fig. 9.7. Herpes simplex infection on the lips and pseudomembranous candidosis on the tongue in an HIV patient

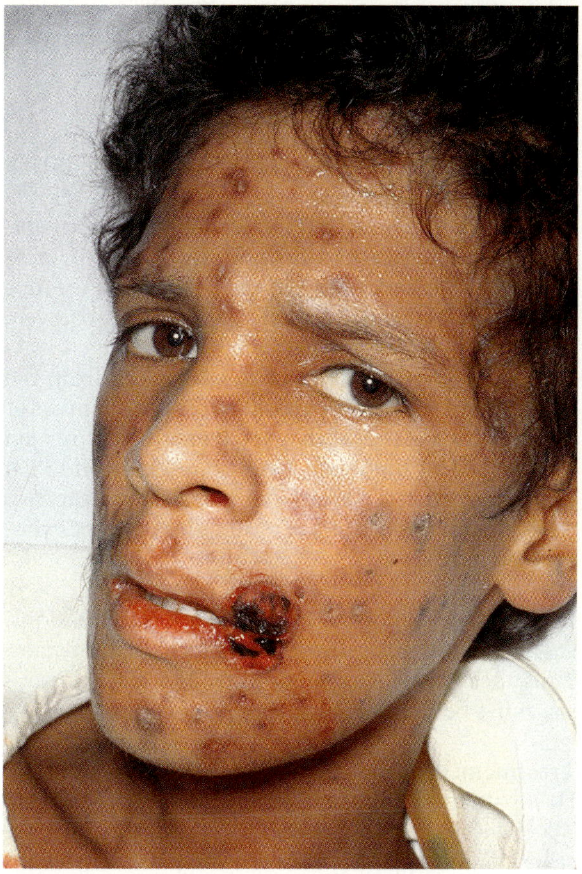

Fig. 9.8. Herpetic ulcerations on the lips and histoplasmosis on the face in an HIV patient

Pathogenesis. After primary infection, there is a latency period, probably due to persistence of virus in the ganglion, and relapses may occur. There are many factors that precipitate recurrences, such as exposure to sun, immunosuppression, upper respiratory tract infection, local trauma, and emotional stress.

Oral Manifestations. The characteristic lesions are crops of short-lived vesicles on an erythematous and swollen base. These vesicles rupture and turn into superficial erosions that heal within 7–10 days. Intraoral lesions can be self-limiting, but frequently progresss to a large nonhealing ulcer, especially in HIV-infected patients (Fig. 9.8), who often show more severe local destruction and persistent mucosal herpes simplex lesions with marked crust formation. Predilection sites are the vermillion border, the hard palate, the gingiva, and the dorsum of the tongue.

Associated Findings. Local lymph node enlargement and pain are usually present. Depending on the localization and severity, there may be fever, malaise, dysphagia, and weight loss. Lesions may be co-infected by other micro-organisms, including cytomegalovirus.

Microscopic Findings. Histology shows infected epithelial cells with edematous cytoplasm, producing ballooning degeneration of the epidermis. Thick-walled vesicles, intra- and intercellular edema in epidermis and inflammatory infiltrate with polymorphonuclear leukocytes and giant cells in dermis are present. Intranuclear inclusions can be observed.

Diagnosis. Cytodiagnosis in smears taken from the vesicle fluid and histopathology can be helpful for the diagnosis. Clinical diagnosis may be confirmed by culture, immunohistochemical method, and PCR technology. Serial serum samples taken over two weeks reveal rising titers of antibodies to herpes simplex viruses.

Differential Diagnosis. Persistent ulcerated lesions, such as aphthous ulcers, candidosis, cytomegalovirus ulcerations, cryptococcosis, and histoplasmosis, must be ruled out.

Treatment. Lesions are usually self-limited, but in HIV-patients systemic therapy is often required. Acyclovir is the drug of choice. Depending on the severity a dosage of 1000–2000 mg per day (five intakes/day), from 5 to 10 days, is given. Longer regimen or intravenous acyclovir may be required. Valaciclovir and famciclovir have proven activity for herpes simplex infection and foscarnet is now considered the drug of choice for acyclovir-resistant cases.

9.3 Fungal Infections

Superficial fungal diseases, especially candidosis, are common in AIDS patients. Oral candidosis is, in general, the first opportunistic manifestation and may suggest the possibility of HIV infection. It is usually asymptomatic and, in most cases, it is diagnosed during a routine exam. Because of its predictive value, oral examination must be included in all routine physical examinations.

Deep mycoses are less frequent and they usually appear in the context of the dissemination of the fungal disease. Oral lesions are usually clinically not specific.

Treatment of these diseases, when associated with HIV infection, has to be maintained for long periods, sometimes for life. Dosage, length of therapy, and prognosis depend on the immunological status of the patient.

9.3.1 Candidosis (Candidiasis, Moniliasis)

Definition. Candidosis, the so-called disease of the diseased, is caused by fungi of the genus *Candida*. In HIV-infected patients, oral candidosis is the most common opportunistic manifestation and is frequently the first sign of AIDS. Almost all patients develop this mycosis at some time during HIV disease. It belongs to group 1 of the EC Clearinghouse classification [1].

Etiology. Although the most prevalent species involved is *Candida albicans*, the disease can, in rare cases, be caused by other species. This genus *Candida* is a member of the family Cryptococcaceae.

Pathogenesis. *Candida albicans* is a saprophyte found in skin folds and in the mouth, genital area and, perianal area. It usually affects the skin and/or mucous membranes when the patient has some type of immunosupression, such as diabetes, neoplasia, or AIDS.

Oral Manifestations. All areas of the oral cavity may be affected. Different clinical manifestations can be seen in the same patient. In AIDS, the most frequent forms are pseudomembranous and erythematous. Other manifestations associated with oral candidal infection, such as angular cheilitis and denture-induced stomatitis, may be observed.

In pseudomembranous candidosis, lesions are white or yellowish plaques (Figs. 9.9, 9.10) that are easily wiped off, revealing an area of erythema, which may bleed.

Erythematous candidosis is characterized by red patches, usually on the dorsum of the tongue, where there is loss of papillae with a glossy appearance, and occasionally on the buccal mucosa. The palate may be affected due to contact with the tongue. White

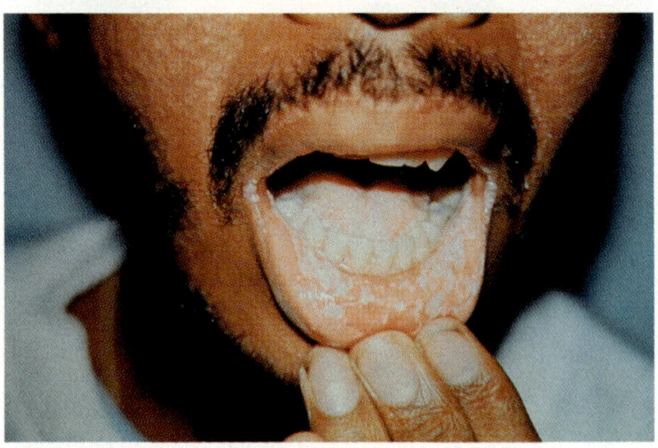

Fig. 9.9. Pseudomembranous candidosis in an HIV patient

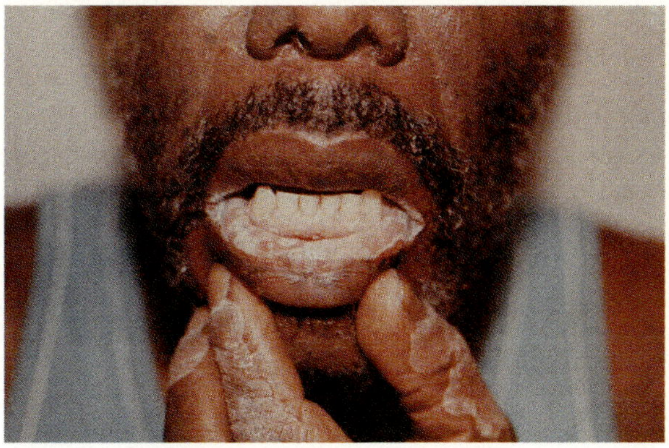

Fig. 9.10. Pseudomembranous candidosis in an HIV patient

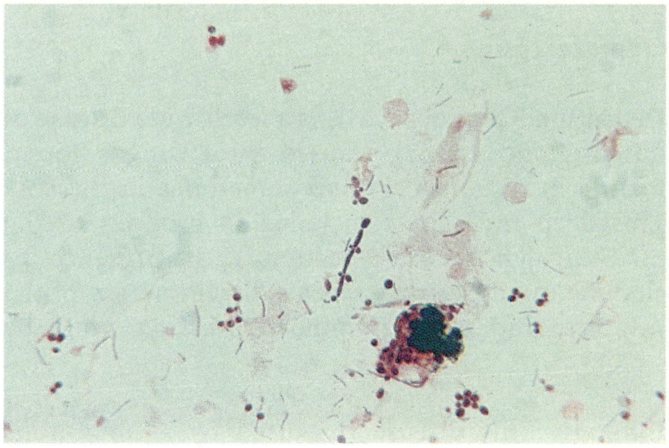

Fig. 9.11. *Candida* sp., direct examination. Gram stain

areas and plaques can also be seen, although erythema predominates.

Associated Findings. In HIV patients, oral candidosis may extend to the lower portions of the gastrointestinal tract, especially the esophagus. In this case, there is dysphagia and lack of taste sense, leading to weight loss, thus differing from the exclusively oral infection in which there are few or no symptoms.

Microscopic Findings. In candidosis, hyphae are more easily detected by PAS stain and silver impregnation techniques, such as Grocott and methenamine silver.

In pseudomembranous candidosis, hyphae of the superior epithelium may be observed as deep as the spinous cell layer. Parakeratosis, acanthosis, and spongiosis may be seen. Intraepithelial microabscesses are characteristic. Inflammatory changes are minimal or absent due to the immunodeficiency.

Erythematous form shows an epithelial atrophy with loss of rete ridges, subepithelial inflammatory infiltration, and vascular ectasia. Microabscesses are occasionally observed. Hyphae do not usually penetrate the epithelium.

Diagnosis. Detection of *Candida* by direct mycology and culture may help to establish the diagnosis, although it must be remembered that this fungus is a saprophyte of the oral cavity and, as such, can be found in up to 50 % of normal individuals (Figs. 9.11, 9.12). The response to antifungal therapy may be helpful.

Differential Diagnosis. Oral candidosis, depending on the clinical presentation, must be distinguished from leukoplakia, erythroplakia, hairy leukoplakia, and squamous cell carcinoma, among others.

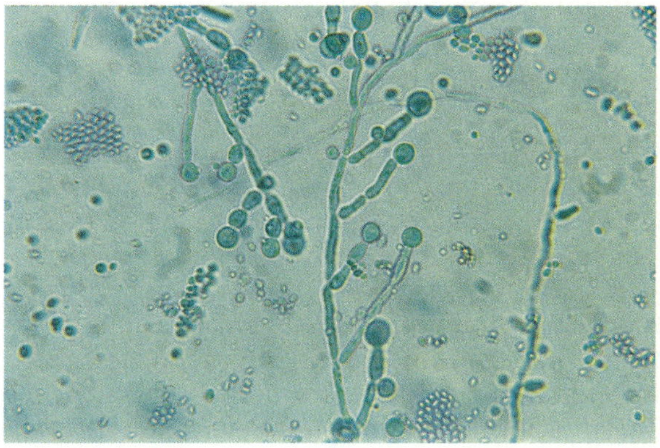

Fig. 9.12. *Candida* sp., culture. Corn meal medium

Treatment. Nystatin in oral suspension may be used as a mouth rinse. Oral azoles, such as ketoconazole (200–400 mg/day) and particularly itraconazole (100–200 mg/day) and fluconazole (50–150 mg/day) are the drugs of choice, although in the final stage of AIDS they may not help.

Systemic amphotericin, in intravenous doses of 0.7–1.0 mg/kg per day given slowly in 5 % dextrose over 4–6 h, is usually effective. The dose is around 2 g, and the maximum daily dose should not exceed 50 mg. Adverse effects of amphotericin B may include thrombophlebitis, nephrotoxicity, chills, nausea, anemia, and hypokalemia, some of which may be avoided by the association of hydrocortisone (100 mg) and heparin (5000 IU) in the intravenous infusion, as well as oral administration of promethazine (50 mg) and paracetamol (500 mg), or acetylsalicyclic acid (500 mg) 30 min before the infusion.

The exact dosage and length of therapy sometimes has to be determined by the infection's severity, the patients response to medication, and the possibility of adverse effects.

9.3.2 Cryptococcosis

Definition. Cryptococcosis is a worldwide disease of humans and animals caused by a fungus found mainly in pigeon feces and sometimes in the soil. This deep mycosis is included in group 3 of the EC Clearinghouse classification [1]. Its presence inside the mouth usually reveals dissemination of the mycosis, and thus immunosuppression must be sought.

Etiology. This disease is caused by a ubiquitous yeast. *Cryptococcus neoformans*, of which there are two varieties, var. *neoformans* and var. *gatti.*

Pathogenesis. Infection in otherwise healthy individuals is usually subclinical. Some have pulmonary disease, but dissemination occurs especially in immunodepressed patients.

Oral Manifestations. Oral cases have been reported as nonspecific persistent lesions, usually nonhealing extraction wounds or chronic ulceration on the palate, maxillary gingiva or tongue.

Associated Findings. In immunocompromised patients, oral cryptococcosis is, in general, associated with disseminated disease, mainly affecting the lungs, meninges, heart, spleen, pancreas, adrenals, ovaries, muscles, bones, liver, and gastrointestinal tract.

Microscopic Findings. Granulomas are seen in hematoxylin-eosin stain, and periodic acid-Schiff, mucicarmine or methenamine silver may reveal the fungi.

Diagnosis. Diagnosis may be confirmed by the finding of the yeast in smears stained with India ink, in histological sections, and in culture. *Cryptococcus neoformans* are usually numerous in lesions, appearing as round clear yeast cells with a typical wide carminophilic capsule.

Differential Diagnosis. All other causes of persistent oral ulcers must be excluded.

Treatment. Intravenous amphotericin, oral ketoconazole, itraconazole, or fluconazole can be used in the same dosage as for candidosis.

9.3.3 Histoplasmosis

Definition. Histoplasmosis is a disease caused by a fungus that produces mainly pulmonary alterations. It is the most frequently diagnosed deep mycosis in the United States, and is included in group 3 of the EC Clearinghouse classification [1].

Etiology. *Histoplasma capsulatum* is a soil saprophyte found in the Americas, India, the Far East, and Australia.

Pathogenesis. In AIDS, histoplasmosis usually arises from reactivated previous infections, especially in patients from endemic areas.

Oral Manifestations. The lesions are usually ulcerative or nodular, located on the tongue, palate, buccal mucosa, or gingiva (Fig. 9.13), rarely invading the mandible or maxilla.

Associated Findings. The oral lesion is sometimes isolated and may appear in apparently healthy persons, although it is often associated with acute or chronic pulmonary and cutaneous infection. Disseminated and potentially lethal forms affecting the reticuloendothelial system, lungs, kidneys, and gastrointestinal tract may typically be seen in the immunocompromised patient.

Microscopic Findings. Microscopy shows chronic granulomatous infiltration with micro-abscesses. Periodic acid-Schiff staining, silver impregnation techniques, and immunofluorescence with specific antisera may permit observation of the tiny and numerous fungi, especially inside macrophages.

Diagnosis. For confirmation of this mycosis, the fungus must be found either on microscopy or in

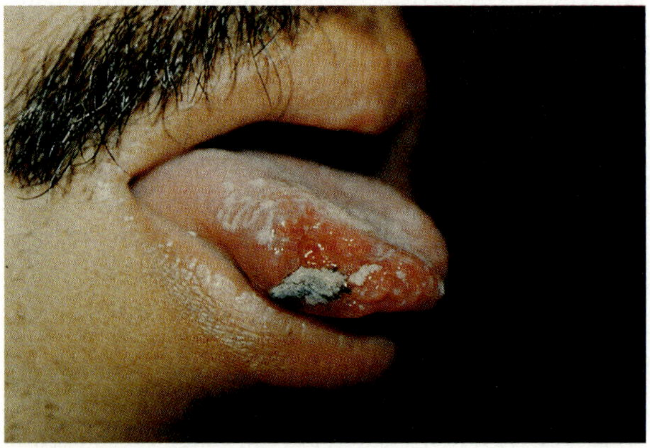

Fig. 9.13. Histoplasmosis in an HIV patient

agar Sabouraud culture. The histoplasmin intradermal test does not help in the diagnosis, because it is also positive in normal individuals from endemic areas.

Differential Diagnosis. All diseases that cause oral ulceration or nodules must be considered in this differential diagnosis.

Treatment. Intravenous amphotericin B, oral ketoconazole or itraconazole must be prescribed.

9.4 Periodontal Diseases

Periodontal diseases, which are still a subject of controversy, belong in group 1 of the EC Clearinghouse classification [1]. Like candidosis, they can appear in early stages of the immunodeficiency. Their clinical presentation, which includes linear gingival erythema, necrotizing gingivitis, and periodontitis, may be altered or exaggerated as a result of immunosuppression. Some authors consider these diseases the same as those seen in HIV-negative individuals without extreme features, while others see them as specific diseases of HIV infection or AIDS.

Tobacco smoking is very important as a risk factor for periodontal breakdown in the general population. For HIV-positive patients, this is true not only for periodontal diseases but also for other forms of oral manifestations, such as candidosis and hairy leukoplakia.

9.4.1 Linear Gingival Erythema

Definition. Linear gingival erythema is clinically typical: a fiery red line along the gingival margin.

Etiology. The cause is unknown and, as with other features, the microbiology of the lesions is still controversial, although *Candida albicans* might be involved in its etiology.

Pathogenesis. The pathogenesis of this type of alteration is unknown.

Oral Manifestations. This lesion is clinically characterized by a distinct red band along the margin of the gingiva. There is no ulceration and no evidence of pockets or attachment loss. Erythema is disproportionately intense for the existing plaque.

Associated Findings. Dental plaques may be found in association with this condition, although they may be discrete.

Microscopic Findings. It is stated by some authors that biopsy should not be performed because the findings are not specific and it is therefore not useful in establishing a definite diagnosis.

Diagnosis. Linear gingival erythema is a clinical diagnosis, and currently there are no definite criteria and no laboratory examinations for its confirmation.

Differential Diagnosis. Mild forms of marginal gingivitis and of desquamative gingivitis from other causes may have a similar clinical appearance.

Treatment. There is no specific treatment, and it has been suggested that the absence of a good response to oral hygiene measures and to removal of dental plaques and calculus is characteristic of linear gingival erythema.

9.4.2 Necrotizing Ulcerative Gingivitis and Periodontitis

Definition. Necrotizing ulcerative gingivitis is the term used for the destruction of one or more interdental papillae, while necrotizing ulcerative periodontitis, a more severe stage of the same process, involves periodontal soft tissue loss as a result of ulceration and necrosis. As periodontal diseases, both are included in group 1 [1]. A less severe form, conventional gingivitis, is also more prevalent, extensive, and severe in HIV infection.

Etiology. The full range of microorganisms observed in HIV-negative adult periodontitis is present in gingival plaque of HIV-infected patients, associated or not with atypical pathogens, such as enterococci and mycoplasm.

Pathogenesis. It is already known that, besides age, dental plaque levels, tobacco use, HIV infection, and decreased CD_4^+ counts predict the presence, extent and severity of loss of periodontal attachment, which facilitates infection by the saprophytic and pathogenic biota, leading to periodontal tissue destruction.

Oral Manifestations. A distinctive red marginal zone at the free gingiva and punctate erythema of the alveolar gingiva, even in patients with excellent oral hygiene and little or no plaque accumulation, are the initial features of HIV-associated gingivitis. Hemorrhage occurring spontaneously or after brushing and swollen, irregularly distributed interdental papillae may be associated.

In necrotizing periodontitis, there is severe ulceration and necrosis with consequent bone exposure. In more aggressive lesions, bone destruction or sequestration, and also tooth loss may occur.

Associated Findings. Necrotizing gingivitis and periodontitis show a tendency to rapid progression in HIV-positive patients and can be associated with complications far more severe and frequent than in the general population. Pain, fever, weight loss, malaise, and other general signs and symptoms are usual.

Microscopic Findings. Microscopy shows an acute, nonspecific inflammatory process with ulceration and necrosis.

Diagnosis. There are no definite criteria and the diagnosis can only be presumptive. Differentiation between necrotizing gingivitis and periodontitis is difficult, as they may be considered two different stages of the same process.

Differential Diagnosis. All specific causes of ulceration and necrosis of gingiva or periodontal areas, such as histoplasmosis and herpes simplex infection, among others, must be eliminated.

Treatment. Poor response to conventional antibiotic therapy is characteristic. Improvement of oral hygiene measures may be attempted as prophylaxis against periodontal disease, as in seronegative patients.

9.5 Malignant Tumors

Immunosuppressed individuals are at greater risk of developing malignant growths. Among these, Kaposi's sarcoma and non-Hodgkin's lymphoma are regarded as AIDS-defining diagnoses. They are considered opportunistic neoplasms, possibly activated by opportunistic oncogenic viruses. Kaposi's sarcoma is the most common neoplastic disease and the most frequent oral neoplasia in seropositive patients. Its frequency seems to be declining, especially since the advent of antiviral drugs.

Among the epidermal tumors of the oral mucosa, the most important is squamous cell carcinoma. In association with AIDS it usually shows a more aggressive and rapid course.

9.5.1 Kaposi's Sarcoma

Definition. Epidemic Kaposi's sarcoma associated with AIDS is a multicentric vascular proliferation and is far more frequent in male homosexual patients than in other AIDS risk groups. This tumor is an AIDS-defining lesion and its oral presentation is classified in group 1 of the EC Clearinghouse classification [1].

Etiology. The etiology is still controversial, but human herpesviruses, especially a newly identified gamma-herpesvirus, KSHV (Kaposi's sarcoma-associated herpesvirus or HHV-8), have recently been implicated.

Pathogenesis. There is still controversy over whether it is a clonal malignant neoplastic or a hyperplastic growth.

Oral Manifestations. Single or multiple erythematous, slightly bluish or violaceous macules or swellings are seen predominantly on the palate (Figs. 9.14–9.18). The most common oral presentations are macular and papulonodular lesions. Eventually, they may become tumorous and ulcerate.

Associated Findings. In general, there are no symptoms, and there may be associated cutaneous, and/or visceral lesions. Because it is a defining diagnosis, is may be associated with other opportunistic infections, as well as other features of AIDS. Upper gastrointestinal and respiratory tract Kaposi's sarcomas must be searched for in the presence of oral lesions.

Microscopic Findings. The histological appearance of Kaposi's sarcoma is characteristic: a vascular proliferation showing interweaving bands of spindle and/or "plump" endothelial cells and atypical vascular channels. Endothelial cells may protrude into the vascular lumen. Erythrocyte extravasation and scattered mononuclear inflammatory infiltrate are present.

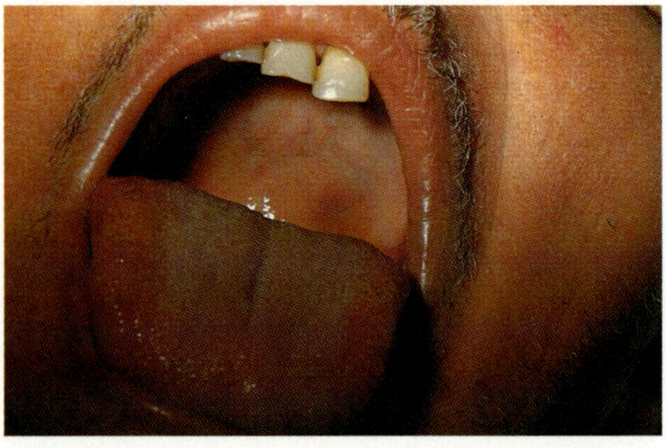

Fig. 9.14. Kaposi's sarcoma of the palate in an HIV patient

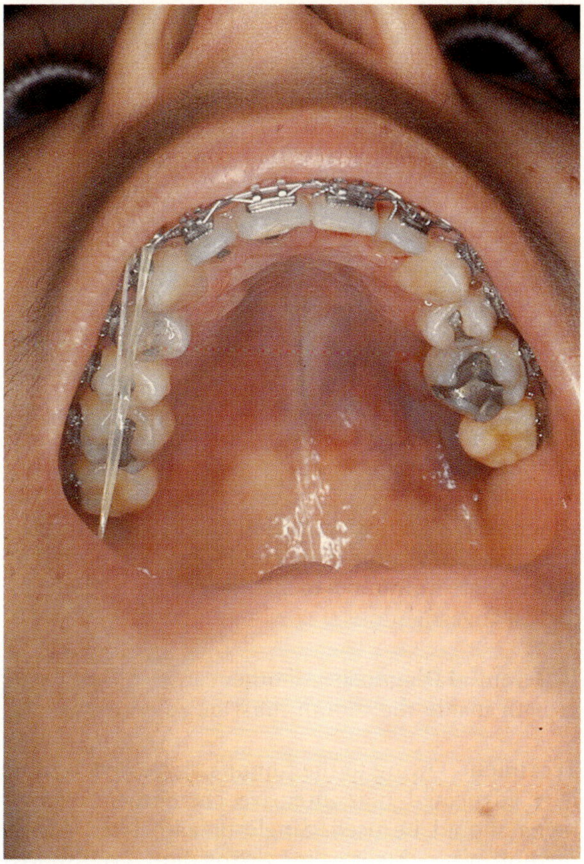

Fig. 9.15. Kaposi's sarcoma of the palate in an HIV patient. Courtesy of Dr. Sandra Torres, Brazil

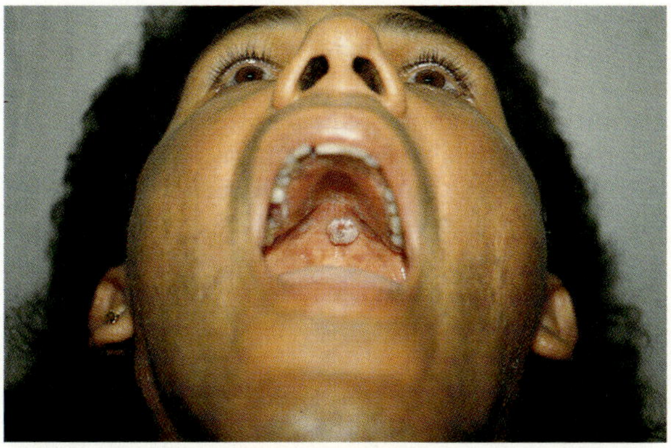

Fig. 9.16. Kaposi's sarcoma of the palate in an HIV patient

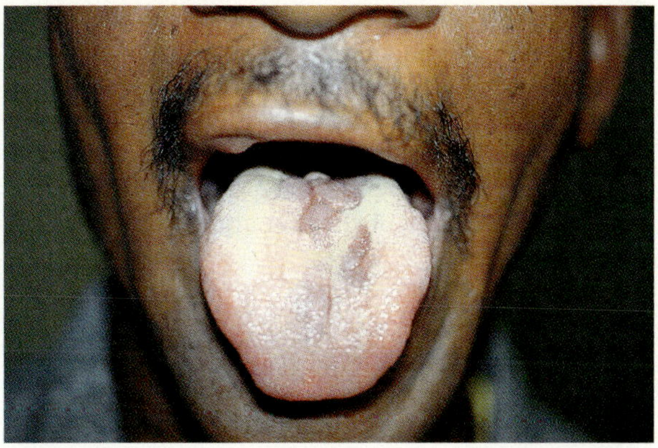

Fig. 9.17. Kaposi's sarcoma of the tongue in an HIV patient

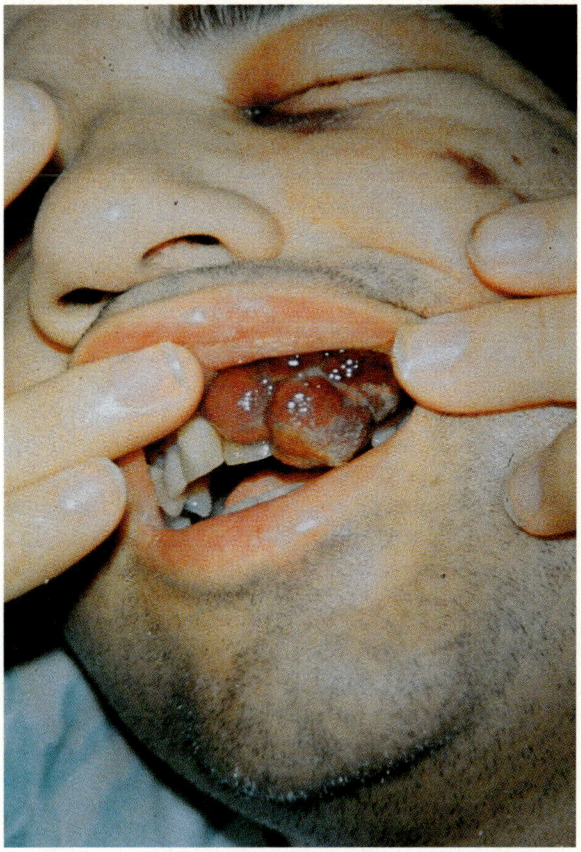

Fig. 9.18. Kaposi's sarcoma of the gingiva in an HIV patient

Diagnosis. Clinical suspicion should be confirmed by histology, because of the importance of this diagnosis.

Differential Diagnosis. Macular lesions must be differentiated from fixed drug eruption, amalgam tattoo, and ecchymosis, while papulonodular lesions should be distinguished especially from angioproliferative processes, such as pyogenic granuloma, angiomas, epitheloid angiomatosis, and hematoma.

Treatment. There are reports of tumor involution without specific treatment, especially since the advent of combined antiretroviral therapy. Local excision, intralesional chemotherapy, especially with vinblastine (1 mg in 0.5 ml of distilled water every

7 or 15 days, with 1–2 mg in each application), regional radiotherapy, and single- or multiagent systemic chemotherapy including vinblastine, vincristine, doxorubicin, and bleomycin can be used. Interferon-α can act as an immunomodulator. Cytokines and photodynamic therapy have recently been advocated. Treatment is not curative and remission is seldom complete.

9.5.2 Non-Hodgkin's Lymphoma

Definition. Oral non-Hodgkin's lymphoma is usually a B-cell lymphoma, either a small Burkitt's lymphoma, or, more commonly, a large cell immunoblastic lymphoma. These tumors belong to group 1 of the EC Clearinghouse classification [1], although moving them to group 2 or 3 has been suggested.

Etiology. These tumors are known to occur in immunosuppression such as occurs in some congenital diseases and in iatrogenic immunosuppression in organ transplant recipients and AIDS. The etiology of these lymphomas remains controversial: some authors attribute their cause to Epstein-Barr virus, while others see them as due to direct activation of B-cell proliferation by HIV infection. The recently discovered human herpesvirus 8 may also have a role in this process.

Pathogenesis. It seems that polyclonal B-lymphocytic activation with consequent B-cell proliferation is induced by immunosuppression, thus leading to tumor formation. Only a minority of non-Hodgkin's lymphomas show an undetermined or T-cell phenotype.

Oral Manifestations. This lymphoma is an oral soft tissue tumefaction, usually a firm, elastic, and often somewhat reddish or purplish swelling, with or without ulceration. Preferential sites are gingiva, palate, and throat (Fig. 9.19).

Associated Findings. Oral non-Hodgkin's lymphoma is usually associated with lesions elsewhere, especially in the central nervous system, gastrointestinal tract, bone marrow, and liver. Most patients present with fever, malaise, night sweats, weight loss, and lymph node involvement.

Microscopic Findings. These tumors have heterogeneous histologic features, with a "blastic" cell morphology. Most of them consist of immunoblastic sarcoma, small non-cleaved-cell lymphoma, or typical Burkitt's lymphoma and their variants.

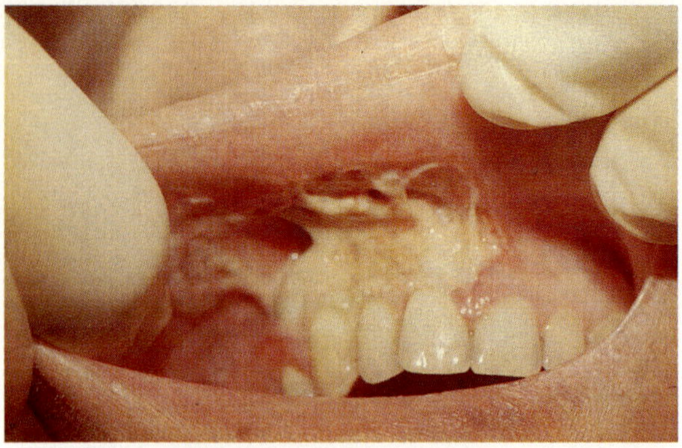

Fig. 9.19. Non-Hodgkin's lymphoma in an HIV patient. Courtesy of Dr. Sonia Ferreira, Brazil

Diagnosis. A clinical suspicion can be confirmed by the histological appearance on biopsy, supported by appropriate immunocytochemical or molecular biological investigations.

Differential Diagnosis. All other causes of soft tissue growth inside the mouth must be ruled out.

Treatment. Owing to the tumor's aggressive course, it is advocated that intensive chemotherapy regimens should be used. Single or associated use of methotrexate, bleomycin, doxorubin, cyclosphosphamide, vincristine, dexamethasone, and zidovudine is suggested.

9.5.3 Squamous Cell Carcinoma

Definition. Squamous cell carcinoma is a malignant tumor that is relatively frequent in the oral mucosa. Although it is the most common malignant lesion of the mouth, it is not even cited as a lesion associated with AIDS in the EC Clearinghouse classification [1]. Present opinion includes it in group 3 of the EC Clearinghouse classification.

Etiology. This is a multifactorial disease in which incidence and/or severity can be increased by immunosuppression of varying etiology, including HIV-infection. Tobacco use is one of the major causes of this neoplasm in the mouth. Others factors involved are exposure to sun, genetic predisposition, alcohol and other chemical agents, human papillomavirus, and local trauma.

Pathogenesis. This tumor is derived from the squamous epithelium and, in many cases, grows from a pre-existing precancerous lesion, especially erythroplakia or leukoplakia in the mouth.

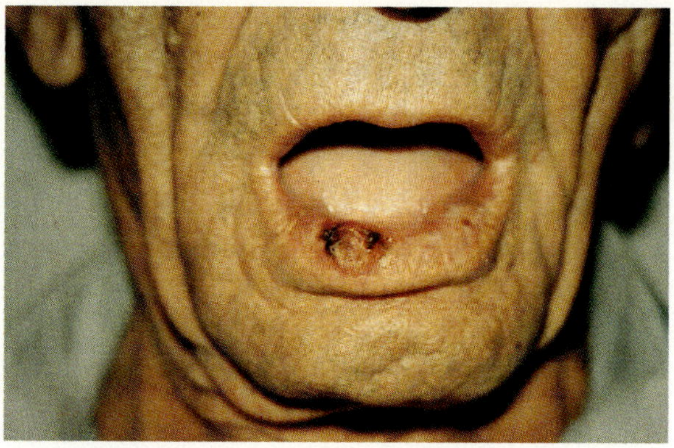

Fig. 9.20. Squamous cell carcinoma in an HIV patient

Oral Manifestations. Clinical presentation of squamous cell carcinoma includes a wide variety of types of lesions: white patches, erythematous areas, ulcers, nodules, and vegetations, among others (Fig. 9.20).

Associated Findings. Oral squamous cell carcinoma is frequently associated with early regional lymph node metastases.

Microscopic Findings. There is keratinocyte proliferation, with lobules, ribbons and trabeculae of neoplastic cells, sometimes with high cellular pleomorphism, high mitotic rate, and many atypical nuclei. Keratin pearl formation is usually present.

Diagnosis. Diagnosis is based on clinical and microscopic findings. Biopsy is mandatory when a squamous cell carcinoma is suspected, and histology confirms the diagnosis in most cases.

Differential Diagnosis. Leukoplakia, erythroplakia, and diseases that cause oral persistent ulcers or vegetations must be considered in the differental diagnosis.

Treatment. Squamous cell carcinoma has to be well evaluated before therapy is decided on. This evaluation concerns its size, and the presence or absence of affected lymph nodes and distant metastases in other organs. Depending on this evaluation, it must be treated by surgery, radiotherapy, or chemotherapy, either singly or in combination.

References

1. Boshoff C, Whitby D, Talbot S, Weiss RA. Etiology of AIDS-related Kaposi's sarcoma and lymphoma. Oral Dis 1997; 3[Suppl 1]:S129–S132
2. Dobleman TJ, Scher N, Goldman M. Invasive histoplasmosis of the mandible. Head Neck 1989; 11:81–84
3. Epstein JB Management of oral Kaposi's sarcoma and a proposal for clinical staging. Oral Dis 1997; 3[Suppl 1]:S124–S128
4. Epstein JB, Silverman S Jr. Head and neck malignancies associated with HIV infection. Oral Surg Oral Med Oral Pathol 1992; 73:193–200
5. Epstein JB, Lozada-Nur F, McLeod A, Spinelli J. Oral Kaposi's sarcoma in acquired immunodeficiency syndrome. Cancer 1989; 64:2424–2430
6. Epstein JB, Fatahzadeh M, Matisic J, Anderson G. Exfoliative cytology and electron microscopy in the diagnosis of hairy leukoplakia. Oral Surg Oral Med Oral Pathol 1995; 79:564–569
7. Flaitz CM, Nichols CM, Adler-Storthz K, Hicks MJ. Intraoral squamous cell carcinoma in human immunodeficiency virus infection. Oral Surg Oral Med Oral Pathol Oral Radiol Endod 1995; 80:55–62
8. Grbric JT, Mitchell-Lewis DA, Fine JB et al. The relationship of candidiasis to linear gingival erythema in HIV-infected homosexual men and parenteral drug users. J Periodontal 1995; 66:30–37
9. Green TL, Eversole LR. Oral lymphomas in HIV-infected patients: association with Epstein-Barr virus DNA. Oral Surg Oral Med Oral Pathol 1989; 67:437–442
10. Greenspan D, Greenspan JS, Schiodt M, Pindborg JJ. Aids and the mouth – diagnosis and management of oral lesions. Copenhagen: Munsksgaard, 1990; 85–145
11. Itin PH, Lautenschlager S. Viral lesions of the mouth in HIV-infected patients. Dermatology, 1997; 194:1–7
12. Johnson NW. Essential questions concerning periodontal diseases in HIV infection. Oral Dis 1997; 3[Suppl 1]:S138–S140
13. Mabruk MJEMF, Flint SR, Toner M et al. In situ hybridization and the polymerase chain reaction (PCR) in the analysis of biopsies and exfoliative cytology specimens for definitive diagnosis of oral hairy leukoplakia. J Oral Pathol Med 1994; 23:302–308
14. Mao EJ, Smith CJ. Detection of Epstein-Barr virus (EBV) by the polymerase chain reaction (PCR) in oral smears from healthy individuals and patients with squamous cell carcinoma. J Oral Pathol Med 1993; 22:12–17
15. Ravina A, Ficarra G, Chiolo M et al. Relationship of circulating CD_4^+ T lymphocytes and p24 antigenemia to the risk of developing AIDS in HIV-infected subjects with oral hairy leukoplakia. J Oral Pathol Med 1996; 25:108–111
16. Regezi JA, Eversole LR, Barker BF, Rick GM, Silverman S. Herpes simplex and cytomegalovirus coinfected oral ulcers in HIV-positive patients. Oral Surg Oral Med Oral Pathol Oral Radiol Endod 1996; 81:55–62
17. Reichart PA. Oral pathology of acquired immunodeficiency syndrome and oro-facial Kaposi's sarcoma. Curr Top Pathol 1996; 90:97–123
18. Reichhart PA, Langford-Kuntz A, Pohle H-D. Epidemic orofacial Kaposi's sarcoma (eKS) – report on 124 cases. Oral Oncol Eur J Cancer 1993; 29B:187–189
19. Robinson PG, Challacombe SJ, Sheimann JM, Zakrzewska JM. Is erythematous candidiasis associated with advanced HIV disease? Oral Dis 1997; 3[Suppl 1]:S116–S118
20. Scully C, de Almeida OP, Sposto MR. The deep mycoses in HIV infection. Oral Dis 1997; 3[Suppl 1]:S200–S207
21. Tirelli U, Franceschi S, Carbone A. Malignant tumours in patients with HIV infection. Br Med J 1994; 308:1148–1153
22. Van der Waal I. Some unusual oral lesions in HIV infection: comments on the current classification. Oral Dis 1997; 3[Suppl 1]:S197–S199
23. Zakrzewska JM. Overview: Kaposi's sarcoma, oral neoplasms. Oral Dis 1997; 3[Suppl 1]:S122–123

CHAPTER 10

Allergic, Toxic, and Drug-Induced Eruptions of the Oral Mucosa

L.E. Millikan

10.1 Types of Reactions

Traditionally, the allergic types of reactions in the mucous membranes have been classified by the Coombs and Gel system. This includes types I–IV and covers most of the major pathologic events (Figs. 10.1–10.11) [1]. In brief, we can look on these as a useful way to sort out reactions as they occur, and provide insight into future potential problems.

Coombs and Gel type I is a classic anaphylactoid/anaphylactic reaction involving the generation of IgE antibodies. This becomes a significant problem in life-threatening drug eruptions, and is often a preferential immunologic response in patients with atopic dermatitis. Additionally, severe types of urticaria may present with type I reactions.

Briefly, the allergen, when received by the host orally, parenterally or however, stimulates an antibody response to the antigenic stimulus and, in the appropriately primed patient, is subsequently manifest by a proliferation of antibodies, primarily of the IgE classification. IgE antibodies are characterized by their ability to bind with cells in local areas, and the combination of the antigen bridging two IgE molecules results in histamine release, which then mediates the subsequent reaction. The best example of this clinically is the positive scratch test in the skin. When the antigen is given sytematically, the systemic response can be urticarial, with widespread hives, and when this histamine reaction involves the upper airway with swelling it can compromise the airway, resulting in life-threatening consequences. For this reason, a type I reaction in the mucous

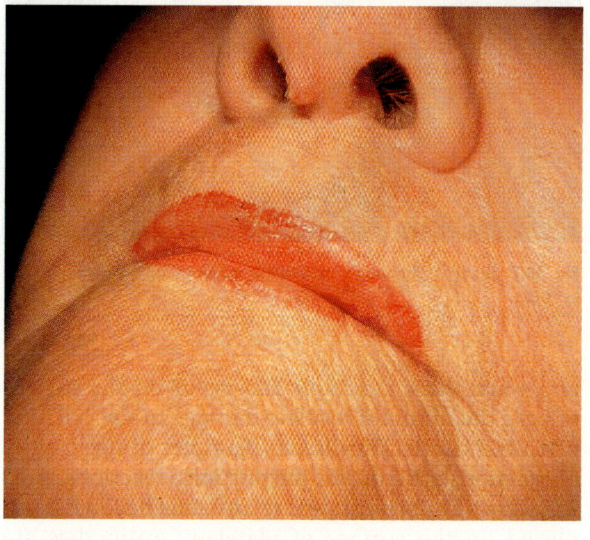

Fig. 10.1. Chronic scarring of the mucocutaneous junction after mucous membrane bullous disease

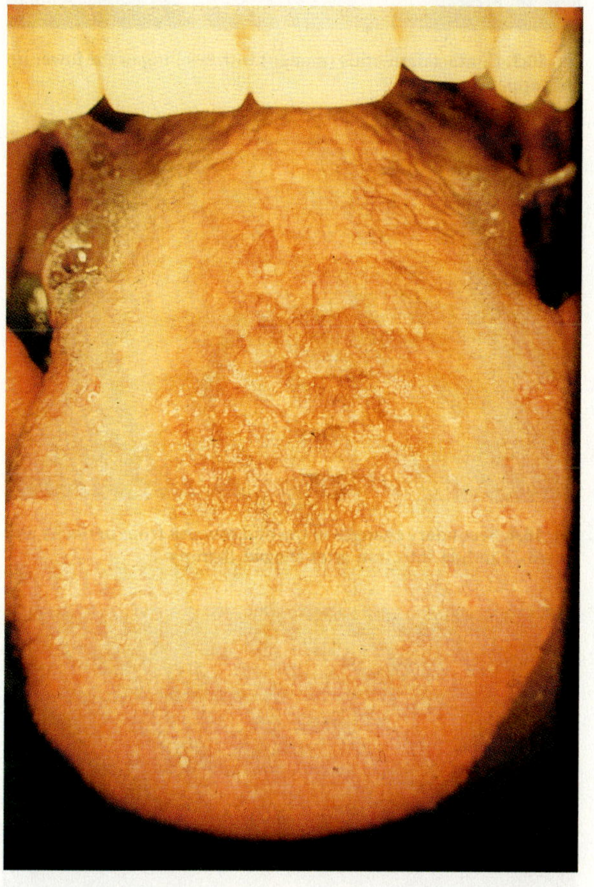

Fig. 10.2. Black hairy tongue, a common complication of antibiotic therapy

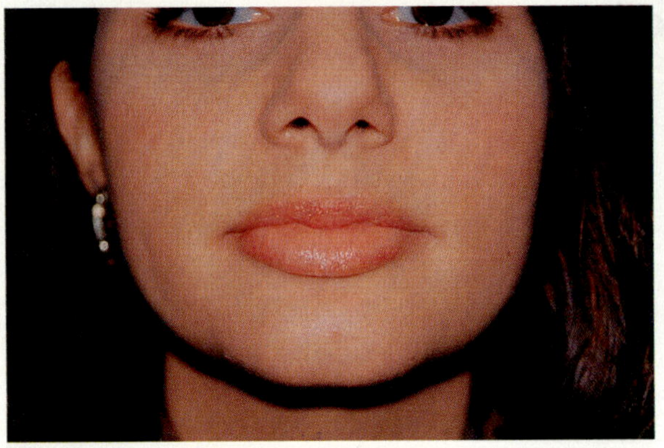

Fig. 10.3. Contact dermatitis (mango) with swelling of the lower lip and upper lip

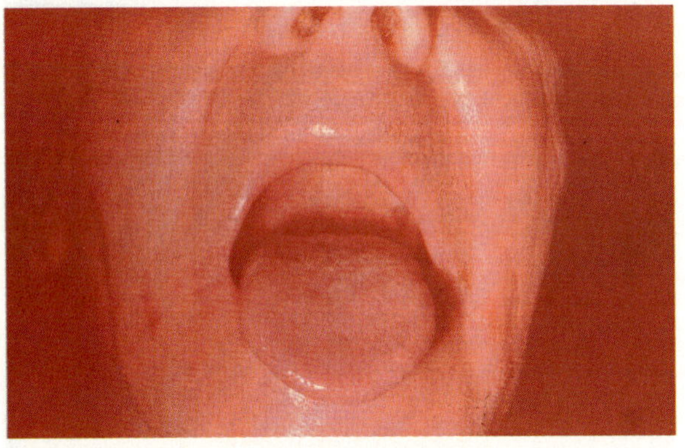

Fig. 10.4. Secondary changes in the oral mucosa from perlèche and thrush, candida infection after steroid therapy

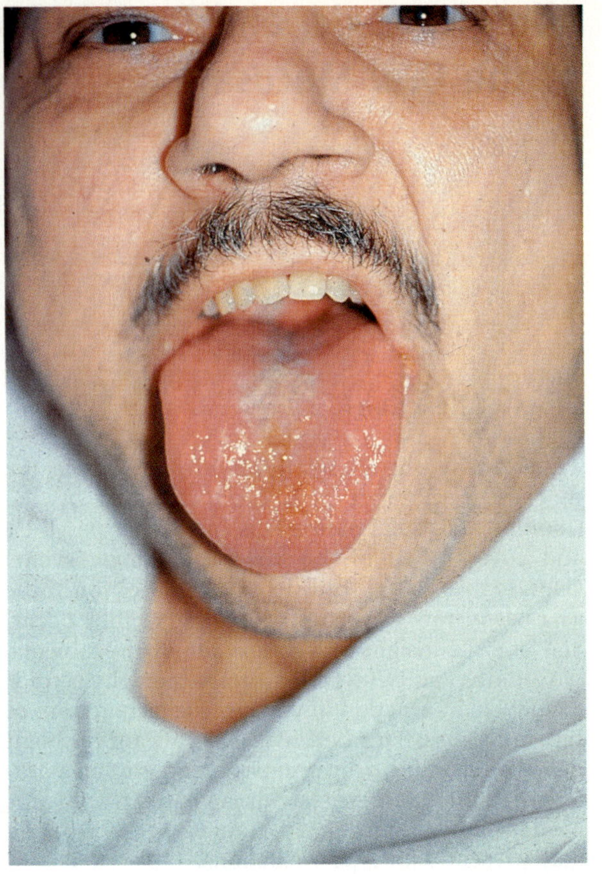

Fig. 10.6. Candidiasis and early black hairy tongue after bactrim therapy

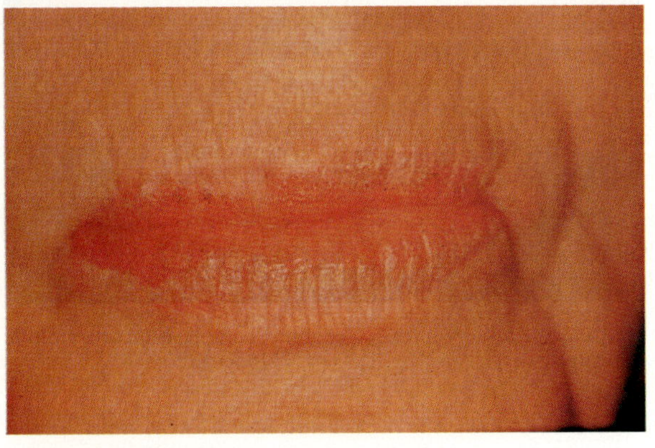

Fig. 10.5. Chronic changes of the lip after lupus erythematosus

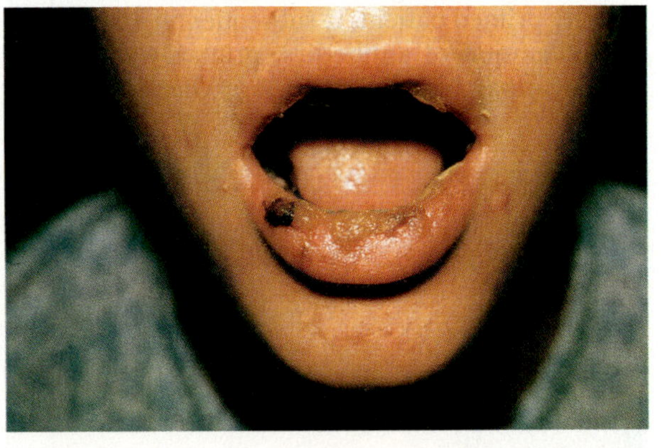

Fig. 10.7. Severe aphthous stomatititis, etiology uncertain, possible herpes

membranes is of great concern because of this potential for swelling and airway problems.

These severe complications make type I reactions clinically the most respected allergic reactions in the mucous membranes.

Type II reactions are generally the result of antibodies initiating complement-mediated sequelae, and when these reactions can occur on the surface of cells the ultimate result is damage to the cell, and often cell death. The classic examples of these types of reactions are some of the purpuric reactions, such as sedormid purpura, where antigens become complexed on the surface of platelets. Antibodies are formed against the drug antigen/hapten, and there

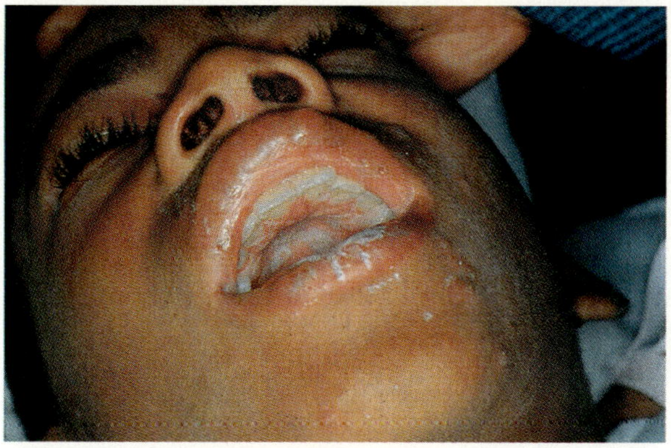

Fig. 10.8. Mucous membrane changes of the Stevens-Johnson syndrome: lip and palate

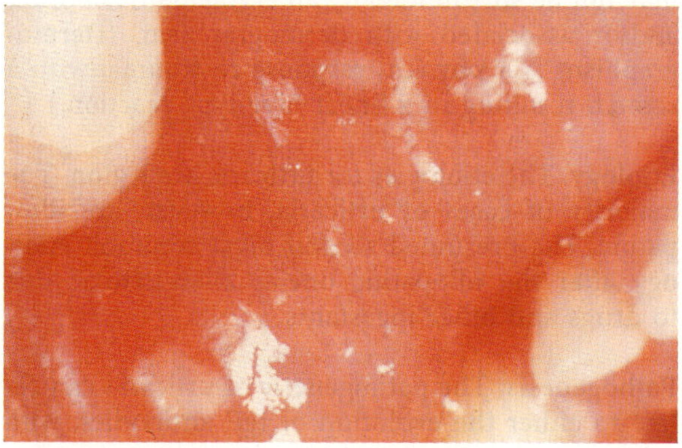

Fig. 10.9. Severe mucous membrane changes with aphthous ulcers

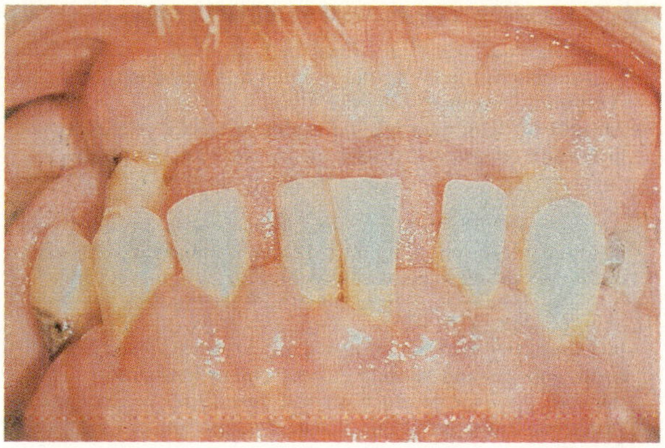

Fig. 10.10. Gingival hyperplasia occurring with the use of Procardia

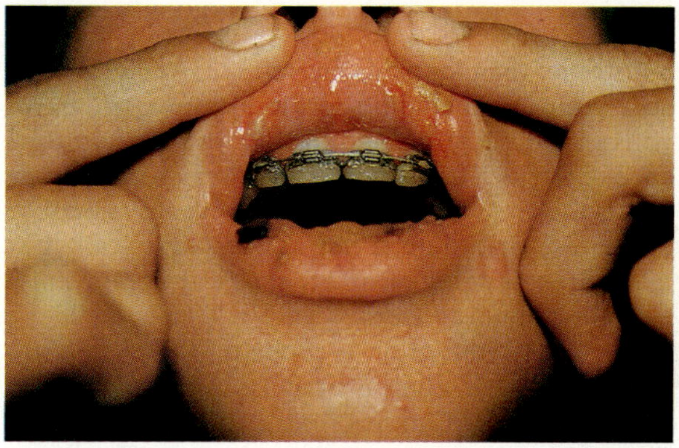

Fig. 10.11. Simple aphthous ulcers (differential diagnosis: other toxic ulcers)

is attachment of the antigen to a cell, such as a platelet. Subsequent drug exposure results in an antigen-antibody reaction on the surface of the cell, and cell destruction. In the case of sedormid, the antibody/antigen platelet reaction results in platelet destruction through the complement pathway, either by complement-mediated cell destruction with the late complement components, or by opsonization and removal of platelets by the reticuloendothelial (RE) system. In both instances, cell destruction or cell opsonization and removal by the RE system, thrombocytopenia results, which clinically gives the picture of purpura. It is estimated that other types of reactions are similar, including the bullous reactions on the mucous membranes and on glabrous skin, and the other cytopenic reactions, including granulocytopenia and allergic hemolytic anemias. This is the possible mechanism of the Stevens-Johnson syndrome and other ulcerative/bullous reactions in the mucous membranes.

Type III is perhaps the most common type of reaction seen in clinical practice according to our current understanding. The type III reaction results from immune complex formation, and this will then clinically present in a variety of ways. Urticaria resulting from drugs is probably the most frequent manifestation of the type III reactions. Beginning with the early studies on serum sickness, this type of reaction has become a standard prototype for various immunologic reactions. The pathophysiology relates to the formation of IgG antibodies to the drug/antigen, and the subsequent amplification of the reaction by the conglomeration of antigen antibody complexes into larger and larger products. General wisdom is that small complexes can often be cleared easily by the body and there is therefore no serious secondary problem. Formation of immune complexes is considered physiologically important to accelerate the clearance of foreign proteins, drugs, etc. When the reaction results in large immune complexes, these can be deposited in the blood vessels, initiating inflammation (vasculitis) and increases in vascular permeability (resulting in urticaria). Tissue necrosis and bullae formation may be another reaction to such immune complexes. The immune complex deposition in parts of the

Table 10.1. Coombs-Gell classification of immunologic reactions

I.	IgE-mediated, anaphylactoid reaction or anaphylaxis, urticarial symptoms, potentially life-threatening Antigen bridging two IgE molecules in cells – results in histamine release, which is a major cause of symptoms
II	IgG cytotoxic Antigen (often hapten) on surface reacts with antibody and yields cell destruction, inflammation mediated by complement and other cytokine activation/generator
III.	Immune complex IgG primarily involves antigen-antibody complexes which form, enlarge, and stimulate complement-mediated cell damage, cytokine production, and opsonization. Urticaria, vasculitis, bulla promotion, tissue dysfunction can all result from this
IV.	Cell-mediated immunity with contact dermatitis as the primary presentation

body other than the skin can result in even more serious sequelae, including serum sickness which involves both the joints and the kidneys. The appearance of a type III reaction in the mucous membrane warns the clinician to evaluate the whole patient to make sure that there is not a more significant systemic process going on and that airway compromise is not a serious concern.

The type IV reaction is probably the most common reaction in clinical practice in the context of the traditional Coombs and Gell classification. Type IV reactions are manifested by the T-cell system and are familiar to dermatologists as contact dermatitis, the most common presentation. This involves the T-cell system, rather than immunoglobulins and the B-cell system, and this then allows for peripheral localization; it can occur on mucous membranes, but is generally considered less common there. Part of this relates to the dilutionary effect of the constant bathing of the mucous membranes with various fluids and may also have something to do with the mucous membrane reservoir of immunoglobulin A antibodies, and the elaboration of immunoglobulin E antibodies, which can interfere with T-cell reactions by histamine release, which tends to blunt T-cell proliferation and T-cell lymphokine elaboration.

Lastly, our understanding of immunologic and immunologic allergic and toxic reactions in the mucous membranes has undergone a significant change with the proliferation of various cytokines in the epidermis and mucous membranes. In many instances, the reactions to certain drugs and chemicals may (especially in the toxic reactions) result primarily from these various substances, stimulating the release of cytokines which may then cause a series of toxic reactions in skin and mucous membranes. (See Table 10.1 on Coombs and Gell reactions.)

Various cytokines can be pro-inflammatory, proproliferative, and cytotoxic to certain cell lines. This is a complex and very dynamic area that is under intensive investigation with continual evolution in our understanding of it.

10.2 Urticaria and Angioedema

10.2.1 Urticaria (Hives, Weal)

Definition. There is superficial edema in the upper dermis and epidermis, resulting in white elevated plaques that are often very pruritic and may or may not be surrounded by an erythematous border and/or associated with dermographism. (Dermographism is a physical response to trauma, with a scratch resulting in a linear hive-type reaction.)

Etiology. The etiologies for urticaria are legion. The majority of cases of urticaria, however, are idiopathic. The presumed second most common etiology after the idiopathic one is allergic/toxic due to drugs and other ingestants.

Pathogenesis. The pathogenesis of urticaria can relate to either the evolution of IgE antibodies, with subsequent exposure to histamine release (see Table 10.1), or local tissue edema and increased vascular permeability [1]. In addition, certain drugs can cause reactions through a type III immune complex reaction, causing local complement-mediated reactions with release of anaphylatoxins, localized cellular edema, and secondary inflammatory infiltrates. Some chemicals, foods/ingestants, can cause a direct reaction with mast cells in the body and subsequent histamine release, with the same ultimate terminal events and urticarial symptoms.

Oral Manifestations. The oral manifestations in urticaria can be amongst the most impressive because of the low tissue pressure in the mucous membranes. Urticarial reactions can result in massive swelling, and the pathologic significance here relates to the edema impinging on airway patency. With a common type of acute urticaria, this waxes and wanes and usually responds to therapy. With the more serious variant, urticarial vasculitis, the edema can be much more long-lasting and is of greater medical significance because of its association with some severe systemic diseases.

Associated Findings. It is rare to find urticaria limited to the mucous membranes, and often the other parts of the body may be involved prior to the mucous membranes.

Urticaria related to physical causes (heat, cold), may primarily appear in the mucous membranes because of the oral exposure to foods and fluids of varying temperatures.

Microscopic Findings. The microscopic findings are related to tissue edema: some perivascular infiltrates and some inflammatory cell infiltration into the tissue, including eosinophils.

Diagnosis. Diagnosis is made on a clinical basis in most instances. Atypical lesions may require biopsy for support of the diagnosis. The diagnosis is usually easily made and not a significant problem.

Treatment. Depending on the severity of the swelling and the potential for airway obstruction, acute therapy is usually parenteral, intravenous, or intramuscular. Epinephrine can be given, 0.3–0.5 ml, 1:1000 (aqueous, SC) in severe episodes. Less severe episodes may respond to intramuscular or intravenous administration of benadryl, 50–75 mg. (Extensive urticaria mandates intravenous and less severe, intramuscular administration.) Steroids may be given in the usual doses of approximately 1.0 ml per kg, but will primarily be effective in long-term correction of the problem, and less so in the short term. Additionally, newer nonsedating antihistamines may be of use, with loratidine, 10 mg once or twice daily, being preferred because of the lesser interaction potential. Astemizole 10 mg may also be used, but serious interactions with many other drugs metabolized by the cytochrome P450 system mandate careful review of concomitant medication. Terfenadine (Seldane) involves a similar problem. Traditionally, hydroxyzine has been the treatment of choice for maintenance control of urticaria, but sedation with atarax has often led to undertreatment and therefore lower efficacy. Dosage should be pushed to 25 mg two or three times daily in a 75-kg patient. A newer alternative for this is the use of cetirizine, which has some residual sedating potential, but significantly less than hydrodoxyzine. Further useful medications for this problem include cyproheptadine, 4–8 mg two to three times daily, and other useful antihistamines are now available over the counter, including oral benadryl and oral chlor-trimeton. The over-the-counter preparations generally need to be pushed in dosage to control the urticaria. The involvement of neuropeptides in this process is an area of increasing knowledge, but effective therapy sytemically for control of substance P release is not yet available, though on occasion capsaicin (OTC) may be useful in controlling those urticarial episodes that are not controlled by antihistamines. The side effects of significant burning require careful patient education, in addition to that provided by the manufacturer [1, 2].

10.2.2 Angioedema (Hereditary Angioedema)

Definition. Angioedema is a particular form of urticaria in which massive swelling occurs in particular areas, especially those with low tissue pressure, i. e., mid-face, around the eyes, neck, and mucous membranes. One of the classic forms of angioedema is the hereditary one and its acquired variant associated with complement abnormalities. In these instances, trauma, infection, temperature changes, etc., initiate activation of the complement cascade in a patient whose normal control mechanisms of complement activation are deficient (C-1 esterase inhibitor). As a result, these patients develop massive urticarial areas after inconsequential events (trauma, infection, menstruation, illness), and airway obstruction is so likely that these patients often require admission to assure prompt tracheotomy if the airway is at risk [3].

Pathogenesis. In both hereditary and acquired forms of angioedema, there is an abnormality of the enzyme C-1 esterase inhibitor, which normally serves as a control over complement activation. In the classic form, the protein is absent, but there are forms in which the enzyme inhibitor is present but nonfunctional and may be positive on screening tests. The hereditary form starts at an early age, but the acquired form may also appear in the second, third, or fourth decade of life.

Oral Manifestations. Angioedema is a more extensive form of urticaria in the mucous membranes.

Associated Findings/Microscopic Findings. Usually, the microscopic findings are similar no those in urticaria.

Diagnosis. For the hereditary forms, the appropriate testing for both structural protein and functional protein can be done, and this will sort out the patients and give some insight into treatment. There is usually little problem in making the diagnosis, as the manifestations are so much more striking than in the more usual type of urticaria that it is rarely missed; the history of recurrent triggering agents is also important in establishing a diagnosis.

Differential Diagnosis. Urticaria is the primary other condition to be considered in the differential diagnosis.

Treatment. Angioedema responds to nearly all the same measures as are used in urticaria (see above). In cases of hereditary or acquired angioedema, with malfunction or absence of the C-1 esterase inhibitor, stimulation of production of the C-1 esterase inhibitor has been demonstrated with various impeded androgens, including stanozolol and danazol. These drugs, while efficacious, have not yet been given definite official approval for this indication; however, no specific therapy has been developed for this condition, and the impeded androgens offer the best therapy. These cases are quite rare and it is important that the treating physician be aware of the literature before therapy with any of these drugs is initiated.

10.3 Atopic Dermatitis

Definition. Atopic dermatitis is a hereditary syndrome aptly described by Sulzberger as "the itch that rashes." The primary symptom, then, is pruritus, often prior to any skin signs. Atopic dermatitis by definition is associated with the atopic diathesis, which also includes airway problems: asthma, hay fever, multiple allergies, and frequent skin infections. In most of the patients affected there is a positive family history of the problem, as well as associated airway signs and symptoms. In most patients there is an elevation of IgE and the level of elevation of the IgE often relates to the severity of the disease, both in the airways/mucous membranes and in the skin.

Etiology. The etiology cannot be simply put. The IgE elevation is undoubtedly a significant factor in the development of the syndrome. The multiple sequelae of the disease can frequently be traced back to the IgE elevation, chronic histamine release, and ongoing hyperhistaminemia, which then results in abnormalities of chemotaxis, inflammation, tissue edema, and pruritus. Other etiologies have been proposed, including changes in skin lipids and changes in the immune system. It is of particular interest that an atopic dermatitis/eczema-type picture is seen in virtually all the congenital immune deficiency syndromes, including Bruton's disease, Fireman's disease, Wiskott-Aldrich syndrome, DiGeorge syndromes, ataxia-telangiectasia, and syndromes presenting with various T-and B-cell abnormalities. These dysfunctions of the immune syndrome are of great interest because of the manifestation of eczema as a common final pathway [1].

Pathogenesis. Exact steps in the development of eczematous lesions relate apparently to the inflammatory cascade from cytokine release after antigen/irritant exposure, IgE release, histamine release, and symptomatic pruritus, which may be the primary step in the development of the eczematous changes and lichenification.

Oral Manifestations. Oral manifestations are often secondary and can be urticarial and sometimes erythematous. Oral manifestations are not a major primary finding in the syndrome, but oral signs and symptoms may be important in the evolving severity of the syndrome.

Associated Findings. A wide number of associated findings are seen in atopic dermatitis, including thinning of the lateral eyebrows (Hertoghe's sign), antecubital and popliteal erythema, lichenification and chronic scaling, changing pigmentation on the chronically involved areas including the midface (the headlight sign), involvement of the eyes and lids with chronic edema, scaling and erythema, and involvement of the rest of the skin to varying degrees, depending on the severity of the syndrome.

Microscopic Findings. There are quite variable findings relating to intensity of infiltrate at extremes resembling a lymphoma, with dermal edema and increasing changes in collagen and ground substance.

Diagnosis. In these patients, there is a propensity for hyperreaction to new substances, but perhaps a decreased response to type IV reaction. With severe disease that is poorly controlled, chronic changes occur in the second and third decade, including severe lichenification and scaling. Severe flares may result in total body erythrodermia.

Differential Diagnosis. Diagnosis is related signs and symptoms modified from to the Rajka Hannafin criteria (see Table 10.2). Additional supportive diagnosis may relate to findings (when present) of elevated IgE, etc.

Table 10.2. Criteria supporting diagnosis of atopic dermatitis

Pruritus
Family history
Typical distribution
Cheeks, face (infants)
Acral (older patients)
Anticubitals
Popliteals
Hands
Nummular eczematous lesions
Respiratory symptoms
Recurrent skin infections
Elevated IgE

Treatment. The treatment of atopic dermatitis primarily centers on the symptomatology. Significant mucous membrane symptoms are infrequent in atopic dermatitis. Urticarial reactions are treated in the same manner as mentioned in Sect. 10.2. The symptoms of local burning and itching may sometimes be relieved by the potential for topical antihistamines, i. e., Zonalon, to cause local hypesthesia. The use of oral benadryl, one to two teaspoons held in the mouth for 1 min or more then swallowed, provides both local relief and systemic benefits. Additionally, more severe reactions may respond to extemporaneously compounded oral/topical agents such as Magic Mouthwash (Benadryl elixir, Tetracycline syrup, Nystatin, and Decadron). Good control of the skin disease usually results in equally good control of the mucous membrane symptoms when present.

10.4 Oculomucocutaneous Syndromes

10.4.1 Erythema Multiforme

Definition. Erythema multiforme is a reactive process, occurring on the skin and mucous membranes. In its mild form, aggressive therapy and removal of etiology results in rapid clinical improvement [4–7].

Etiology. The etiology of erythema multiforme is multiple, and the most treatable forms are the infectious reaction patterns largely due to herpes simplex [8], but occasionally to some other infection, such as mycoplasma [9]. Drug reactions often manifest with erythema multiforme, and a long list of drugs have been implicated [1, 10, 11]. At least 20 %–25 % of cases may never have the etiology determined.

Pathogenesis (see Sect. 10.1). These reactions have been traditionally considered type III reactions related to immune complex formation. In certain specific instances, the infectious agent or drug may activate mechanisms directly through cytokine activation. The exact pathogenesis is not clear in all cases, and hence steroids are used as a broad-spectrum therapeutic agent.

Oral Manifestations. Uncomplicated erythema multiforme results in symptoms of burning, sometimes itching, signs or erythema; sometimes, small ulcerations occur, and on the tongue desquamation may be a significant finding.

Associated Findings. Erythema multiforme is rarely limited to the mucous membranes: classic multiforme lesions on the body can be seen from circinate to bulls-eye, and in more severe cases (see below) the process progresses leading to skin loss through blister formation. These signs and symptoms are distinctly different from the broad sheets of epidermal loss seen in Lyell's disease [6, 7].

Microscopic Findings. There is erythema, a mixed infiltrate, and often vasculitis, which may be lymphocytic, lymphohistiocytic, or leukocytoclastic; later, there is red cell extravasation.

Diagnosis. Diagnosis is directed at the etiology, and a specific test to search for recent infections (ELISA and other specific immunofluorescent tests, especially in herpes simplex) may be most useful. Herpetic lesions are often associated with palmar-plantar vesicular reactions, and this may help in confirming the diagnosis [8]. The drug etiologies are often more difficult to determine because of the paucity of specific tests at present.

Differential Diagnosis. One can differentiate this disease from Lyell's on the basis of the clinical patterns on the skin, but the mucous membrane signs and symptoms may be difficult to separate out. Contact mucositis may also cause similar signs and symptoms.

Treatment. Treatment for erythema multiforme of the mucous membranes should be anticipatory and aggressive. Usually, steroids are effective in controlling the process and given early, parenterally or orally. Dosages are usually 0.75–1.50 mg prednisone (or equivalent) per kilogram. In some instances, there is some benefit from steroid suspensions in the mouth, and on some occasions the use of steroid inhalers, with a quick spray to the oral mucous membranes, may be very beneficial. The specific treatment is removal of the cause. Secondary infections, especially from candidiasis, are to be anticipated and some routinely use anti-*candida* troches. Mild forms of erythema multiforme often resolve without any additional treatment.

10.4.2 Stevens-Johnson Syndrome (Ectodermosis Erosiva Pluriorificialis)

Definition. Stevens-Johnson syndrome is the most extreme form of erythema multiforme. It involves widespread involvement of the skin, often with blister formation, and similar involvement of the mucous membranes. The mucous membrane involvement often connotes a greater degree of severity of Stevens-Johnson syndrome, but is usually present in all cases.

Etiology. Stevens-Johnson syndrome is most frequently associated with drugs, and less often with the other etiologies mentioned for the milder forms of this process [6–8]. A long list is available [1, 11]. Again, as in milder erythema multiforme, it is assumed that the process is an immunologic reaction, with the skin as a primary target.

Pathogenesis. It is assumed that the evolution of the widespread bullous reaction is a type II or type III immunologic reaction, especially in those instances where the etiology seems to be secondary to a drug or an infectious agent [11–14]. The best delineated mechanisms thus far have been associated with herpesvirus, and the work of Huff tends to confirm the immune-associated pathogenesis.

Oral Manifestations. The desquamation of the oral mucous membranes can be extreme, with large areas of loss of mucous membrane, blister formation, and ulcers of varying depth. Extensive involvement of the mucous membranes may often cause very severe symptoms and interfere with normal alimentation.

Associated Findings. The associated findings are widespread across the body; the amount of epidermal loss can parallel that of a third-degree burn and in many cases is treated as such [15].

Microscopic Findings. The primary pathology is obvious in the upper dermis and lower epidermis. Edema causes vasodilatation with an infiltrate that is usually lymphohistiocytic around the blood vessels, and ultimately tissue destruction, with extravasation of red cells.

Treatment. The aggressivity of treatment depends directly on the severity of involvement. Extensive involvement in the skin may mandate treating the patient as a third-degree burn case. Involvement of the mucous membranes alone is uncommon, but aggressive therapy with systemic steroids very early in the process may indeed be beneficial. If one is to abort this process, a significant dosage very early in the process is necessary, in the range of 1.0–2.0 mg/kg prednisone or equivalent per day [9, 15, 16]. With this, one can stop the presumed immunologic reaction or limit its aggression. In the mucous membranes, topical steroid suspensions can be useful, as can aerosol steroids used for upper airway allergic diseases, the aerosol allowing a direct application of preparations such as beclomethasone to the mucous membrane. The aforementioned use of symptomatic oral therapy, such as elixir of benadryl or Magic Mouthwash, will also significantly improve a patient's symptoms. In the case of very severe desquamation and pain, topical anesthetics, including lidocaine viscous, may be very important in minimizing symptoms to the point that the patient can eat and drink normally. Standard treatments for the other denuded areas of the body, including anti-infective and anti-inflammatory agents, are also beneficial for the mucous membrane symptoms.

10.4.3 Lyell's Syndrome (Toxic Epidermal Necrolysis)

Definition. Lyell's syndrome involves widespread desquamation of the skin, and occasionally the mucous membranes.

Etiology. The definition refers primarily to the widespread desquamation due to drug reactions, and sometimes secondary to infections, but is differentiated from the staphylococcal scalded skin syndrome, which is a separate entity of a different mechanism. The most common drugs are antibiotics, with sulfa usually leading, some anticonvulsants, and other antibiotics including amino, penicillin, cephalosporin, and quinolone antibiotics [17–19].

A recent review of this entity suggests that the incidence is less than five cases per million per week [19].

Pathogenesis. This is presumed to be of an immunologic nature, and may well represent a type II or type III reaction. TNF (tumor necrosis factor) has been proposed as a possible mediator in this process, but the exact initiation of the pathogenic steps remains to be worked out [11, 20, 21].

Oral Manifestations. The widespread desquamation of the epidermis may be accompanied by similar changes in the mucous membrane with desquamation and ulceration.

Associated Findings/Microscopic Findings. On biopsy (skin) there is usually epidermal cleavage, with destruction of the basal cell layer, above the PAS-positive basal membrane. There may be a variable infiltrate in the dermis. Biopsy is useful to separate this from staphylococcal scalded skin syndrome (SSSS), in which there is clearly a higher zone separation than with the epidermal bulla formation in TEN/Lyell's [21, 22].

Diagnosis. In cases of uncertainty, the diagnosis is usually sustained by biopsy. Biopsy and frozen section may provide rather rapid differentiation of a drug-induced versus infectious etiology of the widespread epidermal changes.

Differential Diagnosis. Widespread epidermal loss and desquamation can be seen with SSSS and with erythema multiforme, and occasionally there may be difficulty in younger patients in excluding IgA bullous dermatosis. In general, biopsy will differentiate all three, especially when immunofluorescence is used to separate out IgA dermatosis, and the superficial desquamation mentioned above will differentiate SSSS. Some cases of erythema multiforme may be difficult to distinguish from TEN.

Treatment. Treatment is similar to that for erythema multiforme/Stevens Johnson syndrome (sec above). Early use of potent steroids may be useful to slow the process, but the ultimate therapy consists in withdrawal of the offending etiologic agent or drug [23].

10.4.4 Fixed Drug Eruption

Definition. This is a recurrent cutaneous reaction, often in the same site (hence "fixed") with repeated usage of a given drug, primarily affecting the glans penis and mucous membranes and some intertriginous areas, i. e., axilla, groin [1].

Etiology. Various drugs can cause a fixed drug eruption (the list is quite long), but the most common relate to OTC drugs, including laxatives, cold remedies, bromides, etc. Additionally, antimicrobials, especially of the sulfa and tetracycline groups, have been frequent causes [24, 25].

Pathogenesis. This remains obscure, although some workers have proposed a delayed hypersensitivity reaction to explain the localization of the recurrent eruption after drug insult.

Oral Manifestations. The reactions can be primarily on the mucous membranes in the mouth, as well as the areas mentioned above, and range from fixed erythema with subsequent postinflammatory hyperpigmentation, to bulla formation in more severe cases.

Associated Findings/Microscopic Findings. Often erythema and edema are found on biopsy of the skin, and when there is bulla formation it is usually a subepidermal bulla.

Diagnosis. The primary diagnosis is made from a history of repetitive local occurrence of the reactions.

Differential Diagnosis. Some of the older reactions to bromides, arsenicals, etc. Historically these appear to have been similar to fixed drug eruptions, but they are rare today; there is little else that can be confused with the fixed drug eruption.

Treatment. Primary therapy is withdrawal of the drug and avoidance of the drug in the future. Potent topical steroids given early in the erythematous phase may abort the reactions and prevent progression to significant edema of bulla formation and postinflammatory hyperpigmentation.

10.5 Drug Eruptions of Oral Mucosa

Definition. Drug eruptions involving the mucous membrane can include all the above-cited reactions and, most notably, two other possible patterns: mucous membrane desquamation can give the appearance of glossitis areata migrans on the tongue or geographic tongue, and, in addition, certain drugs are noted for their ability to cause gingival hyperplasia [25, 26].

Etiology. By definition, these reactions are all related to drugs as a primary etiology, and in the particular case of gingival hyperplasia, antiseizure medications are amongst the most frequent causes.

Pathogenesis. The evolution of signs and symptoms (edema, bulla formation) will be related to either direct drug release of cytokines, such as TNF, or immunologic factors, as mentioned in Sect. 10.1. The pathogenesis of fixed drug eruptions remains obscure, but it is tempting to equate it with a possible type IV reaction.

Oral Manifestations. Drug eruptions can present in oral mucosa with bulla formation, desquamation, hyperpigmentation, and hypersensitivity. Certain drugs are also noted to cause dysesthesia or dysgeusia which, where extreme, can cause a severe metallic taste in the mouth that is very unpleasant for the patient. The exact mechanism of taste changes on the tongue related to drugs is still unclear. Simple erythema and burning mouth may also be presentations of drug reactions in the mucous membranes [26].

Associated Findings. A fixed drug eruption is often present on other parts of the body, including intertriginous areas and the genitalia. Abnormalities of taste related to drugs are usually limited to the mucous membranes. Most other mucous membrane disorders go hand in hand with similar conditions on the nonmucous membranes of the body.

Microscopic Findings. This is rarely studied by biopsy, but biopsy may show a mixed inflammatory infiltrate, though with a primary proliferation of dermal connective tissue. In the case of desquamation, the pattern is characteristic and is rarely biopsied.

Diagnosis. In the case of geographic tongue, the diagnosis is made clinically, and then the association is made by careful history review. Gingival hyperplasia is very common and obvious as a reaction to medication.

Differential Diagnosis. There are few other disorders that mimic these conditions.

Treatment. With both conditions, very good oral hygiene is essential, and with the geographic tongue, brushing of the tongue with the toothbrush after withdrawal of the drug may help clear up signs and symptoms. Similarly, careful oral hygiene is thought by some to help prevent some of the gingival hyperplasia in cases in which it is thought that oral hygiene and chronic inflammation may play a part in promoting the overgrowth of the gingiva as well as the drug.

Treatment is primarily symptomatic after withdrawal of the drug, if that is appropriate in a given case. With geographic tongue and some of the other types of ulceration, topical therapy, including antibiotics, anti-yeast drugs, and local anesthetics may be useful. Our preference is the Magic Mouthwash (see above).

10.6 Contact Stomatitis and Contact Cheilitis

S. Seidenari

10.6.1 Contact Stomatitis

10.6.1.1 *Irritant Contact Stomatitis*

Oral mucosa is believed to be more resistant than the skin, and irritant stomatitis is considered to be a rare condition. In fact, saliva has neutralizing properties, and it dilutes and disperses substances which come into the oral cavity. The time of exposure to irritants and allergens is also reduced by the rapid absorption provided by the rich vascularization. Contact with hot or spicy food and with improperly used detergents (e.g., as in unrinsed dentures) and antiseptics are the most frequent causes of irritation of the oral mucosa [27, 28].

10.6.1.2 *Allergic Contact Stomatitis*

Contact allergy on the oral mucosa can appear as stomatitis, glossitis, gingivitis, eventually associated with cheilitis and perioral dermatitis [27]. Objective signs include slight to moderate erythema and sometimes edema, and are often less important than subjective symptoms, such as burning sensation and/or pain and loss of taste, the persistence of which may make the patients irritable and anxious [29, 30]. Allergic stomatitis may mimic oral changes due to vitamin A deficiency or certain anemias, uremic stomatitis, stomatitis nicotinica, and candidiasis. When these conditions have been ruled out, the search for contact sensitizing agents has to be carried out by careful clinical history and patch testing [31]. Allergic contact stomatitis may be caused by chemicals used in dentistry, toothpastes and mouthwashes, and even by contact allergens applied to the lips [27] (Table 10.3). Most chemicals used in dentistry may be allergenic, for example, balsam of Peru, colophony, cinnamon, menthol and eugenol which may be found in cements, core pastes, and dental medications. The same substances are also found in foodstuffs, cosmetics, and topical products, so that their intake or application may cause a relapse of skin lesions in sensitive subjects [32]. Resins for dental fillings are obtained by polymerization of different kinds of monomers, like methacrylate and dimethacrylate-urethanes monomers, bisphenol-epoxyresins, and ethylenediammine. These substances may induce contact allergy after release of monomers by the action of saliva and other solutions in the mouth [33]. The role of mercury in sensitive individuals with stomatitis and silver amalgam fillings containing mercury is still controversial [27, 34]. Allergic contact stomatitis from dentures has seldom been reported [29, 30], although it is believed to be quite frequent. Generally, the oral mucosa in contact with the prosthesis is affected, but in some instances the stomatitis extends beyond the borders of the denture involving the palate and the tongue surface which is exposed during speech, chewing, and swallowing. The most frequent sensitizer in dentures is represented by re-

Table 10.3. Products causing allergic contact stomatitis

Toothpastes and mouthwashes
Dental materials
Adhesives for dentures
Topical products for the lips

sidual methyl methacrylate monomer, but also inhibitors (e. g., hydroquinone), plasticizers (e. g., dibutyl phthalate), catalysts (e. g., benzoyl peroxide), or other components may be sensitizing agents [29, 30].

Contact allergy affecting the oral mucosa is occasionally caused by flavoring and coloring agents and preservatives contained in toothpastes [35].

10.6.2 Contact Cheilitis

Inflammation of the lips may be the result of exposure to environmental agents or may represent the expression of a general skin hyperreactivity, as in atopic eczema. The dermatitis may affect the lips alone or may extend to other skin sites.

10.6.2.1 *Irritant Contact Cheilitis*

Irritant contact cheilitis appears with slight erythema, persistent minimal to moderate lip desquamation, slight swelling, and fissuring [27]. Both physical and chemical agents may be involved. Physical agents include cold and dry weather, friction from objects kept between the lips (toothpicks, instruments, etc.), bad habits including biting and lip-licking. Lip-licking cheilitis, which has been reported in children, especially atopics, and in mentally retarded patients, is due both to the physical trauma and to the irritant action of salivary enzymes [36]. Chemical stimuli inducing irritant contact cheilitis include products used for the lips and the oral cavity (Figs. 10.12, 10.13). Identification of the chemical causing irritation is often impossible, and the diagnosis of irritant contact cheilitis is made by exclusion when patch tests give negative results and the search for the sensitizing agent fails.

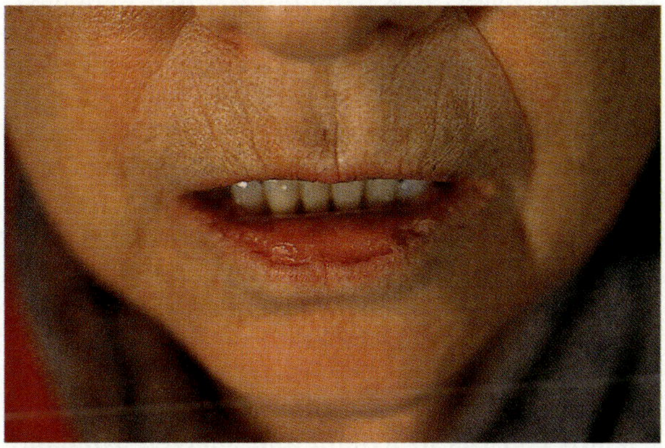

Fig. 10.12. Irritant contact cheilitis from a mouthwash

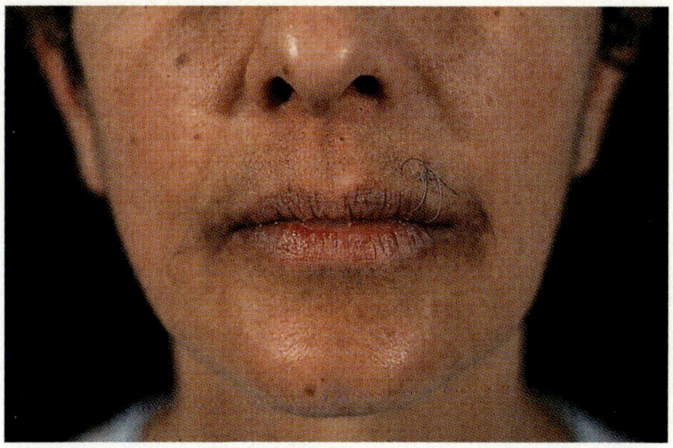

Fig. 10.13. Contact cheilitis from a lip salve containing propolis. Slight edema, erythema, pigmentation, and desquamation are observable

10.6.2.2 *Allergic Contact Cheilitis*

Allergic contact cheilitis appears with erythema and slight to severe edema in the acute phase, and with fissuring, crusting, desquamation, and rarely pigmentation in the chronic phase. Vesicular eruptions on the lips are seldom described. Lesions can extend to the perioral area and the oral mucosa, or may affect labial commissures alone. Products and allergens are listed in Table 10.4.

Toothpastes and mouthwashes can cause both irritation and allergic reactions [35]. The most common allergens in toothpastes are flavoring (e. g., cinnamic aldehyde, cinnamon oil, peppermint, spearmint oil) and preservatives. Moreover, some constituents of toothpastes may cause immediate hypersensitivity reactions. Sainio and Kanerva, examining the composition and labeling of 48 products manufactured in Europe, found that unidentified flavorings were used in 77 % of the toothpastes [35]. At present, it is therefore difficult for allergic consumers to identify suitable products from labels. The most frequent sensitizers in lipsticks and lip salves are listed in Table 10.5 [37–39]. In most cases lesions only affect the lips, while the mouth corners are spared. Contact sensitization to allergens in lipliners appears with dermatitis on the margins of the lips. Nail-enamel cheilitis is caused by contact

Table 10.4. Products and sensitizing agents causing allergic contact cheilitis

Toothpastes and mouthwashes
Dental materials
Topical products for the lips
Sunscreens
Nail enamel
Topical drugs
Metals
Foodstuffs

Table 10.5. Frequent allergens in lipsticks, lip salves and lip liners

Lanolin and lanolin alcohols
Cinnamon
Fragrances
Castor oil
Ricinoleic acid
Microcrystalline wax
Benzoic acid
Propyl gallate and other gallates
Oxybenzone
Eusolex 8021
Salol
C_{18} aliphatic compounds
Sesame oil
Propolis
Vanilla
Colophony
Shellac
Eosin
Para-tertiary-butylphenol

allergy to sulfonamide-formaldehyde resin which occurs when the freshly painted nails come in contact with the lips [27].

Metal-plated pens containing nickel may cause allergic cheilitis in subjects who habitually keep them between the lips [40]. Chewing and sucking plastic pens containing cobalt pigments may lead to the same symptoms in sensitized subjects.

Contact allergy to *Machaerium scleroxylum* and *Arundo donax* wood has been reported in saxophonists and clarinettists with dermatitis of the lips [41, 42].

Photoallergens. Contact dermatitis and photo-contact dermatitis from eosin are now only sporadically reported [43]. Photocheilitis may develop from contact with fruit or vegetables containing photosensitizing agents.

In most patch test-positive cheilitis patients, concomitant sensitizations are observable, sometimes to completely different materials [32]. Therefore, investigations should be continued after the finding of a first sensitizing compound, until a satisfactory list of offending agents is obtained.

10.6.2.3 *Atopic Cheilitis*

Cheilitis, whether or not associated with dermatitis of the perioral area, is frequent in atopic dermatitis patients (Figs. 10.14, 10.15). Skin lesions appear with erythema, edema, cracking, crusting, desquamation, and lichenification in the most severe cases. Continuous moistening or biting of the lips, which is caused by itching and is observed especially in children, can worsen the dermatitis owing to the irritant properties of saliva. Both irritants and allergens may contribute to the pathogenesis of atopic cheilitis. Atopic skin is known to have a particular susceptibility to irritants, and physical and chemical factors may have a role in the maintenance of atopic cheilitis [44]. The protein fractions of animal and vegetable compounds in atopics may cause both immediate urticarial and persistent eczematous lesions [45, 46]. In this case, it is hypothesized that food allergens for type I immediate reactions also bind to IgE molecules on Langerhans' cells, inducing a delayed hypersensitivity response [47]. Food allergens responsible for IgE-mediated cheilitis are listed in Table 10.6. Contact sensitization, especially to topical products employed for lip care, is a frequent complication of atopic dermatitis. Prick-and-scratch chamber tests with food allergens and patch tests with chemical substances are essential diagnostic procedures in atopic cheilitis.

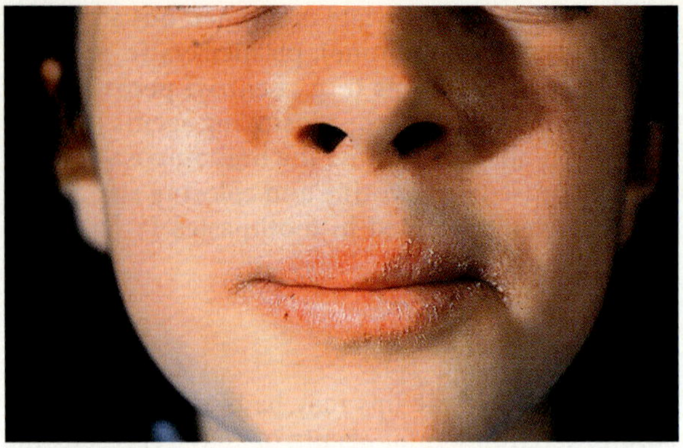

Fig. 10.14. Cheilitis in a girl affected by atopic dermatitis

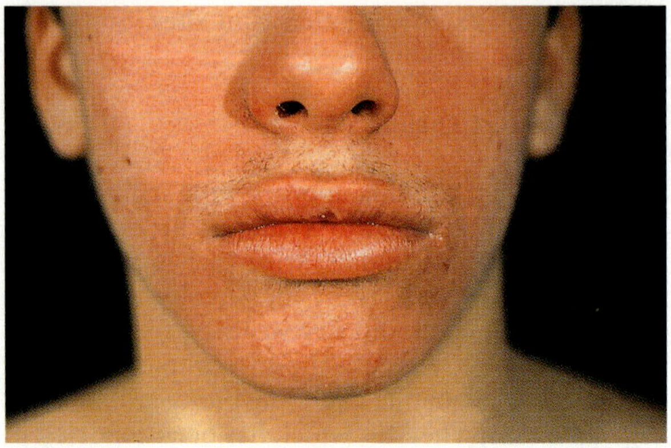

Fig. 10.15. Acute cheilitis appearing after ingestion of raw egg in a boy with atopic dermatitis. Swelling of the lips is associated with erythema of the face

Treatment. The therapy of contact stomatitis and cheilitis consists in irritant and allergen avoidance and in the administration of mild topical corticosteroids and emollients for the lips.

Table 10.6. Frequent foodstuffs causing contact cheilitis

Apple
Kiwi fruit
Garlic
Carrot
Fennel
Parsley
Tomato
Banana
Celery
Orange
Peach
Onion
Pear
Cod
Potato
Plum
Cherry
Parsnip

References

1. Millikan LE. Drug eruptions. In: Moschella and Hurley, 3rd Edn. Philadelphia: Saunders, 1990
2. Roujeau JC SR. Severe adverse cutaneous reactions to drugs. N Engl J Med 1995; 331:1272–1285
3. Wolkenstein PRJ. Drug-induced severe skin reactions. Incidence, management and prevention. Drug Saf 1995; 13:56–68
4. Stewart MG DNr, Franklin DJ, Friedman EM, Sulek M. Head and neck manifestations of erythema multiforme in children. Otolaryngol Head Neck Surg 1994; 111:236–242
5. Wilkins JML, White CR Jr. Oculocutaneous manifestations of the erythema multiforme/Stevens-Johnson syndrome/toxic epidermal necrolysis spectrum. Dermatol Clin 1992; 10:571–582
6. Roujeau JC. The spectrum of Stevens-Johnson syndrome and toxic epidermal necrolysis: a clinical classification. J Invest Dermatol 1994; 102:28S–30S
7. Breathnach SM PW. Epidemiology of bullous drug eruptions. Clin Dermatol 1993; 11:441–447
8. Huff JC Erythema multiforme and latent herpes simplex infection. Semin Dermatol 1992; 11:207–210
9. Cherry JD. Anemia and mucocutaneous lesions due to Mycoplasma pneumoniae infections. Clin Infect Dis 1993; 17[Suppl 1]:S47–51
10. Roujeau JC KJ, Naldi L, Rzany B, et al. Medication use and the risk of Stevens-Johnson syndrome or toxic epidermal necrolysis. N Engl J Med 1995; 333:1600–1607
11. Litt J Drug Eruption Reference Manual (DERM). Cleveland: Wal-Zac Enterprises, 1996
12. Martin Mateos MA PA, Pastor X, Munoz Lopez F. Uncommon serious complications in Stevens-Johnson syndrome: a clinical case. J Investig Allergol Clin Immunol 1992; 2:278–283
13. Schlienger RG HW, Bircher A, Leib SL, Luscher TF. Drug-induced Stevens-Johnson syndrome in a patient with AIDS [German]. Schweiz Rundsch Med Prax 1993; 82:888–892
14. Sharma VK DS. Clinical pattern of cutaneous drug eruption among children and adolescents in north India. Pediatr Dermatol, 1995; 12:178–183
15. Patterson RGL, Greenberger PA, Lawrence ID et al. Stevens-Johnson syndrome (SJS): effectiveness of corticosteroids in management and recurrent SJS. Allergy Proceedings, 1992; 13:89–95
16. Herndon D. Toxic epidermal necrolysis: a systemic and dermatologic disorder best treated with standard treatment protocols in burn intensive care units without the prolonged use of corticosteroids [editorial; comment]. J Am Coll Surg 1995; 180:273–278
17. Friedman PS SI, Pirmohamed M, Park BK. Investigation of mechanisms in toxic epidermal necrolysis induced by carbamazepine. Arch Dermatol 1994; 130:598–604
18. Sturchler DMM, Kerr L. How frequent are notified severe cutaneous adverse reactions to Fansidar? Drug Saf 1993; 8:160–168
19. Bastuji-Garin SRB, Stern RS, Shear NH et al. Clinical classification of cases of toxic epidermal necrolysis, Stevens-Johnson syndrome, and erythema multiforme. Arch Dermatol 1993; 129:92–96
20. Paquet PNA, Arrese JE, Vanderkelen A, Pierard GE. Macrophages and tumor necrosis factor alpha in toxic epidermal necrolysis. Arch Dermatol 1994; 130:605–608
21. Guibal FB-GS, Chosidow O, Saiag P et al. Characteristics of toxic epidermal necrolysis in patients undergoing long-term glucocorticoid therapy. Arch Dermatol 1995; 131:669–672
22. Cribier BPY, Grosshans E. Staphylococcal scalded skin syndrome in adults. A clinical review illustrated with a new case. J Am Acad Dermatol 1994; 30:319–324
23. Kaufman DW. Epidemiologic approaches to the study of toxic epidermal necrolysis. J Invest Dermatol 1994; 102:31S–33S
24. Carstens JWP, Sogaard H, Thestrup-Pedersen K. Toxic epidermal necrolysis and erythema multiforme following therapy with terbinafine. Acta Derm Venereol 1994; 74:391–392
25. Camisa C, Rindler J. Diseases of the oral mucous membranes. Curr Probl Dermatol 1996; 7:41–96
26. Parks ET Lesions associated with drug reaction. Dermatol Clin 1996; 14:327–337
27. Fisher AA. Contact stomatitis and cheilitis. In: Fisher AA (Ed). Contact Dermatitis. Philadelphia: Lea and Febiger, 1986; 773–800
28. Nater JP, De Groot AC. Unwanted effects of cosmetics and drugs used in dermatology, 3rd Ed. Amsterdam: Elsevier Science Publishers, 1993; 187–189
29. Kaaber S, Thulin H, Nielsen E. Skin sensitivity to denture base materials in the burning mouth syndrome. Contact Dermatitis, 1979; 5:90–96
30. Ali A, Bates JF. The burning mouth sensation related to the wearing of acrylic dentures: an investigation. Brit Dent J 1986; 444–447
31. Fisher AA. Contact stomatitis. Dermatol Clinics 5:708–717
32. Angelini G, Vena GA, Grandolfo M, Foti C, Pipoli M, Curatoli G. Contact cheilitis J Appl Cosmetol 1987; 11:91–101
33. Kanzaki T, Kabasawa Y, Jinno T, Isayama K Contact stomatitis due to methyl methacrylate monomer. Contact Dermatitis 1989; 20:146
34. von Mayenburg J, Frosch P, Fuchs T et al. Mercury and amalgam sensitivity. Possible clinical manifestations and sources of contact sensitization. Dermatosen 1996; 5:213–221
35. Sainio EL, Kanerva L. Contact allergens in toothpastes and a review of their hypersensitivity. Contact Dermatitis 1995; 33:100–105
36. Hisa T, Hamada T, Hirachi Y et al. Senile lip licking. Dermatology 1995; 191:339–340
37. Hayakawa R, Matsunaga K, Suzuki M et al. Lipstick dermatitis due to C_{18} aliphatic compounds. Contact Dermatitis 1987; 16:215–219
38. Aguirre A, Izu R, Gardeazabal J et al. Allergic contact cheilitis from a lipstick containing oxybenzone. Contact Dermatitis 1992; 27:267–268
39. Romaguera C, Vilaplana J. Contact dermatitis from gallates. Am J Contact Dermatitis 1993; 2:231–234
40. Bruze M. Allergic contact cheilitis related to university studies. Contact Dermatitis 1994; 30:313
41. Hausen BM. Häufigkeit und Bedeutung toxischer und allergischer Kontaktdermatitiden durch Machaerium scleroxylum Tul. (Pao Ferro), einem Ersatzholz für Palisander (Dalbergia nigra All.) Der Hautarzt 1982; 33:321–328
42. McFadden JP, Ingram MJ, Rycroft RJG. Contact allergy to cane reed in a clarinettist. Contact Dermatitis 1992; 27:117

43. Tomb R. Allergic contact dermatitis from eosin. Contact Dermatitis 1991; 24:27–29
44. Wüthrich B. Minimal forms of atopic eczema. In: Ruzicka T, Ring J, Przybilla B (Eds). Handbook of atopic eczema. Heidelberg: Springer, 1991; 46–53
45. Hannuksela M, Lahti A. Immediate reactions to fruits and vegetables. Contact Dermatitis 3:79–84
46. Lahti A. Immediate contact reactions. In: Rycroft RJG, Menné T, Frosch PJ, Benezra C (eds): Textbook of contact dermatitis. Heidelberg: Springer, 1992; 62–74
47. Bruynzeel-Koomen C. IgE on Langerhans cells: new insights into the pathogenesis of atopic dermatitis. Dermatologica 1986; 72:181–183

CHAPTER 11

Oral Mucosa Signs of Immune, Autoimmune, and Rheumatic Diseases

11.1 Autoimmune Rheumatic Diseases: Oral Manifestations

M. Matucci Cerinic, A. Pignone, A. Lombardi, M. Cagnoni, G. Ferranti, and O. De Pità

11.1.1 Scleroderma

Name. Systemic slcerosis, scleroderma.

Definition. This is a generalized multisystem autoimmune disease characterized by proliferative microcirculatory change leading to fibrosis of skin, lung, heart, kidney, and gastrointestinal tract.

Etiology. This is unknown but immunogenetic events are considered fundamental for the disease development and progression [1].

Pathogenesis. Autoimmune events perturb the endothelium and activate platelets and lead to fibroblast activation, collagen production, and terminal end-point fibrosis [1]. The modification of the connective tissue, and fibrosis in particular, is the main reason leading to the modification of the oral environment and to the most common oral manifestations of scleroderma.

Oral Manifestations. The progression of the disease leads to perioral furrowing creating the "tobacco pouch mouth". Lips are tightly blocked (microcheilia) and oral opening becomes virtual (microstomia). Oral mucosa is usually pale and may become tightened as skin. Gum retraction with teeth pseudowidening becomes progressively evident, as well as thickening of periodontal membrane, loss of lamina dura and gingivitis, teleangectasias of lips and oral mucosa, and atrophy of mucous membrane. The tongue is initially edematous but later develops trophy of papillae, loses its mobility, and becomes stiff in the atrophic phase of the disease. The lingual frenulum shortens and finally disappears. Raynaud's phenomenon of the tip of the tongue may be present. Xerostomia frequently occurs [2, 3].

Associated Findings. Skin fibrosis, Raynaud's phenomenon and fingertip ulcers, kidney insufficiency, lung fibrosis, pulmonary hypertension, myocardial fibrosis, arthropathy and joint retraction, sensorimotor and autonomic neuropathy.

Diagnostic Tests. It is important to identify the presence of Sjögren's syndrome through the determination of lacrimal (Schirmer's test, break up time, rose bengal) and salivary (parotid echography or syalography, Saxon's test) function, as well as a biopsy of minor salivary glands of the lip (to determine the presence of a lymphocytic infiltrate). No other specific tests are required for the oral manifestations. When Raynaud's phenomenon of the tongue is present, in the absence of other symptoms, capillaroscopy, autoantibodies (ANA, ENA and anticentromere), and an esophageal X-ray are mandatory in order to make an early diagnosis of scleroderma.

Differential Diagnosis. Sjögren's syndrome.

Treatment. Treatment is focused mainly on dental care. In particular, artificial saliva may be used to combat xerostomia, and interdental floss and gum prevention are fundamental in order to avoid teeth deterioration: mucolytic drugs may be used to increase lacrimal and parotidal secretion. Administration of large quantities of vitamin E and A may be helpful. Several drugs may be systematically used to treat different disease manifestations (vasodilators, cyclophosphamide, D-penicillamine, antacids, prokinetics, etc).

11.1.2 Lupus Erythematosus

11.1.2.1 *Systemic Lupus Erythematosus (SLE)*

Name. Systemic lupus erythematosus.

Definition. Autoimmune chronic inflammatory disease with periods of remission and acute or chronic relapses, which mainly affects the female sex (female:male ratio, 8:1) and skin, kidney, central nervous system, joints, and serous membranes [4–6].

Etiology. Unknown, multifactorial components have been suggested (viruses, genetic, environmental, hormonal).

Pathogenesis. This is characterized by abnormal immune function. Both B- and T-cell-impaired regulation occurs: tissue damage is produced by the deposition of immune complexes. The size, concentration and solubility of these complexes and their ability to activate the complement cascade are determinant in the development of clinical signs.

Oral Manifestation. Discoid lesions with erythema, atrophy and depigmentation of the lips; irregular white raised plaques; silvery white scarred lesions; areas of erythema on soft and hard palate with punched-out erosions or ulcers around them; vasculitic lesions of the mucosa (Fig. 11.1); gingivitis and xerostomia in patients with cyclosporin A treatment or Sjögren's syndrome, respectively.

Associated Findings. Malar erythema, central nervous system involvement, pleuro-pericarditis, renal and heart involvement.

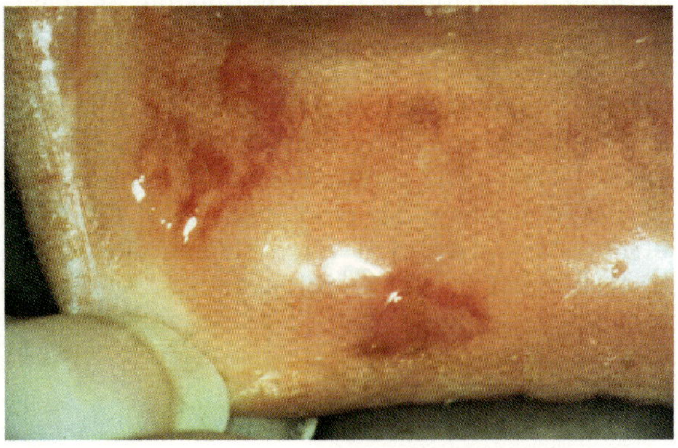

Fig. 11.1. Vasculitic lesions of the oral mucosa in a female patient with severe SLE

Microscopic Findings. In oral lesions, such as discoid lesions, aphthae, or ulcers, the histopathology shows immunoglobulin and complement deposits at the dermal/epidermal junction.

Diagnosis. Diagnosis of oral lesions must consider the presence of Sjögren's syndrome.

Differential Diagnosis. Lichen planus, candidiasis, aphthous stomatitis (Behçet's syndrome), bite marks, leukoplakia, malignancy, Sjögren's syndrome.

Treatment. The lesion usually disappears within a few days after the beginning of steroid use, as well as other immunosuppressants (methotrexate, cyclophosphamide, cyclosporin A).

11.1.2.2 *Discoid Lupus Erythematosus (DLE)*

G. L. Campanile, G. Hautmann, M. Caproni, T. M. Lotti, and P. Fabbri

Name. Discoid lupus erythematosus, Erythematodes.

Definition. Discoid lupus erythematosus (DLE) is the more common form of cutaneous lupus erythematosus, a chronic inflammatory autoimmune disease with a variable spectrum of clinical forms. DLE is rare but, because of its chronic course and the prolonged treatment, it is seen constantly. Frequently, young adults are affected; the disease commences between the ages of 20 and 40 years. All races are affected. Women predominate at 3:1–3:2.

Etiology. This is probably an autoimmune disease in which a genetically determined defect permits the synthesis of autoantibodies and autoreactive T-immunocytes which are normally blocked. Additional exogenous factors such as mechanical trauma, stress, light, cold, or infections are apparently also necessary for the provocation or maintenance of clinical manifestations. There is increased incidence of HLA-B8, especially in women over 40 years of age, and HLA-DR3.

Oral Manifestations. The oral mucosa is involved in 15 %–25 % of cases, usually in association with skin lesions. Persistent erythema is seen. Gray epithelial thickening (Fig. 11.2), fine keratosis, and erosions develop. The typical oral lesion is characterized by a well-defined red area, centrally atrophic, surrounded by a sharp elevated border of irradiating whitish striae. Telangiectasia and small white dots may be present on the erythematous areas. Painful erosions and ulcerations may also be present and progress to atrophic scarring. The vermilion of

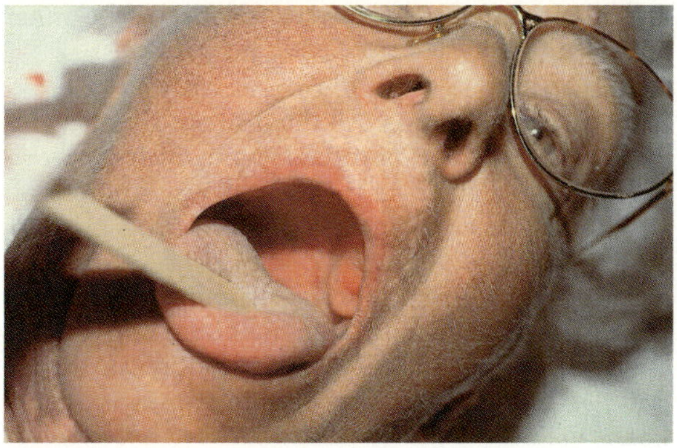

Fig. 11.2. Gray epithelial thickening and roughness localized on the left area between the hard and the soft palate

the lips is often affected, followed by the buccal mucosa, palate, gingiva, and tongue [7, 8].
DLE may predispose to oral carcinoma. Oral ulceration has also been described in drug-induced lupus.

Associated Findings. The disease is usually localized to cheeks, forehead, and nose, but lesions may also be found on the ear, the scalp, or the sternum, more rarely on the rest of the trunk and the extremities. If the disease involves areas above and below the neck, it is characterized as generalized DLE [9]. The disease begins with persistent, sharply demarcated, raised, erythematous plaques less than 1 cm in diameter. Through peripheral growth, the lesions become disk shaped, while the center is covered by firmly adherent, white-yellow scales. Their forceful detachment by scratching causes pain and evidences follicular plugging on the underside originating from the follicular opening, which indicates *follicular keratosis*. The hyperesthesia of the lesions is also of diagnostic importance. Regression commences in the center, resulting in atrophy of the skin. Patches of depigmentation, but also of hyperpigmentation and telangiectasia, may give rise to a poikilodermatous appearance.
Systemic manifestations do not form part of the picture of DLE. If such signs and symptoms should occur, a transition into the systemic form is assumed. This occurs in only 10 %–15 % of cases of DLE.

Diagnosis. Serum antinuclear antibodies are infrequently present at low titers and anti-single-stranded DNA antibodies (ssDNA) are rarely present.
Biopsies taken from affected skin or mucosa show a band of fine granular to coarse plaque-like deposits of immunoglobulins (mostly IgG, but also IgM and IgA) and complement which can be demonstrated in the region of the dermoepidermal junction by direct immunofluorescence. The deposits are described as LE bands or lupus bands and the method as the lupus band test [10, 11]. Histopathologic examination shows an atrophic epidermis. There is orthohyperkeratosis with follicular keratosis, and vacuolar degeneration of the cells of the basal layer. In the upper dermis there is edema, mucin, and later sclerosis. The blood and lymph vessels are dilated; a dense, mostly lymphocytic infiltrate surrounds the vessels of the superficial and deep plexus, and also the adnexa.

Differential Diagnosis. This should include leukoplakia, erythroplakia, lichen planus, actinic cheilitis, syphilis, and cicatricial pemphigoid.

Treatment. The small oral lesions of DLE are treated with local steroids. In case the disease is more extensive, systemic therapy is necessary. Antimalarial drugs have proved of value. The most important side effects are corneal clouding and retinopathy, so that ophthalmological checks are required before and regularly during treatment. Systemic treatment with glucocorticoids additionally or as an alternative is recommended only for exceptional cases.

11.1.3 Mixed Connective Tissue Disease

M. Matucci Cerinic, A. Pignone, A. Lombardi, M. Cagnoni, G. Ferranti, and O. De Pità

Name. Mixed connective tissue disease, Sharp's syndrome.

Definition. Connective tissue disease sharing clinical features of SLE, scleroderma, DPM, and RA with high circulating titers of antinuclear antibodies with specificity for a nuclear ribonucleoprotein antigen (nRNP) [12].

Etiology. Unknown.

Pathogenesis. This is unknown but may combine the varying pathogenesis of different connective autoimmune diseases such as SLE, scleroderma, and DPM.

Oral Manifestations. Buccal ulcerations and xerostomia.

Associated Findings. Clinical manifestations of LES, DPM, and scleroderma.

Diagnosis. Relies on the finding of RNP antibodies.

Differential Diagnosis. Sjögren's syndrome (see below).

Treatment. Steroids, hydroxychloroquine, and specific therapy for the disease that is predominant.

11.1.4 Sjögren's Syndrome

Name. Sjögren's syndrome, sicca syndrome.

Definition. This is an autoimmune inflammatory disease affecting the exocrine glands [13, 14].

Etiology. Unknown.

Pathogenesis. Progressive lymphocyte infiltration of the exocrine glands leads to replacement of the functional epithelium with impairment of secretive capacity.

Oral Manifestations. Xerostomia, caries, atrophy of filiform papillae of the tongue (Fig. 11.3), candidosis.

Associated Findings. Parotid gland enlargement, arthritis, Raynaud's phenomenon, lung and gastrointestinal involvement, peripheral neuropathy, and central nervous system involvement.

Microscopic Findings. In the minor salivary glands of the lips, lymphocytes replace the salivary epithelium: epimyoepithelial islands, composed of keratin-containing epithelial cells, are present.

Diagnosis. The diagnosis is made according to the clinical symptoms (xerophthalmia and xeroostomia) and ocular (Schirmer's test, Rose Bengal stain, and break up time test) and parotidal (syalography, echography, scintigraphy, Saxon's test) function, and biopsy of minor salivary glands of the inner edge of the lip.

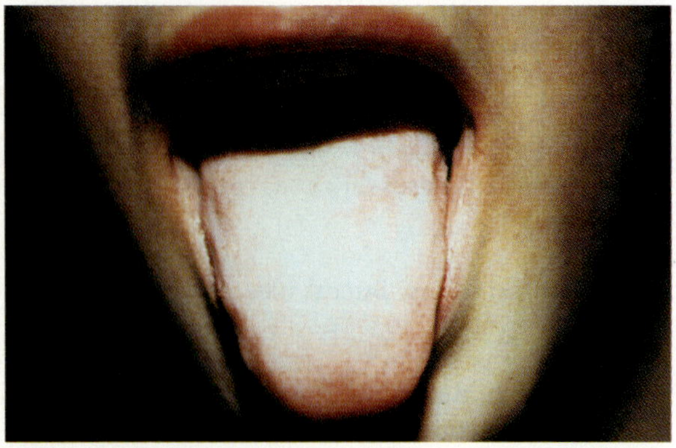

Fig. 11.3. Atrophy of the central part of the tongue in a female patient with Sjögren's syndrome

Differential Diagnosis. All the diseases that may induce enlargement of parotidal glands such as sarcoidosis; lipoproteinemia II, IV, and V; chronic graft versus host disease; and amyloidosis.

Treatment. Hydroxychloroquine and steroids. Special care is needed in order to maintain oral hygiene: antibacterial mouthwashes and toothpaste, long-lasting moisturizing gels, chewing gum, and dental floss.

11.1.5 Dermatomyositis

Name. Dermatomyositis.

Definition. This is an idiopathic inflammatory myopathy involving the skin and the internal organs (heart, lung) [15, 16].

Pathogenesis. It is a vasculitic-like humorally mediated disease. Muscle fibers are necrotic with CD4 and B-lymphocytic infiltrate: an early reduction of capillary density with deposition of immunoglobulin and complement membrane attack on muscle vessels has been clearly described.

Oral Manifestations. Dark and red-bluish erythema; the tongue is edematous at the beginning of the disease and later becomes atrophic.

Associated Findings. Iliac erythema of the eyelids, of the malar area and violaceous, and flat-topped papules of the dorsum of the hands (Gottron's papules). These areas can develop central atrophy, teleangiectasias and hypopigmention. The skin may also be edematous and leave telangiectasias after resolution. The disease is also characterized by profound muscle weakness and pain, fever, and sometimes arthralgia. The heart, gastrointestinal system and lungs are frequently affected.

Diagnosis. This is made according to the clinical picture (muscle weakness and erythema), elevation of muscle enzymes (transaminase, CPK, LDH, aldolase), electromyographic findings, and eventually muscle biopsy. In a small percentage of patients (10 %) anti-Jo1 and -Mi-2 autoantibodies are present [16].

Differential Diagnosis. Tongue atrophy may resemble that observed in Sjögren's syndrome and/or scleroderma.

11.2 Blistering Disorders

S. Brenner, A. Bialy-Golan, and V. Ruocco

11.2.1 Pemphigus

Name. The pemphigus (pemphix = blister) group of diseases comprises several clinical subtypes: pemphigus vulgaris with the pemphigus vegetans variant; pemphigus foliaceus with the variants fogo selvagem and pemphigus erythematosus; and paraneoplastic pemphigus.

Definition. Pemphigus is a chronic, autoimmune, blistering disease involving the skin and mucous membranes. The disease is characterized by the demonstration of circulating and tissue-bound antibodies to the epidermal intercellular substance. These autoantibodies are pathogenic and induce a process known as acantholysis in which epidermal cell cohesion is lost, resulting in intra-epidermal blister formation. The blistering eruption appears insidiously, and the lesions tend to extend peripherally and do not heal spontaneously. Without treatment, the disease is potentially fatal.

Etiology. Pemphigus is a prototype of antibody-mediated autoimmune diseases, and as such is the outcome of interaction between endogenous (genetic) and exogenous (triggering) factors [17]. Certain HLA types are associated with disease susceptibility: A-13, A-10, DR-4 and DR-14, and DQ1 [18–22]. A negative correlation has been shown with HLA DR2 [23], suggesting resistance to the disease. Triggering factors that may induce the disease in predisposed individuals include drugs [17] (especially thiol drugs like penicillamine and captopril, but also non-thiol drugs like penicillin), burns, trauma, viruses, pregnancy, and stress. Fogo selvagem, endemic pemphigus foliaceus, occurring in rural areas in Brazil, has the same epidemiologic distribution as a local black fly suspected of transmitting an as yet unknown triggering factor [23].
Pemphigus appears rarely as a paraneoplastic entity, exhibiting a very severe, often fatal mucocutaneous disease with unique histologic and immunologic characteristics. The sera from paraneoplastic pemphigus patients bind to a variety of epithelia and precipitate a unique complex of four antigens. The underlying malignancy is most often a lymphoproliferative disorder [24].

Pathogenesis. Pemphigus IgG autoantibodies, probably aided by complement components and via mediators like plasminogen activator, bind to disease-specific antigens that are adhesion molecules belonging to the cadherin supergene family and are found on squamous epithelial cell surfaces. These antigens are desmosomal-associated proteins and have been identified by immunoblotting and immunoprecipitation methods. The pemphigus vulgaris antigen is a complex of a 130-kDa glycoprotein, identified as desmoglein 3, and an 85-kDa protein, plakoglobin. The pemphigus foliaceus antigen is a complex of 160-kDa (desmoglein 1) and 85-kDa (plakoglobin) proteins. Disruption of the function of these antigens by autoantibodies interferes with adhesion and induces acantholysis [18–20, 25].

Oral Manifestations. Pemphigus vulgaris, the most common type of pemphigus, presents with oral lesions in 50 %–70 % of patients, in contrast to pemphigus foliaceus, in which mucous membrane involvement is rare. It is uncommon to see intact bullae in the mouth. Painful erosions can involve the entire oral cavity, but are most common on the buccal, palatine, and gingival mucosa (Fig. 11.4). Often, denuded areas are covered with exudate (Fig. 11.5). Lips, gums, and the tongue may be swollen, and hemorrhagic crusts may be seen along the vermilion lip border (Fig. 11.6). In pemphigus vegetans, the tongue may have a distinctive appearance and is described as a cerebriform tongue. Despite early presentation, oral lesions may be late to clear [18–20].

Associated Findings. Lesions may extend from the oral cavity to the larynx, pharynx, and esophagus, resulting in hoarseness, dysphagia, and odynophagia. Other mucous membranes may be involved: conjunctiva, urethra, cervix, and anal mucosa. Several months may elapse between the initial anal manifestations of pemphigus vulgaris and the appearance of skin lesions. They usually start as flaccid bullae arising on normal to erythematous skin, rupture quickly, and result in large denuded areas, eventually covered with crusts (Fig. 11.7) Healing occurs without scarring, sometimes with post-inflammatory hyperpigmentation. The lesions of pemphigus foliaceus are more superifical and tend to occur in a seborrheic distribution (Fig. 11.8). They are characterized by scaling and crusting. In pemphigus erythematosus, a butterfly pattern over the nose and malar area is part of an array of features that are reminiscent of lupus erythematosus. In pemphigus vegetans, lesions heal with hypertrophic granulations (vegetations) and have a predeliction for intertriginous areas. Nail changes are uncommon and nonspecific and include onychoschizia, onychomadesis, cross bridging, pitting, subungual hemorrhages, and discoloration [18–20].

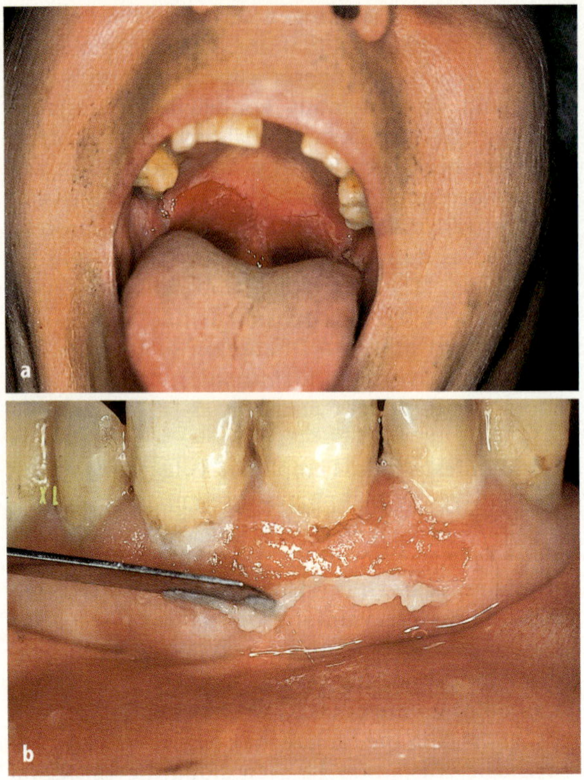

Fig. 11.4 a, b. Oral lesions of PV: **a** palatine erosions, **b** gingival erosions with detached epithelium at the edge

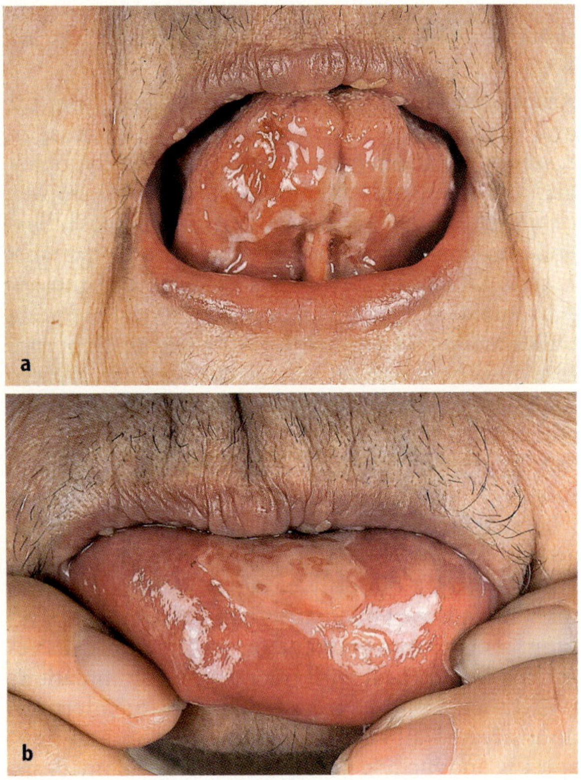

Fig. 11.5 a, b. Oral lesions of PV: **a**, **b** typical erosion on the tongue with detached epithelium, covered with a white exudate

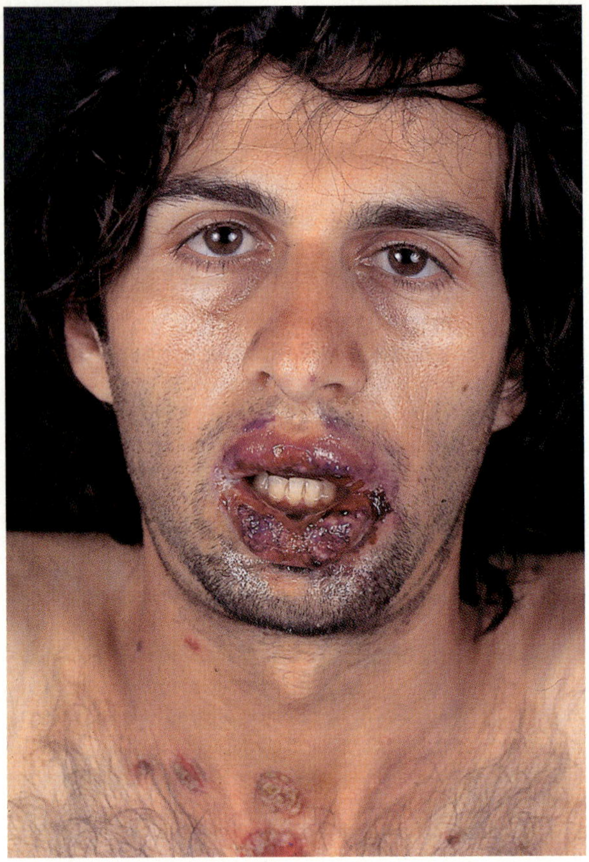

Fig. 11.6. Involvement of the lips in PV: lips are swollen with erosions and hemorrhagic crusting

Microscopic Findings. The hallmark of histologic changes is the intra-epidermal cleft that results from acantholysis, with acantholytic cells in the bullae (Fig. 11.9). The cleft is suprabasal in pemphigus vulgaris and vegetans, and subcorneal in pemphigus foliaceus, erythemathosus, and fogo selvagem. A mild to moderate inflammatory infiltrate may be seen in the upper part of the dermis, basal layer, and bullae. In paraneoplastic pemphigus, dyskeratotic keratinocytes and basal cell vacuolization may be found [18–20].

Diagnosis. Diagnosis is based on the typical clinical picture, clinical signs, and laboratory tests. Nikolsky's sign is produced when lateral pressure is applied to the edge of a blister or to normal-appearing skin, with resultant separation of the epidermis. The Asboe-Hansen sign shows extension of the bullae when direct pressure is applied over an intact bullae. By scraping the base of a bulla or an erosion, acantholytic Tzanck cells may be visualized microscopically (Tzanck test) (Fig. 11.10). The diagnosis is finally established by histology, aided by the demonstration of circulating antibodies against the inter-

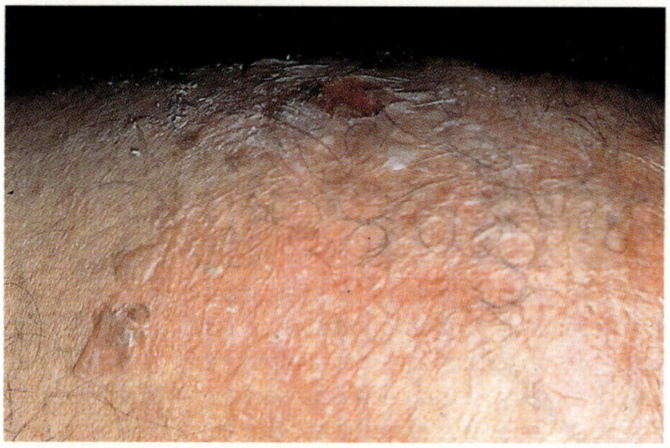

Fig. 11.7. Typical skin lesions of PV: flaccid bullae and erosions, with peripheral extension

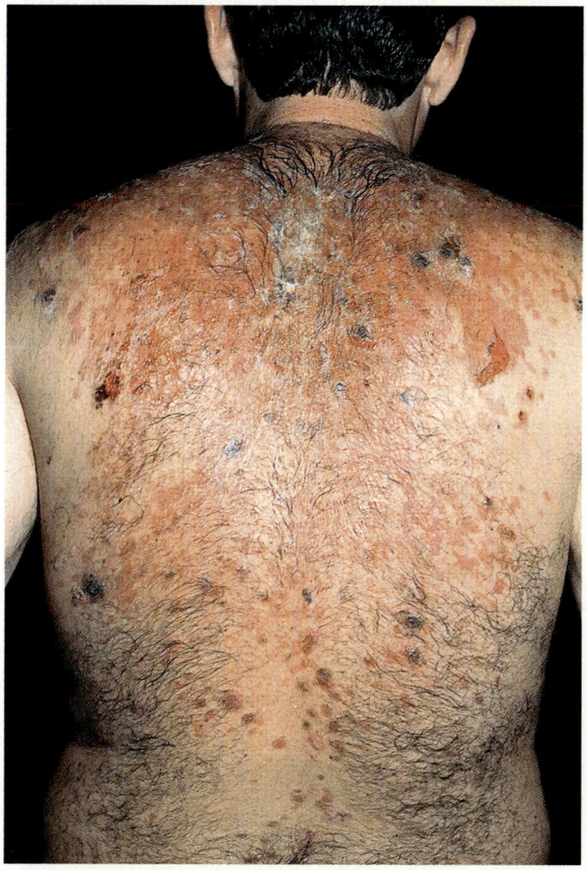

Fig. 11.8. Pemphigus lesions with seborrheic distribution

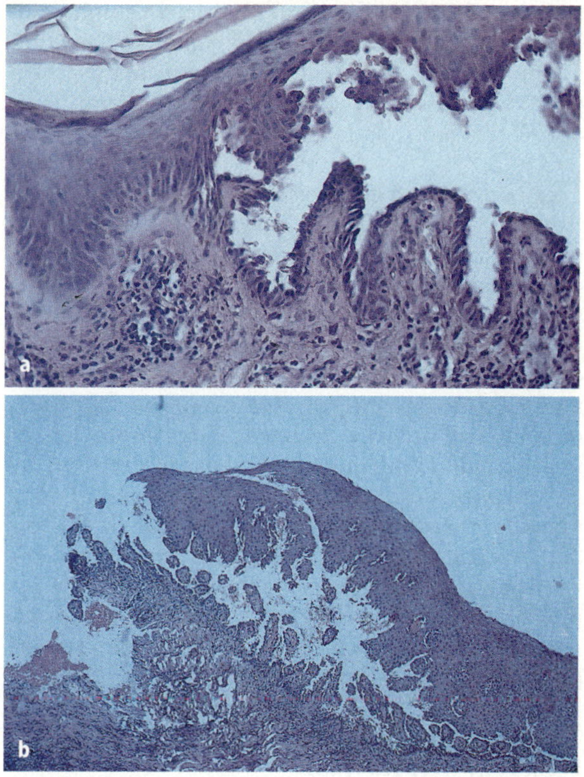

Fig. 11.9 a, b. Typical suprabasal clefting of PV, with aceantholytic cells in bulla. **a** From a skin lesion, × 200. **b** From an oral lesion, × 40

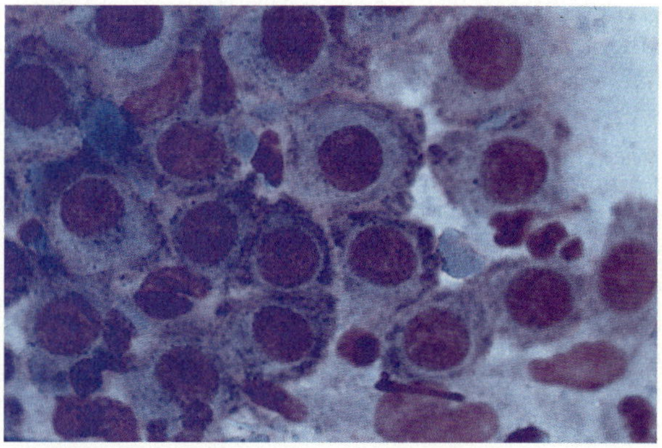

Fig. 11.10. Acantholytic cells in a Tzanck smear, × 1000

cellular substance (by indirect immunofluorescence on monkey esophagus), and by demonstration of tissue bound immunoreactants (IgG, C_3, IgM, IgA) at the intercellular spaces in direct immunofluorescence of perilesional skin. All patients with active disease have IgG deposits in clinically normal and perilesional skin, whereas 80 %–90 % of patients exhibit antibodies in the serum. When the diagnosis cannot be determined by the above standard measures, immunoprecipitation studies should be conducted to identify the antigen [18–20].

Differential Diagnosis. Because diverse oral disease may mimic pemphigus, it is imperative to obtain biopsy specimens for histology and immunofluorescence studies. Pemphigus oral erosions are to be differentiated from bullous and cicatricial pemphigoid, erosive lichen planus, lupus erythematosus, erythema multiforme, recurrent aphthous stomatitis, herpetic stomatitis, Behçet's disease, and other causes of oral ulcers/erosions [18–20].

Treatment. Glucocorticosteroids are the first-line treatment of pemphigus. A well-accepted regimen is a starting dose of 1.5–2 mg/kg/day prednisone, continued for 6–8 weeks until 80 % of the lesions are healed, and then slow tapering is tried down to 80 mg/day, when alternate day tapering is recommended. In mild cases, intralesional therapy may be attempted. If unresponsive, low dose steroids (20 mg) may be initiated. If no improvement is achieved, 80 mg/day is tried, to be increased by 50 % a week until disease is controlled, up to a maximum dose of 240 mg/day [18–20, 26]. Alternative treatment modalities are: corticosteroids with immunosuppressives (azathioprine, cyclophosphamide, cyclosporine), pulse methylprednisolone therapy, corticotropin, plasmapheresis, and extracorporeal photopheresis [18–20, 26–30].

11.2.2 Dermatitis Herpetiformis

Name. Dermatitis herpetiformis (DH), Duhring's disease.

Definition. A chronic, intensely pruritic, papulo-vesicular eruption characterized by the presence of granular deposits of IgA at the dermo-epidermal junction and a usually asymptomatic gluten sensitive enteropathy (GSE), and associated with specific HLA antigens.

Etiology. The etiology is unknown. Genetic susceptibility has been well established with the demonstration of associated genotypes: HLA-DQ2 in 95 % of DH patients, and DR-3 and B-8 in 90 % and 80 % of patients, respectively [31–34]. This susceptibility, possibly in combination with other genes or with inciting factors, results in sensitivity to the dietary protein gluten and in eventual skin eruption.

Pathogenesis. Virtually all patients with DH have some degree of gluten-sensitive enteropathy. It is now well accepted that a cause-effect relationship exists between the ingestion of gluten and the presence of granular IgA and clinical inflammation within the skin. The cutaneous target antigen of the IgA molecule has not been identified, nor has the nature and source of this tissue IgA been characterized. It is speculated, however, that the gastrointestinal immune response to gluten results in the production of IgA antibodies which enter the circulation in small amounts and are deposited in the skin. Over time, the deposition increases sufficiently to cause an overt disease [31–35].

Oral Manifestations. Oral lesions in DH are generally considered rare. In contrast to earlier reports, the oral eruption is primarily non-vesicular in nature. Four main types of lesions are described: (1) an erythematous maculopapular eruption involving lips, buccal mucosa, soft palate, and tongue; (2) pale pseudovesicular lesions surrounded by an erythematous zone, usually on the buccal mucosa at the occlusal plane of the teeth; (3) purpuric lesions, usually under dentures, at the junction of the hard and soft palate, or on the buccal mucosa at the dental occlusal plane; and (4) erosive lesions surrounded by an erythematous zone (Fig. 11.11). The lesions are usually asymptomatic, but may be painful in rare cases. The prediliction for areas affected by trauma (dental closure plane) corresponds to the known affinity of the skin eruption to points of pressure [36, 37].

Associated Findings. *Skin:* The skin eruption of DH is symmetric, with a predilection for the extensor surfaces of the extremities, buttocks, upper aspects of the back, and posterior part of the neck. Facial lesions, particularly perioral, may occur, and palmar or plantar involvement is rare. The primary lesions are pruritic erythematous papules or papulovesicles with secondary excoriations and crusting (Fig. 11.12). Urticarial plaques may sometimes be present, and rarely frank bullae.

Intestinal. Most patients with DH and the associated GSE have no gastrointestinal symptoms; 20 %–30 % have mild steatorrhea, and less than 10 % have the typical symptoms of celiac disease including bloating, diarrhea, and malabsorption. Even when

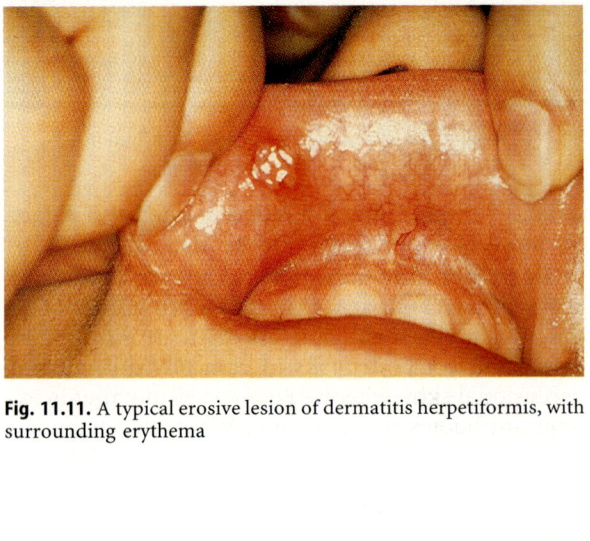

Fig. 11.11. A typical erosive lesion of dermatitis herpetiformis, with surrounding erythema

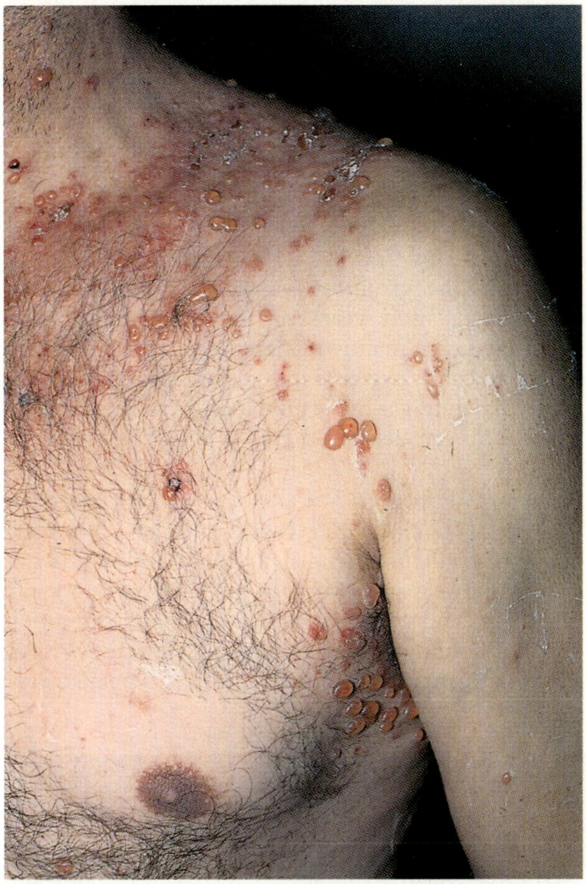

Fig. 11.12. Papulovesicular eruption of dermatitis herpetiformis

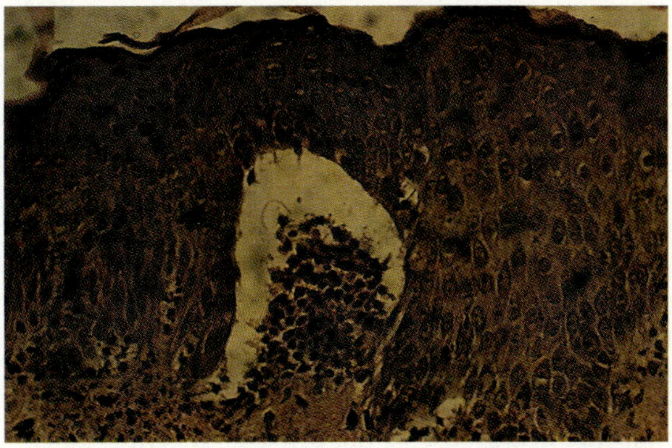

Fig. 11.13. Papillary microabscess in dermatitis herpetiformis, × 400

asymptomatic, laboratory tests may document abnormal intestinal functions.

Associated Disorders. (1) Frequent hypochlorhydria and atrophic gastritis, resulting in pernicious anemia in up to 7 % of patients; (2) high incidence of thyroid abnormalities and detectable thyroid antibodies; and (3) increased incidence of malignancy, predominantly lymphoma [31–38].

Microscopic Findings. In early lesions, the hallmark of histologic findings is the accumulation of neutrophils in the dermal papillae (Fig. 11.13), with an associated perivascular lymphohistiocytic infiltrate. Microabscesses form in the papillae and eventually coalesce to produce a subepidermal blister [31–37].

Diagnosis. Because both the clinical picture and the histologic findings, especially of late lesions, may not be diagnostic, immunofluorescence studies are essential. The biopsy for direct immunofluorescence should be taken from clinically normal appearing skin, in close proximity to active lesions (3–5 mm), in search of the pathognomonic granular IgA deposits in the dermal papillae. Up to 10 % of specimens show a continuous granular pattern along the basement membrane zone. Indirect immunofluorescence is negative for circulating IgA antibodies that bind to dermal papillae. Serologic studies may aid the diagnosis: anti-gluten antibodies were described in 50 %–90 % of DH patients, and anti-endomysial antibodies were found in 5 %–10 % of DH patients; the presence of both correlates well with the severity of the small bowel defect. Topical iodide application on normal skin of DH patients produces lesions that are histologically identical to spontaneous lesions. This is known as the iodide patch test, now only seldom applied as a diagnostic aid [31–37].

Differential Diagnosis. DH and linear IgA bullous dermatosis (LABD) were initially considered variants of the same disorder, and when clinically identical can only be differentiated by the pattern of IgA deposits in the skin (granular in DH, linear in LABD). Patients with systemic lupus erythematosus (SLE) occasionally have bullous skin lesions associated with granular deposition of IgA. Diagnosis of SLE will depend on the criteria for SLE and on the frequent additional immunoglobulins present in the skin. The wide variety of skin lesions in DH may often suggest a long differential diagnosis including erythema multiforme, herpes gestationis, bullous pemphigoid, papular urticaria, scabies, bug bites, and neurotic excoriations [31–37].

Treatment. Dapsone and sulfapyridine are the mainstays of therapy. Dapsone is started with a dose of 50 mg/day and is gradually increased to a maintenance therapy of 100–200 mg/day in a single daily dose. Baseline complete blood count (CBC) and liver functions should be obtained, and G6PD deficiency ruled out prior to treatment. CBC should then be checked weekly for the first month, monthly for the next 5 months, and biannually thereafter. The chemistry profile should be checked every 6 months. If dapsone is not tolerated or contraindicated, treatment with sulfapyridine, 1–4 g/day, is initiated. Topical potent steroid application may provide relief as adjuvant to systemic therapy.

Last but not least, gluten restriction usually results in a significant reduction of dapsone dosage and improvement of gastrointestinal symptoms, and is considered a therapy aimed at the cause rather than the symptoms of the disease [31–35].

11.2.3 Linear IgA Bullous Dermatosis of Adults

Name. Linear IgA bullous dermatosis (LABD).

Definition. A rare chronic bullous disease with clinical presentation and light microscopic findings similar to those of dermatitis herpetiformis or bullous pemphigoid, characterized by linear deposition of IgA at the basement membrane zone (BMZ). LABD is not associated with gluten sensitivity enteropathy, and the associated HLA of dermatitis herpetiformis is not a feature of LABD. Chronic bullous dermatosis of childhood (CBDC) is probably an expression of the same disease process in a different age group [39–41].

Etiology. The etiology of LABD is not known. A genetic background has not been significantly demonstrated: no association was found between the disease and HLA type of the A, B, C, and DR loci. Numerous inciting factors have been implicated, including drugs (vancomycin, lithium, diclophenac, amiodarone, penicillin, contrast intravenous agents), UV radiation, infections (esp. *Staphylococcus aureus*), inflammatory bowel disease, and malignancies [39, 40, 42, 43].

Pathogenesis. The site of production of the IgA deposits and the target structure of this autoimmune process remain to be determined. Anti-basement membrane antibodies of the IgA class are sometimes found in the serum of patients with LABD. These antibodies bind to the basement membrane with a resultant dermoepidermal separation, in a process that does not require complement and is probably mediated via proteinases released by neutrophils [39–41].

Two molecular weights of target antigens have been reported: 97 kDa and 285 kDa; it is not known if the former represents a breakdown product of the latter. The ultrastructural sites of the antigen are probably both the upper lamina lucida and the sublamina densa ("mirror image" deposits) [44]. Corresponding target structures have not been unequivocally identified, but it is speculated that the sublamina densa antigen is collagen VII of the anchoring fibrils [39–41, 45, 46].

Oral Manifestations. Oral lesions are usually a minor or incidental finding of LABD, but a case of oral lesions as the prominent manifestation preceding skin lesions by 5 years has been described. The oral lesions are mainly blisters, erosions, and ulcers and can occur anywhere in the oral mucosa. Erosive gingivitis, gingival hyperplasia, and erosive cheilitis have also been described [39–41, 45, 47].

Associated Findings. The skin lesions are characterized by their clinical diversity: papular, vesicular, bullous, erythematous, edematous, and erythema multiforme-like. The vesicles or bullae may appear on an erythematous or normal appearing skin; they are tense and of different sizes, and sometimes have a herpetiform arrangement (Fig. 11.14). The distribu-

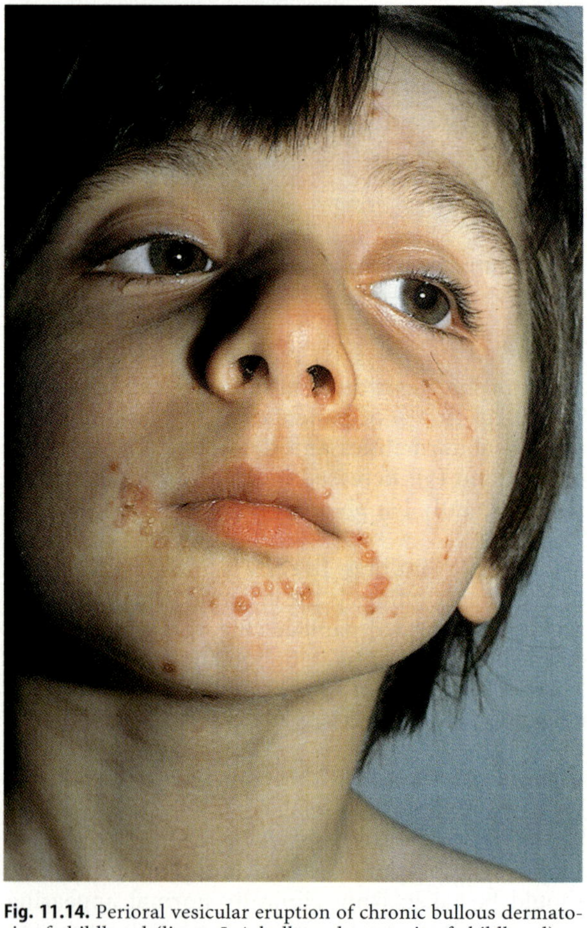

Fig. 11.14. Perioral vesicular eruption of chronic bullous dermatosis of childhood (linear IgA bullous dermatosis of childhood)

tion of the lesions may be symmetric or asymmetric. In CBDC, the lesions are typically located in the lower abdomen and in the anogenital areas (Fig. 11.15). Pruritus may be mild or severe, and sometimes precedes the appearance of skin lesions. It is generally agreed that enteropathy does not occur in LABD: markers for gluten sensitivity (anti-gluten and anti-endomysial antibodies) are negative, and jejunal biopsies are normal [39–41].

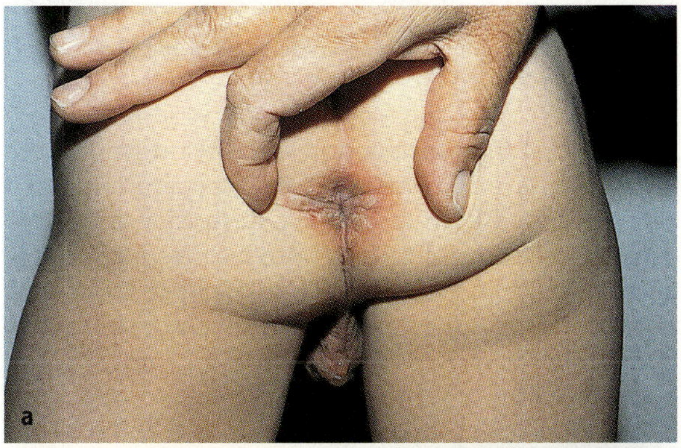

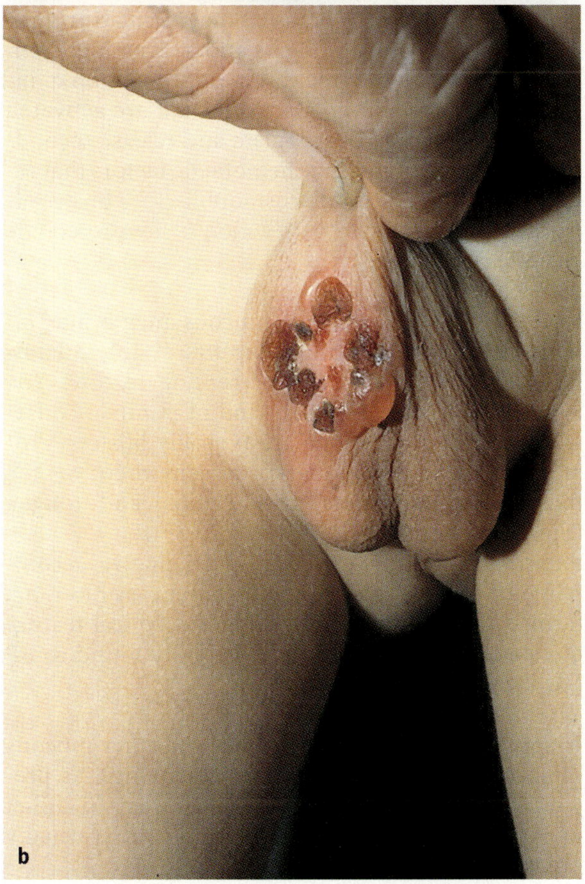

Fig. 11.15 a, b. Typical anogenital distribution of lesions in linear IgA bullous dermatosis of childhood

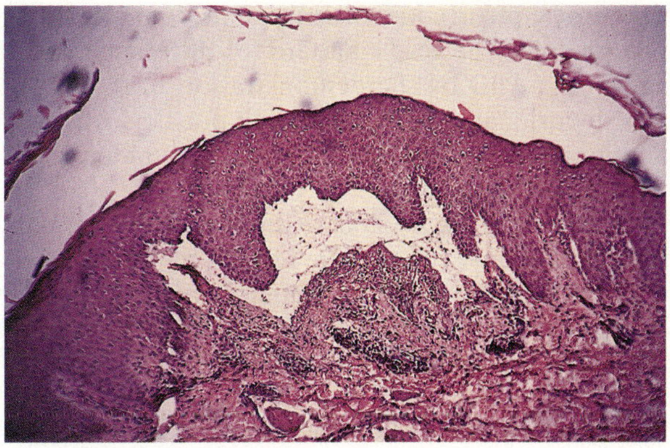

Fig. 11.16. Subepidermal cleft of linear IgA bullous dermatosis

LABD has been reported to be associated with internal malignancies, chiefly lymphomas. Inasmuch as there is no evidence for a causal relationship, it is recommended to evaluate LABD patients with screening measures to detect possible neoplastic disorders [42].

Microscopic Findings. The typical subepidermal bulla is often accompanied by the presence of papillary microabscesses and cutaneous infiltrations of mainly neutrophils and sometimes eosinophils (Fig. 11.16) [39–41].

Diagnosis. Because clinically and microscopically LABD may be identical to dermatitis herpetiformis and to bullous pemphigoid, the hallmark of diagnosis is the linear homogeneous deposits of IgA along the basement membrane zone. The skin biopsy for direct immunofluorescence should be taken from normal appearing skin in close proximity to lesions. Circulating IgA antibodies may be found in the sera of approximately one-third of patients. The serum is studied by indirect immunofluorescent techniques, preferably on salt-split skin, where the immunoreactants bind to either side of the split. Immunoelectron microscopy may demonstrate the diagnostic "mirror image" IgA deposits on both sides of the lamina densa. When the above measures prove insufficient, immunoblotting a 97-kDa antigen confirms the diagnosis [39–42, 44, 46, 48–50].

Differential Diagnosis. LABD may present with a pruritic papulovesicular eruption symmetrically distributed over extensor surfaces indistinguishable from dermatitis herpetiformis, or with tense bullae on erythematous base in clusters mimicking bullous pemphigoid. A herpetiform vesicular presentation might suggest the diagnosis of herpetiform pemphigus. The mucosal oral lesions may be accompanied by symptoms of cicatrizing conjunctivitis, rendering

the clinical picture indistinguishable from cicatritial pemphigoid. The gold standard for differentially diagnosing LABD by the demonstration of the linear IgA deposits along the BMZ may not be sufficient, and immunoelectron studies and antigen identification might be needed.
LABD might be impossible to differentiate from bullous SLE because IgA may be present in the LE band, in addition to other immunoglobulins. Diagnosis should be based on SLE criteria or on identifying the antigen by immunoprecipitation techniques.

Treatment. Sulfones are the therapy of choice: dapsone with average daily doses of 100–150 mg/day, or sulfapyridine at 1–1.5 g/day. When the lesions regress, usually rapidly, the dosage of dapsone is reduced gradually to 50 mg/day, where it is maintained for several weeks or months. If the response is not satisfactory, small doses of corticosteroids should be added (10–30 mg/day). An alternative treatment is sulfamethoxypyridazine (1–1.5 g/day) or salazopyrine (5–6 g/day), in conjunction with small doses of corticosteroids. Gluten-free diet has no impact on the course of the disease [39, 40].

11.2.4 Bullous Pemphigoid

Name. Bullous pemphigoid (BP).

Definitions. BP is an acquired autoimmune disease of the elderly, characterized by subepidermal bullae and circulating and tissue bound autoantibodies directed against components of the basement membrane zone (BMZ). The disease is usually self-limiting and not fatal, and its incidence is estimated to be 1 per 100 000 per year [51].

Etiology. The etiology of this autoimmune process is not known. Patients with BP fail to display any increased incidence of HLA-A, B, C or D locus antigens, suggesting that HLA gene products do not play a role in susceptibility to BP. Several precipitating factors related to disease onset have been described: drugs (mainly furosemide, phenacetin, penicillins), ultraviolet light, and malignancies. The association of BP with malignancy remains controversial. Although it is generally agreed that there is no statistically increased incidence of malignancy in patients with BP, it is possible that subgroups of BP patients (e.g., with figurate erythema or seronegative for anti-BMZ antibodies) are at a greater risk of developing neoplasms [51–53].

Pathogenesis. The autoantibodies, primarily of the IgG class and aided by C_3, are thought to be pathogenic in that their interaction with BP antigens at the BMZ results in dermal-epidermal separation. Two independent BP antigens have been identified, designated BP 180 and BP 230, both localized at the epidermal hemidesmosomes. The BP 180 is a 180-kDa transmembrane protein with the amino-terminal domain in the intracellular hemidesmosomal plaque and the carboxy-terminal half, made up of a long collagenous tail projecting into the extracellular region of the BMZ. It is believed that circulating antibodies bind to these antigens and activate the complement cascade with the resultant production of inflammatory mediators. Mast cells that are activated by these mediators degranulate and release secondary mediators, including chemotactic factors that recruit neutrophils and eosinophils. A blister is formed by direct cytotoxic action or by proteolytic enzymes [51, 52, 54, 55].

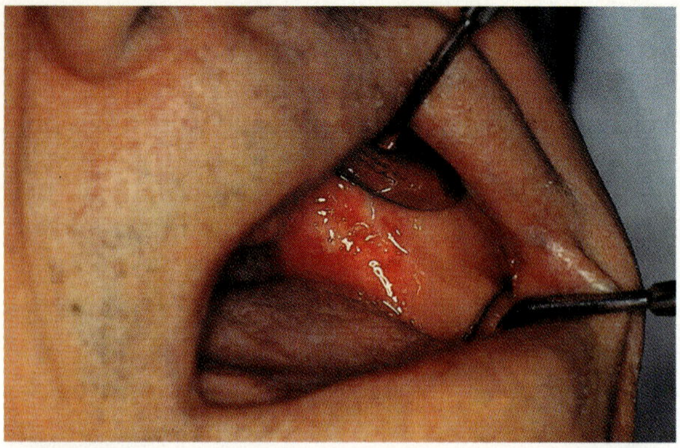

Fig. 11.17. A typical mucosal lesion of bullous pemphigoid: an ulcer surrounded by an erythematous zone

Oral Manifestations. Oral mucous membrane involvement may be found in up to 45 % of patients, but it is usually not the presenting feature. The lesions are usually transient and of minimal consequence. The oral lesions are typically blisters, erosions, or ulcers, and may occur anywhere on the mucosa of the palate, cheeks, lips, and tongue (Fig. 11.17).
Painful swelling and erythema of the gingiva, accompanied by areas of desquamation and easy bleeding, termed desquamative gingivitis, is a typical feature of cicatricial pemphigoid and is rarely found in BP [51, 52, 56, 58].

Associated Findings. Involvement of other mucous membranes is probably not as uncommon as previously believed and has been reported to afflict up to 60 % of patients. The involvement is usually mild and non-scarring.
The characteristic skin lesion is a tense blister appearing on normal or erythematous skin. When

the bulla ruptures, the eroded area does not tend to spread, and if uncomplicated by secondary infection, heals readily. The size of the blister varies greatly from small vesicles to large bullae.

Other common lesions are erythematous macules, papules, or urticarial plaques. These may precede the appearance of blisters and are usually very pruritic. The degree of pruritus in BP varies: it may be the presenting symptom and may persist for a long time without skin lesions, or it may be absent throughout the course of the disease.

Diabetes and psoriasis seem to have an increased association with BP and may pose a problem for choosing systemic corticosteroids for treatment.

The reported association with lichen planus (LP) has been termed lichen planus pemphigoides. It is characterized by the typical LP eruption in conjunction with bullae with the histologic and immunofluorescent features of BP [51, 52, 58].

Microscopic Findings. The characteristic finding is a subepidermal bulla with normal epidermis. The dermis may be "infiltrate-poor" with minimal perivascular infiltrate, corresponding to normal skin at the periphery of the bulla, or "infiltrate-rich", corresponding to an erythematous base. The predominant infiltrate cell type is the eosinophil, but lymphocytes, histiocytes, and neutrophils may also be present. The infiltrate is also typically found in the blister cavity. Ultrastructurally, the dermal-epidermal separation is at the level of the lamina lucida [51, 52, 58].

Diagnosis. Diagnosis is based on the clinical picture, aided by histologic findings and substantiated by immunofluorescence studies. Between 45 % and 90 % of BP patients have linear IgG deposits at the BMZ of perilesional skin (Fig. 11.18), and 80 %–90 % of BP patients have linear C3 deposits. Linear IgM, IgA, IgE, and IgD are less frequently seen. Circulating IgG anti-BMZ antibodies are detectable in 70 % of patients. In order to distinguish BP from other blistering diseases with similar histology and linear immunoreactants along the BMZ, immunoelectron microscopy or indirect immunofluorescence studies on salt-split skin are required. On salt-split skin, BP autoantibodies bind to the roof only, or to the roof and the base of the split skin. When the above measures prove insufficient for substantiating the diagnosis, antigen identification by immunoblotting techniques should be attempted [51, 52, 59–61].

Differential Diagnosis. The main problem is differentiating BP with mucosal involvement from cicatricial pemphigoid (CP) with cutaneous lesions.

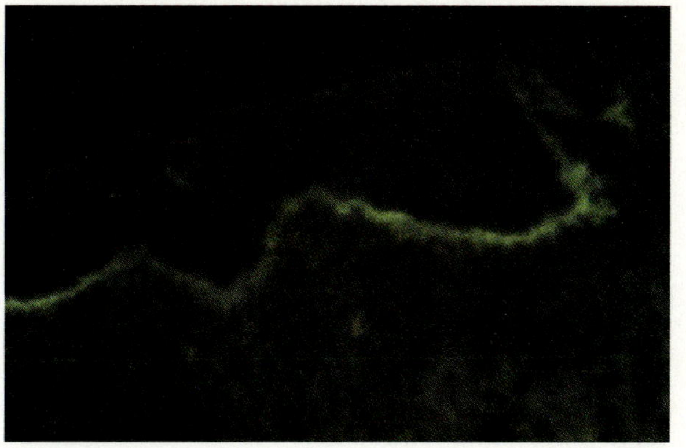

Fig. 11.18. Linear deposition of IgG at BMZ in bullous pemphigoid

The differentiation is usually a clinical one, based on the severity of mucosal involvement in CP and its scarring and disabling nature, but could be aided by salt-split immunofluorescence studies and immunoelectron microscopy, demonstrating immunoreactant depositions at a higher level of the lamina lucida than CP. In addition, circulating autoantibodies in CP, often of the IgA class, do not react with the BP antigens by immunoblotting techniques.

Epidermolysis bullosa and bullous systemic lupus erythematosus, subepidermal dermatoses with BMZ immunoreactants, are also distinguished from BP by the aid of a new salt-split direct immunofluorescence technique, as the immunoreactants are found solely on the dermal side of the split [51, 52, 62].

Differentiating BP with predominant IgA deposits from linear IgA dermatosis (considered by some a subtype of BP) is sometimes possible only by antigen identification.

Treatment. The majority of patients with generalized disease are controlled with 40–80 mg/day prednisone (0.6–1.2 mg/kg/day). When the disease is mild, lower doses (0.5 mg/day) are sufficient, and patients with a localized disease may even respond to topical steroid treatment. When existing lesions heal and new blisters cease to appear, prednisone should be tapered to an alternate day regimen. Failure to respond may be overcome by addition of an immunosuppressive agent like azathioprine or cyclophosphamide [51, 52].

Occasional success has been documented with sulfapyridine or dapsone (especially in patients with neurophil predominance in the infiltrate), and with oral tetracyclines, alone or in combination with niacinamide. Other options for refractory disease are corticoid pulse therapy and plasmapheresis [51, 52, 63].

11.2.5 Cicatricial Pemphigoid

Name. Cicatricial pemphigoid (CP), benign mucous membrane pemphigoid.

Definition. CP is a rare, chronic, autoimmune, subepidermal blistering disease that primarily affects the mucous membranes. As in bullous pemphigoid (BP), patients with CP characteristically have immunoglobulin and complement deposits along the basement membrane zone (BMZ), and some also have circulating antibodies. CP is distinguished from BP by the extent of the mucosal involvement and by the resultant significant scarring that often terminates in permanent loss of function of the involved structures.
Although some authors share the view that CP is actually a variant of BP, it is generally accepted that both disases belong to a clinical spectrum of pemphigoid disorders. The existence of a variant of CP with localized scarring skin lesions and without mucosal involvement (the Brunsting-Perry CP) seems to sever the aforementioned concept [64–66].

Etiology. The etiology of CP is not known. It has been reported to be induced by D-penicillamine by an unclear mechanism. Genetic studies are rare and a genetic predisposition has not been thoroughly established, but an association between CP and a DQβ1 allele has recently been suggested [64, 65, 67].

Pathogenesis. Because CP is a rare disease, and circulating antibodies even rarer to find, the pathogenesis of CP has not been studied, and its understanding is extrapolated from what is known in BP because the two diseases share similar immunopathology. It is believed that the circulating antibodies are pathogenic, and upon binding to the target antigen, fix complement components and thereby induce an inflammatory response. The inflammatory cells degranulate proteolytic enzymes that digest the lamina lucida, leading to dermal-epidermal separation and blister formation. The process that gives rise to scar formation is not known.
Recent studies have identified two subgroups of CP patients:

1. Those with circulating antibodies that bind to the dermal side of salt-split skin and immunoprecipitate a keratinocyte-derived glycoprotein complex termed epiligrin (seemingly identical to laminin 5, an integrin ligand associated with anchoring filaments in the lamina lucida).

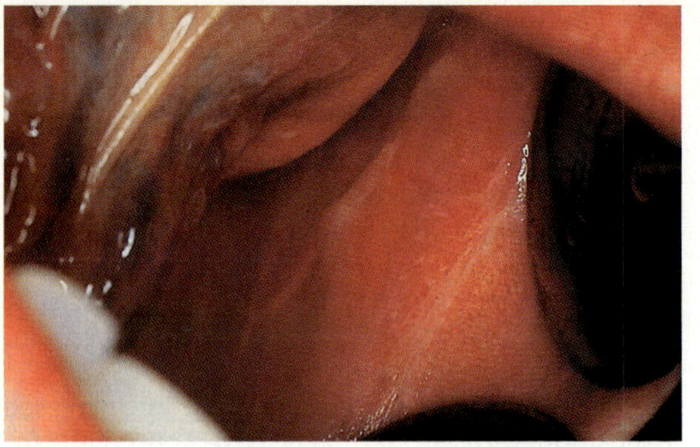

Fig. 11.19. Erosive mucosal lesions of cicatricial pemphigoid

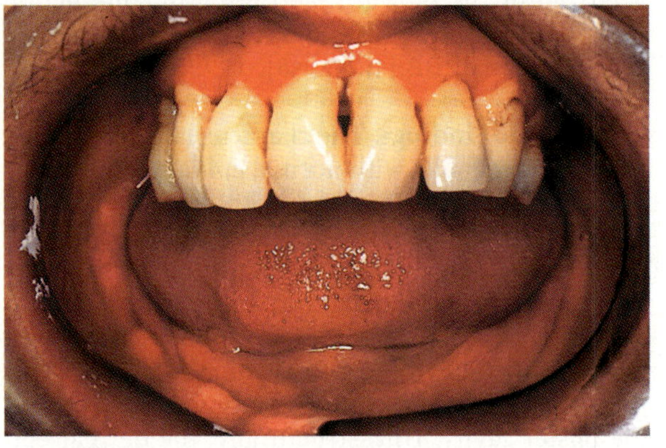

Fig. 11.20. Gingivitis in cicatricial pemphigoid

2. Patients who have circulating antibodies that bind to the epidermal side of salt-split skin, to an unknown antigen, believed by some to be the BP antigen [64, 65, 68–72].

Oral Manifestations. Oral involvement occurs in almost all patients with CP, and is often the only site affected. Oral lesions are believed to develop after local trauma. The primary lesion is a blister that quickly ruptures to form an erosion or an ulcer (Fig. 11.19). These cause little discomfort, heal very slowly, and have a tendency for scar formation upon healing that may lead to a white reticulated pattern resembling lichen planus. Adhesions may form as well, often between the buccal mucosa and the alveolar process.
The oral lesions frequently begin as desquamative gingivitis, characterized by erythema, edema, and desquamation of the gingival mucosa. In the areas of active desquamation, the gingival surface appears raw and hemorrhagic (Fig. 11.20). The desquamation is aggravated by trauma [64, 65, 73–76].

Associated Findings. *Ocular Lesions.* It is estimated that more than half the patients have ocular lesions. The early unilateral chronic conjunctivitis results eventually in conjunctival shrinkage, symblepharon, and less often in ankyloblepharon. Contraction of the conjunctiva results in eyelid inversion (entropion) and eyelash inversion (trichiasis), leading to corneal injury and terminating in blindness.

Other Mucous Involvement. Nasopharynx (in 20 % of patients), larynx (in 8 % of patients), genitalia (20 %), esophagus (4 %), and anus (3 %). Involvement of these organs may be mild or severe, leading to stenosis and may be life-threatening when obstructing the aerodigestive pathway.

Skin. Blistering cutaneous lesions may appear in 10 %–43 % of CP patients, usually on the head, neck, and genitalia. The lesions may be scarring or non-scarring, generalized with a transient nature, or localized but recurrent and chronic. The localized recurrent eruption is typically of scarring nature, and referred to as the Brunsting-Perry type variant when mucosal involvement is absent [64–66, 76].

Microscopic Findings. Histologic examination reveals a subepidermal cleft with a dermal mixed inflammatory infiltrate. Most studies emphasize the higher proportion of neutrophils in comparison to BP infiltrate.
Ultrastructurally, the split occurs in the lamina lucida. It is suggested that the site of separation in the lamina lucida is lower in CP compared to BP. In advanced lesions, the basal lamina may be destroyed [64, 65, 76].

Diagnosis. The presentation of a chronic, blistering, erosive disease of mucosal membrane leading to scarring suggests the diagnosis of CP. Histologic studies are not sufficient to differentially diagnose CP from other subepidermal blistering diseases, especially when skin lesions are present. Direct immunofluorescence reveals immune deposits (mainly IgG and C3, but sometimes IgA or IgM) in the majority of patients. Anti-BMZ antibodies are found in only a third of the patients when using normal skin as a substrate, but the sensitivity of indirect immunofluorescence may reach approximately 88 % when using salt-split, mucosal substrate. Most circulating antibodies are of the IgG class and bind to the epidermal side or to the dermal side of the salt-split. Immunoelectron microscopy studies reveal immune deposits in the lamina lucida and along the lamina densa [64, 65, 69, 71, 72, 74].

Differential Diagnosis. 1. Desquamating gingivitis (DG) as sole manifestation: DG may be the presenting sign of other chronic conditions such as lichen planus (especially when a white lacy scarring is also present), pemphigus vulgaris (PV), or oral epidermolysis bullosa aquisitia (EBA), and of acute conditions such as contact stomatitis.
2. Oral lesions as the sole manifestation: When cutaneous lesions are absent, oral vesicles and erosions are to be differentiated from a variety of diseases, both acute, like herpetic and contact stomatitis, and chronic, like linear IgA bullous dermatosis, PV, and EBA.
3. Mucocutaneous eruption present: The primary differential diagnosis is between CP and BP. BP involves mainly the skin, and mucosal lesions, if existent, are usually non-scarring.
Fifty percent of EBA patients may have oral and ocular lesions associated with scarring, and linear IgA bullous dermatosis, considered by many investigators to be a subtype of pemphigoid, may also present with a scarring mucosal eruption along with cutaneous lesions. An indistinguishable eruption could be the manifestation of bullous systemic lupus erythematosus.
CP is differentiated from all the above with the aid of split skin and immunoelectron techniques to selectively localize the deposits in the BMZ, and when insufficient, antigen identification by immunoblotting is required [64, 65, 70–72, 77].

Treatment. Patients with limited oral disease may be treated with topical steroids and appropriate oral hygiene. With a more extensive disease, systemic treatment is warranted: dapsone should first be attempted, beginning with a dose of 25 mg/day and gradually increasing to 100–150 mg/day. When the response is inadequate, systemic corticosteroids (1 mg/kg/day), preferably combined with immunosuppressive agents like azathioprine (1–2 mg/kg/day) or cyclophosphamide (0.5–2 mg/kg/day), are indicated.
Surgical intervention should not be attempted in active disease [64, 65].

11.2.6 Epidermolysis Bullosa Acquisita

Name. Epidermolysis bullosa acquisita (EBA).

Definition. EBA is a chronic, autoimmune, subepidermal blistering disease affecting the skin and mucous membranes, characterized by tissue-bound and circulating antibodies directed against the anchoring fibril type VII collagen (C7). EBA is a clinicopathologic heterogeneous entity comprising inflammatory and non-inflammatory variants. There is increasing evidence of an association between EBA and bullous systemic lupus erythematosus (BSLE), both diseases of C7 autoimmunity sharing the same genetic susceptibility.

Etiology. HLA-DR_2 has been shown to confer susceptibility to C7 autoimmunity and occurs in about 92% of EBA patients and 90% of BSLE patients. Among DR-2-negative EBA white patients, the incidence of HLA DR5 is significantly increased, and DR-8 is increased in DR-2-negative black patients [78–81]. Triggering factors are believed to exist, and drug-induced EBA has been reported with sulfonamides, sulfamethoxypyridazine, D-penicillamine, and furosemide [82].

Pathogenesis. Blisters are induced by C7 autoantibodies by two hypothesized mechanisms that result in different clinicopathological phenotypes: (1) in situ binding of the antibodies (primarily of the IgG class) results in an inflammatory response via complement activation, culminating in destruction of the anchoring fibrils and in dermal-epidermal separation, and (2) binding of the C7 antibodies to the anchoring fibrils interferes with their function, producing a non-inflammatory dermal-epidermal separation. The target antigen, recognized as C7, is detectable by immunoblotting techniques as two protein bands: a major band of 290-kDa molecular weight, and a 145-kDa minor band [78–81].

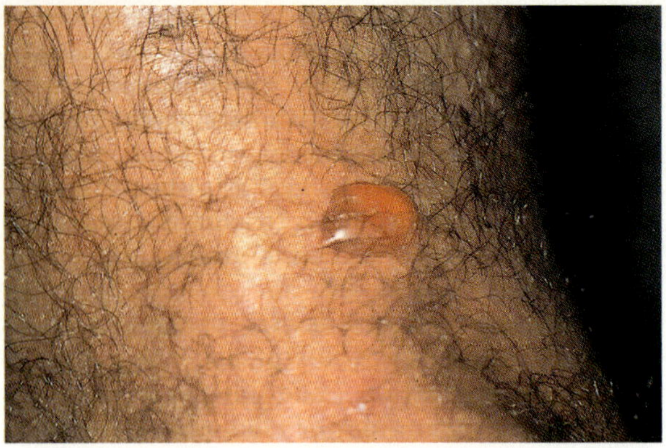

Fig. 11.21. A non-inflammatory bulla of epidermolysis bullosa acquisita

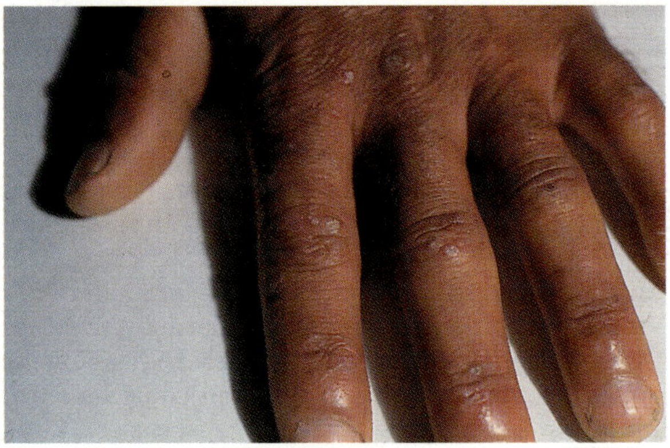

Fig. 11.22. Milia formation at sites of healed lesions of epidermolysis bullosa acquisita

Oral Manifestations. The oral involvement in EBA is manifested in blisters, erosions, and ulcers, with variable degrees of surrounding inflammation. The lesions vary from a non-scarring clinical presentation indistinguishable from bullous pemphigoid, to a severely scarring eruption mimicking cicatricial pemphigoid. Oral EBA may feature desquamative gingivitis, characterized by gingival erythema and edema resulting in desquamation, erosions, and hemorrhage [78–81, 83, 84].

Associated Findings. The diversity of the mucocutaneous eruptions is reflected by the existence of several distinct clinical patterns: (1) the classical phenotype, distinguished by skin fragility and trauma-induced non-inflammatory blisters (Fig. 11.21), mainly on extensor surfaces, that heal with scarring and milia (Fig. 11.22); (2) the bullous pemphigoid phenotype, presenting with inflammatory lesions (erythematous macules, papules, plaques, and blisters on an erythematous base), absence of skin fragility, and usually healing without scarring; and (3) the cicatricial pemphigoid phenotype, featuring a severe scarring mucosal disease resulting in blindness or aerodigestive stenosis, with minimal, if any, skin lesions, confined to the head, neck, and genitalia. The mucous membranes involved are the same as described in cicatricial pemphigoid [78–81].

The association between EBA and BSLE appears to be stronger than the traditional association with inflammatory bowel disease. Patients with EBA may develop SLE, and concurrent SLE and EBA have been described. It is therefore recommended that patients with EBA be monitored for evidence of SLE [78–81].

Microscopic Findings. Lesional skin displays dermal-epidermal separation, with or without dermal infiltration, corresponding to the inflammatory or non-inflammatory clinical subtypes (Fig. 11.23). In the classical phenotype, a sparse dermal infiltrate of mononuclear cells may be found. In the bullous pemphigoid phenotype, the infiltrate may be moderate or dense, of mononuclear cells and granulocytes, with the predominant granulocyte being the neutrophil rather than the eosinophil typical of bul-

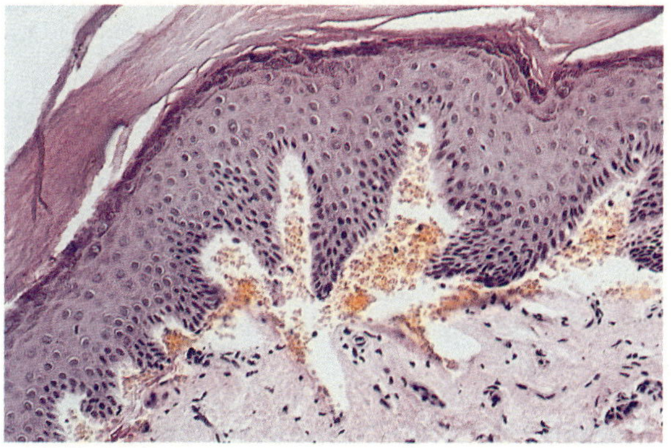

Fig. 11.23. A subepidermal blister of classical epidermolysis bullosa acquisita, with a poor inflammatory response in the dermis and a blister cavity hemorrhage that may have resulted from trauma, × 200

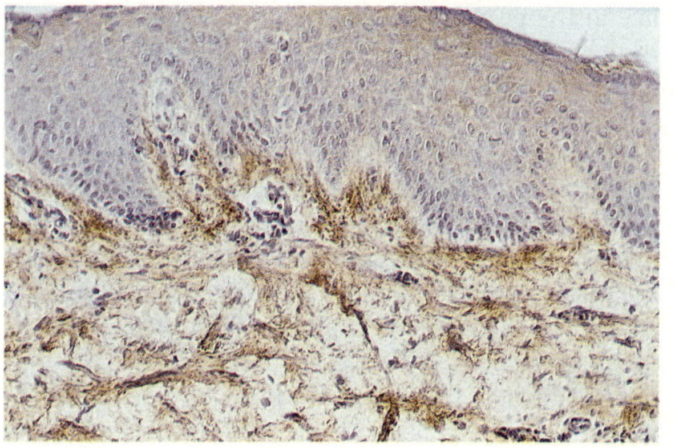

Fig. 11.24. Demonstration of the IgG deposits at the BMZ-dermal papillae level by anti-human IgG serum conjugated with peroxidase, × 200

lous pemphigoid. The electron microscope localizes the level of separation in the upper dermis, just beneath the lamina densa [78–81].

Diagnosis. Inasmuch as the mechanobullous noninflammatory variant is almost diagnostic by virtue of the typical clinical features, other forms of EBA pose a major diagnostic problem as they may be clinically indistinguishable from bullous pemphigoid or cicatricial pemphigoid. The histologic findings do not aid in the diagnosis, except for the neutrophil predominance over eosinophils mentioned above. Immunofluorescence studies on split skin reveal immunodeposits (mainly IgG and C_3, but often also IgA and IgM) on the dermal side of the split (Fig. 11.24). Circulating anti-basement membrane IgG is present in about half the patients. Immunoelectron microscopy is the gold standard for the diagnosis of EBA, showing immune deposits beneath the lamina densa. Because such findings are shared by EBA, BSLE, and some of the linear IgA bullous dermatosis cases, immunoblotting the antigen might be imperative for the final diagnosis [78–81, 85–87].

Differential Diagnosis. EBA should be distinguished from other subepidermal blistering disorders with mucosal involvement. Though clinically indistinguishable, EBA can be differentiated from bullous pemphigoid or cicatricial pemphigoid by indirect immunofluorescence on salt-split skin and immunoelectron microscopy studies. Differentially diagnosing EBA from other diseases of the dermal side of split skin, like BSLE, or some of the linear IgA bullous dermatoses, and of cicatricial pemphigoid, is successfully achieved by antigen identification or by the occurrence of concomitant SLE criteria [78–81].

Treatment. Response to treatment is unpredictable, and some patients are refractory to every treatment modality available. Patients may respond to corticosteroids (prednisone 0.5–1.0 mg/kg/day) alone, or in combination with either azathioprine or cyclophosphamide. Cyclosporine in doses of 3–5 mg/kg/day might be effective in some patients. Because the onset of the disease is sometimes explosive but later activity levels off and the disease becomes milder, pulse corticosteroid therapy might be beneficial. A few patients may respond anecdotally to dapsone or colchicine [78, 81].

11.3 Aphthous and Ulcerative Diseases

M. Caproni and P. Fabbri

11.3.1 Name of Disease

Recurrent Aphthous Stomatitis (RAS), chronic recurrent (habitual) aphthae, Mikulicz's aphthae.

Definition. Recurrent oral ulcers or aphthae (the name comes from an ancient Greek word which means ulcer) are painful, round or ovoid, with loss of mucosa localized, for the most part, on the lining mucosa of the oral cavity, each lasting from 1 to about 4 weeks.

Etiology. Oral aphthae arise in response to unknown stimuli (gastrointestinal disorders, hematological abnormality, immunodeficiency, psychological imbalances, while hormonal influences are only considered as predisposing factors) and the basic lesion is common to a variety of conditions, which is why the classification of these disorders is basically clinical at the present time. Oral aphthae are very common (20 % of the population), especially in higher socioeconomic classes.

Pathogenesis. Cell-mediated and humoral immune mechanisms appear to be involved. The serum immunoglobulin levels are usually normal, though IgA and IgG may be increased and circulating immunocomplexes may be found. In the peripheral blood, a selective activation of cytotoxic T-lymphocytes toward oral epithelial cells has been shown, though CD4 T-helper and CD45R suppressor lymphocyte subsets are depressed. In the mucosa lesions, CD4 and CD8 T, HLA-DR+ cells, 20 % of which express IL-2 and transferrin, predominate and there is evidence for an antibody-dependent cellular cytotoxicity [88–91].

Oral Manifestations. The lesion is a loss of mucosa, the depth of which varies, and it is sharply delineated, covered by a uniform yellowish-white pseudomembraneous fibrin coating, surrounded by a livid red border. A red spot precedes the aphthae and on this spot a small, cloudy blister forms. There are three main clinical types of recurrent aphthous and ulcerative lesions: minor aphthous ulcers (MiAU), major aphthous ulcers (MaAU), and herpetiform ulceration (HAU).

11.3.1.1 *Minor Aphthous Ulcers (MiAU)*

Synonyms. Mikulicz ulcers. The appearance of only a few round ulcers, (one to six) of 2–4 mm in diameter, at a time on the non-keratinized mucosa of the lips (Fig. 11.25), cheeks, and floor of the mouth, define the minor aphthous ulcer form (MiAU). They heal within 7–10 days with no evidence of scarring and recur constantly. The minor form is the most common, comprising 80 % of all forms.

11.3.1.2 *Major Aphthous Ulcers (MaAU)*

Synonyms. Sutton's ulcers. Only a few ulcers, larger (often more than 1 cm), deeper, longer lasting, more painful, more frequently recurrent ulcers than the MiAU, found on any area of the oral mucosa, even on the dorsum of the tongue or palate (Fig. 11.26), define the major aphthous ulcer form (MaAU). They heal slowly within 10–40 days, often with scarring.

Associated Findings. Mastication and phonation difficulty, salivation, and regional lymphadenopathy may be associated.

11.3.1.3 *Herpetiform Ulcers (HAU)*

HAU begin as tiny (2–4 mm), round, with loss of mucosa and then change for coalescence into multiple (10–100), shallow, grouped ulcers (Fig. 11.27). They localize at any oral site but more often on the ventrum of the tongue and persist for 7–10 days, healing with a scar in about one-third of

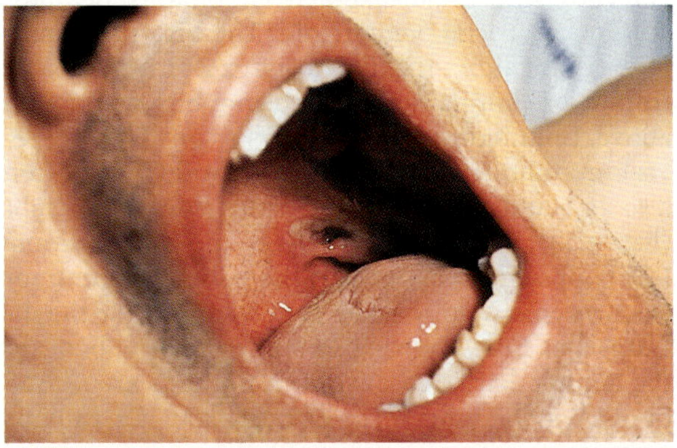

Fig. 11.26. Major aphthous ulcers of the palate left pillar

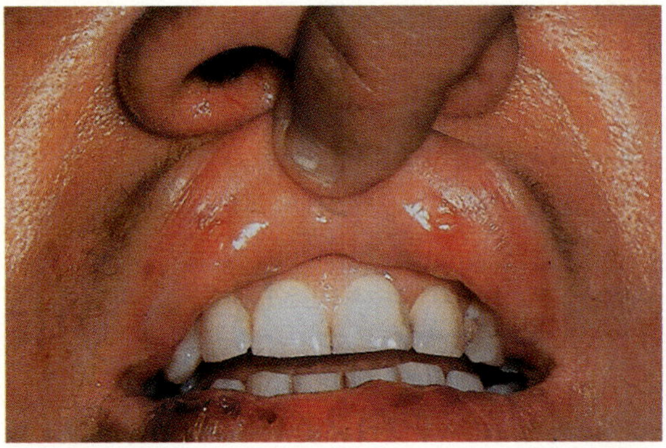

Fig. 11.25. Minor aphthous ulcers of the lip mucosa

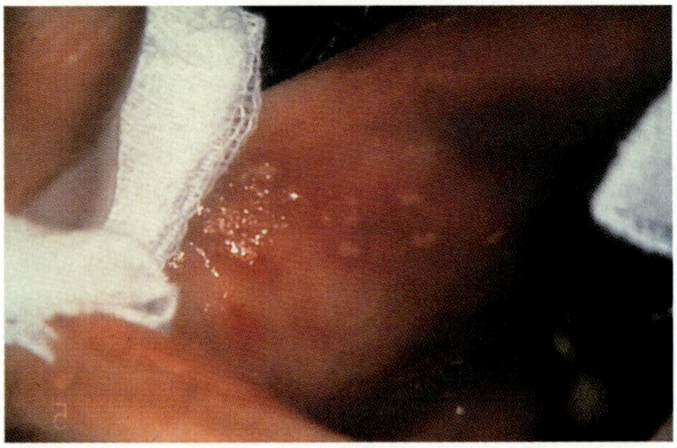

Fig. 11.27. Herpetiform ulcers of the cheek

cases. They are found in a slightly older female group.

Microscopic Findings. The histology is characterized by the presence of dense lymphocytic infiltration of the corium in an angiocentric and interstitial arrangement, often associated with lymphocytic exocytosis in the same sites of degenerative epithelial changes. When the latter are concentrated along the basal layer, the morphology may be cognate to erythema multiforme.

Diagnosis. The diagnosis is clinical. Biopsy is indicated only if other causes of mouth ulcers (malignant neoplasma, local trauma) have to be considered. Investigation should include a full blood count, iron, folate, and serum vitamin B_{12} because coeliac diseases must be excluded.

Treatment
Systemic. Systemic treatment with glucocorticosteroids at a dose of (0.3–0.5 mg/kg/day) can be used in the management of severe aphthae, probably as a first line of systemic therapy [92].
Thalidomide [93], in doses of up to 300 mg daily, induces remission, especially in major aphthae. However, its teratogenic effects and also neurotoxicity in the form of paresthesia, which can progress to permanent sensory or motor dysfunction, must be considered.
Colchicine [94], at 1 mg/day for at least 2 months, seems to significantly reduce the mean number of aphthae per week. Topical corticosteroid or antiinflammatory [95] mouthwashes and analgesic-anesthetic remedies are useful.

11.3.2 Behçet's Disease (BD)

Synonyms. Aphthosis Behçet, bipolar aphthosis, Neumann's bipolar aphthosis.

Definition. Behçet's disease (BD) is a systemic vasculitis, the manifestations which of include orogenital ulcers, uveitis, synovitis, thrombophlebitis, hypersensitivity-related skin lesions, and other symptoms connected to the central nervous system, and gastrointestinal and pulmonary involvement.

Etiology. The etiology of BD is uncertain, but a possible role of *Streptococcus sanguis* (SS) has been suggested. BD patients show a greater frequency of SS in their oral flora, together with serum antibodies against certain serotypes of SS. Also, herpes simplex viruses (HSV-1), being part of HSV-1 DNA integrating in the genome of BD circulating lymphocytes, seem to be involved [96].

Pathogenesis. Viral, bacterial, and genetic factors, as well as immune dysregulation, have all been considered. Moreover, it has been hypothesized that the cells responsible for the lesions of BD are Th1 lymphocytes. In fact, a particular antigen, after being subjected to phagocytosis, processing, and presentation by macrophages or epidermal Langerhans' cells to CD4+ lymphocytes, could activate Tho cells and polarize in the lymph nodes their differentiation, via IL12, towards the Th1 profile (TNF-beta, INF-gamma). The Th1-related cytokines could upregulate the adhesion molecules of the post-capillary venule high endothelial cells, with subsequent entry of lymphocytes and PMN at the site of the lesions [97]. Concerning the role of autoantibodies in BD, the occasional presence of antiphospholipid antibodies [98], and anti-neutrophil cytoplasmic antibodies (AECA) has been described. Between these, AECA are considered the most important, even if their presence is considered a primary event.

Oral Manifestations. Oral lesions in BD appear to be identical to those seen in the more common type of aphthous recurrent stomatitis, and they may have the form of minor, major, or herpetiform ulcers. In fact, aphthous ulcer is found in up to 98 % of patients with BD and is the initial manifestation in 30 %–75 %, but only a very small percentage of patients with oral aphthous ulcers progress to BD.

Associated Findings. Recurrent genital ulcers, which are especially painful in women and may scar on healing, as well as eye involvement (relapsing iridicyclitis, anterior and posterior uveitis, retinal vascular changes, optic atrophy) and skin lesions (erythema nodosum-like nodules, pseudofolliculitis, papulopustular lesions, or acneiform nodules) are held to be diagnostic. There may also be arthralgia or nonmigratory arthritis, especially of the large joints, together with recurrent superficial or deep thrombophlebitis. Systemic manifestations include pneumonitis, gastrointestinal ulcerations, and meningoencephalitis.

Microscopic Findings. According to most observers, the common denominator in all systems is a leukocytoclastic or lymphocytic vasculitis [99]. However, some authors remark that vasculitis would be present only in late lesions [100], while some others even suggest vasculitis could be absent [101].

Diagnosis. Though there are no universally accepted diagnostic criteria, the presence of three major (recurrent oral and genital aphthae, uveitis, and cutaneous lesions such as eythema nodosum-like nodules, pseudofollicolitis, and papulopustolar lesions) or two major and one minor (polyarthritis, gastrointestinal and neurological symptoms) criteria are considered diagnostic. The intracutaneous injection of physiological saline followed by postulation (pathergy test), read by a physician at 24–48 h, is also included in the minor criteria [102].

Treatment. All the local and systemic therapies mentioned for aphthae have been used in BD, with the same variable success. The presence of eye disease or other systemic involvement increases the tendency to employ systemic treatment. Glucocorticosteroids (1 mg/kg/day) given alone or in combination with cytostatics (methotrexate 25 mg/week; azathioprine 1–2 mg/kg/day [103] are effective in disease control. Thalidomide at a dose of up to 400 mg daily may be useful in recalcitrant orogenital ulceration. Cyclosporin (5 mg/kg/day for 6 weeks, to be reduced to 1 mg/kg/day every 4–6 weeks until a dose of 2.0 mg/kg/day is reached) has been utilized in the control of ocular lesions [104]. Glucocorticosteroids can be associated with cyclosporin at a dose of 0.2–0.4 mg/kg/day and reduced to 5 mg every 2 weeks.

11.3.3 Reiter's Syndrome

Synonyms. Fiessinger-Leroy syndrome, keratoderma blenorrhagicum.

Definition. Reiter's syndrome is a complex of urethritis, conjunctivitis, and arthritis, which may also include recurrent oral aphthae.

Etiology. The cause of Reiter's disease is not known, although an antigenic microbial stimulation (*Chlamydia trachomatis, Ureoplasma urealyticum, Shigella, Salmonella, Campylobacter, Yersinia*) [105] is presumed to be responsible for the disease by triggering agents in predisposed individuals (HLA-B27).

Pathogenesis. The pathologic events that give rise to Reiter's disease are obscure. Genetic factors seem to be involved since the disease tends to occur in Caucasian men in whom there is a significantly increased frequency of HLA-B27 (70–80 %).
One possibility is that the HLA-B27 molecule could induce a highly specific immunologic tolerance to some organisms through a process of deleting specific T-cell clones during the formation of the T-cell repertoire, thereby creating a "hole" in the T-cell repertoire. These clones would be necessary for the elimination of the organism, which does not happen in the HLA-B27-positive person. In this model of microbial persistence, the resulting sustained immune response to the organism would be incapable of eliminating the organism, but would be of sufficient intensity to give rise to the clinical disease. A variant of this mechanism involves non-antigen-specific stimulation of T-lymphocytes by bacterial superantigens [106, 107].
The enteric or genitourinary infection that starts Reiter's syndrome is followed by a latent period of 1 week/1 month, after which urethritis and conjunctivitis are usually the first manifestations to appear; they are followed within several days by onset of arthritis. The mucocutaneous involvement sometimes precedes the phase of urethritis and conjunctivitis, and sometimes develops after the onset of arthritis.

Oral Manifestations. The oral lesions spread on the palate, uvula, tongue, buccal mucosa, and lips. They start as small vesicles and evolve into erosions with marginal erythema, tending to be more transient and painless than aphthous ulcers. Larger granular circinate erosions are seen rarely, covered with a whitish epithelium-simulating leukoplakia. They are present in 10 %–15 % of patients with Reiter's disease [108].

Associated Findings
Urethritis and Prostatitis. These may present only as sterile pyuria in the first voided specimen, or range up to moderately severe dysuria with frank mucopurulent discharge. Chronic prostatitis is frequent, and cystitis and pyelonephritis also occur.

Conjunctivitis and Uveitis. Conjunctivitis is present in about half of the cases and is usually bilateral, transient and, being subtarsal, may often be missed. A smaller proportion of patients also exhibit uveitis, initially manifest as acute anterior iritis, which may progress to chronic iridocyclitis and visual impairment [109].

Arthritis. Joint involvement is characteristically non-suppurative and polyarticular and affects predominantly the joints of the lower limbs and sacro-iliac joints. It is present in about 95 % of patients, but radiological changes are detectable in about 40 % of cases. In addition, enthesopathy, mainly of the plantar fascia and Achilles tendon, may be involved.

Skin Lesions. Circinate balanitis is the most common cutaneous finding (36 % of patients). The lesion is initially vesicular with little or no surrounding erythema and may coalesce, giving a circinate distribution.
Keratoderma blenorrhagicum starts as small vesicles or red macules which rapidly become papular, nod-

ular, or even show a horny excresence. A scaly collarette is sometimes present. The localization is most commonly found on the soles, toes, and palms [110]. These psoriasiform skin changes are found in about 10 % of cases, occur some weeks after the urethritis, and are symmetrical.

Microscopic Findings. The histological appearance of Reiter's syndrome is indistinguishable from that of pustular psoriasis, with hyperkeratosis and parakeratosis, elongation and hypertrophy of the rete pegs, epidermal hyperplasia, and neutrophilic infiltration with formation of microabscesses and spongiform pustules. The mouth ulcers have a similar histology but are not keratinized.

Diagnosis. Because specific laboratory tests do not exist to make the diagnosis, the clinical features (the classical triade) are decisive. Great difficulties can arise, however, in oligosymptomatic cases and in women. An important investigation is the examination of the overnight urethral secretion by smear and culture. Accelerated ESR, leukocytosis, and elevation of α_2-globulins occur. The detection of HLA-B27 positivity helps to support the diagnosis and is a useful epidemiological detail.

Differential Diagnosis. The urethritis must be carefully distinguished from gonorrhea by repeated culture tests and also from other types of urethritis [111]. The arthritis is to be distinguished from rheumatoid and psoriatic arthritis.

Treatment. In the absence of a specific known pathogen, well-tolerated doxycycline (100 mg after meals for 14–21 days) or tetracycline (2 g/day for at least 14 days) preparations are approriate in severe recent-onset Reiter's syndrome in HLA-B27-positive patients. Minocycline and erythromycin are other possible alternatives. UVB irradiation and coal tar combined with judicious use of topical steroids form the center of treatment of the psoriasiform lesions. Azathioprine (1.5–2.5 mg/kg body weight daily) and methotrexate (0.2–0.5 mg/kg body weight once weekly) are used for severe involvement [112, 113]. Gold salts, D-penicillamine, and antimalarials do not appear effective. As with any genital infection, the sexual partner should be examined and treated. Conjunctivitis can be managed by nonspecific local therapy or by topical steroids when it is more severe. Anterior uveitis needs to be treated with systemic steroid therapy under specialist ophthalmic advice.

Exercise and physical therapy as frequently as possible [114], together with nonsteroidal anti-inflammatory (NSAID) drug therapy, are the first line of treatment for arthritis and enthesopathy. Indomethacin, naproxen, and phenylbutazone are generally considered the most efficacious of the NSAID class and are started at the lowest dose and then increased. Indomethacin (25 mg two/three times a day) is increased to a total of 225 mg daily for at least 3 weeks. Naproxen (200–350 mg) two or three times a day is increased to the maximum dose of 1500 mg over a 1- to 2-week period. Phenylbutazone is effective in doses of 100–200 mg two to three times a day.

11.3.4 Wegener's Granulomatosis (WG)

Definition. Wegener's granulomatosis (WG) is an idiopathic disease characterized by necrotizing granulomatous inflammation and systemic vasculitis, affecting predominantly small arteries and veins. In its generalized form, there is involvement of the upper and lower respiratory tract, kidney, and often other organs including skin. The disease is probably a continuum.

Etiology. It is not known what triggers this inflammatory process, possibly an infection or some other inciting antigen.

Pathogenesis. The vasculitis of WG has been described as "pauci-immune", meaning that immune deposits are not found in the involved lesions, while neutrophils appear to play a dominant pathogenic role [115]. In fact, antineutrophilic cytoplasmic antibodies (ANCA) directed toward a serine protease (proteinase 3) (C-ANCA) were described as associated with generalized WG [116]. The pathogenic sequence of events may occur in this way: the pathogen may induce the production of cytokines such as TNF-α, IL1, and IL8, which may be able to produce important cytoplasmic changes of polymorphonuclear leukocytes. There might be a migration of the proteinase 3 (PR3) antigen from the cytoplasm to the cell surface and, in this location, PR3 might become antigenic and ANCA might be formed. Cytokines can also stimulate the endothelial cell to express adhesion molecules [115] (LFA1, ICAM1) and these molecules cause adhesion of the PMN to the endothelial cells. The ANCA-activated PMN leukocytes degranulate and release enzymes and toxic oxygen into the microenvironment, causing injury. Autoantibodies to endothelial cells can also be detected by IF in 20 %–60 % of patients with WG [117]. Cellular mechanisms have also been postulated in granuloma formation with sensitized T-lymphocytes releasing lymphokines, leading to recruitment of macrophages and giant cell formation [118].

Oral Manifestations. These are common and not infrequently the first manifestations of WG [119]. A painless, progressive swelling of the gingiva, associated with inflamed papillae, may be the sign of initial WG. The gingival enlargement may have a characteristic "strawberry-like" appearance [120]. WG may also present with oral ulceration or swelling of the lips or salivary gland.

Associated Findings. WG consists of a classic triad: (1) upper respiratory tract inflammation including sinusitis, otitis, rhinitis, ocular inflammation, and epistaxis; (2) lower respiratory tract inflammation including pulmonary infiltrates, cough, and hemoptisis; and (3) rapidly progressive glomerulonephritis [121]. Cutaneous manifestations are reported in 40 %–50 % of cases, commonly as papular or plaque-like and ulcerative lesions, rarely as urticarial, vesicle, or purpura lesions, or subcutaneous nodules.

Microscopic Findings. The pathology of WG is distinctive and shows the features of a granulomatous vasculitis affecting small and medium-sized vessels and granuloma.

Diagnosis. Elevated ESR and C-reactive protein, anemia, and thrombocytosis are found, but the specific laboratory feature of WG is the detection of IgG autoantibodies directed against cytoplasmic components of PMN and monocytes (ANCA). When alcohol-fixed neutrophils are used as substrates, two patterns of ANCA exist: one is a perinuclear staining (P-ANCA) which is associated with antibodies against antigen, contained in the primary granules of PMN (myeloperoxidase); the second is a true cytoplasmic staining (C-ANCA). C-ANCA positivity has been reported to have a sensitivity of 96 % in patients with generalized active WG; sensitivity falls to 41 % in remission patients with generalized WG: In short, ANCA antibody positivity correlates with disease activity in WG.

Differential Diagnosis. Other systemic vasculitis must be considered, such as polyarteritis nodosa and Churg-Strauss syndrome.

Treatment. In the absence of therapy, average survival in WG was 5 months. Oral steroids (prednisone 1 mg/kg/day) associated with cytotoxic agents (cyclophosphamide 2 mg/kg/day i.v.) have more recently become the main treatment for these patients [122]. Steroids are converted to an alternate-day regime and reduced over 3–6 months; cyclophosphamide is maintained for 1 year and then reduced. Some groups have used azathioprine instead of cyclophosphamide with good results.

11.3.5 Lethal Midline Granuloma

Lethal midline granuloma is the term sometimes used to describe a spectrum of conditions including Wegener's granulomatosis, polymorphic reticulosis or lymphomatoid granulomatosis, and idiopathic midline destructive disease (IMDD).

11.3.5.1 *Lymphomatoid Granulomatosis (LG)*

Synonyms. Polymporphic reticulosis. Lymphomatoid granulomatosis (LG) is a systemic disease with characteristics of both inflammatory and neoplastic processes, primarily involving the lung with nodular pulmonary infiltrates.

Etiopathogenesis. This represents an angiocentric immunoproliferative disorder with a wide clinical spectrum ranging from regression to evolution into a T-cell lymphoma.

Oral Manifestations. The most common oral sign of LG is palatal ulceration, but other oral localizations may be present. In HIV disease, painful, aphthous, ulcer-like lesions are described not only in oral mucosa but also in esophageal mucosa [123, 124].

Associated Findings. Extrapulmonary involvement includes the skin, with papules, annular lesions, nodules and plaques, and the central nervous system and the kidney.

Microscopic Findings. The disease is best seen in ulcer margins and deeper submucosal tissues, with perivascular, granulomatous infiltrates of mononuclear cells, some of which are atypical.

Diagnosis. Diagnosis is clinical and immunohistological.

Differential Diagnosis. This includes Wegener's granulomatosis.

Treatment. Untreated LG is a fatal disease; moreover, 20 % of patients develop malignant T-cell lymphomas that are difficult to classify. Prednisone and cyclophosphamide are used in the same way as in WG.

11.3.5.2 *Idiopathic Midline Destructive Disease (IMDD)*

In idiopathic midline destructive disease, palatal necrosis and ulceration may be seen. Occasionally, the disease presents with delayed healing of an extraction socket [125].

11.3.6 Oral Crohn's Disease

Synonyms. Orofacial granulomatosis. Crohn's disease (CD) is an inflammatory granulomatous bowel disease of unknown origin which can involve any part of the gastrointestinal tract, including the oral mucosa.
The term orofacial granulomatosis is preferred in some centers since it is unclear where in the spectrum of Crohn's disease/sarcoidois/allergy these lesions (and related conditions such as Melkersson-Rosenthal syndrome and granulomatous cheilitis) lie [126].

Oral Manifestations. The frequency of nonspecific lesions such as aphthous stomatitis and oral ulcerations is reported to be 4%–9% in patients with CD [127], so investigation of the bowel should be considered in patients with intractable mouth ulcers. Ulcers classically involve the buccal sulcus, where they appear as linear ulcers. Another aspect of oral lesions is granulomata, nodular lesions, which occur both in CD and in ulcerative colitis patients. Granulomata may have a different modality of evolution: (1) they may coalescence to give a "cobblestone" appearance to the mucosa (pyostomatitis vegetans), and (2) they may cause a diffuse granulomatous thickening of the lips (granulomatosis cheilitis with macrocheilia). Not all granulomatous cheilitis is due to Crohn's disease, though this type of lip involvement may predate bowel disease by several years. Granulomata also occur around the anus and vulva, at colostomy and ileostomy sites, and in association with scars, sinuses, and fistulas [128].

Associated Findings. Abdominal pain, gastrointestinal bleeding or diarrhea, pyoderma gangrenosum, erythema nodosum, malnutrition.

Microscopic Findings. Noncaseating granulomas are found in about 10% of patients with oral CD, but, more frequently, there are less specific findings such as focal collections of lymphocytes, lymphoid follicles, and perivascular mononuclear cell infiltration.

Diagnosis. The oral histology is not specific, and investigation of the gastrointestinal tract is mandatory [129]. Investigations such as chest radiography, serum angiotensin converting enzyme, gallium scan, and the Kweim test may be required to exclude sarcoidosis.

Treatment. Topical or intralesional corticosteroids may effectively control the oral lesions but, more frequently, systemic corticosteroids, azathioprine, or salazopyrine are required.

11.4 Kawasaki's Syndrome

F. Falcini and S. Vierucci

Kawasaki syndrome (KS) is an acute mucocutaneous, self-limiting febrile illness of infancy and early childhood, characterized by a systemic vasculitis of small- and medium-sized vessels, predominantly involving the coronary arteries [129].

The clinical symptoms of the disease are: (1) unremittent high fever lasting more than 5 days; (2) bilateral, non-exudative conjunctivitis; (3) changes in the oropharynx, including strawberry tongue, red fissured lips, and oropharyngeal erythema; (4) changes in the extremities including indurative edema of the hands and feet, erythema of palms and soles, and digital peeling; (5) cervical non-suppurative lymphoadenopathy; and (6) polymorphous skin rash [130, 131].

KS occurs worldwide and affects children of all races, with Orientals and Afro-Caribbeans at highest risk; a male preponderance, some seasonality, and occasional epidemics have been reported.

In Japan, the incidence of KS is 150, in the United States approximately 10.3, and in Europe 3.0 per 100 000 children under 5 years of age.

The clinical features of KS are self-limiting, but cardiovascular alterations may be detected by EKG and 2D echocardiography in 30%–35% of patients. Coronary aneurysms, the most severe life-threatening cardiac complication in KS, develop in up to 20%–25% of untreated children, leading to thrombosis or stenosis responsible for myocardial infarction or sudden death in about 1% of cases [132].

The etiology of KS is still unknown, even though many viral, bacterial, and toxic agents have been reported over the years as causative agents. The age distribution, with a peak during the first 2 years of life, the seasonal distribution with a high incidence in late winter and spring, the occurrences of epidemics and the incidence of previous upper respiratory tract infections support the hypothesis that an infectious agent triggers the disease.

The strong similarity with toxic shock syndrome suggests a possible role in KS of new clones of toxic shock syndrome toxin-1-producing staphylococci or pyrogenic exotoxin-producing streptococci, both acting as superantigens [133].

Recently, human parvovirus B19 has been isolated in a small group of KS children, indicating the virus to be a potential etiologic agent [134].

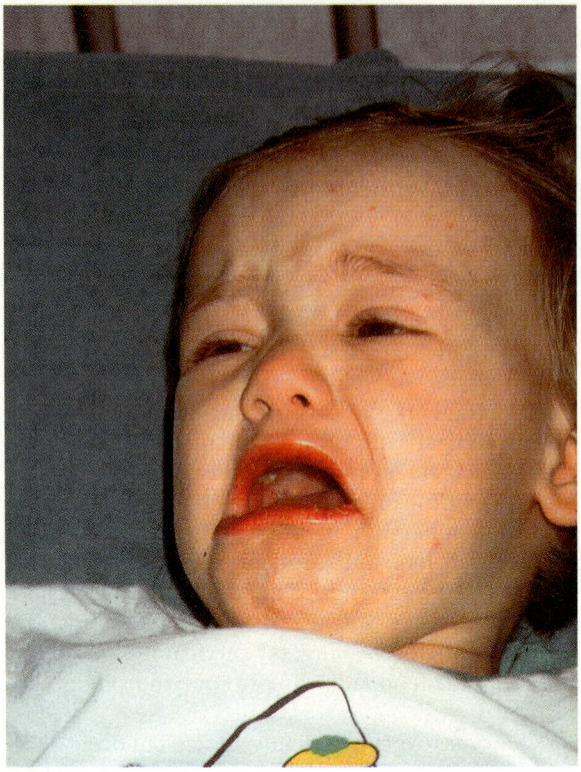

Fig. 11.28. Marked erythema involving the lips in the acute phase of the disease

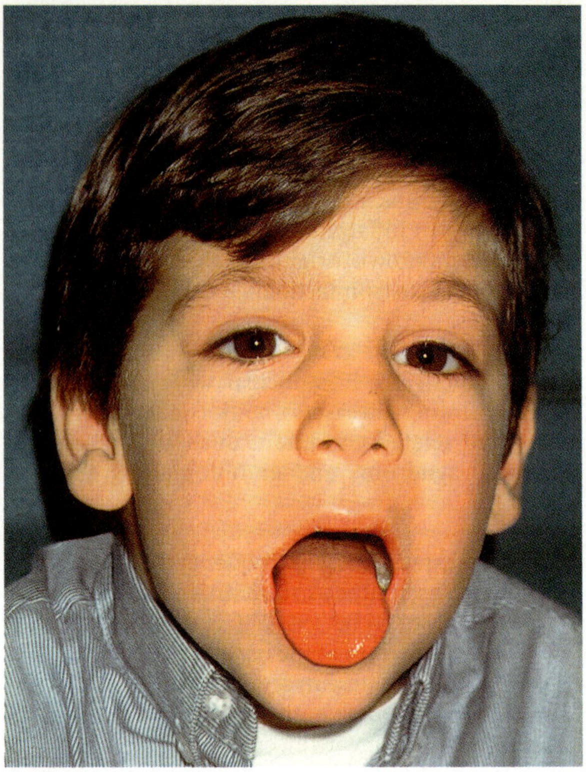

Fig. 11.29. Swollen, fissured, and bright red lips in a child with KS

The pathogenesis of KS is immunologically mediated and the main steps are represented by immune activation and endothelial damage, mainly affecting coronary arteries. KS is associated with activation of T-cells, monocytes and macrophages, and multiple humoral and cellular abnormalities in the acute phase of the disease [135]. The presence of circulating immunocomplexes and lymphocytosis, with a predominance of B-cells secreting IgM and IgG, and an abnormal balance of regulatory T-cells subsets, with increased activation of CD4+ T-cells and reduced or normal CD8+ T-cells have been reported. The activation of CD4+ T-cells leads to an increased production of cytokines; raised levels of IL-1a, IL-6, IL-8, IFN-γ, soluble IL-2 receptors and reduced circulating levels of IL-2 have been detected in KS patients, supporting the role of cytokines in vascular damage [136].

In the acute phase of KS, B-cell activation leads to production of immunoglobulins, as well as of cytotoxic autoantibodies. Antinuclear antibodies, antiendothelial antibodies, antineutrophils, cytoplasmic antibodies, and anticardiolipin antibodies have also been implicated in the pathogenesis of vascular injury [137].

Indices and inflammation (erythrocyte sedimentation rate, white blood cells, and C-reactive protein) are significantly increased early in the course of the disease, while platelet count is markedly raised during the 2nd and 1st week after disease onset. In most children, mild to moderate normocytic, normochromic, or hypochromic anemia, and increased levels of liver enzymes are also observed.

The mouth changes (Table 11.1), characterized by a marked and diffuse erythema involving all the oropharynx (Fig. 11.28), are observed in all KS children

Table 11.1. Differential diagnosis of mouth alterations in KS and other similar diseases

	KS	Streptococcus scarlet fever	Toxic shock syndrome	Staphylococcal scarlet fever
Lips	Red, fissured, cracking, bleeding	Normal	Red	Normal
Oropharynx	Erythematous	Erythematous	Erythematous	Erythematous
Tongue	"Strawberry"	"Strawberry"	Red	Red

in the acute phase of the disease. In the majority of children, this clinical finding follows the fever by 4–5 days and lasts 1–2 weeks in untreated patients. A "strawberry tongue" with prominent papillae is usually associated with oropharynx redness (Fig. 11.29).

The most typical mucous membrane alteration is represented by swollen, fissured, and bright red lips, which easily crack and bleed.

The diagnosis of KS is established according to the Japan Jawasaki Disease Research Committee guidelines, including six clinical criteria; at least five of the six items listed in Table 11.2 should be present for diagnosis, or four items if coronary aneurysms are also detected by 2D echocardiography or coronary angiography [138].

There are now increasing reports of patients with atypical or incomplete KS, at high risk for the development of coronary artery lesions, who do not fulfill the diagnostic guidelines [139].

KS may mimic many conditions; in particular, the differential diagnosis includes scarlet fever, measles, staphylococcal "scalded skin" syndrome, toxic shock syndrome, and juvenile rheumatoid arthritis. However, clinical and laboratory data should help the clinician to distinguish KS from other similar diseases.

The recommended schedule of treatment for KS [140–142] includes:

1. Aspirin, 50–100 mg/kg, antiinflammatory dose, during the acute phase of the disease and 3–5 mg/kg, as an antithrombotic for the convalescence. The drug is usually discontinued by 8–12 weeks from disease onset in the absence of cardiac complications. If coronary aneurysms are detected, aspirin or dypiridamole should be administered up to the normalization of vessel alterations.

2. Intravenous gammaglobulin (IVIG) (2 g/kg) during the first 10 days after disease onset.

Table 11.2. Kawasaki syndrome: diagnostic criteria (From the Center for Disease Control. MMWR 1985; 34:33)

1. Fever	Duration of 5 days or more not responding to antibiotics
2. Conjunctivitis	Bilateral, bulbar, non-purulent, conjunctival congestion
3. Lymph node enlargement	Cervical, acute, non-purulent, > 1.5 cm
4. Rash	Polymorphous, no vesicles or crusts
5. Changes of lips or oral mucosa	Dry, red, vertical fissured lips, "strawberry" tongue, diffuse erythema of oropharynx
6. Changes of extremities	Erythema of palms or soles, indurative edema of hands or feet, digital peeling

The current treatment for KS is shown in Table 11.3.

Table 11.3. Treatment for Kawasaki syndrome

Aspirin	*Acute phase* 50–100 mg/kg/day (antiinflammatory dose) *Convalescence* 3–5 mg/kg/day (antiaggregant dose)
Intravenous γ-globulin	2 g/kg/day i.v. during the first 10–12 days after disease onset
Dipyridamole	2–3 mg/kg/day in children with aspirin intolerance or large or multiple coronary aneurysms

11.5 Vitiligo

G. L. Campanile, G. Hautmann, and T. M. Lotti

Definition. Vitiligo is an acquired heritable melanocytopenic disorder characterized by progressive, well-circumscribed, cutaneous white macules, ocular abnormalities, autoantibodies, and a high incidence of associated disorders.

Etiology. Various theories are suggested. The *immune hypothesis* suggests an aberration of immune surveillance which results in melanocyte destruction and/or dysfunction. The defect may arise as primary autoimmunization with formation of autoantibodies against an antigen of the melanogenic system, or the primary event may be an injury to melanocytes with release of an antigenic substance and subsequent autoimmunization [143, 144]. The *neural hypothesis* theorizes that there is a neurochemical mediator that destroys melanocytes or inhibits melanin production [145]. The *self-destruct hypothesis* proposes that an intermediate or metabolite in melanin synthesis causes melanocyte destruction, or that the normal mechanism for melanosome destruction proceeds unchecked to cause melanocytic dysfunction or death [146]. None of the theories alone is entirely satisfactory. The actual mechanism of inhibition or destruction of melanocytes may, in fact, be much more complex than any of these mechanisms suggests.

Oral Manifestations. Vitiligo may not uncommonly involve the oral mucosa. Areas characteristically involved include lips and gingiva (Fig. 11.30 a, b). Depigmentation of distant digits and the lips produces the *lip-tip syndrome*. Areolar and penile involvement is part of this subtype.

Associated Findings. Hypomelanotic macules are found particularly in areas of skin that are normally

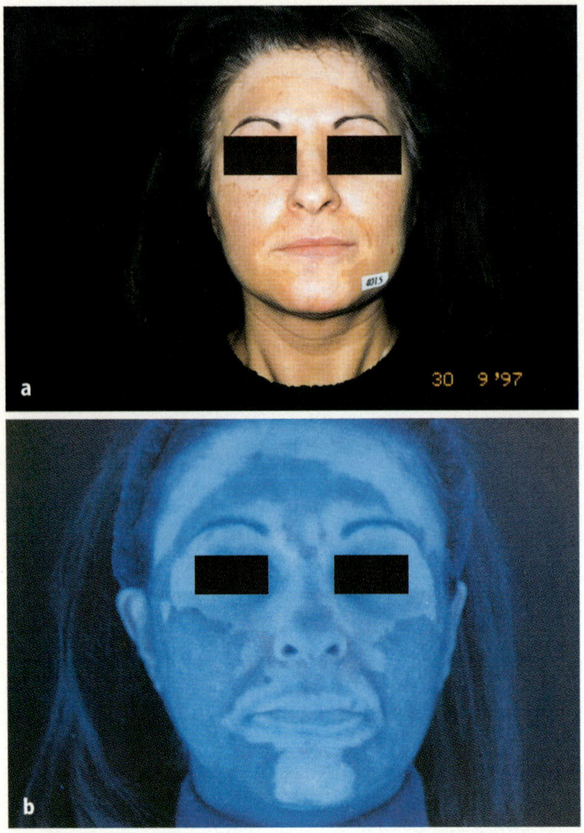

Fig. 11.30 a, b. Vitiligo, facial and perioral involvement. **a** Appearance under normal light conditions. **b** Appearance under Wood's light. Note the sharper demarcation of the perioral achromic areas

hyperpigmented, e. g., the face, axillae, groins, areolae, and genitalia. The distribution of the lesions is usually symmetrical, though sometimes it is unilateral and may have a dermatomal arrangement. Premature grayness of the hair is common in vitiligo. Vitiligo has been associated with uveitis, thyroid disease, diabetes mellitus, Addison's disease, pernicious anemia, alopecia areata, malignant melanoma, and psoriasis [147–149].

Microscopic Findings. Hematoxylin and eosin stains are normal except for an absence of melanocytes and melanin in the epidermis. Histochemical studies show a lack of dopa-positive melanocytes in the basal layer of the epidermis. Electron microscopy studies confirm the loss of melanocytes, which appear to be replaced by Langerhan's cells [150].

Differential Diagnosis. Generalized vitiligo must be distinguished from piebaldism (congenital, stable, with hyperpigmented macules in white patches), Waardenburg's syndrome and Woolf's syndrome (including hearing defects), and Ziprkowski-Margolis syndrome (familial history).

Segmental vitiligo must be distinguished from nevus depigmentosus, tuberous sclerosis, and hypomelanosis of Ito.

Treatment. The treatment is unsatisfactory. Systemic psoralens combined with exposure to sunlight or to light sources is effective in a proportion of cases. In some patients, the more potent topical corticosteroid preparations are effective in producing repigmentation of areas of vitiligo. In those patients with extensive vitiligo, skin bleaching creams are of use [151].

11.6 Oral Lichen Planus

G. L. Campanile, G. Hautmann, B. Lorusso, and T. M. Lotti

Definition. Lichen planus (LP) is a self-limiting mucocutaneous eruption of unknown etiology which, according to current knowledge, may represent a cell-mediated immunological response to induced antigens in the skin and mucosa. Thus, LP may be considered a localized autoimmune disease due to keratinocyte antigen changes.

It is characterized by isolated pruritic violaceous polygonal flat papules, often coalescing in large plaques on the flexural areas with typical localization on the flexural side of the wrists. Mucous membranes are often involved. Oral mucosa has been reported to be involved in about 50 % of cases and in 25 % of patients without skin manifestations.

The skin manifestation resolves generally within a few years, leaving pigmentary sequelae; in contrast, oral lesions often last for many years, presenting therapeutic and prognostic difficulties.

Prevalence of LP in the general population is about 0.9 %–1.2 %; the prevalence of oral lichen planus (OLP) is between 0.1 % and 2.2 % [155]. Although described in children and adolescents, LP is a disease usually occurring at ages ranging from 30 to 70 years, with higher incidence in females. No racial prevalence has been described [152].

Etiology. In this relatively common disorder of unknown etiology, cell-mediated immunity seems to play a major role. Serologic typing studies have demonstrated an association between the HLA-DR1 tissue type and both drug-related and idiopathic lichenoid lesions [153], consistent with the view that a genetic predisposition or susceptibility to the development of LP does exist. It has been proposed that modified keratinocyte surface antigens are the target for cytotoxic cell response, which is further supported by the finding that LP-like eruptions can be observed in graft-versus-host disease where donor-derived lymphocytes destroy the host's tissues. Analysis of the lesional cell infiltrate shows a predominant T-lymphocyte cell type (CD3+) and helper-inducer (CD4+) outnumber suppressor-cytotoxic (CD8+), though activated CD8+ cells have been observed located close to damaged basal cells, suggesting an active role for these cells in the immune response. Some hypothesized antigens of viral, pharmacological, and cellular origin could interact with keratinocytes or Langerhan's cells (numerically increased in the lesional skin). Interleukin-1 produced by Langerhan's cells could activate T-lymphocytes [154]. Activated T-lymphocytes increase their production/release of interferon-gamma, which in turn causes keratinocytes to express HLA-DR antigen and the adhesion molecule ICAM-1, which may represent a binding site for those lymphocytes expressing the LFA-1 ligand [154]. HLA-DR+ keratinocytes are able to release additional interleukin-1 [155], with the consequent amplification of the immunologic process. Lymphokines may cause direct cellular damage themselves or mocal downregulation of CD8+ cells. Mast cells have been recognized in oral lichen planus lesions, increased in number and showing morphological changes consistent with degranulation of cytoplasmic granules, suggesting a possible role in the tissue damage of OLP.

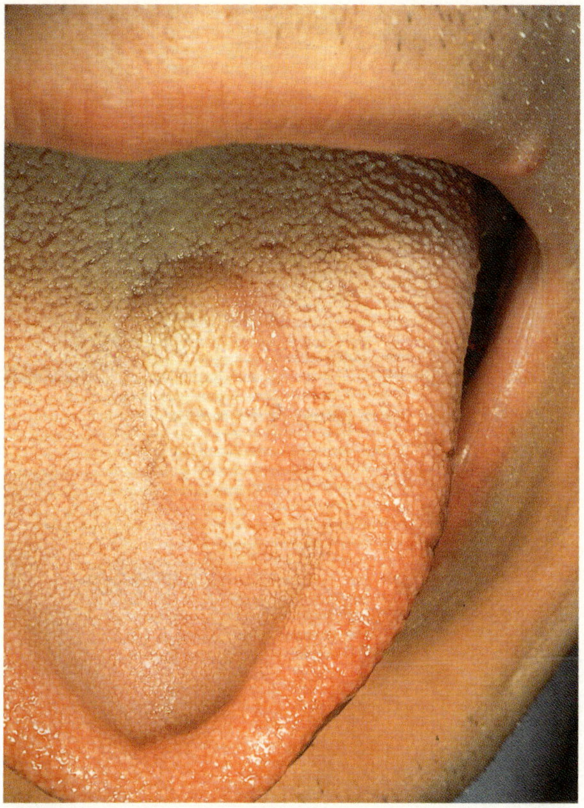

Fig. 11.32. Lichen planus of the tongue

Oral Manifestations. OLP may be found in any area, but favored sites are buccal mucosa, tongue, and gingiva. Palatal and sublingual lesions are uncommon and gingival involvement may lead to a picture of desquamative gingivitis.

The lesions, almost bilateral, present different clinical features: reticular (Figs. 11.31, 11.32), papular, plaque-like (Figs. 11.33, 11.34), bullous, atrophic (Figs. 11.35–11.37), erosive and ulcerative, and pigmented [152]. The *reticular form* is the most common and is characterized by a whitish arborized pattern. Linear and annular distribution of the papules may be seen. The *erosive or ulcerative form* represents the second most frequent variant and is characterized by small or extensive erosions with isolated papules or lines at the periphery. These lesions may provoke a painful or "burning" sensation. A metallic taste in the mouth has been described. The *atrophic form* is less common and usually the result of the erosive form, and is characterized by epithelial atrophy. The lesions have a smooth, red

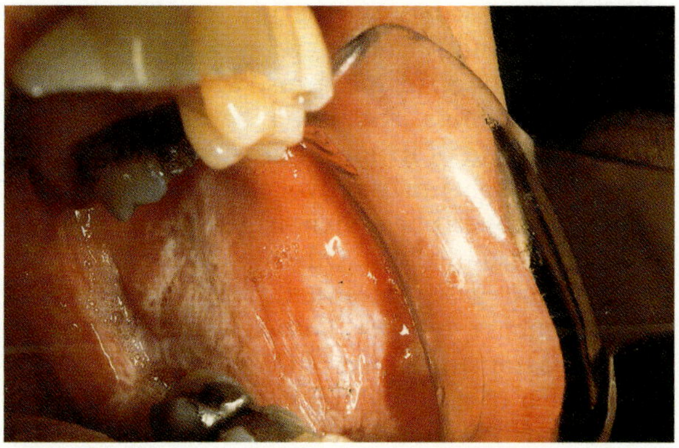

Fig. 11.31. Reticular lichen planus of the buccal mucosa

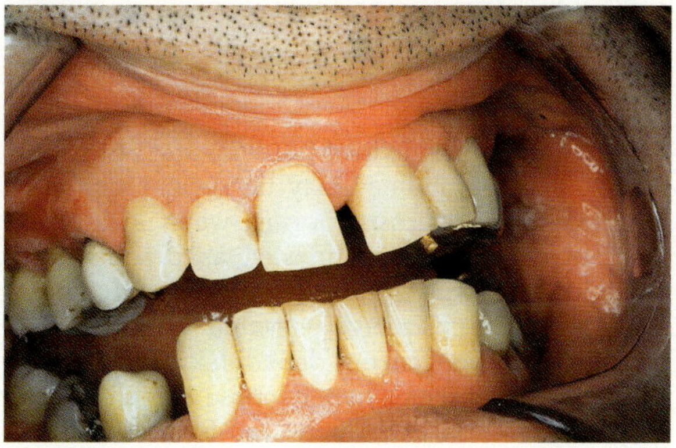

Fig. 11.33. Atrophic and reticular lichen planus of the gingiva

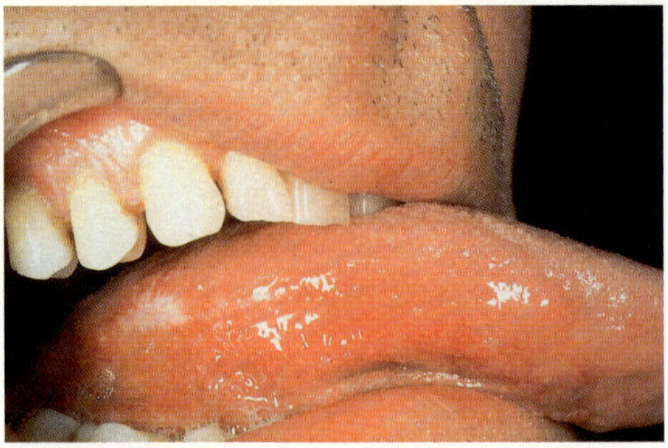

Fig. 11.34. Plaqued lichen planus of the tongue

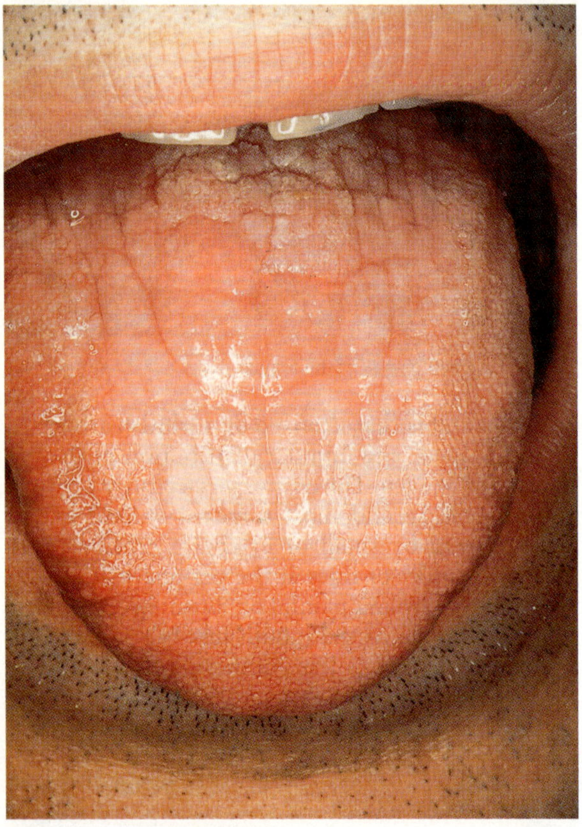

Fig. 11.35. Atrophic lichen planus of the tongue

surface and poorly defined borders, and at the periphery, papules or lines may be seen. Frequently, the atrophic and erosive forms, when located on the gingiva, may be manifested as desquamative gingivitis. The *hypertrophic form* is rare and appears as a well-circumscribed, elevated white plaque resembling homogeneous leukoplakia and is the result of coalescing hypertrophic papules. The rare bullous form is characterized by the presence, on a background of papules or striae, of bullae

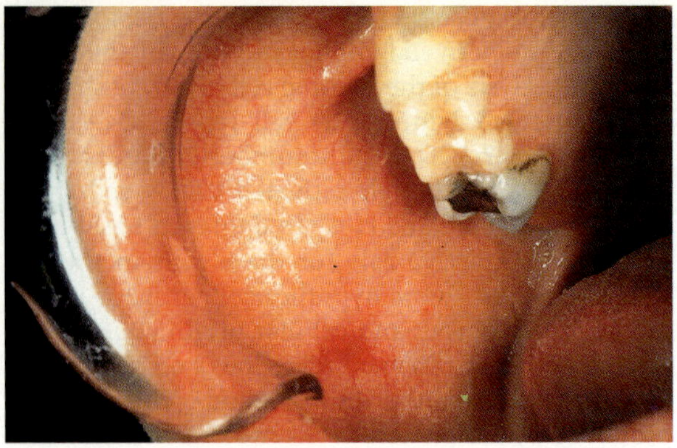

Fig. 11.36. Atrophic lichen planus of the buccal mucosa

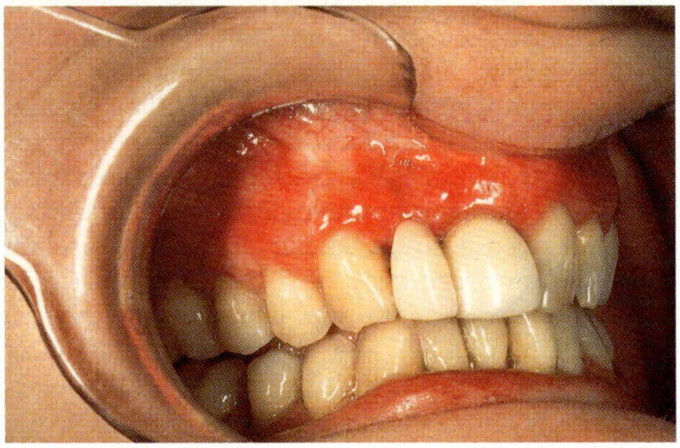

Fig. 11.37. Atrophic lichen planus of the gingiva

of variable size which rapidly leave painful ulcerations. In the *pigmented form*, pigmented papules arranged in a reticular pattern intersperse with whitish lesions. This very rare form is due to local melanin overproduction during the acute phase of disease.

Associated Findings. The skin eruption is characterized by tiny, flat, polygonal pruritic, violaceous, or purple papules. A thin kind of transparent scale or a network of fine white lines or puncta, known as Wickham's striae, can be present. The lesions, symmetrical and bilateral, are usually localized on the flexor surface of the arms, wrists, side of the neck, thighs, shins, and lower back. Trauma and almost any kind of irritant (burns, lacerations, friction, or UV-light) may provoke the isomorphic response (Koebner phenomenon). Genital mucosa is frequently also involved. Other mucous membranes involved are gastrointestinal tract, anal mucosa, vaginal mucosa, bladder, larynx, and conjunctivae. Malignant transformation of OLP has been reported in a number of studies [156]. Follow-up studies [157] demonstrated that less than 1% of OLP cases show malignant transformation. OLP has been found to

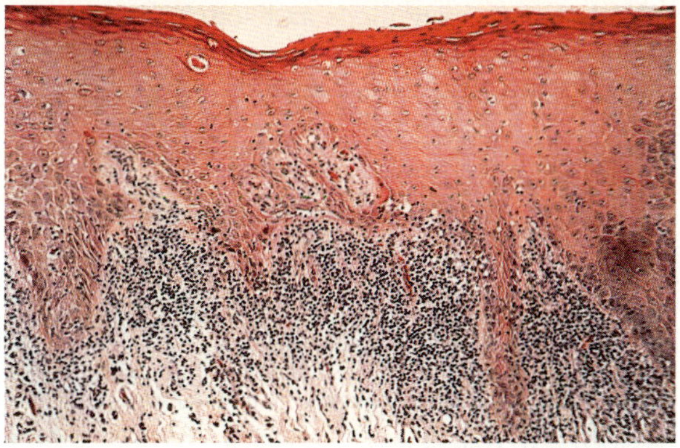

Fig. 11.38. Histologic findings in a case of lichen planus

Table 11.4. Histological features of oral lichen planus

1. Hyperorthokeratosis
2. Parakeratosis
3. Thickening of the granular cell layer
4. Irregular acanthosis ("saw-tooth" appearance)
5. Well-defined band-like inflammatory lymphohistiocytic infiltrate in the upper dermis
6. Liquefaction degeneration of the basal cell layer
7. Colloid bodies (cytoid, hyaline, or Civatte bodies) in the basal epidermis and superficial dermis
8. Detachments between epidermis and dermis may be present (Max Joseph spaces), leading to subepidermal vesicle formation
9. Melanin pigmentary incontinence and melanophages

be associated with diabetes, hypertension, and liver diseases. Associations between LP and chronic active hepatitis have also been reported. Drugs and chemicals such as non-steroidal anti-inflammatory drugs, antihypertensive agents, gold salts, angiotensin converting enzyme inhibitors [152, 158], and amalgam/metals, composite resin, and cyanoacrylate may also induce the so-called oral lichenoid lesions (OLL). Factors that may also precipitate or aggravate OLP are surgery, psychological stress, and viral infections [152].

Microscopic Findings. The histological features of OLP are diagnostic and similar to those of cutaneous LP and OLL. Immunofluorescence microscopy and electron microscopy may be very helpful tools for reaching the diagnosis of OLP, predominantly when the differentiation of OLP from discoid lupus erythematosus and carcinomatous lesions exhibiting dysplastic changes, is difficult.
Typical histopathological findings consist of hyperorthokeratosis or hyperparakeratosis (Fig. 11.38), (Table 11.4). Irregular acanthosis with a rare "saw-tooth" appearance of the rete ridges and a thickening of the granular cell layers are normally found. Moreover, one of the earliest findings in the epithelium is an increased number of Langerhan's cells. The upper connective tissue displays a well-defined band-like inflammatory lymphohistiocytic infiltrate. Moreover, in the very early findings, there is an increased number of Langerhan's cells in the epithelium. In the basal cell layer, liquefaction degeneration is characteristically present. Colloid bodies (also known as cytoid, hyaline, or Civatte bodies) may be seen either in the basal cell layer or in the superficial connective tissue. Detachments between epithelium and connective tissue may be present (Max-Joseph spaces), leading to subepithelial vesicle formation. Furthermore, melanin pigmentary incontinence and melanophages are found.

Ultrastructural Aspects. The changes noted in OLP are mainly in the basement membrane zone (BMZ) and in the basal cell layer, and consist of three major types of figures reflecting the clinical types of OLP [159]:

1. Discrete breaks in BMZ are shown only in reticular OLP;
2. Branched BMZ characterizing both reticular and erosive OLP;
3. Patch-like thickenings are present only in erosive OLP.

The desmosomes and emidesmosomes are decreased in number, while the tonofilaments are increased in the epithelial cells, but do not usually show the original orientation at the desmosomal region.
The colloid bodies, as shown by transmission electron microscopy or direct immunofluorescence, can be considered degenerated keratinocytes.
Ultrastructural study of the inflammatory cells infiltrate shows predominantly typical lymphocytes of the CD8+ subtype, frequently in contact with macrophages in the epithelial layer or in the superficial dermis, whereas CD4+ lymphocytes are found in a cluster in the deeper connective tissue.
Other inflammatory cells are included in the intraepithelial layer such as macrophages, mast cells, and interdigitating reticulum cells. The interdigitating reticulum cells form a rather extended cellular network in the dermal infiltrate, in close apposition to lymphocytes.

Differential Diagnosis. Several dermatological diseases can resemble OLP. Oral mucosa may present the localized form of cutaneous discoid lupus erythematosus as white plaques with an erythematous halo. White sponge nevus and leukoplakia are common white lesions of the oral cavity to differentiate from OLP and may present some clinical aspects of

Table 11.5. Oral lichen planus treatments

Acute form:	
	– Prednisone (per os) 15–20 mg/day, for 2 weeks
	– Triamcinolone acetonide 0.1 % mixed with oral protective base (local use, twice a day, for 2 weeks)
Subacute or chronic form:	
	– Etretinate (0.7 mg/kg/day) for 6–10 weeks
	– Cyclosporin A (4 mg/kg/day) for 12 weeks
	– Topical isotretinoin (twice a day, for 6–10 weeks)
	– Topical cyclosporin A (three times a day, for 6–12 weeks)
Erosive OLP:	
	– As above or:
	– Dapsone (50–150 mg/day, for 12 weeks)
	– Cyclophosphamide

OLP. Cicatricial and bullous pemphigoid must be distinguished, with direct immunofluorescence examination, from erosive or bullous OLP. Even erythema multiforme and the oral lesion of secondary syphilis and overall lichenoid dysplasia can mimic OLP. Often erythroplasia and carcinomas need a histological diagnosis from OLP.

Diagnosis. Histopathologic examination and direct immunofluorescence help in establishing the diagnosis.

Treatment. Several treatments have been tried in OLP. Most of these are purely symptomatic and without any adequate trials such as mercury, bismuth, or arsenic [160]. The use of systemic steroids gives benefit in some acute forms of OLP, i. e., prednisolone or its equivalent, 15–20 mg daily for about 2 weeks and gradual reduction thereafter. In some cases the lesions of OLP are treated with potent corticosteroids such as triamcinolone acetonide mixed with an oral protective base, or used as aerosol or as ointment.

Injectable steroids, e. g., methylprednisolone or bethamethasone, are advocated in numerous trials [160].

Oral etretinate and isotretinoin have been used successfully in severe OLP, but side effects are frequent. Instead, the use of topical etretinate gives greater benefit and fewer side effects.

PUVA treatment has provided clearing of OLP lesions supported by the histological picture. The use of topical and systemic cyclosporin has been advocated with good results in severe forms of OLP [161]. Other treatments for erosive LP include dapsone and cyclophosphamide (Table 11.5).

In the treatment of OLP, as well as pharmacological treatment, the total elimination of local and predisposing factors such as local mechanical, chemical and physical irritants, including alimentary irritants such as hot or spicy foods and sour fruit, is of supreme importance.

References

1. Black CM. The etiopathogenesis of systemic sclerosis. J Int Med 1993; 234:3–8
2. Foster TD, Fairburn EA. Dental involvement in scleroderma. Br Dent J 1968; 124:353–56
3. Rowell NR, Hopper FE. The periodontal membrane in systemic sclerosis. Br J Dermatol 1977; 96:15–20
4. Andreasen JA. Oral manifestations in discoid and systemic lupus erythematosus. Acta Odontol Scand 1964; 22:295–310
5. Schiødt M, Halberg P, Hentzer B. A clinical study of 32 patients with oral discoid lupus erythematosus. Int J Oral Surg 1978; 7:85–94
6. Urmann JD, Lowenstein MB, Abeles M, Weinstein A. Oral mucosal ulceration in systemic lupus erythematosus. Arthritis Rheum 1978; 21:58–61
7. Schiødt M. Oral manifestations of lupus erythematosus. Int J Oral Surg 1984; 13:101–105
8. Schiødt M, Pindborg JJ. Oral discoid lupus erythematosus. I. The validity of previous histopathologic diagnostic criteria. Oral Surg 1984; 57:46–51
9. Gilliam JN, Sontheimer RD. Distinctive cutaneous subsets in the spectrum of lupus erythematosus. J Am Acad Dermatol 1981; 4:471–475
10. Callen JP. Systemic lupus erythematosus in patients with chronic cutaneous (discoid) lupus erythematosus. Clinical and laboratory findings in seventeen patients. J Am Acad Dermatol 1985; 12:278–288
11. Callen JP, Tuffanelli DL, Provost TT. Collagen-vascular disease. An update. J Am Acad Dermatol 1993; 28:477–484
12. Alarcon Segovia D. Mixed connective tissue disease. Clin Dermatol 1994; 12:309–316
13. Bertram U. Xerostomia. Clinical aspects, pathology and pathogenesis. Acta Odontol Scand 1967; 25 suppl 49
14. Moutsopoulos HM, Kordossis T. Sjoegren syndrome revisited: autoimmune epithelitis. Br J Rheumatol 1996; 35:204–206
15. Schuermann H, Greither A, Hornstein O. Krankheiten der Mundschleimhaut und der Lippen. 3. Aufl. Munich: Urban and Schwarzenberg, 1966; 239–240, 305–307
16. Medseger TA, Oddis CV. Inflammatory muscle disease: clinical features. In: Klippel JH, Dieppe PA (Eds). Rheumatology. London: Mosby, 1994; 12.1–12.14
17. Ruocco V, Sacerdoti G. Pemphigus and bullous pemphigoid due to drugs. Int J Dermatol 1991; 30:307–12
18. Thivolet J. Pemphigus: past, present and future. Dermatology 1994; 189 (Suppl 2):26–9
19. Becker BA, Gaspari AA. Pemphigus vulgaris and vegetans. Dermatol Clin 1993; 11:429–52
20. Korman NJ. Pemphigus. Dermatol Clin 1990; 8:689–700
21. Niizeki H, Inoko H, Mizuki N, et al. HLA-DQA1, DQβ1 and DRβ1 genotyping in Japanese pemphigus vulgaris patients by the PCR-RFLP method. Tissue Antigens 1994; 44:248–51
22. Matzner Y, Erlich HA, Brautbar C, et al. Identical HLA class II alleles predispose to drug-triggered and idiopathic pemphigus vulgaris. Acta Derm Venereol (Stockh) 1995; 75:12–4
23. Moraes JR, Moraes ME, Gernadez Vina M, et al. HLA antigens and the risk of development of pemphigus foliaceus ("fogo selvagem") in endemic areas of Brazil. Immunogenetics 1991; 33:388–91
24. Anhalt GJ, Kim SC, Stanley JR, et al. Paraneoplastic pemphigus. An autoimmune mucocutaneous disease associated with neoplasia. N Engl J Med 1990; 323:1729–35
25. Amagai M. Adhesion molecules. I: Keratinocyte-keratinocyte interactions; cadherins and pemphigus. J Invest Dermatol 1995; 104:146–52
26. Bystryn JC. Therapy of pemphigus. Semin Dermatol 1988; 7:186–94

27. Aberer W, Wolff-Schreiner EC, Stingl G, et al. Azathioprine in the treatment of pemphigus vulgaris. J Am Acad Dermatol 1987; 16:527–33
28. Søndergaard K, Carstens J, Jørgensen J, Zachariae H. The steroid-sparing effect of long-term plasmapheresis in pemphigus. Acta Derm Venereol 1995; 75:150–2
29. Barthelemy H, Frappaz A, Cambazard F, et al. Treatment of nine cases of pemphigus vulgaris with cyclosporine. J Am Acad Dermatol 1988; 18:1262–6
30. Rook AH, Jegasothy BV, Heald P, et al. Extracorporeal photochemotherapy for drug-resistant pemphigus vulgaris. Ann Intern Med 1990; 112:303–5
31. Smith EP, Zone JJ. Dermatitis herpetiformis and linear IgA bullous dermatosis. Dermatol Clin 1993; 11:511–26
32. Hall III RP. Dermatitis herpetiformis. J Invest Dermatol 1992; 99:873–81
33. Hall III RP, Otley C. Immunogenetics of dermatitis herpetiformis. Semin Dermatol 1991; 10:240–5
34. Otley C, Hall III RP. Dermatitis herpetiformis. Dermatol Clin 1990; 8:759–69
35. Katz SI. Dermatitis herpetiformis. Clinical, histologic, therapeutic and laboratory clues. Int J Dermatol 1978; 17:529–35
36. Fraser NG, Kerr NW, Donald D. Oral lesions in dermatitis herpetiformis. Br J Dermatol 1973; 89:439–50
37. Economopoulou P, Laskaris G. Dermatitis herpetiformis: oral lesions as an early manifestation. Oral Surg Oral Med Oral Pathol 1986; 62:77–80
38. Ahmed AR, Hameed A. Bullous pemphigoid and dermatitis herpetiformis. Clin Dermatol 1993; 11:47–52
39. Chorzelski TP, Jablonska S, Maciejowska E. Linear IgA bullous dermatosis of adults. Clin Dermatol 1992; 9:383–92
40. Jablonska S, Chorzelski TP, Rosinska D, Maciejowska E. Linear IgA bullous dermatosis of childhood (chronic bullous dermatosis of childhood). Clin Dermatol 1992; 9:393–401
41. Smith EP, Zone JJ. Dermatitis herpetiformis and linear IgA bullous dermatosis. Dermatol Clin 1993; 11:511–26
42. McEvoy MT, Connolly SM. Linear IgA dermatosis: association with malignancy. J Am Acad Dermatol 1990; 22:59–63
43. Smith JB, Hogan DJ. Factors that exacerbate linear IgA disease (Correspondence). J Am Acad Dermatol (Correspondence) 1995; 33:320–21
44. Prost C, De Leca AC, Combemale P, et al. Diagnosis of adult linear IgA dermatosis by immunoelectronmicroscopy in 16 patients with linear IgA deposits. J Invest Dermatol 1989; 92:39–45
45. Kelly SE, Frith PA, Millard PR, Wojnarowska F, Black MM. A clinicopathological study of mucosal involvement in linear IgA disease. Br J Dermatol 1988; 119:161–70
46. Wojnarowska F, Collier PM, Allen J, Millard PR. The localization of the target antigens and antibodies in linear IgA disease is heterogeneous, and dependent on the methods used. Br J Dermatol 1995; 132:750–7
47. Chan LS, Regezi JA, Cooper KD. Oral manifestations of linear IgA disease. J Am Acad Dermatol 1990; 22:362–5
48. Gammon WR, Fine JD, Forbes M, Briggaman RA. Immunofluorescence on split skin for the detection and differentiation of basement membrane zone autoantibodies. J Am Acad Dermatol 1992; 27:79–87
49. Flowers FP, Sherertz EF. Immunologic disorders of the skin and mucous membranes. Med Clin N Am 1985; 69:657–73
50. Gately III LE, Nesbitt LT. Update on immunofluorescent testing in bullous diseases and lupus erythematosus. Dermatol Clin 1994; 12:133–42.
51. Anhalt GJ. Pemphigoid. Bullous and cicatricial. Dermatol Clin 1990; 8:701–16
52. Korman NJ. Bullous pemphigoid. Dermatol Clin 1993; 11:483–98
53. Ahmed AR, Hameed A. Bullous pemphigoid and dermatitis herpetiformis. Clin Dermatol 1993; 11:47–52
54. Hopkinson SB, Baker SE, Jones JCR. Molecular genetic studies of human epidermal autoantigen (the 180-kd bullous pemphigoid antigen/BP 180): identification of functionally important sequences within the BP 180 molecule and evidence for an interaction between BP 180 and $\alpha 6$ integrin. J Cell Biol 1995; 130:117–25
55. Liu Z, Giudice GJ, Swartz SJ, et al. The role of complement in experimental bullous pemphigoid. J Clin Invest 1995; 95:1539–44
56. Shklar G, Meyer I, Zacarian SA. Oral lesions in bullous pemphigoid. Arch Dermatol 1969; 99:663–70
57. Venning VA, Frith PA, Baron AJ, Millard RP, Wojnarowska F. Mucosal involvement in bullous and cicatricial pemphigoid. A clinical and immunopathological study. Br J Dermatol 1988; 118:7–15
58. Person JR, Rogers RS. Bullous and cicatricial pemphigoid. Clinical, histopathologic and immunopathologic correlations. Mayo Clin Proc 1977; 52:54–66
59. Gammon WR, Fine JD, Forbes M, Briggaman RA. Immunofluorescence on split skin for the detection and differentiation of basement membrane zone autoantibodies. J Am Acad Dermatol 1992; 27:79–87
60. Flowers FP, Sherertz EF. Immunologic disorders of the skin and mucous membranes. Med Clin N Am 1985; 69:657–73
61. Gately LE, Nesbitt LT. Update on immunofluorescent testing in bullous diseases and lupus erythematosus. Dermatol Clin 1994; 12:133–42
62. Chan LS, Yancey KB, Hammerberg C, et al. Immune-mediated subepithelial blistering diseases of mucous membranes. Pure ocular cicatricial pemphigoid is a unique clinical and immunopathological entity distinct from bullous pemphigoid and other subsets identified by antigenic specificity of autoantibodies. Arch Dermatol 1993; 129:448–55
63. Pereyo NG, Davis LS. Generalized bullous pemphigoid controlled by tetracycline therapy alone. J Am Acad Dermatol 1995; 32:138–9
64. Ahmed AR, Kurgis BS, Rogers III RS. Cicatricial pemphigoid. J Am Acad Dermatol 1991; 24:987–1001
65. Mutasim DF, Pelc NJ, Anhalt GJ. Cicatricial pemphigoid. Dermatol Clin 1993; 11:499–510
66. Kurzhals G, Stolz W, Maciejewski W, et al. Localized cicatricial pemphigoid of the Brunsting-Perry type with transition into disseminated cicatricial pemphigoid. Report of a case proved by preembedding immunogold electron microscopy. Arch Dermatol 1995; 131:580–5
67. Yunis JJ, Mobini N, Yunis EJ, et al. Common major histocompatibility complex class II markers in clinical variants of cicatricial pemphigoid. Proc Natl Acad Sci USA 1994; 91:7747–51
68. Bédane C, Prost C, Bernard P, et al. Cicatricial pemphigoid antigen differs from bullous pemphigoid antigen by its exclusive extracellular localization: a study by indirect immunoelectronmicroscopy. J Invest Dermatol 1991; 97:3–9
69. Shimizu H, Masunaga T, Ishiko A, et al. Autoantibodies from patients with cicatricial pemphigoid target different sites in epidermal basement membrane. J Invest Dermatol 1995; 104:370–3
70. Chan LS, Yancey KB, Hammerberg C, et al. Immune-mediated subepithelial blistering diseases of mucous membranes. Pure ocular cicatricial pemphigoid is a unique clinical and immunopathological entity distinct from bullous pemphigoid and other subsets identified by antigenic specificity of autoantibodies. Arch Dermatol 1993; 129:448–55
71. Gammon WR, Fine JD, Forbes M, Briggaman RA. Immunofluorescence on split skin for the detection and differentiation of basement membrane zone autoantibodies. J Am Acad Dermatol 1992; 27:79–87
72. Gately LE, Nesbitt LT. Update on immunofluorescent testing in bullous diseases and lupus erythematosus. Dermatol Clin 1994; 12:133–42.
73. Shklar G, Meyer I, Zacarian SA. Oral lesions in bullous pemphigoid. Arch Dermatol 1969; 99:663–70
74. Venning VA, Frith PA, Bron AJ, et al. Mucosal involvement in bullous and cicatricial pemphigoid. A clinical and immunopathological study. Br J Dermatol 1988; 118:7–15
75. Williams DM. Non-infectious diseases of the oral soft tissue: a new approach. Adv Dent Res 1993; 7:213–9
76. Person JR, Rogers RS. Bullous and cicatricial pemphigoid. Clinical, histopathologic and immunopathologic correlations. Mayo Clin Proc 1977; 52:54–66

77. Flowers FP, Sherertz EF. Immunologic disorders of the skin and mucous membranes. Med Clin N Am 1985; 69:657–73
78. Gammon WR, Briggaman RA. Epidermolysis bullosa acquisita and bullous systemic lupus erythematosus. Diseases of autoimmunity to type VII collagen. Dermatol Clin 1993; 11:535–47
79. Woodley DT, Briggaman RA, Gammon WR. Acquired epidermolysis bullosa. A bullous disease associated with autoimmunity to type VII (anchoring fibril) collagen. Dermatol Clin 1990; 8:717–26
80. Woodley DT, Sarret Y, Briggaman RA. Autoimmunity to type VII collagen. Semin Dermatol 1991; 10:232–9
81. Gammon WR. Epidermolysis bullosa acquisita: a disease of autoimmunity to type VII collagen. J Autoimmunity 1991; 4:59–71
82. Van Joost T, Van't Veen AJ. Drug induced cicatricial pemphigoid and acquired epidermolysis bullosa. Clin Dermatol 1993; 11:521–7
83. Rubenstein R, Esterly NB, Fine JD. Childhood epidermolysis bullosa acquisita. Arch Dermatol 1987; 123:772–6
84. Williams DM. Non infectious diseases of the oral soft tissue: a new approach. Adv Dent Res 1993; 7:213–9
85. Gammon WR, Fine JD, Forbes M, Briggaman RA. Immunofluorescence on split skin for the detection and differentiation of basement membrane zone autoantibodies. J Am Acad Dermatol 1992; 27:79–87
86. Flowers FP, Sherertz EF. Immunologic disorders of the skin and mucous membranes. Med Clin N Am 1985; 69:657–73
87. Gately LE, Nesbitt LT. Update on immunofluorescent testing in bullous diseases and lupus erythematosus. Dermatol Clin 1994; 12:133–42
88. Eversole LR. Immunopathology of oral mucosal ulcerative, desquamative, and bullous diseases. Oral Surg Oral Med Oral Pathol 1994; 77:555–71
89. Poulter LW, Lehener T. Immunohistology of oral lesions from patients with recurrent oral ulcers and Behet's syndrome. Clin Exp Immunol 1989; 78:189–95
90. Fischman SL. Oral ulcerations. Semin Dermatol 1994; 13:74–7
91. Pederson A. Recurrent aphthous ulceration: virological and immunological aspects. APMIS 1993; 37:1–37
92. Boisnic S, Tovaru S. Evaluation and treatment of aphthous ulcerations of the mouth. Ann Dermatol Venereol 1991; 118:53–9
93. Peterson DL, Georghion PR, Allworth AM, Kemp RJ. Thalidomide as treatment of refractory aphthous ulceration related to human immunodeficiency virus infection. Clin Infect Dis 1995; 20:250–4
94. Katz J, Langevitz P, Shermer J, et al. Prevention of recurrent aphthous stomatitis with colchicine: an open trial. J Am Acad Dermatol 1994; 31:459–61
95. Turnbull RS. Benzydamine hydrochloride (tantum) in the management of oral inflammatory conditions. J Can Dent Assoc 1995; 61:127–34
96. Fabbri P. Immunodermatologia. Brescia: ISED, 1993: 201
97. Emmi L, Brugnolo F, Salvati G, Marchione T. Immunopathological aspects of Behcet's disease. Clin Exp Rheum 1995; 13:687–91
98. Aydintug AO, Tokgoz G, D'Cruz DP et al. Antibodies to endothelial cells in Behcet's disease. Clin Immunol Immunopathol 1993; 67:157–62
99. James DG. Behcet's syndrome. N Engl J Med 1979; 301:431–2
100. Civatte J, Belaich S. Histopathologie des aphtes cutanes au cours du syndrome de Behcet. Ann Dermatol Syph 1976; 103:135–40
101. Haim S. The pathogenesis of lesions in Behcet's disease. Dermatologica 1979; 158:31–7
102. International Study Group for Behcet's disease: Criteria for diagnosis of Behcet's disease. Lancet 1990; 1:1078–80
103. Yazici H, Pazarli H, Barnes CG, et al. A controlled trial of azathioprine in Behcet's syndrome. N Engl J Med 1990; 322:281–5
104. Muftuoglu AU, Pazarli H, Yardakul S et al. Short term cyclosporin-A treatment of Behcet's disease. Br J Ophthalmol 1987; 71:387–90
105. Khan MA, van der Linden SM. A wider spectrum of spondyloarthropathies. Semin Arthritis Rheum 1990; 20:107–13
106. Schumacher HR. Light and electron microscopic studies on the synovial membrane in Reiter's syndrome. Immunocytochemical identification of chlamydial antigen in patients with early disease. Arthritis Rheum 1990; 33:s26
107. Hammer RE. Spontaneous inflammatory disease in transgenic rats expressing HLA-B27 and human beta2m: an animal model of HLA-B27-associated human disorders. Cell 1990; 63:1099
108. Arnet GF. Reiter syndrome: report of case. J Oral Surg 1980; 38:382
109. Calin A, Fries JF. An "experimental" epidemic of Reiter's syndrome revisited: follow-up evidence on genetic and environmental factors. Ann Intern Med 1976; 84:564
110. Calin A. Keratoderma blenorrhagicum and mucocutaneous manifestations of Reiter's syndrome. Ann Rheum Dis 1979; 38 (suppl): 68–72
111. Dunlop EM. Venereal disease: chlamydial genital infection and its complications. Br J Hosp Med 1983; 29:6–11
112. Calin A. A placebo controlled crossover study of azothioprine. Ann Rheum Dis 1986; 45:653–35
113. Chu SM. Reiter's syndrome. treatment with methotrexate. Singapore Med 1976; 17:101–3
114. Yunus MB. Current therapeutic practices in spondyloarthropathies. Compr Ther 1988; 14:54
115. Valente RM, Conn DL. Influence of pathogenesis on therapeutic choices in systemic vasculitis. Ann Med Interne 1994; 145:517–52
116. Gross WL, Hauschild S, Mistry N. The clinical relevance of ANCA in vasculitis. 5th International ANCA Workshop 7–10. 1993
117. Kallenberg CGM. Autoantibodies in vasculitis: current perspectives. Clin Exp Rheumatol 1993; 11:355–60
118. Leavitt RY, Fauci AS. Pulmonary vasculitis. Ann Rev Respir Dis 1986; 134:149–154
119. Abraham-Inpijn L. Oral and otal manifestations as the primary symptoms in Wegener's granulomatosis. J Head Neck Pathol 1983; 2:20–2
120. Israelson H, Binnie WH, Hurt WC. The hyperplastic gingivitis of Wegener's granulomatosis. J Periodontal 1981; 52:81–7
121. Alpern RJ. Southwestern internal medicine conference: vasculitis – it's time to reclassify. Am J Med Sci 1995; 309:235–248
122. Hoffman GS, Kerr GS, Leavitr RY. Wegener granulomatosis: an analysis of 158 patients. Ann Intern Med 1992; 116:488–98
123. Najjar T, Gadol C, Khan MY. Immune deficiency with polymorphic reticulosis. Oral Surg 1989; 67:322–6
124. Sloan P, Fanibunda K, Proctor S. Polymorphic reticulosis with oral lesions: a case report. Br J Oral Surg 1986; 24:426–32
125. Crissman JD, Weiss MA, Gluckman J. Midline granuloma syndrome. Aclinicopathologic study of 13 patients. Am J Surg Pathol 1982; 6:335–8
126. Shehade SA, Foulds IS. Granulomatous cheilitis and a positive Kweim test. Br J Dermatol 1986; 115:619–22
127. Greenstein AJ, Janowitz HD, Sachar DB. The extraintestinal complications of Crohn's disease and ulcerative colitis: a study of 700 patients. Medicine 1976; 55:401–12
128. Worsal N, Christensen KO, Bondensen S et al. Melkersson-Rosenthal syndrome and Crohn's disease. Br J Oral Surg 1980; 18:254–8
129. Kawasaki T. Acute febrile mucocutaneous syndrome with lymphoid involvement with specific desquamation of the fingers and the toes in children. Jap J Allergy 1967; 16:178–222
130. Tizard EJ, Suzuki A, Levin M and Dillon MJ. Clinical aspects of 100 patients with Kawasaki disease. Arch Dis Child 1991; 66:185–88
131. Rooley AH, Gonzalez-Crussi F, Shulman ST. Kawasaki syndrome. Adv Pediatr 1991; 38:51–74
132. Kato H, Inoue O, Akagi T. Kawasaki disease: cardiac problems and management. Pediatr Rev 1988; 9:209–217
133. Leung DJM, Meissner HC, Fulton DR, Murray DL, Kotzin BL, Schlievert PM. Toxic shock syndrome toxin-secreting Staphylococcus aureus in Kawasaki syndrome. Lancet 1993, 342:1385–1388

134. Nigro G, Zerbini M, Krzysztofiak A, Gentilomi G, Porcaro MA, Mango T, Musiani M. Active or recent parvovirus B19 infection in children with Kawasaki disease. Lancet 1994; 343:1260–1261
135. Arav-Boger R, Assia A, Jurgenson U, Spirer Z. The immunology of Kawasaki disease. Adv Pediatr 1994; 41:359–67
136. Rider LG, Wener MH, French J, Sherry DD, Mendelman PM. Autoantibody production in Kawasaki syndrome. Clin Exp Rheumatol 1993; 11:445–449
137. Lin CY, Lin CC, Hwang B, Chiang BN. Cytokines predict coronary aneurysm formation in Kawasaki disease patients. Eur J Pediatr 1993; 152:309–312
138. Japan Kawasaki Disease Research Committee. Diagnostic guidelines of Kawasaki disease: 4th Revision. Tokyo: Kawasaki Disease. Research Committee, 1984
139. Fukushige J, Takahashi N, Ueda Y, Ueda K. Incidence and clinical features of incomplete Kawasaki disease. Acta Paediatr 1994; 83:1057–1060
140. Committee on Rheumatic Fever, Endocarditis and Kawasaki disease, American Heart Association. Guidelines for long-term management of patients with Kawasaki disease. Circulation 1994; 89:916–22
141. Newburger JW. Treatment of Kawasaki disease. Lancet 1996; 347:1128
142. Salo E, Wangel AG, Pelkonen PI. Intravenous immune globulin reduces the IgG antiendothelial cell antibody response in Kawasaki disease. Endothelium 1993; 1:61–66
143. Naughton GK, et al. Detection of antibodies to melanocytes in vitiligo by specific immunoprecipitation. J Invest Dermatol 1983; 81:540
144. Morohashi M, et al. Ultrastructural studies of vitiligo, Vogt-Koyanagi syndrome, and incontinentia pigmenti achromians. Arch Dermatol 1977; 113:755
145. Voulot C. Mecanisme de controle de l'extension pigmentaire liee aux autogreffes de la peau. Ann Dermatol Syphiligr (Paris) 1970; 97:549
146. Lerner AB. Neural control of pigment cells. In: Kawamura T, et al. (Eds). The biology of normal and abnormal melanocytes. Tokyo: University Park Press, 1971: 3
147. Miklaszewska M, et al. Clinical and immunologic aspects of the relation of acquired leukoderma (vitiligo) to thyroid diseases. Arch Immunol Ther Exp (Warsz) 1972; 20:855
148. Koh HK, et al. Malignant melanoma and vitiligo-like leukoderma: an electron microscopic study. J Am Acad Dermatol 1983; 9:696
149. Chapman RS. Coincident vitiligo and psoriasis in the same individual. Arch Dermatol 1973, 107:776
150. Bhawan J, Butain LK. Keratinocyte damage in vitiligo. Cutan Pathol 1983; 10:207
151. Lassus A, et al. Treatment of vitiligo with oral methoxsalen and UVA. Photodermatology 1984; 1:170
152. Lissia M, Lugliè PF, Bandettini MV. Lichen planus of oral mucosa: clinical consideration. Ital Gen Rev Dermatol 1988; 25:60–68
153. Valsecchi R, Bontempelli M, Rossi A, et al. HLA DR and DQ antigens in lichen planus. Acta Derm Venereol 1988; 68:77–80
154. Morhenn VB. Etiology of lichen planus. Am J Dermatopathol 1986; 8:154–156
155. Shioara T, Moriya N, Nagashima M. The lichenoid tissue reaction. Int J Dermatol 1988; 27:365–374
156. Marder MZ, Deesen KC. Transformation of oral lichen planus to squamous cell carcinoma: a literature review and report of case. J Am Dent Assoc 1982; 105:55–60
157. Fulling HJ. Cancer development in oral lichen planus. Arch Dermatol 1973; 108:667–669
158. Firth NA, Reade PC. Angiotensin-converting enzyme inhibitors implicated in oral mucosa lichenoid reactions. Oral Surg Oral Med Oral Pathol 1989; 67:41–44
159. Jungell P, Malmstrom M, Wartiovaara J, Konttinen YT. Ultrastructure of oral leukoplakia and lichen planus. I. Basal region and inflammatory cells. J Oral Pathol 1987; 16:170–178
160. Jungell P. Oral lichen planus: a review. Int J Oral Maxillofac Surg 1991; 20:129–135
161. Grattan CEH, Boon AP, Gregory J. A preliminary open study of topical cyclosporin for hypertrophic lichen planus. J Dermatol Treatment 1989; 1:39–41

CHAPTER 12

Traumatic Lesions of Oral Mucosa

F. Ayala and E. Bucci

12.1 Introduction

Despite the frequent occurrence of traumatic lesions of the oral mucosa, patients suffering from these conditions seldom refer to the clinician. This is due to the easy recognition of aetiologic agents, thus enabling patients to eliminate them.

The most common cause is generally that of self-induced trauma, such as involuntary chewing, biting, or sucking on the buccal mucosa, tongue, or lip. Other common causes are accidents, acute crushing types of trauma, chronic mechanical trauma, and chemical burns. *Self-induced trauma* generally includes erosions or small ulcers that heal in a few days or weeks, frequently requiring no treatment. Rarely, gums, palate, or other areas of the oral mucosa can be the site of *accidents* such as punctures induced by pencils, pens, pins, toothpicks, and fish bones.

Crushing types of trauma clinically manifest in different forms: red patches or necrotic areas surrounded by an erythematous halo are probably the most common types. At times, focal areas of hemorrhage can occur.

Mechanical *trauma chronic or moderate*, for example resulting from compulsive cheek chewing, can lead to grayish-white, irregularly elevated lines along the occlusal plane, or to patches clinically resembling leukoplakia. Despite its resemblance to this latter condition, as a rule diagnosis is easily made on the basis of history. Besides, the condition is often bilateral. *Chemical burns* may be caused by erroneous use of a variety of drugs and chemical agents. Iatrogenic burns induced by the chemicals used in dental therapy (silver nitrate, phenol, oxidizing and bleaching agents, etc.) may also occur.

Other causes of traumatic lesions include jagged teeth, ill-fitting dentures, toothbrush trauma, and food (e.g., toast). Dental or surgical procedures (e.g., intubation) account for most iatrogenic injuries, which are strictly related to the instrument and/or technique used.

In most cases, elimination of the cause is the best way to allow normal healing to occur.

12.2 Traumatic Ulcers

Traumatic ulcers may occur on any site of the oral mucosa, even if they are more frequently observed on the lateral borders of the tongue, cheeks, and lips. Their size varies and this may be related to the intensity, length, and type of trauma. Sometimes, secondary infections modify the primary aspect of the lesion. Palpation usually reveals a lesion of soft consistency. Long lasting ulcers may have elevated borders and a hard consistency. Broken teeth, carious teeth (Fig. 12.1), dental prostheses (Figs. 12.2, 12.3), inappropriate use of toothbrush (Fig. 12.4) or chemicals, surgical instrumentation and odontological treatments (Fig. 12.5), foods and various items may cause injury to oral mucosa leading to ulceration. It is worth remembering that an ulcer that fails to heal may necessitate biopsy to rule out the possibility of malignancy. In addition, the clinician should always consider the possibility of a self-inflicted injury as an expression of mental disturbance. Differential diagnosis includes various neoplasias, aphthous stomatitis, syphilis, tuberculosis, and fungal infections. When necessary, these will be excluded by specific laboratory investigations.

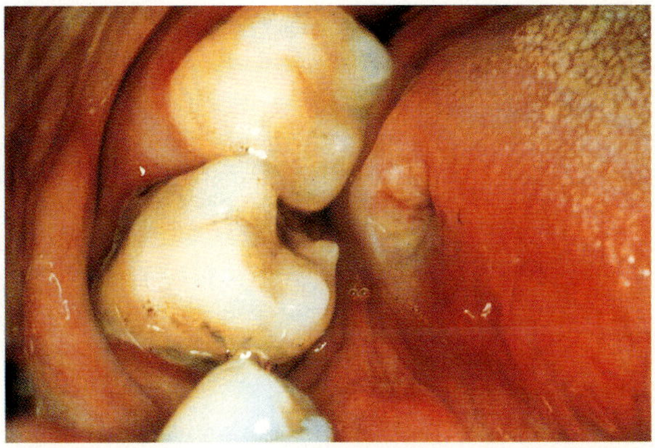

Fig. 12.1. "Decubitus" ulcer of the tongue caused by a carious tooth

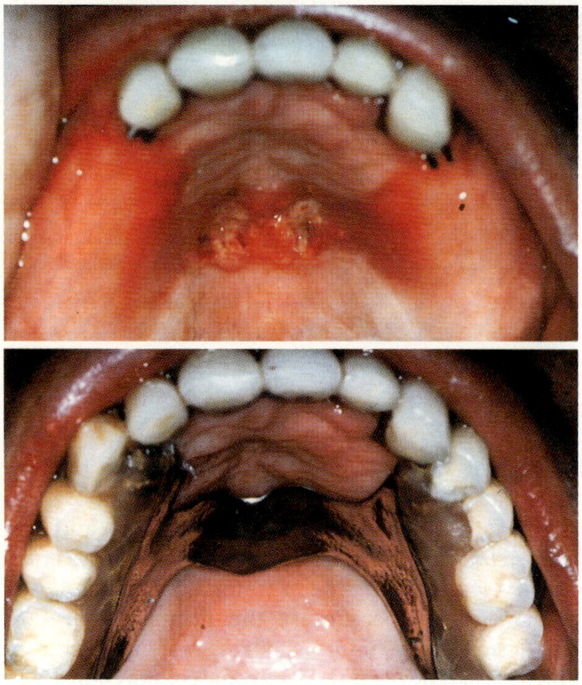

Fig. 12.2. Palatal ulcer secondary to traumatic pressure induced by the metal arch of a denture

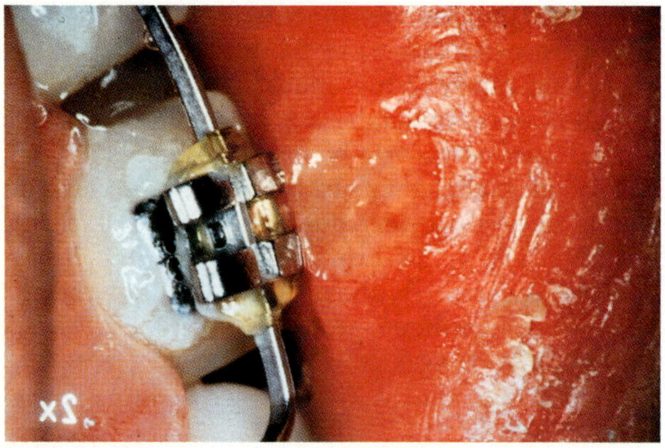

Fig. 12.3. Ulcer induced by mechanical trauma at the site of contact with a metal bracket

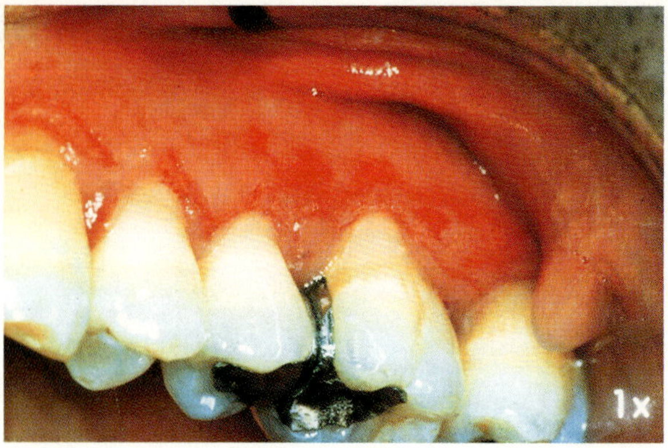

Fig. 12.4. Erosions caused by vigorous use of the toothbrush

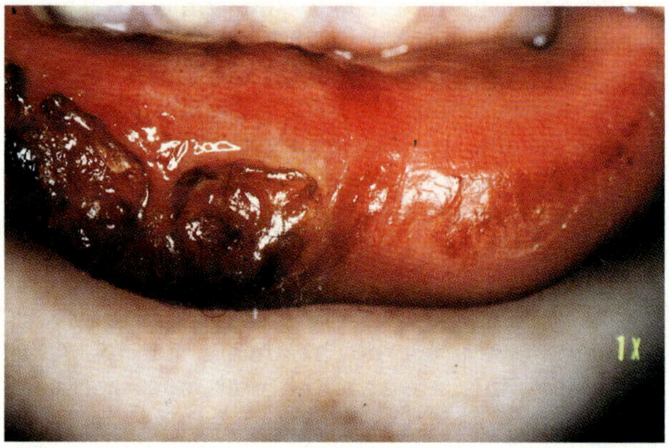

Fig. 12.5. Lip erosion covered by a crust. The lesion was the effect of strongly biting the lip due to loss of sensitivity immediately after a tooth extraction done under local anesthesia

Reference

Laskaris G. Color atlas of oral diseases. New York: Thieme, 1994

CHAPTER 13

Endocrine, Nutritional, and Amino Acid Metabolism Diseases

G. Hautmann, G. L. Campanile, and T. M. Lotti

13.1 Endocrine Disease

13.1.1 Diabetes Mellitus

Definition. Diabetes mellitus is a chronic metabolic syndrome caused by a relative or absolute insulin deficiency. Its most typical characteristics are fasting hyperglycemia, atherosclerotic and microvascular changes, and neuropathy.

Oral Manifestations. The oral effects of diabetes mellitus include xerostomia, glossodynia, cheilitis, benign migratory glossitis, an increase in the incidence and severity of fungal (Fig. 13.1) and bacterial infections, taste change and delayed wound healing [1]. Any one or a combination of these signs and symptoms may indicate diabetes. The dehydration caused by diabetes also affects the salivary glands, with a reduction in salivary flow and an increase in the glucose concentration in saliva. Oral sensory disorders such as altered taste (dysgeusia) or tactile response, difficulty in speech, and dysphagia all occur as the result of a decrease in saliva. Other problems such as dental caries, periodontal disease, and mucositis occur commonly. For denture wearers, such involvement of the oral mucosal barrier may lead to denture irritation and painful ulcerations which heal slowly. Another common finding in patients with diabetes mellitus is asymptomatic bilateral enlargement of the parotid glands. This phenomenon does not appear to be influenced by the duration of diabetes, and in certain cases the enlargement precedes the onset of diabetes. The cause of this enlargement is unclear, but it may be a compensatory mechanism that results from xerostomia secondary to dehydration in diabetes. Sialograms are invariably normal, and histopathologic examination reveals fatty infiltration of the interstitium with normal acini and ducts. Glossodynia may occur secondary to diabetic neuropathy and microangiopathy. The neuropathic and microangiopathic manifestations of diabetes may occur in the genetically pre-diabetic patient who has minimal glucose intolerance and none of the classic symptoms of diabetes [2]. Also, patients with glucose intolerance and the classic symptoms of diabetes have neuropathic and microangiopathic manifestations that may result in the burning mouth syndrome. Several mechanisms have been suggested to account for the burning sensation in diabetes mellitus. It may be an oral manifestation of peripheral neuropathy or microangiopathy (or a combination of these two factors) or result from the increased incidence of oral candidiasis in diabetics. Alternatively, it has been suggested that the lack of insulin may produce a catabolic process within the mucosa in response to previously insignificant trauma.

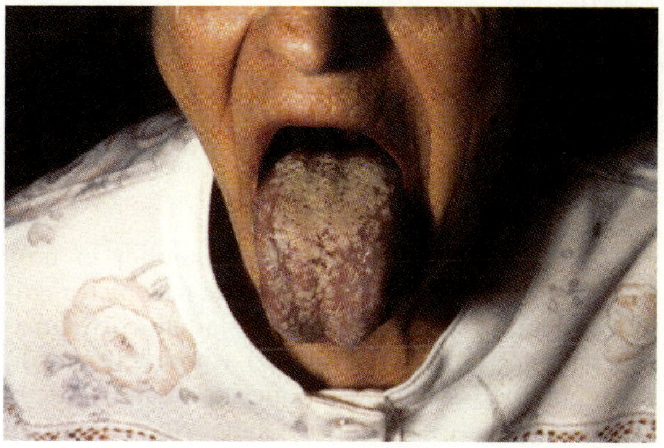

Fig. 13.1. *Candida* infection of the tongue in a diabetic patient

Associated Findings. Its overt symptoms are usually polydipsia with polyuria, generalized weakness, and weight loss.

Diagnosis. When diabetes is suspected as the source of the glossodynia and xerostomia, appropriate blood tests must be ordered. A fasting blood glucose test and a 2-h post-prandial blood glucose level are recommended.

Treatment. The treatment of the oral manifestations of diabetes mellitus ideally should be based on the treatment of the disease itself. It is not known whether the symptoms of xerostomia and glossodynia will be reversed with the proper control of the diabetes. The treatment of patients with glossodynia and elevated glucose tolerance levels with hypoglycemic agents has met with very limited success. However, certain patients may have their glossodynia reversed with diet control. A suggested cause of the oral dryness in these patients is the neuropathy and basement membrane changes in small blood vessels. The poor response to treatment could be caused by irreversible nerve or blood vessel damage. It is not known whether the parotid gland enlargement seen in diabetics can be altered with control of the disease.

13.1.2 Hypophysis Disorders

These disorders are related to a number of hormones of hypophyseal origin, some of which regulate endocrine structures (such as adenocorticotropin, gonadotropins, thyrotropin), whereas others do not appear to stimulate endocrine tissue directly (such as growth hormone, melanocyte-stimulating hormone). The effects of pituitary dysfunction on the skin and oral mucosa result from actions mediated via targeted endocrine gland hormones whose elaboration is regulated by tropic stimulation from the pituitary. The latter introduces multiple potentialities, so that the alterations of the skin in pituitary disorders usually present a composite of endocrine effects. For example, too much hormone of one sort may be accompanied by too little of another variety [3].

13.1.2.1 *Panhypopituitarism*

Etiology. Several conditions may compromise the anterior pituitary and, thereby, the elaboration of all pituitary hormones (Sheehan's syndrome, syphilis, tuberculosis, granulomatous inflammation, neoplastic invasion, etc.).

Clinical Features. Cutaneous pallor is prominent; melanin content is apparently diminished. Lack of normal capillary flush of the face, ear lobes, and palms contributes to the pallor, but mucous membranes retain their normal hue unless there is concomitant anemia. The normal facial folds are diminished and there is frequently some puffiness of the face, which is expressionless. The thinness of the face and subcutaneous tissues results in fine wrinkling around the eyes and mouth, giving the appearance of advanced age. Sweat and sebaceous secretions are diminished. Loss of body hair occurs in all patients and is noted early. Beard growth diminishes but is not lost altogether in adult males [3].

13.1.2.2 *Acromegaly*

Etiology. Acromegaly is an uncommon disease caused by growth hormone (GH) excess in adults, usually from a benign pituitary adenoma. Excessive GH elaboration is commonly associated with eosinophilic adenomas of the pituitary. Although pituitary elaboration of other hormones, such as the gonadotropins, may be compromised, the preponderant changes in the skin, mucosa, and the rest of the body are those of excessive stimulation with GH.

Oral Manifestations. Oral involvement is manifested in the lower lip, which is enlarged and protruding. There is macroglossia [4]. The enlargement of the lower jaw (prognathism) makes the teeth more widely spaced.

Associated Findings. Acromegaly is grossly characterized by enlarged feet and hands, nasal bone hypertrophy, frontal bossing, and coarsening of facial features (hence, acromegaly). There are also neurologic disturbances, decreased vision, musculoskeletal symptoms, cardiorespiratory and genitourinary disorders, myopathy, and fatigue. The cutaneous changes are most pronounced in the dermal connective tissue. The amount of glycosaminoglycans (in particular, chondroitin and dermatan sulfate) is increased. These substances are hygroscopic and, consequently, retain a significant amount of water. Thus, there is characteristic hyperplasia. In acromegaly, there is also hyperplasia of the epidermis and dermal appendages. Clinically, the effect on the integument can be described as "too much skin". The entire skin is thickened and has a doughy feel; this is most marked over the face and on the extremities, where the skeletal changes are also most prominent. Increased sweating and heat intolerance are common. Furrowing and accentuation of the folds contribute to the coarsening of the features. Deepening of creases on the forehead and in the nasolabial area gives the patient a scowling, somber expression. Usually, the eyelids appear thick and edematous; the nose becomes enlongated, and the increased soft tissue in the alae nasi gives the nose a characteristic triangular configuration.

Differential Diagnosis. The oral involvement must be differentiated from amyloidosis, lipoid proteinosis, Down's syndrome, and hypothyroidism.

Diagnosis. The diagnosis may be confirmed by measurement of basal serum GH level. Radiologic examination to localize the adenoma may be useful.

Treatment. Treatment should be left to the endocrinologist; in severe cases, surgical correction of the enlarged jaw and tongue have been suggested.

13.1.3 Thyroid Disorders

An altered secretion of thyroid hormones may cause oral manifestations.

13.1.3.1 *Hypothyroidism*

Etiology. Hypothyroidism, congenital or acquired, may be primary, due to failure of the thyroid to secrete sufficient amounts of hormones, secondary, due to insufficient stimulation of this gland by thyroid stimulating hormone (TSH), or tertiary, due to a hypothalamic disorder resulting in insufficient pituitary secretion of TSH.

Oral Manifestations. The oral manifestations of the congenital type include macroglossia, enamel dysplasia, and delayed eruption of the teeth. The acquired type of the adult may present oral involvement. There is a myxedematous infiltration of the tongue, with subsequent macroglossia that causes difficulties in speech and mastication [5].

Associated Findings. The congenital type is characterized by severe mental deficiency (cretinism), delayed skeletal growth, myxedema, protracted neonatal jaundice, and sluggishness. The acquired type of the adult is characterized by bradycardia, constipation, susceptibility to cold, myxedema, and carotenemia.

Diagnosis. Diagnosis consists of measurement of serum levels of thyroid hormones (in bound and free form) and TSH.

13.1.4 Parathyroid Hormone Disorders

This hormone regulates the flux of calcium and phosphate between extra- and intracellular compartments in responsive tissues (such as bone and renal tubules) and the metabolism of vitamin D. The exact role of this hormone in the skin and oral mucosa is still debated, but abnormal serum levels of calcium and/or phosphate produce changes in the skin, attesting to the importance of circulating levels of these ions in normal skin physiology [6].

13.1.4.1 *Hyperparathyroidism*

Etiology. Primary hyperparathyroidism is usually due to parathyroid hyperplasia, adenoma, or carcinoma.

Oral Manifestations. "Brown" giant cell tumors located in the lower or upper jaws may be an early sign of disease. The protrusion of the tumor as a soft mass in the oral cavity (due to bone destruction) is very rare.

Associated Findings. Clinically, the disease is characterized by polydipsia, polyuria, muscular weakness, lassitude, osteoporosis, mental dysfunction, renal calculi, and urinary concentration.

Differential Diagnosis. The disease may simulate Kaposi's sarcoma, pyogenic granuloma, hemangioendothelioma, or hemangiopericytoma.

Diagnosis. Laboratory tests (such as histologic examination, measurement of parathyroid hormone levels, serum calcium and phosphate levels, alkaline phosphatase, skeletal and dental radiograms) are useful for the diagnosis.

Treatment. The excision of the "brown" tumor is curative only if the underlying disease is treated.

13.1.4.2 *Hypoparathyroidism*

Etiology. Hypoparathyroidism is usually due to ablation of the parathyroids as a complication of thyroidectomy; in fact, parathyroid failure is a very uncommon cause.

Oral Manifestations. This condition seems to predispose to chronic candidiasis; the infection commonly affects oral mucosae, but vulvovaginitis and infections of intertriginous areas are also frequent [7]. This infection is not altered by regulation of blood calcium and phosphorus levels and is accompanied by defects in cellular immunity.

Associated Findings. In hypoparathyroidism the skin appears dry, scaly, hyperkeratotic, and puffy. Nails are opaque and brittle, and have transverse ridges. Eczematous dermatitis, exfoliative dermatitis, hyperkeratotic, papular, and macular eruptions have been reported. Hair is coarse and sparse.

13.1.5
Sex Hormones, Menstrual Cycle, and Pregnancy Disorders

Etiology and Pathogenesis. Hormones in saliva and oral tissue affect overall dental and oral mucosal health. Evidence of a relationship between oral symptoms and sex steroid hormone activity comes from several sources [8, 9]. Although the evidence is not conclusive, the data demonstrate a strong association between these hormones and some oral symptoms, such as burning mouth sensation. The physiologic effects of sex steroids depend on the absolute concentration of one hormone compared to absolute concentrations of other sex steroids. The concentration of steroid hormones in the saliva is in proportion to blood levels. Because the majority (90 %–98 %) of plasma sex steroids are bound, or inactive, changes in the unbound, or active, hormone may not be measurable by clinically available hormone assays. Hormone concentrations in the saliva reflect the unbound, or active, hormone levels in the serum. Sex steroids, such as androgens, estrogens, or progesterone, and cortisol levels in saliva fluctuate with diurnal and menstrual alterations, and the oral tissues are affected by the salivary levels, as well as systemic levels of these hormones. Sex steroids have been detected bound to receptors in the gingiva, parotid glands, and minor salivary glands following administration of triturated hormones. Thus, the presence of these receptors suggests hormone action on the oral tissues [1].

Testosterone stimulates oral epithelial growth through receptors located within the oral tissues, particularly in the gingiva. Phenytoin provokes an increase in testosterone receptor sites that induce gingival hyperplasia. Inflamed gingivae in both men and women metabolize testosterone. However, when the gingivae are healthy, testosterone is metabolized only in men [10]. Testosterone increases protease activity and inhibits calcification, thereby decreasing inflammation; however, it also stimulates fibroblast and leukocyte migration that may contribute to inflammation [10].

It has also been demonstrated that *progesterone* has the ability to augment the exudative leukocyte migration stimulated previously by local factors within the oral environment [11]. In humans, elevated serum progesterone concentrations accompany periodontal inflammation in men and women [10]. In women, progesterone causes a change in gingival microflora and microvasculature. Increased serum progesterone during pregnancy or oral contraceptive use causes a 50-fold increase in *Bacteroides* species (*Bacteroides intermedium*, in particular). The organism causes stomatopyrosis and gingivitis, and it is most abundant during the second trimester of pregnancy, when gingivitis scores are highest. Elevated progesterone increases androgen metabolism to the more active form and may stimulate epithelial growth [10]. *Estrogen* and *progesterone* regulate prostanoid synthesis in oral tissues. Estradiol stimulates prostacycline formation and leukotriene production, and progesterone prevents the formation of these two inflammatory mediators. Estrogen stimulates synthesis of salivary peroxidase and an increase in inflammatory products. Different relative concentrations of progesterone either augment or suppress some effects of estrogen. Estrogen metabolism that occurs in oral tissues results in the formation of an estrogen that is more potent. In inflamed tissues, this leads to a three-fold increase in estrogen potency, and metabolism of progesterone proceeds more rapidly [12].

Oral Manifestations. Oral inflammation and glossodynia may sometimes occur during puberty, pregnancy, menses, and therapy with hormones (especially oral contraceptive agents) and other medications, such as phenytoin. Alterations in sex hormone levels are manifested primarily in the gingival tissues as exaggerated reactions to the minor irritants usually present around the teeth.

In pregnancy, gingivitis is the more commonly encountered condition. It increases in severity from the 2nd month to a maximum in the 8th month, with a reduction in the postpartum period. Furthermore, during pregnancy, oral granulomas (*pregnancy granulomas*) may occur which are clinically and histopathologically identical to pyogenic granulomas. This condition is localized to the gingiva and appears after the first trimester. It usually appears as a single, pedunculated lesion with a smooth, red-colored surface. Multiple lesions are rare. The mass may regress spontaneously and disappear. It must be differentiated from pyogenic granuloma and peripheral giant cell granuloma.

Menopausal and postmenopausal oral lesions include atrophic mucositis or stomatitis, glossitis, and desquamative gingivitis. Oral symptoms, such as glossodynia, glossopyrosis, and dysgeusia are particularly common.

13.1.6
Adrenocortical Gland Insufficiency

Etiology. Deficient production of glucocorticoids (i. e., Addison's disease) occurs because of insufficient parenchyma (atrophy, adrenalectomy), inadequate stimulation by ACTH (e. g., secondary adrenal failure), or endogenous blockade of the biosynthetic sequence (e. g., adrenogenital syndrome).

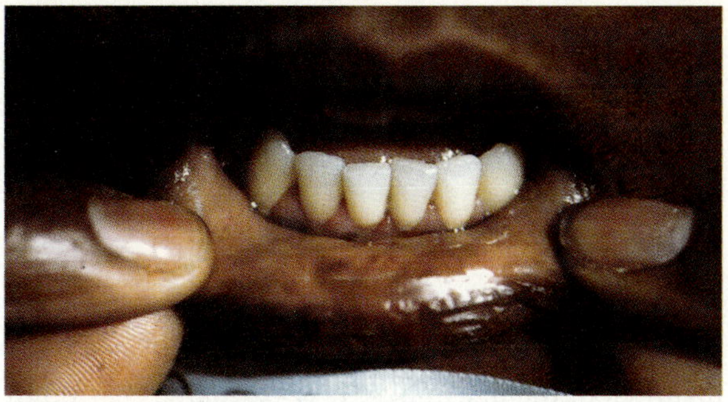

Fig. 13.2. Pigmentation of the lip in a patient with Addison's disease

Oral Manifestations. Pigmentation appears on mucosal surfaces (Fig. 13.2), especially the buccal mucosa, gums, and tongue. It is a pale to dark brown pigment usually seen on the buccal mucosa bilaterally; it eventually involves most lining mucosal sites, as well as gingiva. The oral pigmentation, along with malaise and lowered blood pressure, may be the earliest signs of the disease. When hypoadrenocorticism results from pituitary failure, the pigmentary changes do not occur [13].

Associated Findings. The most striking change is cutaneous hyperpigmentation, which is generalized and represents an accentuation of the normal distribution of melanin in the skin. It is always darker in sun-exposed areas. Darkening occurs in areas of trauma, points of pressure and friction, sexual areas, hair, and nails.

Treatment. Replacement therapy with corticosteroids produces a gradual diminution of the hyperpigmentation [3].

13.2 Deficiency of Vitamins and Altered Mineral Metabolism

It is well known that macroscopic changes in the tongue (swelling of the tongue, papillary atrophy, surface ulceration) can occur as a result of deficiencies of iron, folic acid, or vitamin B_{12}, but it is less well appreciated that a prodromal glossodynia can precede any macroscopic change [14].

13.2.1 Vitamin A

Deficiency of vitamin A provokes a keratinizing metaplasia of major and minor salivary glands with resultant xerostomia. Hypervitaminosis A may produce dry and scaly lips, tender, swollen, and bleeding marginal gingivae, and sore tongue and mouth.

13.2.2 Vitamin B

13.2.2.1 *Vitamin B_1 (Thiamine)*

Deficient intake of thiamine may provoke small vesicles on the buccal mucosa, ventral tongue, or palate.

13.2.2.2 *Vitamin B_2 (Riboflavin)*

Oral Manifestations. The most frequent oral manifestation is angular cheilitis, which may be unilateral or bilateral. The lips appear dry and cracked. There may be swelling of the fungiform papillae and a granular glossal surface. A continued deficiency may lead to papillary atrophy and irregular areas of surface denudation [15]. Generally, the color of the tongue is a magenta or purple-red color.

Associated Findings. Deficiency may result in seborrheic dermatitis, corneal vascularization, and, in advanced stages, keratitis (oro-ocular-genital syndrome with burning mouth sensation).

Diagnosis. This vitamin deficiency is marked by urinary excretion of less than 50 μg/day of riboflavin.

Treatment. Treatment of vitamin B_2 deficiency consists of 10 mg/day of riboflavin administered orally.

13.2.2.3 *Vitamin B_3 (Niacin)*

Etiology. Niacin deficiency is the cause of pellagra. The pathogenesis of the lesions of pellagra is still not entirely clear. It may result from a diet deficient in niacin or tryphtophan (which can be converted in the body to niacin), or more commonly both, and amino acid imbalance may also play a part. Besides the dermatosis, there are important gastrointestinal and nervous system changes.

Oral Manifestations. Oral involvement may occur as enlargement of the papillae on the tip and margins of the tongue. Glossal reddening, swelling, and noticeable discomfort may occur; persistence of the deficiency can lead to total papillary atrophy that creates a smooth, bald, and beefy red glossal surface [16]. Gingivitis, dry and fissured lips, angular cheilitis, and dysphagia may be present. A common complication is Vincent's infection, a necrotizing infection of the gingiva.

Diagnosis. Measurement of urinary excretion of methylated metabolites of nicotinic acid does not provide unequivocal evidence of deficiency. Therefore, the diagnosis of niacin deficiency is largely based on clinical findings.

Treatment. Specific therapy consists of the oral administration of 100–300 mg niacinamide daily in divided doses. The amide is preferable since it does not precipitate the vasomotor disturbances resulting from administration of niacin in large doses.

13.2.2.4
Vitamin B_6 (Pyridoxine)

The main symptom of pyridoxine deficiency is a painful, swollen, purplish tongue; glossopyrosis may be present. The swelling can obscure the structure of the filiform papillae. Papillary atrophy can occur.

13.2.2.5
Vitamin B_{12} (Cyanocobalamin)

Etiology. The most common cause of vitamin B_{12} deficiency is pernicious anemia [17], a megaloblastic anemia usually caused by a gastric mucosal defect that decreases the synthesis of intrinsic factor, which is required for intestinal uptake of vitamin B_{12}. Other less frequent causes of pernicious anemia are total gastrectomy, pancreatic dysfunction, parasitic diseases, and diseases of the ileum.

Oral Manifestations. Burning sensation of the tongue and taste loss are early symptoms. The tongue may show glossitis and varying degrees of papillary atrophy (filiform and fungiform papillae). Initially, only the tip and lateral margins of the tongue are red and atrophic; if left untreated, total papillary atrophy, which results in a smooth, bald, fiery-red surface, can occur. Dorsal surface lobulations, generalized surface ulcerations, and dysgeusia may also occur.

Associated Findings. Symptoms may include glossodynia, neurologic abnormalities, tingling and numbness of the extremities, weakness, difficulty in walking, pallor, malaise, lassitude, weight loss, and gastrointestinal upset.

Diagnosis. Laboratory tests generally reveal macrocytic anemia (mean corpuscular volume greater than 100 mm^3), low serum vitamin B_{12} (less than 100 pg/ml), and absence of intrinsic factor as determined by the Schilling test. In pernicious anemia, urinary excretion of radioactive B_{12} without intrinsic factor will be less than 5 %.

Treatment. Treatment consists of regular parenteral administration of vitamin B_{12} every 2 months for life. The oral signs and symptoms of the disease may resolve 48 h after the first administration of vitamin B_{12}.

13.2.3
Folic Acid

Etiology. Folic acid deficiency is usually the result of insufficient dietary intake. It is estimated that up to 20 % of pregnant women suffer from this deficiency [18]. Other patients at risk include alcoholics, hemodialysis patients, the elderly, and patients taking certain drugs such as phenytoin and oral contraceptives, which interfere with the absorption and storage of folate in tissues. Malabsorption states, such as tropical and non-tropical sprue, can also cause folic acid deficiency.

Oral Manifestations. The glossal changes related to folic acid deficiency are indistinguishable from those caused by deficiency of vitamin B_{12}. Thus, the clinician may observe glossitis with papillary atrophy; there are reports of early glossal swelling with pallor, followed by atrophy of filiform papillae and reddening of the fungiform papillae. Occasionally, there are aphthous-like ulcerations. As the deficiency persists, the dorsal surface of the tongue may develop a typical bald, shiny, smooth, raw appearance.

Diagnosis. The patient with folic acid deficiency commonly presents with a macrocytic anemia that resembles pernicious anemia. However, intrinsic factor is not absent in folic acid deficiency.

Treatment. Folic acid deficiency treatment consists of 0.1–30 mg/day folic acid administered orally. Inappropriate administration of folic acid can mask the progression of vitamin B_{12} deficiency, and even exacerbate existing vitamin B_{12} deficiency, since it is not uncommon for a patient to present both folic acid and vitamin B_{12} deficiencies.

13.2.4
Biotin

Biotin deficiency may cause "geographic tongue" due to patchy atrophy of the papillae and pale tongue color.

13.2.5
Pantothenic Acid

This deficiency may provoke glossitis and cheilosis.

13.2.6 Vitamin C (Ascorbic Acid)

Etiology. Vitamin C deficiency causes scurvy. In vitamin C deficiency, collagen formation is impaired as a result of failure of hydroxylation of protocollagen, proline, and lysine.

Oral Manifestations. Gum changes are often very marked. The earliest signs are reddening, swelling, and tiny hemorrhages in the tips of the interdental papillae. More advanced changes are a purplish, swollen, and spongy appearance of the gums; part of the tissue becomes necrotic with some bleeding. Aphthous ulcers (Fig. 13.3), pain, tenderness, and enamel hypoplasia of developing teeth may occur.

Associated Findings. Clinical manifestations may include malaise, susceptibility to infection, hematomas, hemorrhages, delayed wound healing, mental symptoms, anemia, pain, and edema of the lower extremities. The first cutaneous changes are enlargement and keratosis of hair follicles, chiefly on the outer aspect of the upper arm, back, buttocks, back of thighs, calves, and shins.

Treatment. Scurvy responds dramatically to the administration of vitamin C. Infants should receive 150–300 mg vitamin C daily, orally administered in divided doses for 10 days, followed by 150 mg daily for 1 month. Adults should receive up to 800 mg daily in divided doses for 1 week and half this amount daily until complete recovery [19].

13.2.7 Iron Deficiency

Etiology. Iron deficiency may result from inadequate dietary iron intake, malabsorption, blood

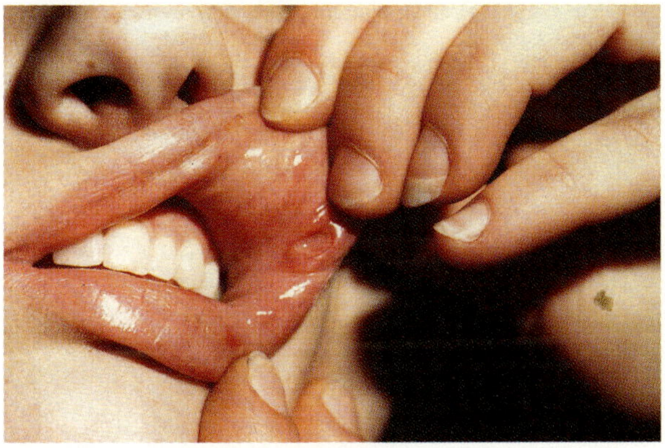

Fig. 13.3. Aphtous ulcer of the buccal mucosa in a patient with vitamin C deficiency

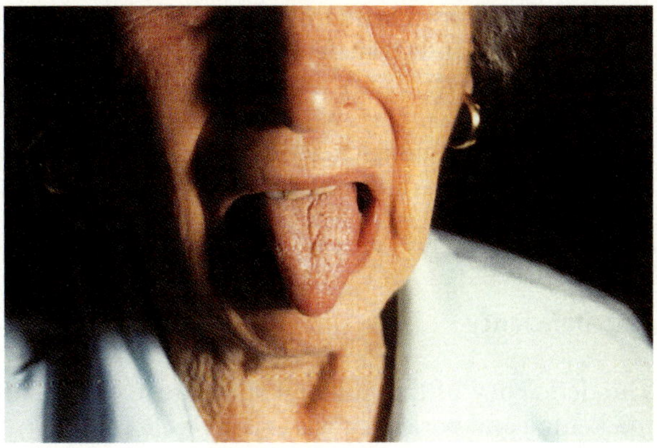

Fig. 13.4. Atrophic and smooth tongue in an anemic patient

loss, or rarely, intravascular hemolysis with hemoglobinuria. The most common cause of anemia is iron deficiency. The prevalence of this deficiency among women is related to the increased need for iron during pregnancy and menstruation.

Oral Manifestations. Burning or soreness of the tongue is reported to occur in about 39 % of cases [20]. Typically, the tongue of an anemic patient will exhibit papillary atrophy (filiform and fungiform papillae) and a smooth surface (Fig. 13.4); progressively, the dorsal surface of the tongue becomes smooth and glistening. The tongue atrophy may be patchy or generalized. Candidiasis and angular cheilitis are common findings, but rarely do leukoplakia or superficial erosions develop.

Associated Findings. The patient with iron deficiency may also experience fatigue and weakness, anorexia, headache, and pallor of skin and mucosae. About 7 % of patients with iron deficiency anemia will develop Plummer-Vinson syndrome [1, 17]. The syndrome is marked by the presence of dysphagia caused by an esophageal stricture or web, koilonychia (spoon-shaped nails), and glossitis.

Differential Diagnosis. These tongue manifestations must be differentiated from those found in the course of pernicious anemia, geographic tongue, atrophic lichen planus, atrophic glossitis of tertiary syphilis, and other malnutrition disorders.

Diagnosis. Early recognition and treatment is important because patients with Plummer-Vinson syndrome have a 10 % risk of developing eosophageal carcinoma. The diagnosis of iron deficiency is based on several available laboratory tests. A peripheral blood smear will show hypochromic, microcytic erythrocytes. Plasma ferritin will be less than 40 μg/100 ml, and transferrin saturation will be less than 10% [1].

Treatment. Iron deficiency is generally corrected with oral administration of ferrous sulfate, 300 mg three times/day.

13.2.8 Zinc Deficiency

The deficiency of this mineral may cause epithelial thickening and parakeratosis [13], as well as the syndrome of acrodermatitis enteropathica.

13.3 Uremic Stomatitis

Etiology. Uremia is a metabolic disorder due to accumulation of nitrogenous waste products in the blood. It may be the result of acute or chronic renal failure.

Oral Manifestations. Oral manifestations include xerostomia, unpleasant taste, gingival friability, and ulcerative stomatitis [21]. Xerostomia is most common and is probably secondary to mouth breathing or dehydration in most patients. Stomatitis rarely appears before the blood urea level reaches 300 mg/dl, responds promptly to dialysis, and is probably an ammoniacal burn due to bacterial decomposition of salivary urea. Two forms of uremic stomatitis are recognized: *ulcerative*, characterized by painful superficial ulcers covered by a pseudomembrane, and *nonulcerative*, characterized by a painful diffuse edematous erythema and a thick grayish pseudomembrane on the oral mucosa.

Treatment. The oral lesions improve after hemodialysis.

References

1. Hautmann G, Panconesi E. Glossodynia. J Eur Acad Dermatol Venereol 1996; 7:207–227
2. Wysocki GP, Daley TD. Benign migratory glossitis in patients with juvenile diabetes. Oral Surg 1987; 63:68–70
3. Freinkel RK, Freinkel N. Cutaneous manifestations of endocrine disorders. In: Fitzpatrick TB, Eisen AZ, Wolff K, Freedberg IM, Austen KF (Eds). Dermatology in general medicine. New York: McGraw-Hill, 1987
4. Davidoff LM. Studies in acromegaly. III. The anamnesis and symptomatology in one hundred cases. Endocrinology 1926; 10:461–472
5. Dyrbe MO. Effect of thyroxine, thyrotrophic and somatotrophic hormones on skin of dwarf mice. Proc Soc Exp Biol Med 1959; 102:417–426
6. Hirano K. Cutaneous manifestations in idiopathic hypoparathyroidism. Arch Dermatol 1975; 109:242
7. Sutphin A. Five cases (three in siblings) of idopathic hypoparathyroidism associated with moniliasis. J Clin Endocrinol 1943; 3:625–631
8. Myers A, Naylor GD. Glossodynia as an oral manifestation of sex hormone alterations. Ear Nose Throat J 1989; 7:786–790
9. Hung W, August GP. Pediatric endocrinology. Garden City: Medical Examination Publishing Co, 1984: 213–215
10. Vittek J, Rappaport Sc, Gordon GG. Concentration of circulating hormones and metabolism of androgens by human gingiva. J Perio 1977; 50:254–264
11. Lindhe J, Hellden L, Lundren D. Exudation and leukocyte emigration on progesterone and estrogen treated rats. Scand J Dent Res 1972; 80:434–439
12. El Attar TM, Hugoson A. The in vitro conversion of female sex steroid, estrogen, in normal and inflamed human gingiva. Arch Oral Biol 1974; 19:425–429
13. Dolby AE (Ed). Oral mucosa in health and disease. Oxford: Blackwell, 1975
14. Jackson AA, Golden MHN. In: Weatherall DJ, Ledingham JGG, Warrell DA (Eds). Oxford textbook of medicine. 2nd Ed. Oxford: Oxford Univ Press, 1987: 8–23
15. Shafer WG, Hine MK, Levy BM. Textbook of oral pathology, 4th Ed. Philadelphia: WB Saunders 1983
16. Dreizen S. Oral indications of the deficiency states. Postgrad Med 1971; 49:97–102
17. Hendler BH, Steinberg BJ, Brown S. Dental correlations. In: Rose LF, Kaye D (Eds). Internal medicine for dentistry. St. Louis: C. V. Mosby Co. 1983: 1090–1113
18. Wallerstein RO. Blood. In: Krupp MA, Chatton MJ. (Eds). Current medical diagnosis and treatment. Los Alton: Lange Medical Publications, 1983: 289–336
19. Bartley W. Vitamin C requirement of human adults. Medical Research Council Special Report Series no 280, vol 28. London: Her Majesty's Stationery Office, 1953
20. Dayal PK, Mani NJ. Clinical aspects of the tongue in anemia. Ann Dent 1979; 38:21–26
21. Grunskin SE, et al. Oral manifestations of uremia. Minn Med 1970; 53:495

CHAPTER 14

Diseases of the Tongue, Lips, and Salivary Glands

14.1 Diseases of the Tongue

R. S. Rogers, III

14.1.1 Macroglossia

Name of Disease. Macroglossia; enlarged tongue.

Definition. Macroglossia is a tongue enlarged out of proportion to the jaws and mouth [1].

Etiology. There are numerous causes for macroglossia. These are listed in Table 14.1.

Oral Manifestation. The edges of the tongue may be scalloped by pressure on the lingual aspect of the upper and lower teeth. If a few teeth are missing, the tongue may expand into the available space to produce a pseudotumor-like mass. If all the lower teeth are absent, the tongue will expand into the vacated area. This causes difficulty with adaptation to a denture. Depending upon the cause of the macroglossia, changes can occur in the tongue including surface morphology and changes noted by palpation, such as woody induration.

Associated Findings. These depend upon the condition. For example, with amyloidosis of the tongue, there may be purpura elsewhere in the skin or on examination of mucous membranes.

Table 14.1. Causes of macroglossia

Developmental	Congenital hypothyroidism, Down's syndrome
Tumors	Various mesenchymal tumors such as neurofibromas, lymphangiomas, hemangiomas, granular cell myoblastomas, and Kaposi's sarcoma, and squamous cell carcinoma
Infections	Syphilis, actinomycosis, histoplasmosis, tuberculosis
Metabolic	Hypothyroidism, amyloidosis
Miscellaneous	Sarcoidosis, angioedema, Melkersson-Rosenthal syndrome

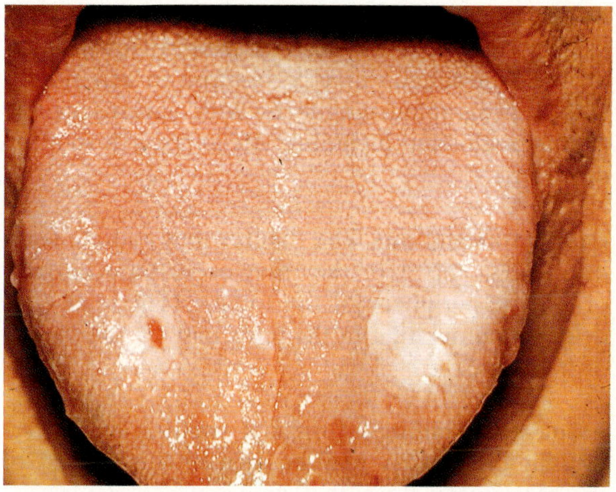

Fig. 14.1. Macroglossia. Note the enlarged tongue with purpuric macules and plaques of the anterior dorsal and ventral surface. This is the characteristic pattern for amyloidosis of the tongue

Microscopic Findings. This is dependent upon the cause of the macroglossia.

Diagnosis. In order to determine the cause of macroglossia, tests to exclude the various causes must be conducted. A biopsy specimen is often very helpful.

Differential Diagnosis. Enlargement of the tongue with few physical findings may be seen as a congenital condition, in association with Down's syndrome, or with congenital hypothyroidism. Purpura of the tongue is often associated with amyloidosis (Fig. 14.1). Erythema, edema, and hyperkeratosis may be seen in an enlarged tongue of a patient with Melkersson-Rosenthal syndrome.

Treatment. This depends upon the cause of the macroglossia.

14.1.2 Fissured Tongue

Name of Disease. Fissured tongue; lingua plicata; lingua scrotalis; grooved tongue.

Definition. The fissured tongue is thrown into deep fissures and folds which are lined by epithelium [2, 3].

Etiology: Fissured tongue may occur as a developmental defect. It is rare in neonates and increases in prevalence in the general population with each passing decade. It may also be seen in Down's syndrome. The tongue may be fissured in association with a geographic tongue or with various causes of macroglossia, including Melkersson-Rosenthal syndrome.

Oral Manifestations. The fissures may radiate from the median raphe, or they may occur paracentrally or on the periphery of the tongue (Fig. 14.2). The debris accumulating in the folds may be the source of halitosis.

Associated Findings. Orofacial swelling and intermittent facial palsy may be seen in the context of the Melkersson-Rosenthal syndrome.

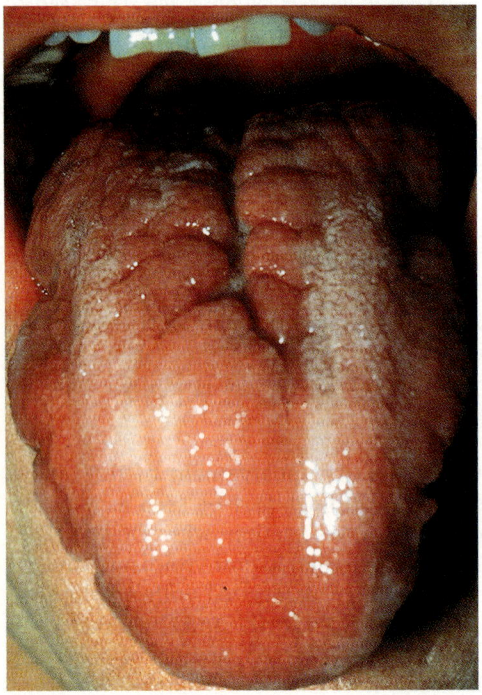

Fig. 14.2. Fissured tongue. Note the enlarged tongue with the scalloped lateral surface and the deep groove along the median raphe with radiating grooves. The tongue is also furred

Microscopic Findings. Non-caseating granulomas may be seen in the fissured tongue associated with Melkersson-Rosenthal syndrome.

Diagnosis. The clinician should examine the patient for signs of Down's syndrome or Melkersson-Rosenthal syndrome.

Differential Diagnosis. The fissured tongue may occur as an isolated defect, in families, or in association with medical conditions such as Down's syndrome or Melkersson-Rosenthal syndrome.

Treatment. The patient should brush with a dentifrice and a soft-bristled toothbrush. Care should be taken to brush down into the folds to reduce debris which can lead to halitosis.

14.1.3 Median Rhomboid Glossitis

Name of Disease. Median rhomboid glossitis; glossitis mediana rhomboidica; central papillary atrophy.

Definition: Median rhomboid glossitis is a disorder of the tongue characterized by a rhomboidal plaque in the central portion of the tongue, with surface changes of hypertrophy or atrophy [4, 5].

Etiology. Traditionally, median rhomboid glossitis has been considered a developmental defect of the tuberculum of the impar. Some authors believe that this is a site of chronic hyperplastic or atrophic candidiasis.

Oral Manifestations. In the central and middle third of the tongue, a rhomboidal or geometrically regular plaque is noted. The plaque can be elevated or depressed and can be covered by an atrophic or hyperplastic epithelium. The area may be reddened or pale. There may be fissures or even erosions present in the plaque (Fig. 14.3). Palpation can reveal a distinct firmness compared to the rest of the tongue tissue.

Associated Findings. The examiner should seek evidence of chronic candidiasis elsewhere in the skin and mucous membranes.

Microscopic Findings. The epithelium shows pseudoepitheliomatous hyperplasia. PAS stains will reveal invading hyphae of *Candida*. An inflammatory reaction of round cells is seen in the lamina propria, with inflammatory cells abutting and invading the epithelium.

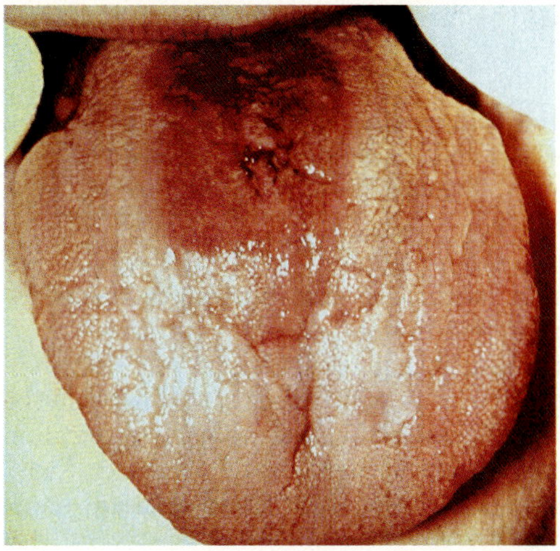

Fig. 14.3. Median rhomboid glossitis. Note the atrophic red plaque in the dorsal midline of the tongue. There is an erosion in the center of the plaque. The overall architecture of the changes extend anteriorly in a rhomboidal shape

Diagnosis. A biopsy specimen may be necessary to exclude squamous cell carcinoma. A scrub culture for *Candida* may be obtained.

Differential Diagnosis. Most clinicians and patients are concerned about the possibility of oral cancer. Chronic hyperplastic candidiasis should be considered in the differential diagnosis and treatment. No treatment is necessary once the diagnosis is established. The condition tends to be chronic, although it may spontaneously resolve. Topical or systemic anti-candidal treatment is only of moderate efficacy.

14.1.4 Black Hairy Tongue

Name of Disease. Black hairy tongue; lingua villosa nigra.

Definition. The papillae of the tongue are seen as long (hairy) and pigmented (black). The condition is more likely to occur in the central and middle third of the tongue [6, 7].

Etiology. The black pigment is due to overproduction of pigment byproducts by bacteria which flourish in situations of ecological imbalance such as following antibiotic therapy. Occasionally, there is hyperplasia of the filiform papillae (hairy tongue), which may be secondary to the chronic irritation.

Oral Manifestations. The surface of the tongue may be black to brown in color. The pigment appears to be superimposed upon the filiform papillae, which may be overly long. The tongue may also be furred (Fig. 14.4).

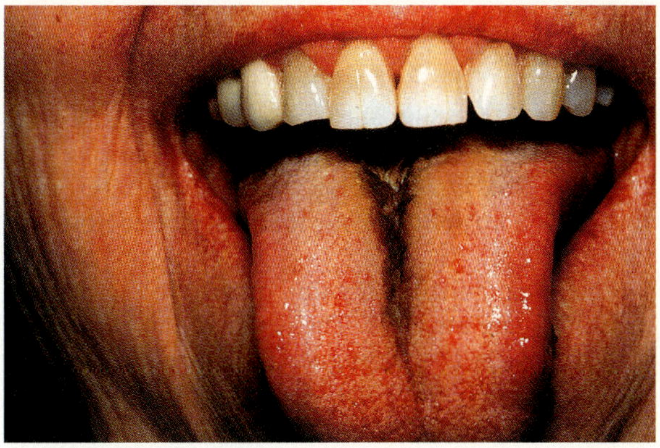

Fig. 14.4. Black hairy tongue. The median raphe is hyperplastic with elongated filiform papillae which are dark brown in color. The tongue is also furred

Associated Findings. None.

Microscopic Findings. The black color is due to byproducts of bacterial proliferation, and the papillae show long columns of epithelial cells covered by stratum corneum.

Diagnosis. The diagnosis is readily apparent upon inspection.

Differential Diagnosis. One must exclude the color changes of bismuth-containing products such as Pepto-Bismol. The patient should be reassured regarding the benign nature of this condition. The tongue may be brushed with 1% hydrogen peroxide to bleach the pigment. The tongue may be brushed with a dentifrice to reduce some of the fur and the pigment.

14.1.5 Geographic Tongue

Name of Disease. Geographic tongue; glossitis areata migrans; benign transitory plaques of the tongue.

Definition. The surface of the tongue reveals annular or arcuate lesions which appear similar to a bas-relief map [8, 9].

Etiology. Geographic tongue is a common glossitis affecting 2% of the population. It is the result of migratory transient atrophy of some filiform papillae with adjacent heavy exudate or hyperplasia of other filiform papillae. The base is erythematous from vasodilatation.

Oral Manifestations. The geographic tongue is characterized by alternating areas of hypertrophy and atrophy. The hypertrophic borders are white and raised. The atrophic adjacent areas are red and flatter (Fig. 14.5).
Fungiform papillae may stand out as the filiform papillae become atrophic. The lesions may be present on a small area of the tongue, or may be present over an extensive area of the tongue. The lesions may change in their position, migrating over the tongue in a matter of hours or days.

Associated Findings. Some believe that annulus migrans is a variant of geographic tongue and can occur in association with psoriasis. Other authors believe that the geographic tongue is seen more commonly in the atopic state.

Microscopic Findings. The microscopic picture of geographic tongue shows a tremendous inflammatory reaction with findings similar to pustular psoriasis of the skin with intraepithelial neutrophilic microabscesses and pseudoepitheliomatous hyperplasia, as well as a round-cell inflammatory infiltrate and vasodilatation of the lamina propria.

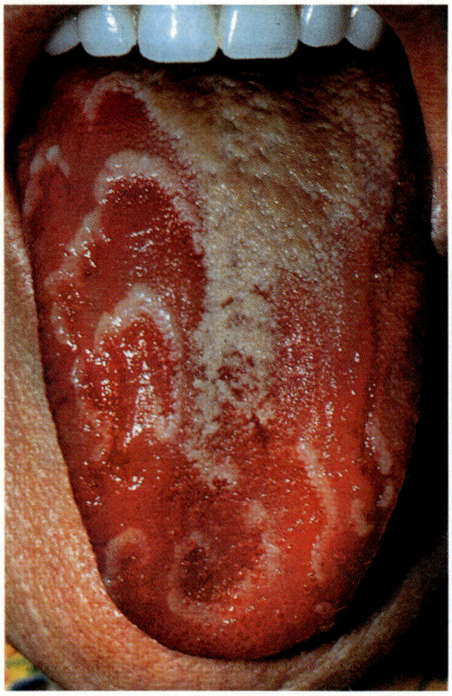

Fig. 14.5. Geographic tongue. The dorsum of the tongue is involved by alternating atrophic and hypertrophic changes, producing a bas-relief pattern. The atrophic areas are erythematous and tender

Diagnosis. The diagnosis is made by clinical inspection.

Differential Diagnosis. The potential association with psoriasis and atopic dermatitis should be considered.

Treatment. Most patients accept reassurance. For those patients with a sore burning tongue, the avoidance of spicy foods, gentle brushing of the tongue, the avoidance of harsh anti-bacterial mouthwashes, and soothing rinses with saline solutions may be considered. Occasionally, the topical application of fluorinated corticosteroids or treatment with mycostatin oral suspension may benefit some patients.

14.1.6 Glossodynia

Name of Disease. Glossodynia; stomatodynia; burning tongue; burning mouth syndrome.

Definition. Glossodynia is a syndrome of burning or stinging sensations of the tongue. Many patients have no physical findings, and other patients may have evidence of a geographic tongue, a smooth tongue, or a fissured tongue [10–12].

Etiology. Glossodynia is a multifactorial condition. Often, one or more potential causes may be identified by a careful clinical evaluation. Many patients suffer from psychiatric disease such as anxiety or depression. Other patients have cancerophobia. Still other patients have hematinic deficiencies, candidiasis, diabetes, xerostomia, or contact stomatitis.

Oral Manifestations. The tongue may be completely normal. Some patients with a tongue-thrusting habit will have a scalloped border of the tongue (Fig. 14.6). Other patients with nutritional deficiencies will show changes typical of those deficiencies. Some patients may have a geographic, fissured, or furred tongue.

Associated Findings. Glossodynia is a condition with many potential causes. The associated factors are traced back to the specific causes which are identified in Table 14.2.

Microscopic Findings. Microscopic findings depend on the specific causes.

Diagnosis. Table 14.3 depicts the diagnostic workup for a patient with glossodynia.

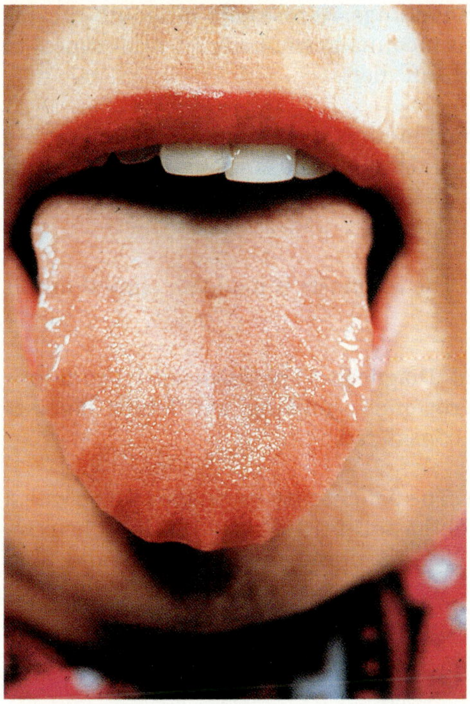

Fig. 14.6. Glossodynia. Note the scalloped edges of the lateral tongue. These result from a tongue-thrusting habit

Table 14.2. Differential diagnosis of glossodynia

1. Trauma: habits, dentures
2. Candidiasis: dentures, diabetes, antibiotics
3. Menopause: one-fourth complain of glossodynia
4. Diabetes: 10 % complain of glossodynia, need to change therapy
5. Nutritional: deficiency of iron, folic acid, vitamin B_{12}, B_6, zinc, anemia
6. Drugs: lithium, griseofulvin, antibiotics, metronidazole
7. Xerostomia: Sjögren's syndrome, age, drugs
8. Cancerophobia: careful exam, reassurance
9. Psychological: depression, anxiety
10. Miscellaneous: mercurialism, hiatus hernia, angina, neuralgia, dental disease, contact stomatitis

Table 14.3. Assessment of glossodynia

1. Evaluation for organic disease – seek more than one cause
a) Trauma: dentures, oral habits
b) Candidiasis: dentures, diabetes, antibiotics
c) Menopause: estrogen, FSH levels, bone loss
d) Diabetes: plasma glucose, medications
e) Nutritonal: iron, folic acid, vitamin B_{12}, B_6, zinc, anemia
f) Xerostomia: Sjögren's syndrome, drugs, age

Differential Diagnosis. The differential diagnosis includes those conditions associated with glossodynia or the burning mouth syndrome.

Treatment. Treatment is dependent upon identifying one or more underlying causes and addressing them. At least 70 % of patients with glossodynia experience sustantial improvement when all identifiable causes are corrected or treated.

14.1.7 Smooth Tongue

Name of Disease. Smooth tongue; bald tongue; atrophic tongue.

Definition. Smooth tongue results from atrophy of the filiform papillae. The background color may be pink, red, or magenta [13].

Etiology. The smooth tongue is due to nutritional deficiencies such as vitamin B_{12}, folic acid, or iron deficiencies. It may be seen in the context of a malabsorption state or in the Riley-Day dysautonia syndrome.

Oral Manifestations. The tongue is smooth and the papillae are absent. The underlying color of the tongue may show through, or the tongue may be pale (iron deficiency), red (folate deficiency), or magenta (vitamin B_{12} deficiency) (Fig. 14.7).

Associated Findings. Koilonychia with iron deficiency; tremulousness with vitamin B_{12} deficiency; pèrleche with other vitamin deficiencies.

Microscopic Findings. Biopsy of the tongue reveals a thinned epithelium which has a smooth surface no longer thrown into the large folds typical of the papillae of the tongue.

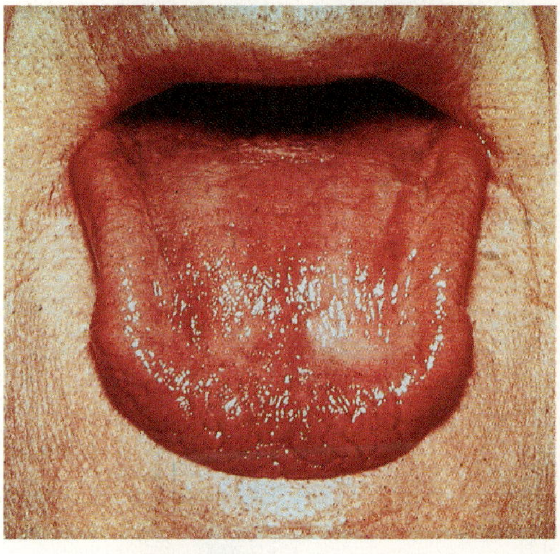

Fig. 14.7. Smooth tongue. Note the atrophic and erythematous tongue dorsum plus the muscle atrophy in this patient with pernicious anemia. Pèrleche is also present at the labial commissures

Diagnosis. A smooth tongue should indicate to the clinician the need to search for nutritional deficiencies or associated conditions.

Differential Diagnosis. Differential diagnosis of smooth tongue includes nutritional deficiencies, gluten-sensitive enteropathy, and the Riley-Day dysautonia syndrome.

Treatment. The nutritional deficiencies should be identified and replaced. The diet should be soft and limited in hot or spicy foods in order to reduce the symptoms secondary to the atrophic tongue surface.

14.1.8 Furred Tongue

Name of Disease. Furred tongue; hairy tongue.

Definition. The surface of the tongue is thickened. The color may be variable from white to black [14].

Etiology. The furred tongue results from hypertrophy of the filiform papillae. Desquamated epithelium is trapped next to the hypertrophic filiform papillae, producing a large plaque. Halitosis can result from degeneration of the food and epithelial debris collecting in the plaque. The furred tongue is noted with febrile illnesses and in smokers. It is noted in patients who have a soft diet and who do not eat a diet high in roughage and fiber.

Oral Manifestations. The surface of the tongue is thickened. The color may be variable from white to black (Fig. 14.8).

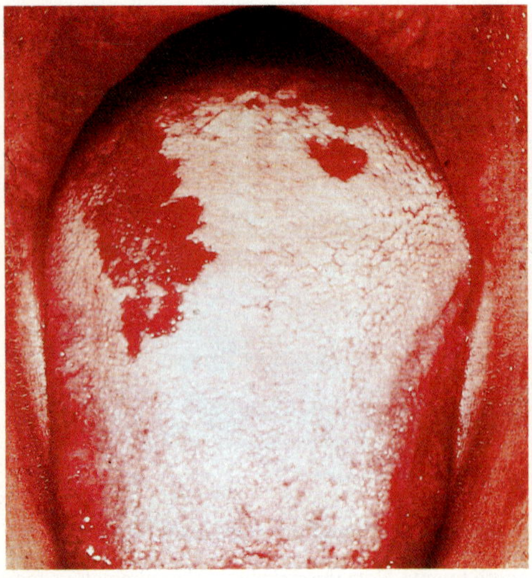

Fig. 14.8. Furred tongue. Note the hypertrophic white plaque covering the tongue dorsum

Associated Findings. Xerostomia in mouth-breathers. Palatitis nicotina in smokers. Edentulousness in patients on soft diets.

Microscopic Findings. The filiform papillae are hypertrophic, and the stratum corneum is covered with debris. Minimal inflammation is noted in the lamina propria.

Diagnosis. The diagnosis is made on clinical examination.

Differential Diagnosis. The associated conditions such as xerostomia, smoking, and febrile illnesses should be considered.

Treatment. The patient may brush the tongue with a dentifrice and a soft-bristled toothbrush to help remove the "fur". A diet high in roughage and fiber will reduce the fur on the surface of the tongue.

14.1.9 Varices of the Tongue

Name of Disease. Varices of the tongue; sublingual varices.

Definition. Tortuous veins are noted on the undersurface of the tongue bilaterally.

Etiology. Vasodilatation and venous ectasia occur with aging.

Oral Manifestations. Tortuous veins are noted on the ventral surface of the tongue. Occasionally, a single varix may be noted as a soft purple papule which indents with firm palpation (Fig. 14.9).

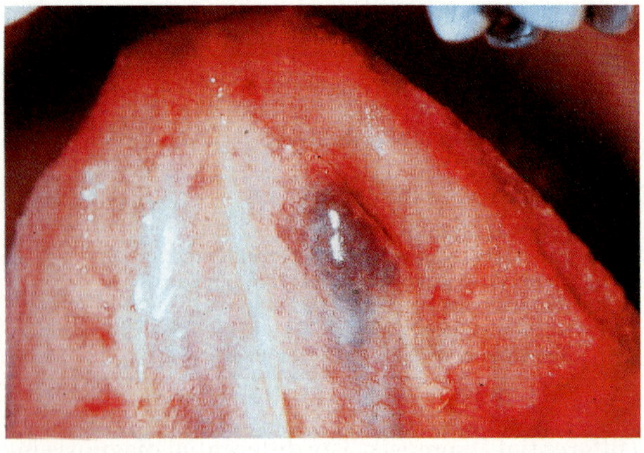

Fig. 14.9. Varices of the tongue. Note the large purple varix of the right ventral tongue and the smaller linear erythematous macules of the right ventral tongue

Associated Findings. Occasionally with a similar appearance to the lateral border or the tongue or on the labial mucosa.

Microscopic Findings. Dilated venous blood vessels are noted in the lamina propria.

Diagnosis. Sublingual varices is a clinical differential.

Differential Diagnosis. The clinician should be sure to exclude hereditary hemorrhagic telangiectasia syndrome. These lesions are small punctate telangiectatic mats which can occasionally be a 1.0–2.0-mm papule. The sublingual varices are larger, longer, compressible papules and nodules.

Treatment. No treatment is necessary once the proper diagnosis has been established.

14.1.10 Herpetic Geometric Glossitis

Name. Herpetic geometric glossitis.

Definition. Painful linear fissured glossitis caused by the herpes simplex virus occurring in immunocompromised hosts [15].

Etiology. Herpes simplex virus.

Oral Manifestations. Painful linear fissures on the central tongue dorsum which have a geometric pattern with right angle radiations. The presentation is atypical since vesicles are rare, ulcerations occur rapidly, the lateral tongue borders are spared, and other oral lesions are absent (Fig. 14.10).

Associated Findings. Immunodeficiency.

Microscopic Findings. Intraepithelial vesicles with multinucleated giant cells and superficial ulcerations.

Diagnosis. Typical pattern. Positive culture for herpes simplex virus.

Differential Diagnosis. The clinician should exclude other infections such as candidiasis.

Treatment. Herpetic geometric glossitis responds promptly to systemic antiviral therapy such as acyclovir 200 mg every 4 h for 7–10 days. It may recur after clearing.

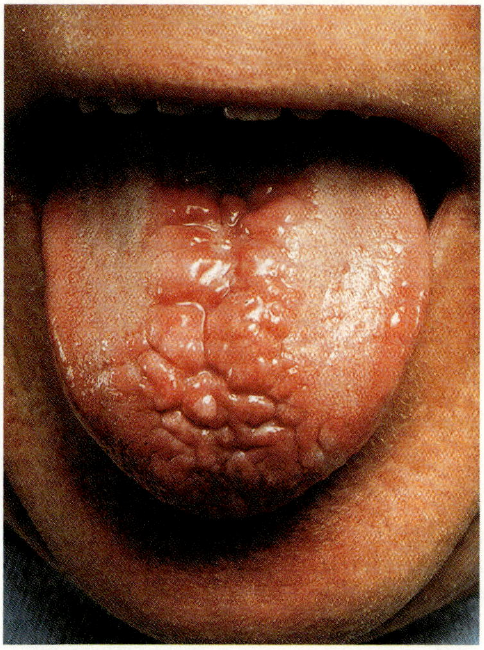

Fig. 14.10. Herpetic geometric glossitis. Note the lobulated, grooved dorsal tongue with radiating grooves and a vesicle of the anterior tongue dorsum

14.1.11 Microglossia

D. Ioannides and D. Antoniades

Definition/Etiology. Microglossia or hypoglossia is a rare developmental condition characterized by an abnormally small tongue (Fig. 14.11). Rarely, the entire tongue may be missing [16, 17].

Oral Manifestations/Associated Findings. Mild degrees of microglossia may be difficult to diagnose. However, most cases are associated with one of

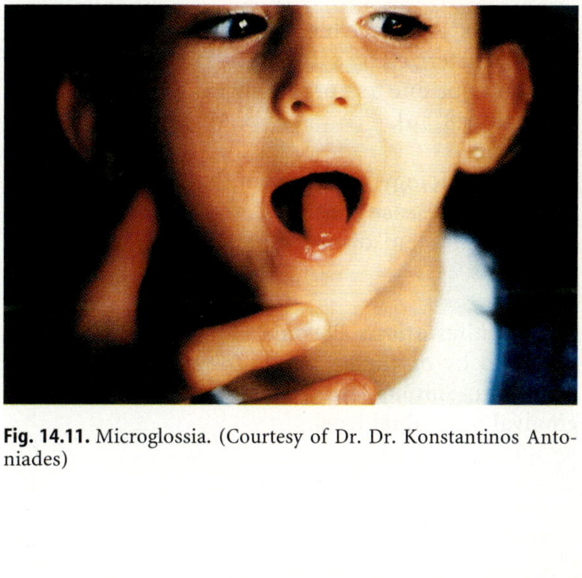

Fig. 14.11. Microglossia. (Courtesy of Dr. Dr. Konstantinos Antoniades)

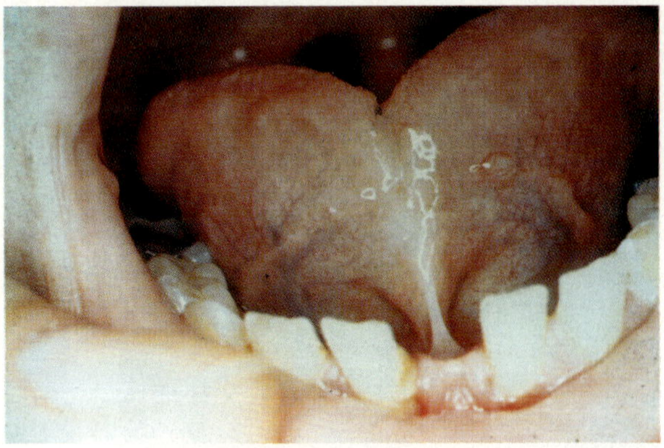

Fig. 14.12. Ankyloglossia in an adult

the oromandibular limb hypogenesis syndromes. Microglossia is also frequently related to hypoplasia of the mandible. Speech development is usually normal.

Treatment. Surgery and orthodontics may improve oral function.

14.1.12 Ankyloglossia

Ankyloglossia or tongue-tie (Fig. 14.12) is a symptomless congenital abnormality of little consequence. The tongue is difficult to use to cleanse food away from the vestibules and teeth and this is sometimes annoying to the patient. Ankyloglossia does not seem to interfere with speech [16, 17].

14.1.13 Plasmacellular Glossitis

I. Ghersetich and T. M. Lotti

Definition. Plasmacellular glossitis is a rare condition characterized by a diffuse or localized erythema of the tongue due to a predominantly plasmacellular infiltrate [18, 19].

Etiology. Etiology is unknown, but major risk factors for this disease are considered allergic reactions, endocrine system disorders, and *Candida albicans* infections.

Oral Manifestations. Plasmacellular glossitis is characterized by erythema of the tongue with burning sensation. Similar lesions may develop also at the gingival and labial level.

Differential Diagnosis. Differential diagnosis includes candidiasis, geographic tongue, and allergic reactions.

Diagnosis. Biopsy and microscopic examination is the only method to make a certain diagnosis.

Treatment. Plasmacellular glossitis may last for a long time. Only symptomatic therapy is required, but sometimes antihistamine drugs or topical nystatin may be helpful.

14.1.14 Hypertrophy of Papillae

14.1.14.1 *Hypertrophy of Foliate Papillae*

Foliate papillae consist of 4–11 parallel ridges, alternating with deep grooves in the mucosa, on the lateral margins on the posterior part of the tongue. There are taste buds on their lateral walls. These papillae may enlarge and become inflamed after chronic local irritant factors or infections [20]. The patient may feel burning and may be worried by the development of a cancer. No therapy is required, but the patient should be reassured of the benign course of this affection.

14.1.14.2 *Hypertrophy of Circumvallate Papillae*

Circumvallate papillae are localized on the posterior part of the dorsum of the tongue, they number 8–12, in a V formation. Each papilla is surrounded by a deep groove into which open the ducts of serous minor salivary glands. Hypertrophy of such papillae determines the appearance of well-circumscribed, usually asymptomatic, red nodules which may be noticed by the patient and be a cause of worry. No therapy is required [21].

14.1.14.3 *Hypertrophy of Fungiform Papillae*

Fungiform papillae are mushroom-shaped, red structures covered by non-keratinized epithelium and localized along the anterior side of the dorsum of the tongue.

These papillae may occasionally become inflamed and enlarged, producing a sensation of burning and pain, especially at the tip of the tongue. Smoking and alcohol abuse, hot or spicy food, or mechanical trauma may predispose to this condition. The only therapy is the avoidance of such predisposing factors [22].

14.2 Diseases of the Lips

R. S. Rogers, III

14.2.1 Angular Cheilitis

Name of Disease. Angular cheilitis; pèrleche.

Definition. Inflammation in the form of atrophy, erythema, ulceration, crusting, scaling, and fissures may be noted at the commissures of the lips [23–26].

Etiology. Angular cheilitis is a multifactorial condition. It is frequently seen in HIV-infected patients where one in ten develop an opportunistic infection due to *Candida albicans*. It is often seen in the elderly and the immunoincompetent host where *Candida* and *Staphylococcus aureus* are often isolated from lesions as a primary or mixed infection. This situation may be exacerbated by diabetes mellitus, internal malignancy, and anemia. Angular cheilitis may also be a non-infectious entity such as intertrigo, which is the result of mechanical irritation. Finally, angular cheilitis may be the result of a nutritional deficiency or another dermatological condition such as atopic dermatitis.

Oral Manifestations. The clinical manifestations may be confined to the corners of the mouth, or extend beyond the vermilion border onto the skin in the form of fissures. Atrophy, erythema, ulceration, crusting, and scaling are clinical findings with or without fissures (Fig. 14.13). In long-standing lesions, suppuration and granulation tissue may develop. Unilateral lesions are usually induced by trauma and are short-lived. Bilateral lesions often represent infectious etiology or an underlying disease process and may be long standing.

Associated Findings. In immunoincompetent individuals, other manifestations of immunodeficiencies such as oral candidiasis, oral hairy leukoplakia, and Kaposi's sarcoma may be noted in the oral examination. In patients with single or mixed infections as a cause for angular cheilitis, there are usually no associated findings. In those patients whose angular cheilitis is due to a nutritional deficiency, careful examination of the tongue may reveal helpful clues. Atrophy of the epithelium with a depapillated pale tongue often indicates iron deficiency. A depapillated, glossy, red tongue may indicate a folic acid deficiency. Angular cheilitis is characteristic of ariboflavinosis and is accompanied by a reddish-purple tongue with flattened filiform and enlarged fungiform papillae. A vitamin B_{12} deficiency may also be accompanied by a magenta atrophic tongue and angular cheilitis. In the primary irritant form of angular cheilitis, there may be evidence of excessive salivation, loss of vertical dimension seen in denture wearers, denture stomatitis, overhanging skin folds due to the aging process, dry mouth, or perioral dermatitis.

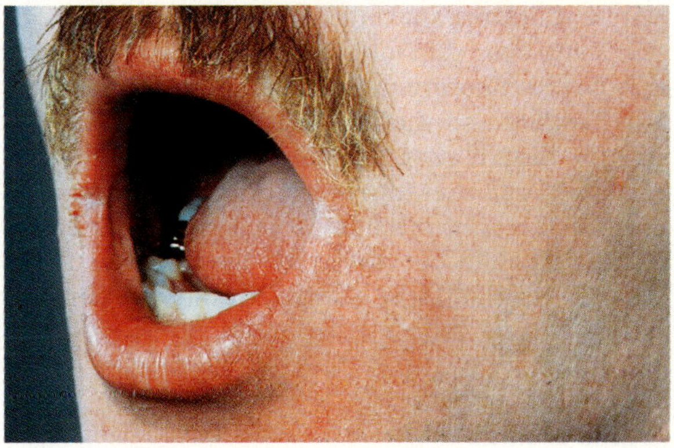

Fig. 14.13. Angular cheilitis. Note the atrophy with hyperkeratosis of the left labial commissure and the fissured dermatitic changes of the right labial commissure

Microscopic Findings. There are no specific histopathologic findings other than identifying microorganisms in special stains.

Diagnosis. The clinician should consider immunocompetency and evaluate patients with appropriate testing for HIV infection and immunocompetency. Cultures may be utilized to identify *Candida albicans* and/or *Staphylococcus aureus* organisms. Sensitivities may be ordered on the cultures. For those patients with nutritional deficiencies, serum or red blood cell assays for the specific hematinic levels may be ordered.

Differential Diagnosis. Patch testing may be helpful in excluding allergic contact dermatitis. The major elements of the differential diagnosis are included in the separation of the different forms of angular cheilitis from each other. As treatment for those patients who are immunoincompetent and suffering from a chronic, low-grade infectious process, anti-yeast therapy in the form of mycostatin or miconazole cream after meals and at bedtime, may be used. For mixed infections with both *Candida* and *Staphylococcus aureus*, topical miconazole after meals and at bedtime is appropriate. Topical mupirocin or Polysporin may be effective in staphylococcal-induced angular cheilitis.

Habitual licking, sucking on objects, or seepage of saliva into deep skin folds at the corner of the mouth may be contributory to pèrleche. Dentures may harbor *Candida* and should be properly cleaned. Rinsing the mouth after treatment with inhalant corticosteroids can prevent recurrent episodes of candidiasis. Sources of mechanical factors leading to intertrigo should be corrected. Specific hematinic deficiencies should be identified and the hematin should be replaced.

14.2.2 Actinic Cheilitis

Name of Disease. Actinic cheilitis; solar cheilitis; squamous cell carcinoma in situ of the lips.

Definition. Actinic cheilitis is a premalignant condition involving the lower lip [27–32].

Etiology. Actinic cheilitis is the result of long-term damage with ultraviolet light. For this reason, it usually affects the lower lip and not the upper lip.

Oral Manifestation. Actinic cheilitis is manifested by a hyperkeratotic, desquamating disorder with erythema, crusting, erosions, and intermittent bleeding. It may appear as a smooth or scaly friable patch, or can involve the entire lip. At times, the border between the vermilion and the skin or mucosa becomes indistinct (Fig. 14.14). The adjacent mucosal epithelium may display leukoplakia, atrophy, and fissures. The lip is dry and wrinkled with gray to white changes in pigmentation. There is sparing of the oral commissures, and the upper lip is seldom involved.

Associated Findings. Actinic keratoses or skin cancers elsewhere on the head and neck areas.

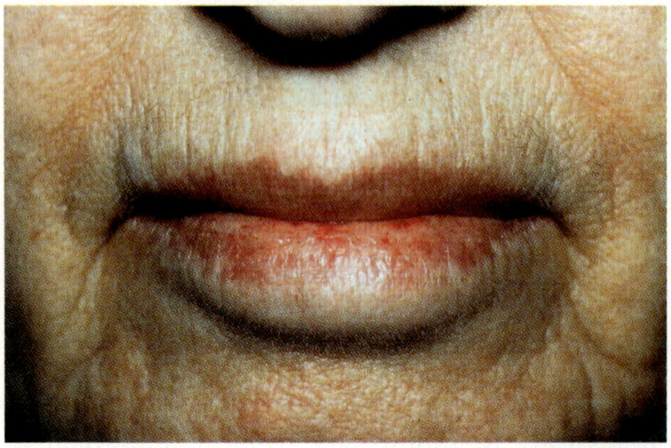

Fig. 14.14. Actinic cheilitis. Note the erythematous, atrophic, and scaly vermilion involving the lower lip exclusively. The border between the vermilion and lower lip skin is indistinct

Microscopic Findings. The histologic picture of epithelial hyperkeratosis, parakeratosis and acanthosis, along with dysplastic changes ranging from atypia to carcinoma in situ of the epithelium, may be noted. Basophilic degeneration of collagen and elastic fibers, along with an infiltration of lymphocytes and plasma cells scattered in the epidermis, suggest actinic damage.

Diagnosis. A lip biopsy may be necessary to establish the nature of the condition and the degree of dysplasia.

Differential Diagnosis. Allergic contact or photocontact cheilitis may be considered. Contact cheilitis is usually more acute than actinic cheilitis. Lichen planus should be considered, along with lupus erythematosus. A biopsy will usually differentiate these conditions from actinic cheilitis.

Treatment. Treatment rests on the successful removal of the premalignant epithelium and replacing it with healthy tissue. This could be accomplished by various modalities employing two methods: Re-epithelialization by secondary intention healing, or by surgical excision with advancement of a mucosal flap. Induction of re-epithelialization is accomplished with chemoexfoliants such as topical 5FU and topical tretinoin, trichloracetic acid, electrodesiccation and currettage, and CO_2-laser ablation. CO_2-laser ablation offers the advantages of being simple and easy to use, with excellent postoperative results. The rigorous and regular use of sunscreen should be encouraged to prevent further actinic damage.

14.2.3 Exfoliative Cheilitis

Name of Disease. Exfoliative cheilitis.

Definition. Exfoliative cheilitis is a peculiar chronic inflammatory disorder characterized by hyperkeratosis and desquamation of the vermilion epithelium [33–35].

Etiology. Exfoliative cheilitis is often attributed to factitious activity resulting in self-induced trauma such as repetitive biting, picking, or unconscious licking of the lips. An underlying psychiatric disturbance or personality disorder is suspected. A preoccupation with the lips is prevalent in some individuals, while others may exhibit a state of denial. Treatment is difficult and patient denial of potential factitial causes is common. A psychiatric consultation may be beneficial or may not be acceptable

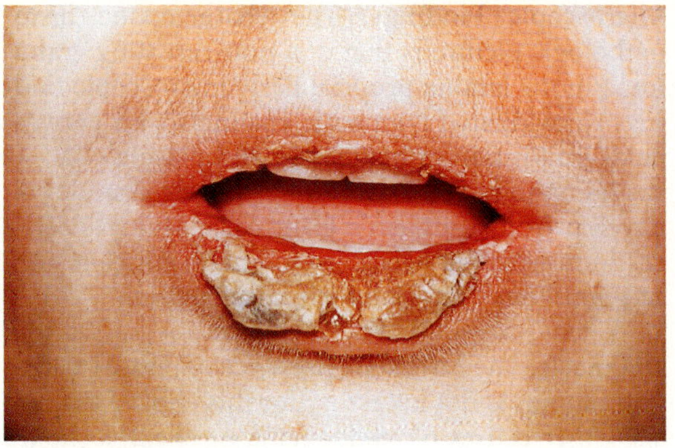

Fig. 14.15. Exfoliative cheilitis. Note the heavy scale-crust of both lips with sparing of the perioral skin

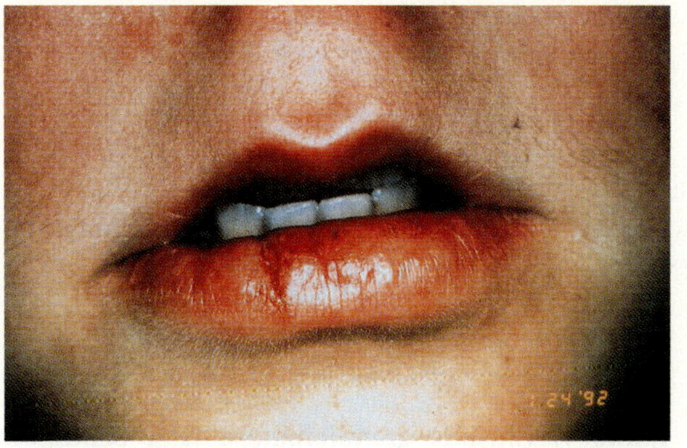

Fig. 14.16. Cheilitis glandularis. Note the erythema, edema, and fissuring limited to the lower lip vermilion

to the patient. Exacerbations have been associated with stress and have been shown to regress with psychotherapy or anti-anxiolytic or antidepressant treatment.

Oral Manifestations. Scaling and desquamation of the vermilion epithelium, along with crusting and erosions may be seen. There may be bizarre yellow hyperkeratotic or thick hemorrhagic crusts (Fig. 14.15).

Associated Findings. None.

Microscopic Findings. Nonspecific cheilitis may be noted.

Diagnosis. A biopsy of the specimen may be indicated to exclude other potential causes of cheilitis. A MMPI may direct the clinician toward a psychiatric disturbance or personality disorder.

14.2.4 Cheilitis Glandularis

Name of Disease. Cheilitis glandularis; simple cheilitis glandularis; superficial suppurative cheilitis glandularis (Baelz); deep suppurative cheilitis glandularis (Volkman).

Definition. Cheilitis glandularis is a rare, chronic inflammatory disorder of labial salivary glands in which there his hypersecretion and ductal ectasia present in the affected lip [36–39].

Etiology. Sunlight exposure, emotional problems, the atopic diathesis, and familial macrocheilia have been identified as exacerbating factors.

Oral Manifestations. The lower lip of adult males is usually affected. The lip appears swollen, enlarged, and everted, exposing superficial puncta of the salivary ducts along the mucosal vermilion border. Fissuring may be present (Fig. 14.16). The puncta may be macular or papular in appearance and may be topped with red, white, or black dots. The salivary ducts release a thick, sticky substance that forms a crust on the lip surface as it dries. If the lip is manipulated, nodularity may be felt and droplets of the viscous fluid may be expressed from the ductal openings. Ruptured ducts appear as mucocysts and depending upon the degree of inflammation, the lip may be nontender to painful with a decrease in mobility.

Associated Findings. No specific associated findings are present.

Microscopic Findings. Nonspecific findings are present, ranging from no changes to hypertrophy and hyperplasia of the minor salivary glands with ductal ectasia.

Diagnosis. The diagnosis of cheilitis glandularis is a diagnosis of exclusion of other causes of cheilitis. The simple type consists of multiple asymptomatic papular lesions containing dilated minor salivary gland ducts. The superficial suppurative type (Baelz) also contains asymptomatic lesions; however, these are indurated with crust formation and may exhibit superficial erosions. The deep suppurative type (Volkman) includes an infectious component with abscesses and fistulous tract formation.

Treatment. A wide range of treatments have been used with limited success. Systemic antibiotics and systemic corticosteroid therapy are palliative and provide symptomatic relief. Other conservative approaches such as systemic antihistamines, lip balms, sunscreens, and cryosurgery have been tried with limited success. Some authors advocate vermilionectomy to re-establish esthetics and function. Surgery is the treatment of choice in advanced disease because of the risk of squamous cell carcinoma developing in association with this disorder.

14.2.5 Cheilitis Granulomatosa

Name of Disease. Cheilitis granulomatosa; Miescher's cheilitis granulomatosa.

Definition. Cheilitis granulomatosa is a rare idiopathic inflammatory disorder of the lips [40–46].

Etiology. Cheilitis granulomatosa is a condition which may have several causes or for which no cause may be identified. The clinician should consider inflammatory bowel disease, sarcoidosis, contact cheilitis, and tooth-associated infections in the differential diagnosis. Cheilitis granulomatosa is one element of orofacial granulomatosis and of the Melkersson-Rosenthal syndrome.

Oral Manifestation. Cheilitis granulomatosa is an episodic, non-tender, swelling and enlargement of one or both lips. The upper lip is involved slightly more often than the lower lip. The lip may feel soft or firm, or even nodular on palpation. The normal lip architecture is altered by the presence of lymphedema and the non-caseating granulomas in the lamina propria. Involvement of the sublingual, palatal, gingival, and buccal mucosa may be seen. The swelling eventually becomes permanent, resulting in facial distortion and functional disability. Scaling and a ruddy color to the lip are present at this time (Fig. 14.17).

Associated Findings. Intermittent facial palsy and lingua plicata are the two other components of the Melkersson-Rosenthal syndrome. Inflammatory bowel disease may be noted in patients.

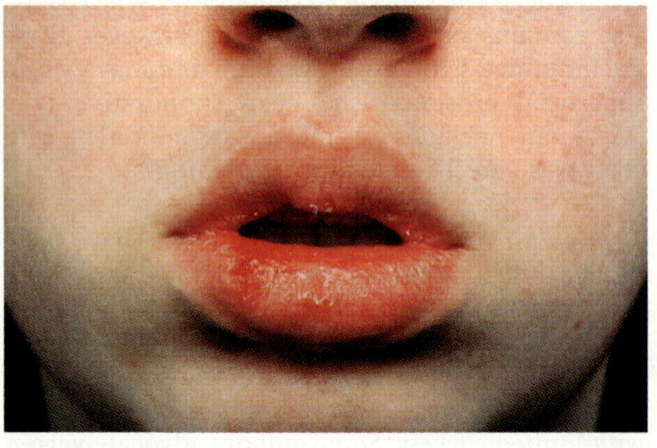

Fig. 14.17. Cheilitis granulomatosa. Note the erythema and edema of both lips with prominent perioral ridges. Also note the fine scaling of the vermilion

Microscopic Findings. The characteristic histopathologic picture is that of a non-caseating granuloma in the lamina propria. Early microscopic findings show dilated lymphatic channels with perivascular infiltration of histiocytes and plasma cells. As the lesion matures, small non-caseating granulomas develop from Langhan's giant cells. Multiple serial sections are often necessary to obtain a higher yield of granulomas for histologic confirmation.

Diagnosis. The histologic presence of non-caseating granulomas is not necessary for this clinical diagnosis. Other causes of angioedema or cheilitis should be excluded.

Differential Diagnosis. Other elements of Melkersson-Rosenthal syndrome should be sought: intermittent facial palsy, and lingua plicata. The firm induration of the lip is characteristic.

Treatment. The obscure pathophysiology has led to various trials of therapy that have resulted in success in some patients. Intralesional corticosteroid injections, a variety of nonsteroidal anti-inflammatory agents, and systemic administration of antibiotics and corticosteroids have all resulted in improvement. At times, facial nerve decompression may be necessary to relieve the associated facial palsy. The removal of odontogenic infectious foci has been shown to shorten the duration of the disease. Patch testing with identification of specific allergens and the removal of those allergens has resulted in a clearing of this condition.

Reduction cheiloplasty followed by intralesional triamcinolone and systemic tetracycline, 500 mg t.i.d., may improve the cosmetic deformity. Surgery should be withheld until the disease is stable. Many authors believe that a combination of systemic corticosteroids and tetracycline is considered more efficacious than either alone. Recently, metroindazole has been reported to be effective in some patients with Crohn's disease.

14.2.6 Plasma Cell Cheilitis

Name of Condition. Plasma cell cheilitis; plasma cell orificial mucositis.

Definition. Plasma cell cheilitis is a rare inflammatory disorder with a characteristic band-like infiltrate of plasma cells in the upper dermis or lamina propria [47–50].

Etiology. This is a benign idiopathic disorder which is not associated with any known dermatosis, although

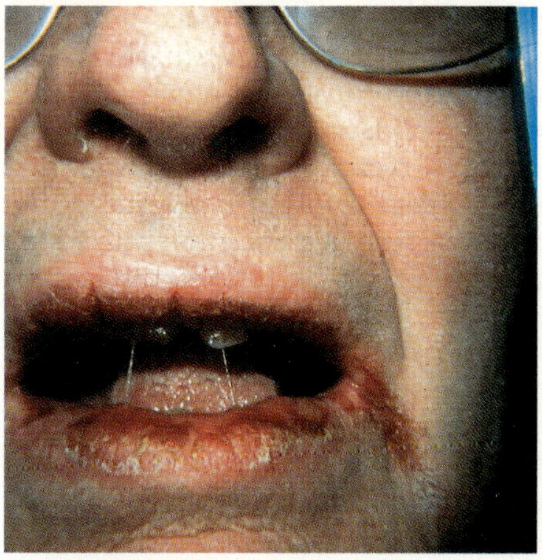

Fig. 14.18. Plasma cell cheilitis. Note the erythema, edema, scale, and fissuring of both the upper and lower lip with extension to the commissures and perioral skin

the histologic pictures are shared with neoplasms, chronic infections, and allergic contact cheilitis.

Oral Manifestations. The lip shows a glistening, red lower lip which may extend onto the oral mucosa. The lip may be thick and fissured with ulceration, and may be accompanied by tenderness and sensitivity to certain foods (Fig. 14.18). The rare tumor-like variant, plasmoacanthoma, is a warty manifestation reportedly following trauma.

Microscopic Findings. The characteristic histopathology is that of a band-like inflammatory infiltrate, consisting largely of plasma cells which abut and then invade the epithelium.

Associated Findings. The clinician should consider plasma cell dyscrasias and underlying myeloma, as well as other hematologic diseases.

Diagnosis. The erythematous squamous swollen lip and periorificial tissue is rather distinctive.

Differential Diagnosis. Patch tests should be performed to exclude contact hypersensitivity. Infections such as candidiasis should be sought. A denture may be a source of seeding of a chronic candidal cheilitis.

Treatment. Intralesional or topical corticosteroids are beneficial in controlling the process in some patients, or topical or systemic treatment of candidiasis, when appropriate, can be helpful. Identification and removal of contact hypersensitivity allergens is important.

14.3 Diseases of the Salivary Glands

J. M. Hall and R. S. Rogers, III

14.3.1 Necrotizing Sialometaplasia

Name of Disease. Necrotizing sialometaplasia.

Definition. Necrotizing sialometaplasia (NS) is a benign, reactive, inflammatory disease of salivary glands that mimics malignancy both clinically and microscopically [51–57].

Etiology. Any factor that disrupts the flow of blood to a major or minor salivary gland or mucoserous gland of the upper respiratory tract may cause NS. Based on microscopic changes, it appears that ischemia is the underlying cause. These findings have been reproduced in experimental animals. Traumatic injury from dental injections or ill-fitting dentures, swelling due to upper respiratory infections, association with local tumors or cysts, or prior surgical procedures have been implicated as predisposing factors. On the hard palate, the most common site of NS, any agent, physical, chemical, or infectious, which can cause swelling around the greater palatine foramen may compromise the blood supply and lead to ischemic necrosis. In the major salivary glands, disruption of the vascular supply after surgery accounts for 86 % of cases.

Pathogenesis. Infarction of the salivary gland results in necrosis and resultant inflammation. Sequestration of the necrotic tissue occurs with ulcer formation. Healing of the epithelial defect is seen as pseudoepitheliomatous hyperplasia and downward proliferation of rete pegs that can be seen fusing with the salivary ducts and mucous acini undergoing squamous metaplasia. Repair of the salivary glands is initially accomplished by ductal and acinar squamous metaplasia, and finally by replacement with fibrous connective tissue.

Oral Manifestations. NS can involve any mucous gland of the respiratory tract. The original description was of seven ulcerative lesions involving the hard palate. The posterior hard palate remains the primary site, followed by the junction of the hard and soft palate. The parotid is the most likely site for major salivary gland involvement, which is seen in 10 % of cases. Other oral locations reported include the lower lip, retromolar area, and the tongue. A deep-seated ulcer is the most common sign (Fig. 14.19, 14.20); however, a non-ulcerated swelling

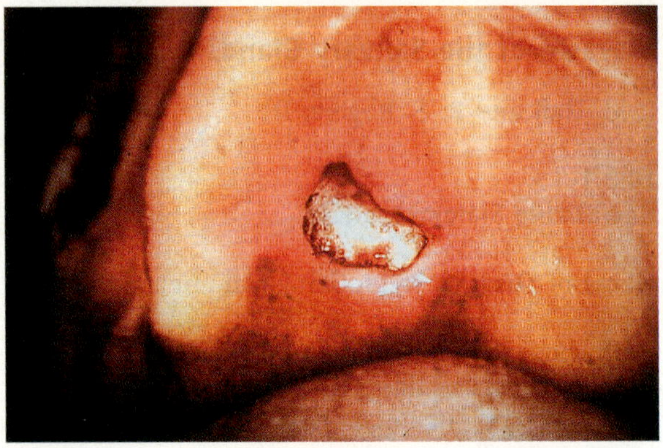

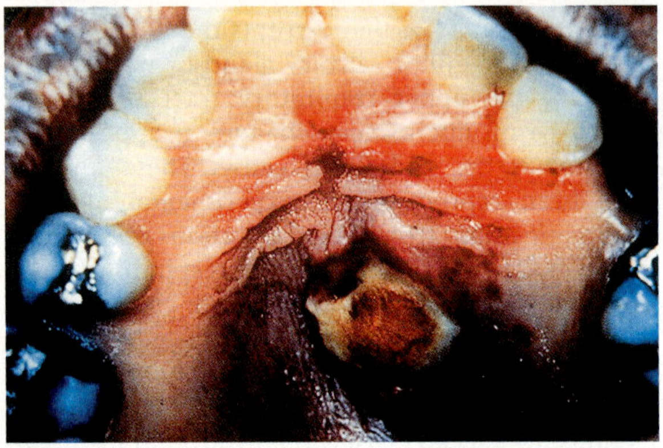

Fig. 14.19, 14.20. Necrotizing sialometaplasia. Deep necrotic ulcer on the hard palate. (Photographic credit, Michael Kahn, DDS)

or mass may be seen in one-third to one-half of patients with an average size of 1.8 cm. The lesions are usually accompanied by pain, although some lesions can be asymptomatic. Men develop NS twice as often as women at an average age of 46 years.

Associated Findings. NS is a local process without systemic manifestations. Saucerization of underlying palatal bone is a possible radiographic finding but not common. NS has also been found in conjunction with another lesion in 19 % of cases where the tumor or cyst probably caused a disruption of the blood supply, resulting in ischemic necrosis and sialometaplasia.

Microscopic Findings. Specific diagnostic criteria exist for the diagnosis of NS. These include: (1) lobular necrosis of salivary tissue, (2) granulation tissue with acute and chronic inflammation, (3) squamous metaplasia of ducts and acini, and (4) maintenance of salivary gland globular morphology. Earlier lesions are most apt to exhibit coagulation necrosis of glandular acini, with later development of squamous metaplasia and reactive fibrosis. Serous and mucous salivary glands and sinonasal glands are not as likely to show acinar necrosis, but often display changes that suggest acinar atrophy. Squamous metaplasia is a constant finding. Pseudoepitheliomatous hyperplasia of the surface epithelium will sometimes merge with the ductal squamous metaplasia. Bland cytology is the norm, but reactive atypia can be seen in association with severe inflammation.

Diagnosis. A history of trauma might suggest a reactive rather than neoplastic process, but histologic examination is the only reliable method of diagnosis. Because of the spectrum of microscopic findings, the diagnosis of NS requires recognition, even in the absence of acinar necrosis.

Differential Diagnosis. NS is most often mistaken for a tumorous process, usually a salivary gland neoplasm or squamous cell carcinoma. Over 50 % of cases are clinically presumed to be neoplasms. The microscopic diagnosis can also prove problematic, with mucoepidermoid carcinoma or squamous cell carcinoma being the most likely misdiagnoses. Helpful criteria for distinguishing NS from malignancy are: (1) maintenance of the overall lobular architecture, (2) bland appearance of the squamous epithelium, (3) simultaneous metaplasia of ducts and mucinous acini, and (4) inflammatory response. The preservation of the lobular morphology is the most important criterion for the diagnosis of NS. Healed NS can present the same histopathologic characteristics as chronic sialadenitis or degenerative changes seen with aging.

Treatment. Surgical management consisting of excisional or incisional biopsy is the recommended treatment. After diagnosis, no further therapy is required. The average healing time is 5–6 weeks. Follow-up is advised until healing is complete.

14.3.2 Sialolithiasis

Name of Disease. Sialolithiasis; salivary duct stone; salivary duct calculus.

Definition. Sialoliths are calcifications that develop within the ductal system of salivary glands [58–61].

Etiology. The cause of sialolithiasis is unknown. The formation of ductal calculi does not appear to be related to any systemic defect in calcium or phosphorus metabolism. Infection or inflammation may produce a change in the mucoid elements in saliva that favors the deposition of calcium. Stones develop in about 60 % of patients with chronic sialadenitis.

Pathogenesis. Salivary stones form from the accumulation of debris that is eventually transformed into a resinous mass. Mineral salts, composed largely of calcium phosphate, are deposited in the matrix, which grows by addition of concentric layers of organic material. The central nidus may consist of mucin, foreign bodies, bacteria, or ductal epithelial cells.

Oral Manifestations. Characteristic to this disease in the major salivary glands are recurrent bouts of pain, possibly severe, and swelling of the involved gland. This is typically concurrent with meals due to the stimulation of salivary flow. Swelling gradually subsides as secretions escape. Severity varies with the degree of obstruction and amount of resultant back pressure; symptoms, however, are more marked when the stone is in the duct rather than in the substance of the gland. Most cases involve the submandibular (submaxillary) gland where the long tortuous path of Wharton's duct and the viscous mucoid secretions contribute to the formation of salivary calculi (Fig. 14.21). Sialoliths of the minor salivary glands are not seen with the frequency of those in the major salivary glands. When present, they are almost always in the upper lip or buccal mucosa. Salivary stones of the minor glands are firm, freely movable, small masses that usually remain asymptomatic unless secondarily infected. Sialolithiasis is most often a process seen in middle age.

Associated Findings. A previous history of sialolithiasis can be found in 18 % of patients. Diffuse cellulitis or abscess formation may be seen as complicating factors in sialolithiasis of the major salivary glands. Patients with a long history of recurrent sialadenitis often have fibrosis of the gland.

Microscopic Findings. Sialoliths are round to cylindrical masses that may be white or yellow-brown.

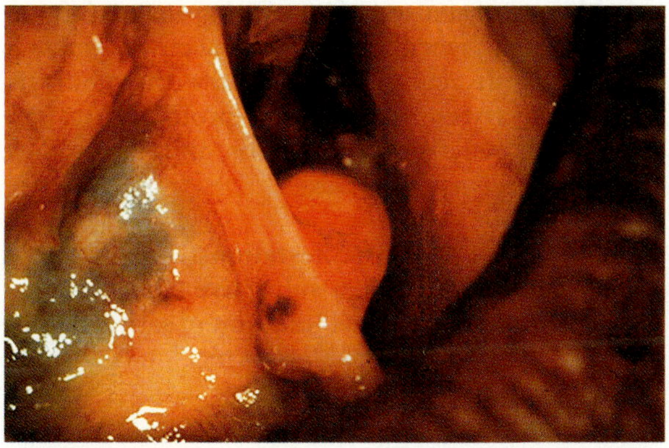

Fig. 14.21. Sialolithiasis. Salivary stone producing swelling of the submandibular duct

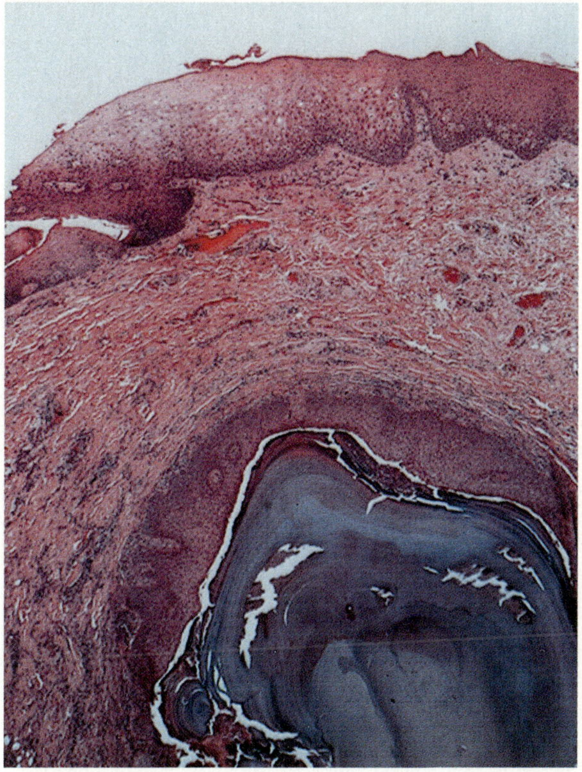

Fig. 14.22. Sialolithiasis. A salivary duct occluded by a sialolith. The concentric laminations of dystrophic calcification are produced by layers of calcium phosphate added to a central nidus

The calcified specimen microscopically presents as concentric laminations surrounding a central area of amorphous debris. The associated duct may exhibit squamous or mucous cell metaplasia, as well as periductal inflammation with chronic sialadenitis of the gland (Fig. 14.22).

Diagnosis. A patient complaint of pain and swelling, especially at meal times, is highly suggestive of major salivary gland duct obstruction. In many cases, the stone can be palpated during physical examination. One of the greatest aids to diagnosis is radiographic visualization of the calcified mass. Some reports have roentgenographically demonstrated submandibular gland calculi in 9 % of cases (Fig. 14.23).

Differential Diagnosis. Salivary stones located at the periphery of a gland, rather than the distal duct, have been mistaken as tumorous masses. Multiple calculi may radiographically appear to be calcified parotid lymph nodes, such as might be seen in tuberculosis.

Treatment. Small sialoliths can sometimes be massaged through the duct orifice. Forceps delivery after infiltration with local anesthesia may be attempted if

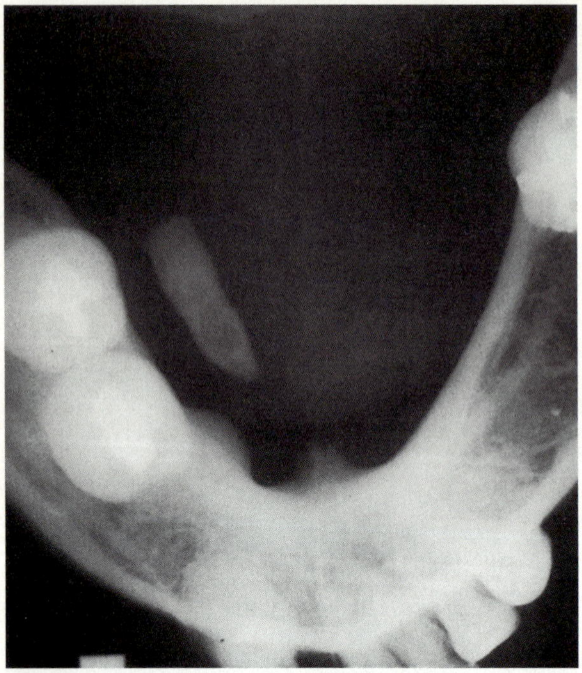

Fig. 14.23. Sialolithiasis. Salivary stone in Wharton's duct demonstrated by occlusal radiograph. Radiographic evidence of a sialolith in this location is present in the great majority of cases and a valuable diagnostic aid. (Photographic credit, Brad Potter, DDS)

the stone is close enough to the opening. Sialogogues, moist heat, and increased fluid intake might also promote passage of the stone. Larger calculi usually require surgical removal. Patients with persistent symptoms, recurrent infections, or multiple recurrent sialoliths often benefit by removal of the entire salivary gland.

14.3.3 Sialoadenosis

G. Hautmann, G. L. Campanile, and T. M. Lotti

Definition. Sialoadenosis represents a rare enlargement of the parotid and, less frequently, of the submandibular glands. It is neither an inflammatory process, nor a neoplastic growth. The exact cause of this increase in dimensions is still unclear and under debate.

Oral Manifestations. Clinically, it presents as a bilateral painless, usually recurrent, swelling of the parotids: the swelling is soft and a decreased salivary secretion with xerostomia and glossodynia may be present [62].

Associated Findings. It may be associated with liver cirrhosis, diabetes mellitus, chronic alcoholism, malnutrition, and thyroid and ovarian failures.

Diagnosis. This is primarily based on histopathologic findings.

Differential Diagnosis. The disease has to be differentiated from Sjögren's syndrome, Mikulicz's and Heerfordt's syndromes, chronic recurrent sialoadenitis, and salivary gland tumors.

Treatment. Therapy is essentially symptomatic; therapy of associated conditions sometimes improves the sialoadenosis.

14.3.4 Xerostomia

Changes in Saliva Quantity and Quality. The fluid component of saliva primarily acts to protect the oral epithelium from drying, but it also acts as a mechanical cleansing solution that aids in the removal of food, cellular debris, and microorganisms. The fluid is the vehicle for the glycoproteins and mucoids from a protective hydrochloric acid produced therein. These proteins add lubrication to mimize the abrasive action of foods, aid in speech, provide a buffer to neutralize acids, encourage antibacterial activity, and aid in the remineralization of the teeth. Any change in saliva quantity or quality will affect these functions. A change in quantity also will affect a change in quality; therefore, as salivary flow diminishes, all protective functions are reduced. The most obvious effect on the patient is a decrease in the lubrication of affected tissues and an increase in friction that may present as a burning sensation. In addition, a decrease in saliva alters the efficient removal of normally growing organisms, reduces the buffering and antibacterial activity, and alters the mechanical removal of debris, which, if not removed, provides a medium for organisms. All of these changes alter the microflora of the oral cavity and allow the proliferation of unwanted organisms such as *Candida albicans*, a fungal organism implicated in mucosal discomfort when growth is left unchecked. Thus, when the normal oral environment is altered by a decrease in salivary flow or a modification of salivary composition, the probability of caries, periodontal disease, mucositis, and many other, serious problems increases.

Definition and Oral Manifestations. Xerostomia is the term used to define a subjective clinical condition of less than a "normal" amount of saliva, but the amount that constitutes "abnormal" has yet not been defined.

Dry and cracking oral mucosa and soft tissues, ulcerations, opportunistic bacterial infections, glossodynia, periodontal atrophy and deterioration, and extreme difficulty in lubricating, tasting, masticating, and swallowing certain foods are among the many manifestations of xerostomia.

Etiology and Pathomechanism. The causes of xerostomia include radiation damage to the salivary glands, certain systemic diseases (such as diabetes mellitus and autoimmune disorders such as scleroderma, systemic lupus erythematosus, Sjögren's syndrome), and pharmacologic agents. Xerostomia caused by radiation therapy has been studied extensively, as has xerostomia resulting from Sjögren's syndrome. In both of these conditions, the damage to the salivary glands may be complete and irreversible. The amount of saliva loss caused by pharmacologic agents, on the other hand, varies quantitatively, depending on the pharmacologic agent, its dosage, the time interval between dosages, and the individual effect on the patient, as these drugs affect the neural pathway of secretion, not the glandular structure itself. Their quantitative variations make pharmacologic agents a difficult group to study, although they are probably the most common cause of xerostomia, especially in the elderly [63–70].

The primary mechanism of action of drugs that cause xerostomia involves an interference of the parasympathetic pathways of the autonomic nervous system. These pathways contain chiefly cholinergic fibers, which, when stimulated, cause an increase in the salivary secretions. Anticholinergic agents, therefore, are the primary offenders in a reduction in salivary flow. Alpha- and beta-adrenergic receptors in the sympathetic nervous system also contribute to flow, so alpha- or beta-blockers will have some effect on the amount of saliva secreted, but much less so than anticholinergic agents. Beta-adrenergic blockers appear to affect primarily the protein content of saliva. Although the effects appear to be reversible on removal of the offending agents, no studies have been made to determine if permanent changes occur with long-term use of certain pharmacologic agents in man.

Medications with xerostomic side effects are categorized in Table 14.1. Some of these groups overlap with others in terms of their pharmacologic agents; however, the grouping illustrates the different indications for which a drug with xerostomic side effects may be prescribed.

Many of these drugs, such as the antihypertensives and diuretics taken by patiens with hypertension, are used by patients as life-saving agents. Others, such as appetite suppressants or antidepressants, may be abused or overprescribed. Regardless of why they are prescribed, the practitioner must be aware of xerostomic side effects so that if patients develop glossodynia, the medication can be evaluated. Xerostomia may also not be recognized as a side effect worth noting. A better indicator of possible xerostomic side effects may be the classification of the drug (see Table 14.1) [70, 71].

It is even more difficult to evaluate nonprescription medications than prescription medications because patients often do not consider these drugs to be medications and therefore will not list them in their medical history. If the patient does list an over-the-counter medication, it is difficult to find the additional information on side effects unless one has a reference volume such as the *Handbook of Nonprescription Drugs*.

Three groups of over-the-counter medications have great potential for abuse, precisely because they are nonprescription and may be used improperly. These drugs include laxatives, cold and allergy products, and weight-control products.

All laxatives have the potential for causing xerostomia because of the dehydrating effect of long-term use. Patients suspected of having anorexia nervosa need to be evaluated for this type of abuse. Self-medication for colds and the symptoms of allergies is common. Included in this group are decongestants, whether oral, topical, or nasal, antitussives, expectorants, and analgesics. All of these drugs may contain agents with powerful xerostomic side effects. Many weight-control over-the-counter medications contain phenylpropanolamine hydrochloride and caffeine, both of which have xerostomic side effects.

Less used medications with xerostomic side effects are the antidiarrheal agents, some of which contain a belladonna alkaloid, or anticholinergic, in doses equivalent to 0.6–1.0 mg atropine, and the antihelminthic products used to treat worms, such as metronidazole [63–71].

Caffeine and alcohol are generally not considered to be drugs, but are, in fact, pharmacologic agents with xerostomic side effects. Both are found in a number of prescription preparations.

Although most people probably do not ingest enough analgesics, vitamins, or chocolate on a daily basis to cause noticeable xerostomia, there are many people who consume large quantities of caffeinated beverages every day, and this consumption results in some xerostomia. Alcohol, besides being a beverage, may also be an ingredient in a pharmacologic preparation. Some vitamin products contain from 1.5 % to 18 % alcohol. The alcoholic or the heavy social drinker may suffer from noticeable xerostomia.

Drugs such as marijuana or cocaine have severe xerostomic side effects, but information on the use of these drugs by the patient may not be elicited easily;

this makes the task of tracking down xerostomia as the cause of glossodynia more difficult.

Thus, patients with glossodynia should have a thorough medical evaluation, after which the physician should evaluate the patient's use of medications, whether prescription or nonprescription, diet, recreational drug or alcohol habits, and level of hydration.

In evaluating the patient's prescription medications, if there is a choice between equally effective drugs, the xerostomic potential of each should be considered in the therapeutic decision. One example is a change to trazodone hydrochloride for those patients taking tricyclic antidepressants. Trazodone hydrochloride has less xerostomic side effects, yet has been shown to be as effective as other antidepressants [63–71].

Diagnosis. When evaluating the patient's over-the-counter medications, look especially for chronic allergy symptoms, a self-perceived weight problem, long-term pain, or a history of heart problems that causes the patient to take an aspirin preparation daily. Any over-the-counter medication for the above-mentioned conditions may include powerful anticholinergic agents.

The patient's diet should also be evaluated. Alcohol and caffeine must be consumed in large quantities to be primary offenders; however, when patients are required to take medications with xerostomic side effects, an alteration in the diet may make the difference between comfort and discomfort.

In part, salivary flow rate is regulated by masticatory forces; therefore, a diet that encourages chewing is important. Patients should refrain from dry, bulky, or spicy foods. A diet that restricts all but proteins and fats will cause xerostomia because of its potent antidiuretic effect. The prescription of sugarless gum or candy, or a toothpick on which to chew between meals, should be helpful in stimulating salivary flow.

The examiner should evaluate the patient's habits to determine if "recreational" drugs are being used frequently. It so, the patient must be educated about the contributing factors of these habits to glossodynia. The patient with xerostomia may perceive a bad taste in the mounth that he or she may try to alleviate with mouthwash. These products usually contain a large amount of alcohol and will aggravate an existing problem. Smoking also dries the oral mucosa and aggravates an existing problem.

The patient's state of hydration in terms of fluid intake and environment should also be considered. Dehydration from inadequate fluid intake or from very low humidity will magnify the problem.

All of the above factors must be evaluated together, as each may contribute in a small way to a large problem. The determination of where alterations can be made to solve the problem of glossodynia or other discomfort related to xerostomia requires an in-depth review of the patient's lifestyle.

Table 14.4. Drugs with xerostomic side effects

Analgesic mixtures	Diuretics
Anticonvulsants	Expectorants
Antiemetics	Muscle relaxants
Antihistamines	Psychotropic drugs:
Antihypertensives	Central nervous system depressants
Antinauseants	Dibenzoxazepine derivatives
Antiparkinson agents	Phenothiazine derivatives
Antipruritics	Monoamine oxidase inhibitors
Antispasmotics	Tranquilizers – major
Appetite suppressants	Tranquilizers – minor
Cold medications	Sedatives

Treatment. Methods of managing xerostomia include palliative mouthwashes such as warm salt water rinses or a combination of bicarbonate of soda and water. The bicarbonate rinses are beneficial to the teeth in those patients with xerostomia resulting from the dehydration of chronic vomiting. This type of xerostomia is commonly seen in patients taking chemotherapeutic agents. Cholinergic drugs have been prescribed in severe cases of xerostomia; however, caution must be used in administering yet another prescription drug.

References

1. Mc Nally MA, Langlais RP. Conditions peculiar to the tongue. Dermatol Clin 1996; 14: 257–272
2. Redman RS. Prevalence of geographic tongue, fissured tongue, median rhomboid glossitis, and hairy tongue among 3,611 Minnesota schoolchildren. Oral Surg Oral Med Oral Pathol 1970; 30: 390–395
3. Darwazeh AM, Pilai K. Prevalence of tongue lesions in 1013 Jordanian dental outpatients. Community Dent Oral Epidemiol 1993; 21: 323–324
4. Cooke BED. Median rhomboid glossitis: Candidiasis and not a developmental anomaly. Brit J Dermatol 1975; 93: 399–405
5. Farman AG, VanWyck CW, Staz H, et al. Central papillary atrophy of the tongue. Oral Surg 1977; 43: 48–58
6. Darwazeh AM, Pilai K. Prevalence of tongue lesions in 1013 Jordanian dental outpatients. Community Dent Oral Epidemiol 1993; 21: 323–324.
7. McNally MA, Langlais RP. Conditions peculiar to the tongue. Dermatol Clin 1996; 14: 257–272
8. Marks R, Simons MJ. Geographic tongue – a manifestation of atopy. Brit J Dermatol 1979; 101: 159–162
9. Sigal MJ, Mock D. Symptomatic benign migratory glossitis: report of two cases and literature review. Pediatric Dentistry 1992; 14: 392–396
10. Lamey PJ. Burning mouth syndrome. Dermatol Clin 1996; 14: 339–354
11. Lamey PJ, Allam BF. Vitamin status of patients with burning mouth syndrome and response to replacement therapy. Br Dent J 1986; 160: 81–84

12. Drage LA, Rogers RS III. Burning mouth syndrome (submitted for publication)
13. Beaven DW, Brooks SE. Color atlas of the tongue in clinical diagnosis. Year Book Medical Publishers, 1988: 256
14. Beaven DW, Brooks SE. Color atlas of the tongue in clinical diagnosis. Year Book Medical Publishers, 1988: 256
15. Grossman ME, Stevens AW, Cohen PR. Herpetic geometric glossitis. N Eng J Med 1993; 329: 1859–1860
16. Neville B, Damm D, Allen C, Bouquot J. Oral and maxillofacial pathology. Philadelphia: W.B. Saunders, 1995
17. Scully C, Flint S, Porter S. Oral diseases. An illustrated guide to diagnosis and management of diseases of the oral mucosa, gingivae, teeth, salivary glands, bones and joints. London: Martin Dunitz, 1996
18. Matthews JB, Basu MK. Plasma cell lesions within the oral tissues: immunoperoxidase staining of routinely fixed and processed tissue. Oral Surg 1982; 54: 414
19. Regezi JA, Zarbo RJ, Keren DF. Plasma cell lesions of the head and neck: immunofluorescent determination of clonality from formalin-fixed paraffin-embedded tissue. Oral Surg 1983; 56: 616
20. Simpson HE. Lymphoid hyperplasia in foliate papillitis. J Oral Surg 1964; 22: 209
21. Laskaris G. Color atlas of oral diseases. New York: Thieme, 1994: 98
22. Laskaris G. Color atlas of oral diseases. New York: Thieme, 1994: 100
23. Samaranayake LP. Oral mycoses in HIV infection. Oral Surg 1992; 73: 171–180
24. Lamey PJ, Lewis MAO. Oral medicine in practice: angular cheilitis. Br Dent J 1989; 176: 15–18
25. Ohman SC, Dahlen G, Moller A, et al. Angular cheilitis: a clinical and microbial study. J Oral Pathol 1986; 15: 213–217
26. Konstantinidis AB, Hatziotis JH. Angular cheilosis: an analysis of 156 cases. J Oral Med 1984; 39: 199–205
27. Cataldo E, Duko C. Solar cheilitis. J Dermatol Surg Oncol 1981; 7: 989–995
28. Stanley RJ, Roenigk RK. Actinic cheilitis: treatment with the carbon dioxide laser. Mayo Clinic Proc 1988; 63: 230–235
29. Epstein E. Treatment of lips keratoses (actinic cheilitis) with topical fluorouracil. Arch Dermatol 1977; 113: 906–908
30. Birt BD. The "lip shave" operation for pre-malignant conditions and micro-invasive carcinoma of the lower lip. J Otolaryngol 1977; 6: 407–411
31. Field LM. An improved design for vermilionectomy with a mucous-membrane advancement flap. J Dermatol Surg Oncol 1991; 17: 833–834
32. Kugman A. Topical tretinoin: indications, safety, and effectiveness. Cutis 1987; 39: 486–488
33. Crotty CP, Dicken CH. Factitious lip crusting. Arch Dermatol 1981; 117: 338–340
34. Reade PC, Sim R. Exfoliative cheilitis – a factitious disorder. J Oral Maxillofac Surg 1986; 15: 313–317
35. Postlethwaite KR, Hendrickse NM. A case of exfoliative cheilitis. Br Dent J 1988; 165: 23
36. Winchester L, Scully C, Prime SS, et al. Cheilitis glandularis: a case affecting the upper lip. Oral Surg Oral Med Oral Pathol 1986; 62: 654–656
37. Yacobi R, Brown DA. Cheilitis glandularis: a pediatric case report. J Am Dental Assoc 1989; 228: 317–318
38. Cohen DM, Green JG, Diekmann SL. Current anomalies: cheilitis glandularis and double lip. Oral Surg 1988; 66: 397–399
39. Joshi HN, Dayal PK. Cheilitis glandularis. Oral Med 1984; 39: 183–185
40. Miescher G. Uber essentielle granulomatose makrocheilie (cheilitis granulomatosa). Dermatologica 1945; 91: 57–85
41. Allen CM, Camisa C, Hamzeh S, et al. Cheilitis granulomatosa: report of six cases and review of the literature. J Amer Acad Dermatol 1990; 23: 444–450
42. Worsaae N, Christensen KC, Schiodt M, et al. Melkersson-Rosenthal syndrome and cheilitis granulomatosa. Oral Surg 1982; 54: 404–413
43. Williams PM, Greenberg MS. Management of cheilitis granulomatosa. Oral Surg 1991; 71: 436–439
44. Rogers RS III. Melkersson-Rosenthal syndrome and orofacial granulomatosis. Dermatol Clin 1996; 14: 371–379
45. Zimmer WM, Rogers RS III, Reeve CM, et al. Orofacial manifestations of Melkersson-Rosenthal syndrome. Oral Surg 1992; 74: 610–619
46. Camacho F, Garcia-Bravo B, Carrizosa A. Treatment of the Miescher's cheilitis granulomatosa in the Melkersson-Rosenthal syndrome (personal communication)
47. Baughman RD, Berger P, Pringle WM. Plasma cell cheilitis. Arch Dermatol 1974; 110: 725–726
48. White JW Jr, Olson KD, Banks PM. Plasma cell orificial mucositis. Arch Dermatol 1986; 122: 1321–1324
49. Aiba S, Tagami H. Immunoglobulin-producing cells in plasma cell orificial mucositis. J Cutan Pathol 1989, 16: 207–210
50. Tamaki K, Lsada A, Tsukamoto K, et al. Treatment of plasma cell cheilitis with griseofulvin. J Am Acad Dermatol 1994; 30: 789–790
51. Abrams AM, Melrose RJ, Howell FV. Necrotizing sialometaplasia; a disease simulating malignancy. Cancer 1973; 32: 130–135
52. Brannon RB, Fowler CB, Hartman KS. Necrotizing sialometaplasia: a clinicopathologic study of sixty-nine cases and review of the literature. Oral Surg Oral Med Oral Pathol 1991; 72: 317–325
53. Sneige N, Batsakis JG. Pathology consultation; necrotizing sialometaplasia. Ann Otol Rhinol Laryngol 1992; 101: 282–284
54. Anneroth G, Hansen LS. Necrotizing sialometaplasia; the relationship of its pathogenesis to its clinical characteristics. Int J Oral Surg 1982; 11: 238–291
55. Arguelles MT. Necrotizing sialometaplasia. Oral Surg 1976; 42: 86–90.
56. Batsakis JG, Manning JT. Necrotizing sialometaplasia of major salivary glands. J Laryngol Otol 1987; 101: 962–966
57. Standish SM, Shafer WG. Serial histologic effects of rat submaxillary and sublingual salivary gland duct and blood vessel ligation. J Dent Res 1957; 36: 866–879
58. Neville BW, Damm DD, Allen CW, Bouquot JE. Oral and maxillofacial pathology. Philadelphia: WB Saunders, 1995; 326–327
59. Jensen JL, et al. Minor salivary gland calculi. Oral Surg 1979; 47: 44–50
60. Levy DM, ReMine WH, Devine KD. Salivary gland calculi. JAMA 1962; 181: 99–1119
61. Shafer WG, Hine MK, Levy BM. A textbook of oral pathology. 4th Ed. Philadelphia, WB Saunders, 1983; 561–562
62. Seifert G, Miehlke A, Haubrich J, et al. Diseases of the salivary glands. Pathology, diagnosis, treatment, facial surgery. Stuttgart-New York: Thieme, 1986
63. Glass BJ, Van Dis ML, Langlais RP, et al. Xerostomia: diagnosis and treatment planning considerations. Oral Surg 1984; 58(2): 248–252
64. Menaker L. Biologic basis of dental caries. New York: Harper and Row, 1980: 33–36
65. Rankow RM, Polayes IM. Diseases of the salivary glands. Philadelphia, 1976: 32–51
66. Glass BJ, Kuhei RF, Langlais RP. Management of common oral conditions. In: Terezhalmy C (Ed). Urgent care. Dent Clin North Am, 1986; 30(3): 421–6
67. Kohler PF, Winter ME. A quantitative test for xerostomia. Arthritis Rheum 1985; 28(10): 1128–1132
68. Handelman SL, Baric JM, Espeland MA, et al. Prevalence of drugs causing hyposalivation in an institutionalized population. Oral Surg 1986; 62(1): 26–31
69. Bahn SL. Drug-related dental destruction. Oral Surg 1972; 33(1): 49–54
70. Hautmann G, Panconesi E. Glossodynia J Eur Acad Dermatol Venereol, 1996; 7: 207–227
71. Glass BJ. Drug-induced xerostomia as a cause of glossodynia. Ear Nose Throat J 1989; 68: 776–781

CHAPTER 15

Periodontal Diseases

G. Pini Prato, P. Cortellini, B. Lorusso, and D. Saletta

15.1 Periodontal Anatomy

The periodontium is made up of tissues that invest and support the teeth, including gingiva, cementum, periodontal ligament, and supporting bone (Fig. 15.1). Gingiva surrounds a tooth and is contiguous with the periodontal ligament and with the mucosal tissues of the mouth. Attached gingiva is the portion that is firm, dense, stippled, and tightly bound with connective fibers to the underlying periosteum, cementum, and bone. The free gingiva, constituted by marginal and papillary gingiva, surrounds the tooth and is not directly attached to the tooth surface. A gingival sulcus (S) surrounds the tooth.

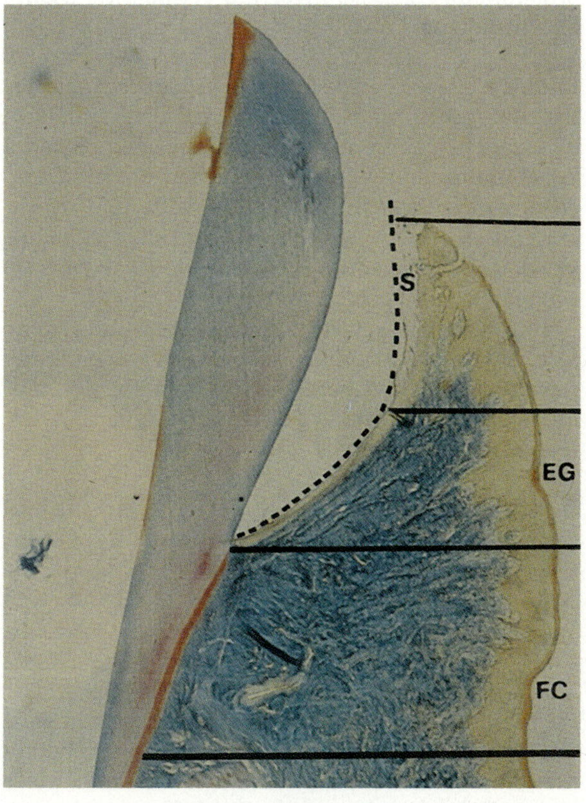

Fig. 15.1. Periodontium: bucco-lingual section. S, sulcus; EG, junctional epithelium; FC, connective fibers

Gingiva is a fibrous tissue covered by epithelium, which reflects at the gingival margin to limit the sulcus. The sulcular epithelium continues apically in the junctional epithelium (EG) attached to the tooth surface. Apically to the junctional epithelium, connective fibers (FC) are inserted into cementum (connective tissue attachment).

Cementum is the thin, calcified tissue of ectomesenchymal origin covering the roots of teeth. A complex system of fibers strictly links cementum to the periodontal ligament. Alveolar bone surrounds the tooth. A complex of inserting connective fibers, functionally oriented, connects cementum to alveolare bone.

15.2 Periodontal Diseases

Periodontal diseases are a group of pathologies involving the periodontal tissues, described as follows: (1) gingivitis, (2) periodontitis, (3) oral hygiene-related gingival lesions, and (4) gingival enlargement.

15.2.1 Gingivitis

Definition. Gingivitis is the inflammation of the gingiva without apical migration of the junctional epithelium.

Etiology. Microbial plaque is the cause of gingivitis. Several factors such as calculus, improper restoration, tooth malposition, and deficient salivary glands may contribute to plaque accumulation. Accumulation of bacteria at the gingiva/tooth surface induces an inflammatory response of the marginal gingiva consisting of blood vessel alterations and proliferation of inflammatory cells [1, 2]. Polymorphonuclear leukocytes, lymphocytes, plasma cells, and macrophages infiltrate the gingival connective tissue.

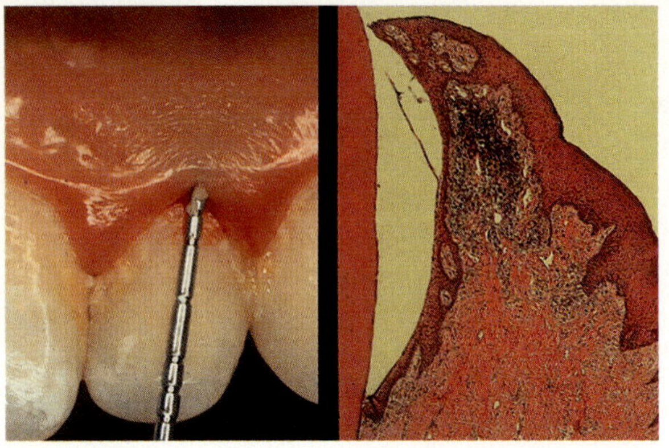

Fig. 15.2. Gingivitis

Oral Manifestations. Inflammation is mainly located at the marginal gingiva and the interdental papillae. The gingiva appears red, swollen, and sometimes hyperplastic. The flow of crevicular fluid is increased. A common feature is bleeding on gentle probing (Fig. 15.2).

Microscopic Findings. The initial inflammatory lesion appears within 4 days of plaque accumulation, and is characterized by migration of polymorphonuclear leukocytes from the vascular plexus subjacent to the junctional and the sulcular epithelia [2]. After 7 days of plaque accumulation, lymphocytes and macrophages are the predominating cells in the underlying gingival connective tissue. Sparse plasma cells are located at the periphery of the lesion. After 2–3 weeks, plasma cells and lymphocytes predominate at the periphery of the lesion. Neutrophil, macrophages, and lymphocytes are present in the lamina propria of the gingival sulcus. There is no destruction of connective fibers inserted into the root cementum and apical migration of the attachment apparatus [3].

Diagnosis. Diagnosis of gingivitis is based on detection of clinical signs.

Differential Diagnosis. The more common disorders are herpetic gingivostomatitis, recurrent aphthous stomatitis, desquamative gingivitis secondary to lichen planus, mucous membrane pemphigoid, and pemphigus vulgaris. All the above diseases frequently also involve oral mucosa, and plaque removal does not result in re-establishment of gingival health.

Treatment. Gingivitis is reversible. Bacterial plaque removal results in complete resolution of the gingival inflammation.

15.2.2 Periodontitis

Definition. Periodontitis is an inflammation of the supporting tissues of the tooth, associated with destruction of the attachment apparatus, apical migration of junctional epithelium, and alveolar bone resorption.

Classification. According to the Proceedings of the AAP, 1989 World Workshop in Clinical Periodontics [4], the classification distinguishes:

- Adult periodontitis
- Early onset periodontitis:
  - A. Prepubertal periodontitis (generalized, localized)
  - B. Juvenile periodontitis (generalized, localized)
  - C. Rapidly progressive periodontitis
- Periodontitis associated with systemic disease
- Necrotizing ulcerative periodontitis
- Refractory periodontitis

15.2.2.1 *Adult Periodontitis*

Definition. Adult periodontitis (AP) is a chronic inflammatory disease involving periodontal tissues and usually has onset after 35 years of age [5].

Etiology. Recent experimental evidence indicates that AP is a complex, multifactorial disease caused by local environmental factors (associated bacterial flora) and retentive factors [6]. A few bacterial species are most frequently associated with AP: *Porphiromonas gingivalis, Actinobacillus actinomycetemcomitans, P. intermedia, F. nucleatum, B. forsytus, E. corrodens*, and *Spirochetes*.

It is likely that specific environmental and genetic factors determine both site and subject susceptibility to colonization by a pathogenic flora to the development of infection and to destructive inflammatory response [7].

Oral Manifestations. AP is characterized by the presence of recessions and/or periodontal pockets, associated with attachment loss and radiographic bone resorption (Fig. 15.3). Gingival inflammation and bleeding on probing can be present.

Microscopic Findings. The lesion is characterized by the presence of all features of an established gingival inflammatory lesion, accompanied by destruction of the connective tissue attachment to the root surface and apical migration of the epithelial attachment. Though the inflammatory infiltrate is confined to

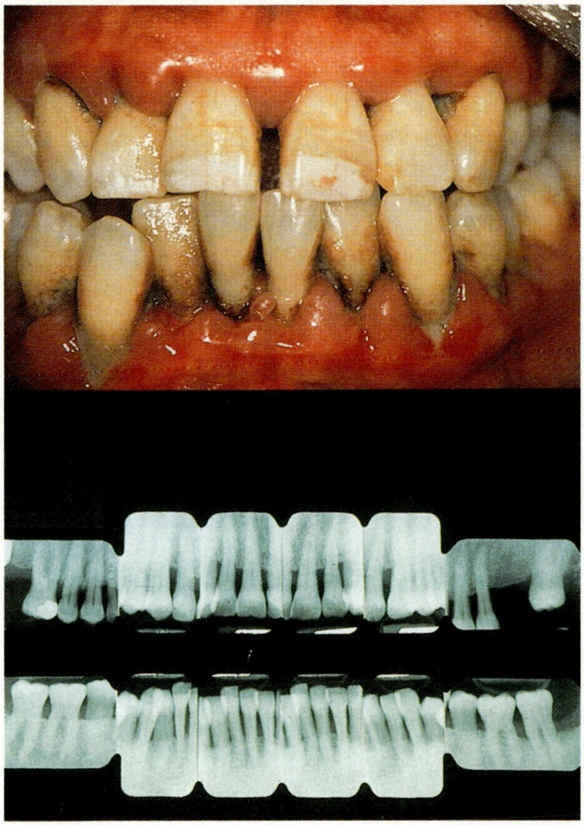

Fig. 15.3. Adult periodontitis

the gingiva and does not extend into the alveolar bone, the connective tissue attachment loss is associated with crestal resorption.

Diagnosis. The clinical diagnosis of AP is based on detection of clinical attachment and radiographic bone loss. Bleeding on probing occurs if gingivitis is present.

Treatment. Oral hygiene instructions, scaling, and root planing with or without flap access are indicated for proper root débridement, and to establish conditions which favor healing of lesions caused by AP. The subgingival instrumentation is probably the single most important therapeutic act. If surgical intervention is required, different surgical techniques may be employed for pocket reduction and pocket elimination. Regenerative treatment methods may be employed [8].

The maintenance of optimal supragingival plaque control by the patient mechanically and/or chemically (chlorhexidine mouth rinses), and periodic professional controls tailored to individual needs, is of paramount importance to prevent recurrent disease.

15.2.2.2 *Prepubertal Periodontitis*

Definition. Prepubertal periodontitis (PP) is a rare form that occurs in children and involves the primary dentition extending to periodontal permanent teeth [9].

Etiology. *A. actinomycetemcomitans, P. intermedia, E. corrodens,* and *Capnocitophaga* are putative microbial agents often associated with the disease. In PP blood peripheral granulocytes and monocytes have been found with an abnormal chemotactic response [10].

Oral Manifestations. PP may be localized or generalized, and clinical signs are acute inflammation, gingival tissue proliferation, and deep periodontal pockets. Rapid destruction and demineralization of the alveolar bone are a frequent occurrence in the generalized form.

Associated Findings. Recurrent otitis and other infectious diseases of the high respiratory tract.

Diagnosis. Based on clinical and radiographic examinations.

Treatment. See adult periodontitis. Systemic antibiotics can be prescribed.

15.2.2.3 *Juvenile Periodontitis*

Definition. Juvenile periodontitis (JP) is an inflammatory periodontal disease occurring in young people (12–20 years of age).

Etiology. Etiologic agents involved are *A. actinomycetemcomitans* (especially in the localized form) and other common periodontal pathogens [11]. Abnormalities of leukocyte chemotaxis are the basis of altered responsiveness to microbiota [12].

Oral Manifestations. Loss of periodontal connective tissue attachment and alveolar bone resorption, localized at first molars and incisors (Fig. 15.4), with symmetric lesions (LJP). Generalized forms involve other teeth in different sites of the mouth. The localized form can become generalized if not treated. In JP, plaque accumulation and gingival inflammation are not relevant findings.

Associate Findings. Hypophosphatasia is commonly detected.

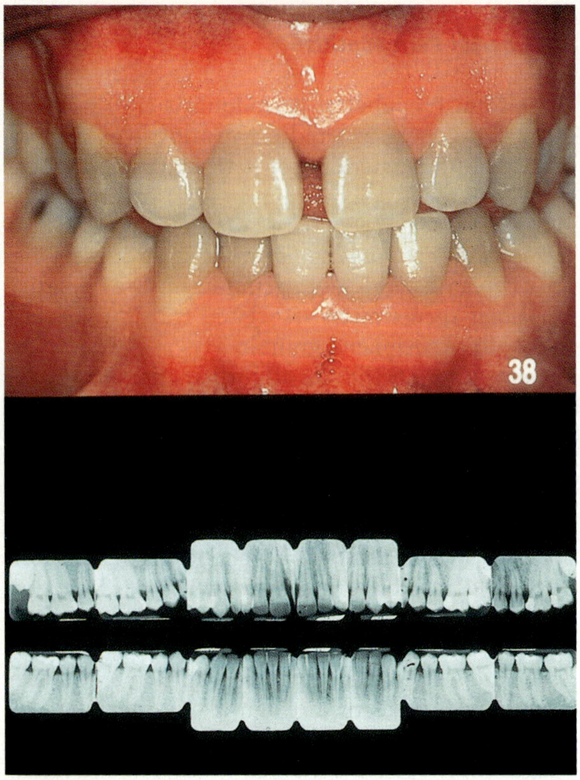

Fig. 15.4. Localized juvenile periodontitis

Diagnosis. Clinical and radiographic examinations are required for diagnosis.

Differential Diagnosis. Hypophosphatasia, resulting in disturbed cementogenesis and resultant failure to provide periodontal attachment. Papillon-Lefèvre syndrome showing hyperkeratosis of the palms and soles.

Treatment. See adult periodontitis. Systemic antibiotic administration (1 g/day of tetracycline for 3 weeks) has been found to be beneficial.

15.2.2.4
Rapidly Progressive Periodontitis

Definition. Rapidly progressive periodontitis (RPP) is a particular form of periodontitis seen mostly in individuals in their twenties, although the onset may be between puberty and 30–35 years of age [13]. Sometimes, juvenile periodontitis may precede RPP, while in other cases there is no evidence of previous disease.

Etiology. *P. gingivalis* and *A. actinomycetemcomitans* are the most important involved pathogens. Disease progression is episodic and cyclic, with exacerbation and quiescence. Most patients who develop RPP manifest abnormalities in their peripheral blood cells or in their serum. The relationship between RPP and juvenile periodontitis is not clear.

Oral Manifestations. Lesions are generalized, affecting most teeth (Fig. 15.5). The extent of clinical signs of inflammation may be less than expected. The most typical clinical characteristics are florid, acute inflammation with bleeding periodontal abscesses, and proliferation of the marginal gingiva. Alveolar bone resorption and destruction of periodontal ligament occur rapidly.

Diagnosis. Diagnosis is based on history, clinical, and radiographic features.

Treatment. See adult periodontitis.

15.2.2.5
Periodontitis Associated with Systemic Disease

Several systemic, congenital, and acquired diseases predispose the patient to periodontitis, which may be of the early-onset type, but which may differ

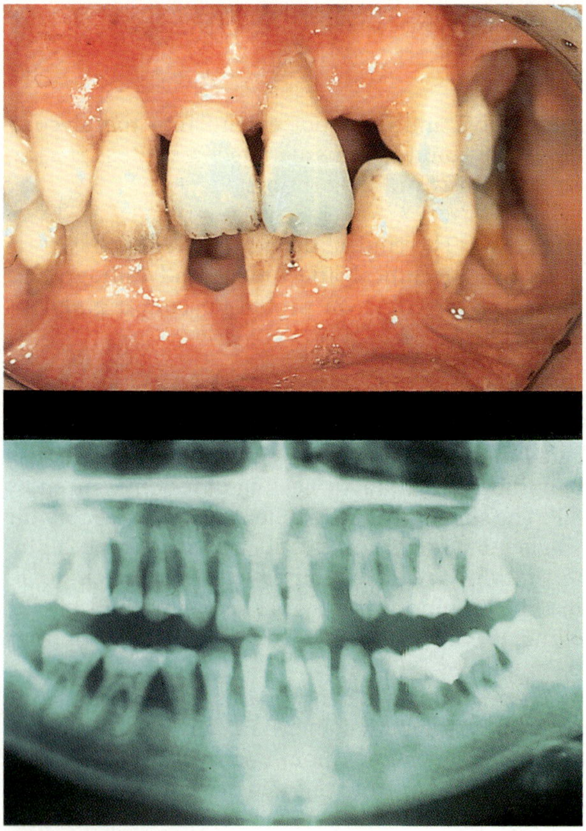

Fig. 15.5. Rapidly progressive periodontitis

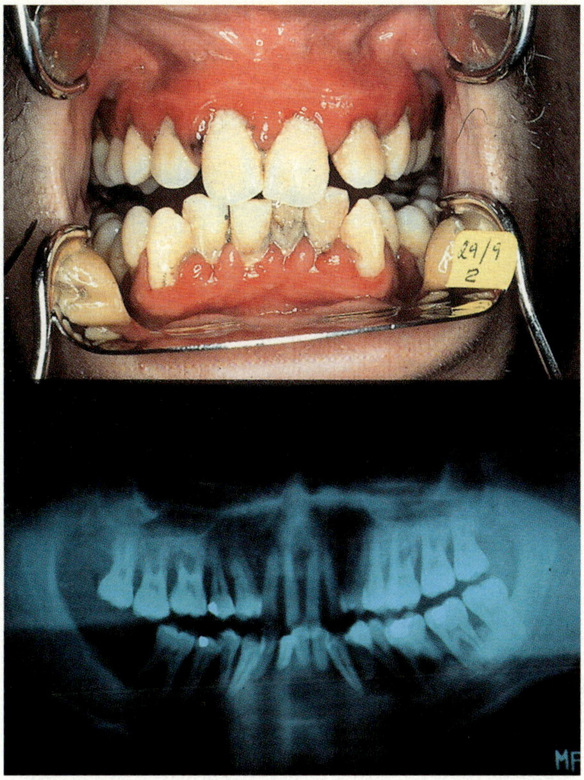

Fig. 15.6. Cyclic neutropenia

from the early onset described above. Many diseases present disorders of cellular immunity. Among these are Down's syndrome with multiple immune dysfunctions and anatomical/structural dysplasias; cyclic neutropenia (Fig. 15.6), Papillon-Lefèvre syndrome with structural abnormalities, usually the main susceptibility factor; and diabetes mellitus (Fig. 15.7) presenting depressed neutrophil functions [7].

15.2.2.6
Necrotizing Ulcerative Periodontitis

Definition. Necrotizing ulcerative periodontitis (NUP), also called acute necrotizing ulcerative gingivitis, is an acute inflammatory periodontal disease characterized by the rapid destruction of gingiva [14].

Etiology. Poor attention to oral hygiene and previous chronic marginal gingivitis are frequently found in patients with NUP. In addition, NUP is associated with smoking and mental or physical stress. Perhaps, neuroimmunological mechanisms are involved, but there is no evidence for this aspect [15]. NUP seems to be a manifestation of mixed bacterial infection modified by particular systemic determinants. Spirochetes, *Fusobacterium*, and other common periodontal pathogens are always found in plaque.

Oral Manifestations. Necrotic lesions start from the gingival margin (Fig. 15.8). Destruction especially involves interdental papillae, which appear to be split up in a buccal and lingual area separated by a crater. Ulcerated gingival margins and pain are presenting signs. Malodor and a pseudomembrane over affected areas of the gingiva are usually present.

Associated Findings. NUP is more common in HIV seropositives than in the general population, and is associated with lymphoadenopathy and fever.

Microscopic Findings. The histopathology picture is that of a nonspecific inflammation with necrosis involving either epithelium or connective tissue.

Diagnosis. Ulcerations, necrosis of papillae, pain, and other clinical signs, together with radiographs, permit diagnosis.

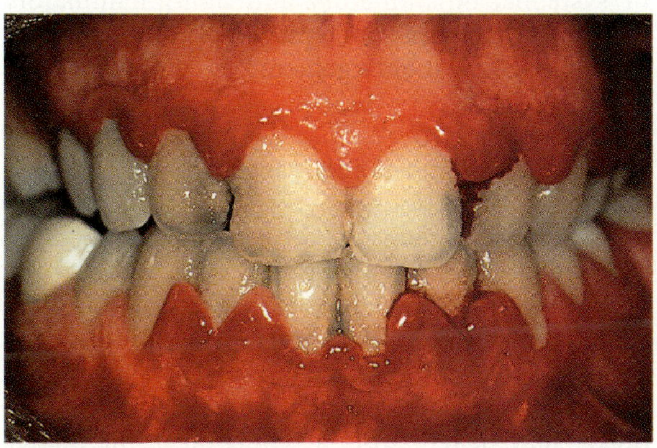

Fig. 15.7. Diabetes mellitus

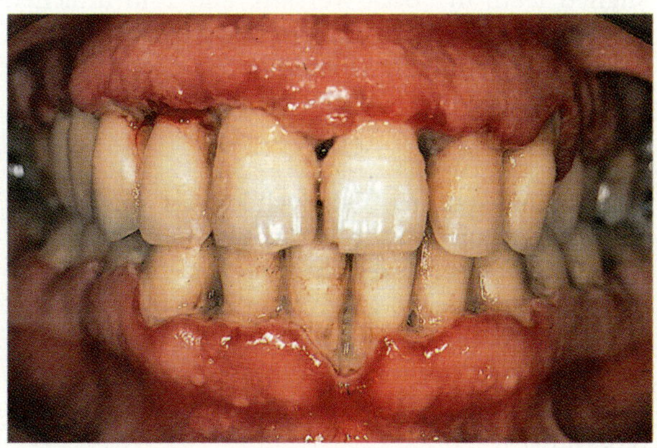

Fig. 15.8. Necrotizing ulcerative periodontitis

Differential Diagnosis. The more common disorders are herpetic gingivostomatitis and desquamative gingivitis secondary to mucous membrane pemphigus. Herpetic gingivostomatitis usually involves other areas than the gingival margin, and erythema is more widespread including all the gingiva and alveolar mucosa. Desquamative gingivitis frequently involves also oral mucosa, and plaque removal does not result in the re-establishment of gingival health.

Treatment. See adult periodontitis. In the acute phase, systemic metronidazole, 250 mg three times a day for 1 week, is frequently prescribed.

15.2.2.7
Refractory Periodontitis

Refractory periodontitis, including patients unresponsive to any treatment provided, as well as patients with very frequent episodes of disease recurrence, represents a disease entity of acknowledged heterogeneity. It is not certain that the refractory form is a real nosologic entity; poor patient compliance may be the major cause.

15.2.3
Oral Hygiene-Related Gingival Lesions

Definition. Oral hygiene-related gingival lesions (recessions, abrasions) are quite common conditions caused by improper use of oral hygienic measures and showing signs of traumatism.

Etiology. The most likely cause of gingival lesions is trauma caused by improper oral hygiene techniques [16]. Gingival lesions may be ascribed to poor toothbrushing techniques, direction, frequency, and magnitude of toothbrushing.

Moreover, shape of the toothbrush, type of bristles, frena in proximity of the gingival margin, malaligned teeth in buccal version, and thin attached gingiva appear to be related to gingival lesions. An improper flossing technique can produce a cut lesion localized to the parabolic gingival margin of the papilla.

Oral Manifestations. Gingival lesions may occur anywhere, especially on canines and bicuspids (Fig. 15.9). Sites of lesions are the free gingival margin, the attached gingiva, and the oral mucosa. Often, tooth abrasions are associated with gingival lesions. When the total thickness of the gingiva is destroyed and the root is evident, the lesion is a recession.

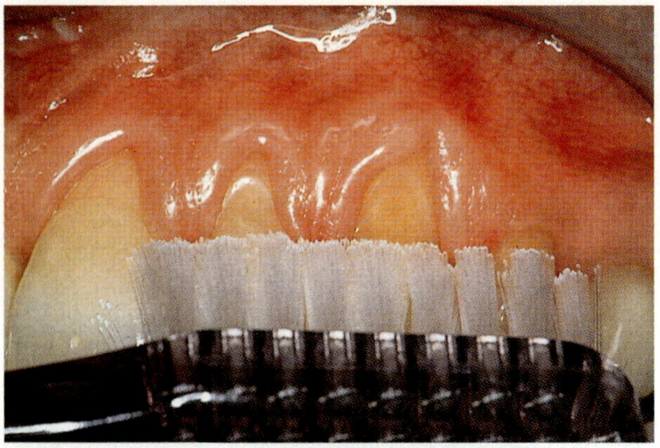

Fig. 15.9. Oral hygiene-related gingival lesions

Microscopic Findings. Gingival lesions can be restricted to the keratinized superficial layer of the epithelium, or involve the basal layer and the underlying connective tissue corium. At a higher magnification, cells in the active phases of mitosis can be clearly detected. Epithelial proliferation during the wound phase is observed.

Diagnosis. Clinical aspect of lesions associated with tooth abrasions and history are sufficient for diagnosis.

Treatment. Early recognition of gingival lesions followed by a modification of oral hygiene measures according to the patient's needs. Sometimes, interruption of toothbrushing is advisable. Plaque control with clorhexidine mouthrinses is supplemented. In advanced phases, when damage leads to important recession, mucogingival surgery and GTR therapy should be taken into account [17].

15.2.4
Gingival Enlargement

Gingival enlargement is a sign of different localized or systemic, inflammatory and non-inflammatory diseases. Drug use and epulis are very common causes of gingival enlargement.

15.2.4.1
Drug-Induced Gingival Enlargement

Gingival enlargement [18, 19] has been described in patients receiving phenytoin (Fig. 15.10), cyclosporin, and nifedipine. The degree of hyperplasia does not significantly correlate with serum levels of the drugs. Plaque control and removal of local irritants can improve the gingival health of some patients, while others may benefit from a reduction in the dosage

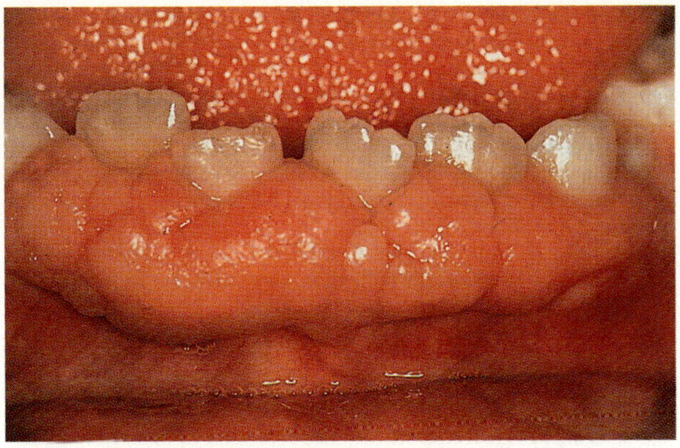

Fig. 15.10. Phenytoin-induced gingival enlargement

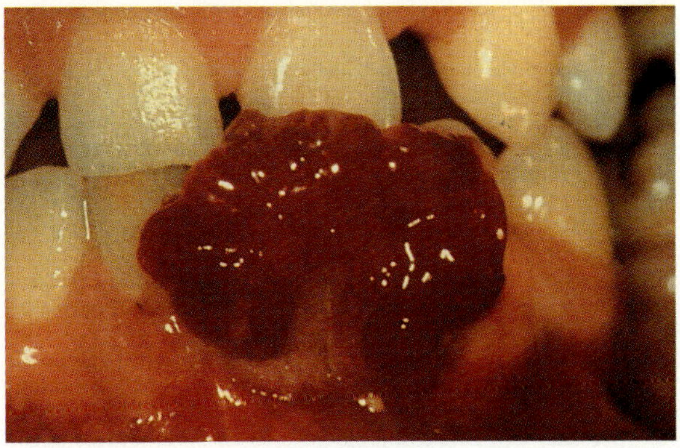

Fig. 15.11. Peripheral giant cell granuloma

of the drug. Gingivectomy or gingivoplasty is required when there is extensive gingival enlargement.

15.2.4.2 *Epulis*

The Greek term "epulis" is a topographic descriptive lesion of a common localized overgrowth, not considered a neoplasm, but a nonspecific hyperplastic benign and inflammatory reaction. Local excision is the preferred treatment. Recurrence may occur.

The histologic classification [20] used is: (1) pyogenic granuloma, (2) peripheral giant cell granuloma, (3) fibrous hyperplasia, and (4) peripheral fibroma with calcification.

Pyogenic granuloma represents an exuberant tissue response to a nonspecific irritant. It usually appears in the gingiva between two teeth, but is also found on the lips, tongue, and palate. Clinically, it is an elevated, pedunculated or sessile, smooth or ulcerated mass. Histologically, the lesion is composed of endothelium-lined vascular spaces, an infiltrate of lymphocytes, plasma cells, and frequently polymorphonuclear neutrophils, and is covered by a thin layer of stratified squamous epithelium.

Peripheral giant cell granuloma occurs on the gingiva or alveolar mucosa in edentulous areas. Clinically, it is sessile or pedunculated and bleeds easily (Fig. 15.11). Histologically, the consistent findings are a non-encapsulated mass of tissue containing large numbers of young connective tissue cells and multinucleated giant cells in an architectural pattern of focal nodules of giant cells separated by fibrous septa.

Fibrous hyperplasia is often related to irritation. Clinically, the lesion is asymptomatic with a variable rate of growth. It usually appears in the interdental papilla as a result of calculus, caries, or restorations with improper margins. Histologically, fibrous hyperplasia shows a layer of keratinized squamous cell epithelium and bundles of collagen fibers running in all directions, sometimes forming a pseudocapsule.

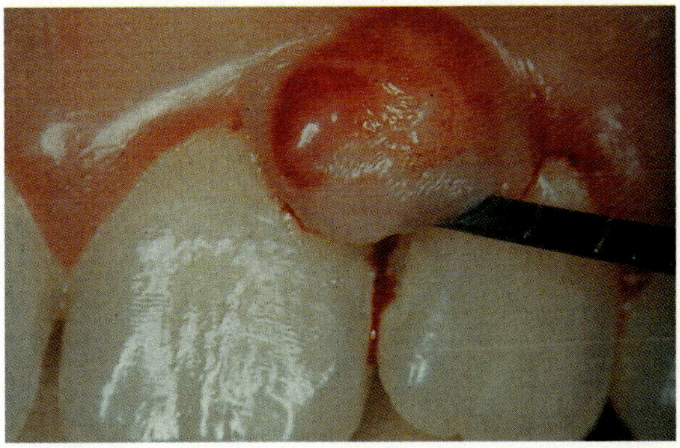

Fig. 15.12. Peripheral fibroma with calcification

Peripheral fibroma with calcification appears pedunculated, pink, and involves the anterior segment of the dental arches (Fig. 15.12). Histologically, it consists of bundles of collagen fibers running in all directions in a dense stroma. Focal deposits of calcified material or osseous lamellae or trabeculae are common findings.

References

1. Page RC, Schroeder HE. Pathogenesis of inflammatory periodontal disease. A summary of current work. Lab Invest 1976; 33:235–249
2. Löe H, Theilade E, Jensen SB. Experimental gingivitis in man. J Periodontol 1965; 36:177–187
3. Haffajee AD, Socransky SS, Lindhe J et al. Clinical risk indicators for periodontal attachment loss. J Periodontol 1991; 18:117–125
4. Consensus report, discussion section I. In: Nevins M, Becker W, Kornman K (Eds). World workshop in clinical periodon-

tics. Princeton: American Academy of Periodontology 1989; 23:1–31
5. Listgarten MA. Pathogenesis of periodontitis. J Clin Periodontol 1986; 13:418–425
6. Caton J. Periodontal diagnosis and diagnostic aids. In: Nevins M, Becker W, Kornman K (Ed). World Workshop in Clin Periodontics. Princeton: American Academy of Periodontology 1989 I:1–22
7. Genco RJ. Host responses in periodontal diseases: current concepts. J Periodontol 1992; 63:338–355
8. Cortellini P, Pini Prato GP, Tonetti M. Periodontal regeneration of human infrabony defects. I–II. J Periodontol 1993; 254–268
9. Watanabe K. Prepubertal periodontitis: a review of diagnostic criteria, pathogenesis, and differential diagnosis. J Periodont Res 1990; 25:31–48
10. Crossner CG, Carlsson J, Sjödin B, et al. Periodontitis in the primary dentition associated with Actinobacillus actinomycetemcomitans infection and leukocyte dysfunction. A 3 1/2-year follow-up. J Clin Periodontol 1990; 17:264–267
11. Gunsolley JC, Ranney RR, Zambon JJ, et al. Actinobacillus actinomycetemcomitans in families afflicted with periodontitis. J Periodontol 1990; 61:643–648
12. Bimstein E, Lustmann J, Sela MN, et al. Periodontitis associated with Papillon-Lefèvre syndrome. J Periodontol 1990; 61:373–377
13. Page RC, Altman LC, Ebersole JL, et al. Rapidly progressive periodontitis: a distinct clinical condition. J Periodontol 1983; 54:197–205
14 Kristoffersen T, Lie T. Necrotizing gingivitis. In: Lindhe (Ed). Textbook of clinical periodontology. Copenhagen: Munksgaard, 1989: 221–234
15. Johnson BD, Engel D. Acute necrotizing ulcerative gingivitis: a review of diagnosis, etiology and treatment. J Periodontol 1986; 57:141–150
16. Agudio G, Pini Prato G, Cortellini P, et al. Gingival lesions caused by improper oral hygiene measures. Int J Periodontics Restorative Dent 1987; 53–65
17. Pini Prato G, Tinti C, Vincenzi G, et al. Guided tissue regeneration versus mucogingival surgery in the treatment of human buccal gingival recession. J Periodontol 1992; 63:919–928
18. Barber MT, Savage N, Seymour GJ. The effect of cyclosporin and lipopolysaccharide on fibroblasts: implications for cyclosporin-induced gingival overgrowth. J Periodontol 1992; 63: 397–404
19. Barclay S, Thomason JM, Idle JR, Seymour RA. The incidence and severity of nifedipine-induced gingival overgrowth. J Clin Periodontol 1992; 19:311–314
20. Kfir Y, Buchner A, Hansen SL. Reactive lesions of the gingiva. A clinicopathological study of 741 cases. J Periodontol 1980; 51:655–661

CHAPTER 16

Labial Melanotic Macules

F. C. Powell

Definition. These are asymptomatic, discrete, benign, acquired tan to black-pigmented macular lesions, usually measuring 2–15 mm in size, which may be single (commonly) or multiple, and appear usually on the vermilion surface with some extension onto the mucosal aspect of the lower (80 %) lip. Approximately 3 % of the population develop these lesions, with peak onset in the 3rd decade of life [1].

Etiology. The etiology is unknown. There is a family history of similar lesions in 15 % of patients. The majority of affected individuals are female. Children and the elderly can develop these lesions.

Pathogenesis. There may be faulty transfer of melanosomes to keratinocytes after melanisation in melanocytes. This is supported by the lack of melanosomes in keratinocytes of the upper epidermis and pigment incontinence and melanophages in the dermis.

Oral Manifestations. The typical presentation is of an asymptomatic, well-defined tan oval-shaped macule on the vermilion border of the lower lip of a female patient (Fig. 16.1a, b). Variations in size, shape, colour and location occur (Fig. 16.2a, b). Progressive change in size or alteration in shape may be

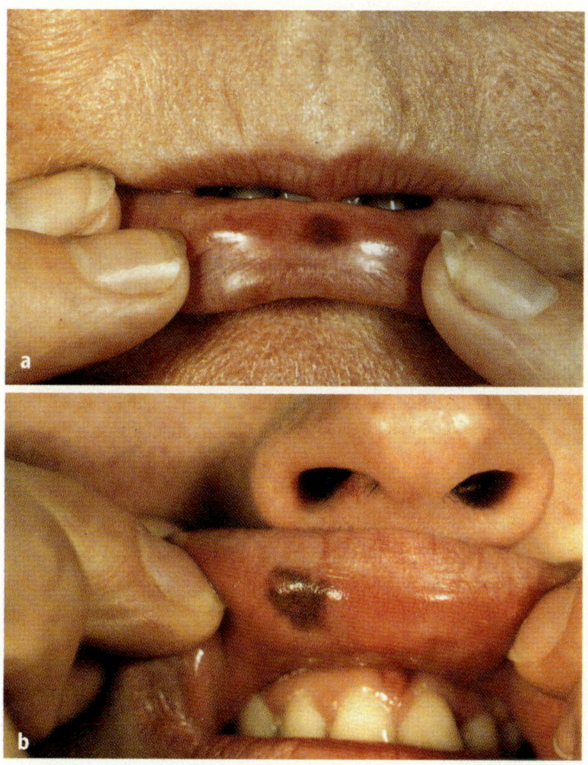

Fig. 16.1. a Discrete light brown macular pigmented lesion on the lower lip, typical of labial melanotic macule. **b** Similar but larger lesion on the upper lip with slightly irregular border extending onto the mucosal aspect of the labial surface. This labial melanotic macule had slowly been extending in size

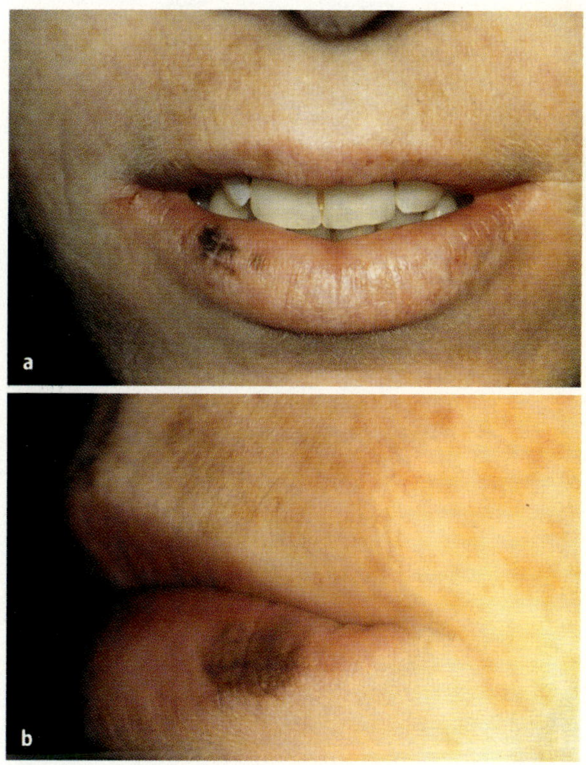

Fig. 16.2. a Labial melanotic macule on the lower lip showing irregularity in outline and pigmentation. Biopsy confirmed the benign nature of this lesion. **b** Irregular labial melanotic macule extending to the vermilion border of the lower lip with good skin markings

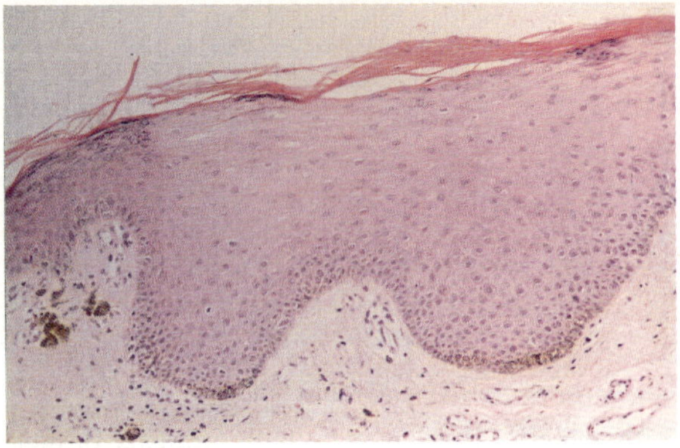

Fig. 16.3. Typical histology of a labial melanotic macule showing hyperpigmentation at the tips of the rete ridges with relative sparing of the remainder of the basal layer. Note also prominent melanophages in the left upper dermal region

reported by the patient. Mucosal lesions are usually absent, but extension of pigmentation onto the labial mucosal surface may occur.

Associated Findings. Usually none. Linear hyperpigmentation of nails (longitudinal melanychia) occur in the Laugier-Hunziker syndrome. Similar pigmented macules are rarely found on the genital mucosa (genital melanotic macules) in association with labial melanotic macules.

Microscopic Findings. Increased melanin pigmentation of the basal layer of the epidermis is noted, especially at the tips of the rete ridges with sparing of the interpapillary areas (Fig. 16.3). Prominent melanophages are present in the basal papillary dermis. The number of basal melanocytes is within normal limits. HMB-45 staining is negative, supportive of the benign nature of the melanocytes.

Diagnosis. The discrete size, well-defined regular outline and uniform pigmentation makes the diagnosis of typical lesions simple. Irregular lesions or those with alteration of pigmentation should be biopsied. Peutz-Jegher's syndrome shows multiplicity of lesions in a perioral distribution with prominent mucosal pigmentation (Fig. 16.4a, b). Perioral and pigmented lesions of the vermilion border tend to fade with increasing age in Peutz-Jegher's syndrome. Malignant melanoma of the labial surface is rare but should be considered in irregular or changing lesions and histological samples taken.

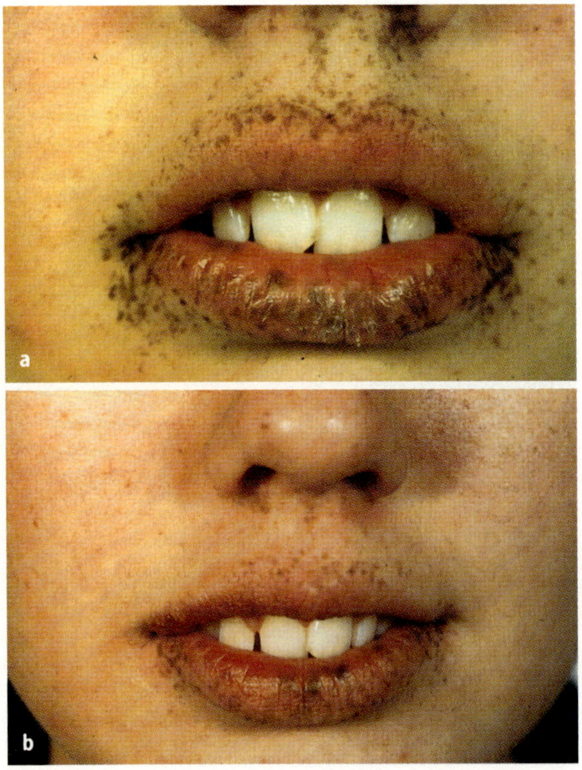

Fig. 16.4. **a** Peutz-Jegher's syndrome showing multiple labial and perioral macular area pigmentation in a 12-year-old girl. **b** The same patient 5 years later showing marked reduction in the number of cutaneous and labial macular pigmented spots. The degree of mucosal pigmentation remained static

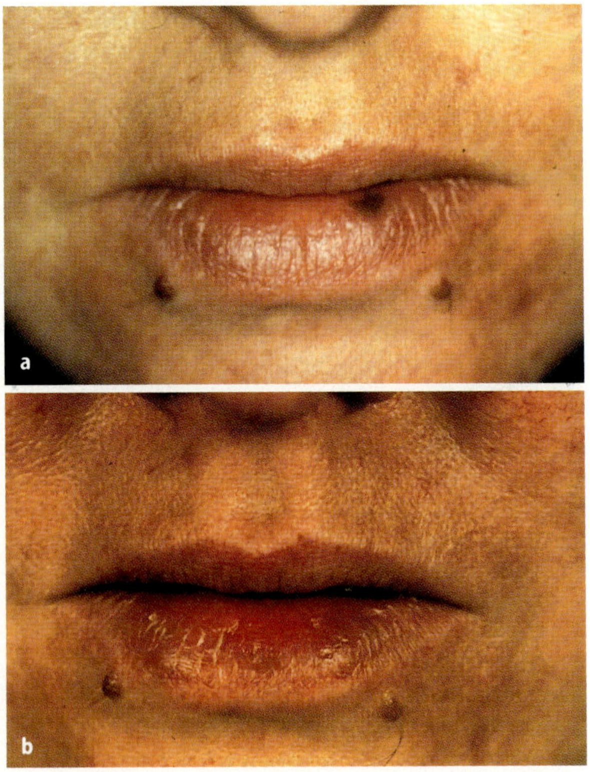

Fig. 16.5. **a** Labial melanotic macule on the left side of the lower lip before surgical excision. **b** Same patient after surgery showing complete healing of area of excision without perceptible scarring

Treatment. Usually none required. May be excised with good cosmetic results (Fig. 16.5a, b). Liquid nitrogen application may also be effective in removing established labial melanotic macules.

Reference

1. Ho KL, Dervan P, O'Loughlin S, Powell FC. Labial melanotic macule: a clinical, histopathologic and ultrastructural study. J Am Acad Dermatol 1993; 28: 33–39

CHAPTER 17

Psychosomatic Medicine, Orality and Disorders of the Oral Cavity Related to Psychoemotional Factors

G. Hautmann and E. Panconesi

17.1 Psychosomatic Medicine as a Premise for Understanding the Patient

The difficulties of being human oblige one to create a great psychic structure to bond or in some way cope with the inevitable physical and mental pain to be encountered during one's lifetime. The individual must start doing this shortly after birth and is able to do it only because of a unique phylogenetic heritage: the capacity for symbolic functioning.

In the earliest attempt to deal with physical pain, frustration, and absence, psychically one must make that first "mysterious leap" from body to mind. We know very little about this. Considerably more knowledge has been garnered by psychoanalysis about that even more mysterious leap in the other direction, the leap from mind to body which underlies hysterical conversion and the various inhibitions of bodily functioning. Long before such complicated psychic creations are absorbed, the baby must first have been seduced into life by its mother, for herein lies the initial movement which stirs the first glimmerings of psychic life. This much we know: the structuring of the psyche is a creative process destined to give each individual his unique identity. It provides a bulwark against psychic loss in traumatic circumstances and in the long run man's psychic creativity may well contain essential elements of protection against his biological destruction.

This brings us to a very important consideration: the importance of man's innate capacity for symbolic activity and psychic creation and, in particular, the *heterogeneous character* of these creations. In the attempt to maintain some form of psychic equilibrium under any circumstance, every human being is capable of creating a neurosis, a psychosis, a pathological character pattern, a sexual perversion, or a "*psychosomatic disease.*" In spite of the human tendency to maintain a relatively stable psychic economy, thus guaranteeing a more-or-less enduring personality pattern, the individual is liable to produce any or all of these diverse creations at different periods in life. Although the various results of psychic productions do not all have the same psychological social value, they are all the product of man's mind and their forms are determined by the way the individual psyche has been structured. They all have inherent meaning in relation to one's wish to live and to get along as well as possible. From this point of view, it is evident that the *psychosomatic creations* appear the most mysterious since they are at least appropriate to the overall desire to live. If their psychological function is conspicuous by its absence, their biological meaning also eludes us. In many respects, psychosomatic creations are the antithesis of neurotic or psychotic manifestations. Indeed, frequently when the latter cease psychosomatic (as opposed to psychological) illness becomes manifest.

Moreover, we believe that man's irrepressible psychic fertility of whatever order is coexistent with life itself. If we admit that something like psychic death may occur, then it is possible that when psychic creation faulters or comes to a halt, man may be threatened with biological death. The psychic processes that create and maintain psychic health, as well as those responsible for maintaining psychic ill-health, are nevertheless on the side of life. When we, for any reason, fail to create some form of mental management to deal with psychic pain, a *psychosomatic process* may take over.

Research into the meaning and treatment of psychosomatic illness (including the presence of certain parameters such as chronicity, involvement of a psychic stress, and characteristic and constant personality traits) is at the crossroads of various scientific disciplines. We focus mainly on the psychosomatic features that can be evidenced through that very peculiar viewpoint, psychoanalytic interpretation; this is a highly specific instrument, concerned with psychic and symbolic functioning rather than somatic transformations. We prefer to use the "psychoanalytic microscope," also because of our use of liaison consultation with psychoanalysts and psychodynamically oriented psychiatrists. Moreover, the term "psychosomatic" embodies the concept of the immaterial "psyche," in contrast to the material "brain." The mind (psyche) cannot send impulses directly to body tissues (soma): such impulses originate in the diencephalon, from which projection fibers extend to all organs of the body. Therefore, the term "psychosomatic" is imprecise as it does not explain the disease, from either an anatomic or a physiologic viewpoint.

We note that people suffering from disorders, which, according to the literature, may be of psychosomatic origin or may be aggravated by psychic stress, usually seek a physician rather than a psychiatrist or an analyst for their somatic ills, unless of course they consider they have psychological problems as well. Sometimes, however, patients who are unaware of suffering from psychological symptoms do turn up in the psychiatrist's or analyst's consulting room, complaining for example of skin disorders (urticaria, itching, contact dermatitis, etc.), gastric symptoms, or cardiopathology, because a psychoanalytic or psychiatric consultation has been suggested by the consulting physician.

The uses and abuses of man's body by his mind are so varied and so extensive that it is important to define what the term *psychosomatic* means, and we want to delineate, in particular, the distinction between psychosomatic disorders and hysterical or other somatic manifestations. We might recall that Freud designated two types of somatization: *conversion hysteria* and *real neurosis*. In a sense, one was the antithesis of the other [1]. Whereas in hysterical conversion we witness the "mysterious leap" from mind to body, in the concept of actual neurosis there is a leap in the opposite direction, from the somatic to the psychic sphere. In either case, an invisible barrier is crossed. The problems raised by this transition have, to date, still lost very little of their mystery.

Although "actual neurosis" as a nosographical entity is little used nowadays, it is pertinent to our enquiry to note, as Laplanche and Pontalis [2] pointed out, that in Freud's conception, the "actual" symptoms (neurasthenia and anxiety neurosis) were principally somatic ones. Being of a physiological order, they were considered by Freud to be devoid of symbolic meaning and therefore not truly within the scope of psychoanalytic treatment. Freud's belief that real neurosis is brought about as a reaction to actual everyday tension, and in particular to the blocking of libidinal satisfactions, is closely related to certain modern conceptions of psychosomatic reactions, although today the notion of "psychic pressure" would lay equal emphasis on the blocking of aggressive impulses and on all that might be included in the term "environmental stress." Freud believed that conversion hysteria and real neurosis both arose from sexual sources, but whereas the latter was related to the present sexual problems, the former stemmed from the sexual conflicts of early childhood, and the physical symptoms retained their symbolic significance, i. e., they appeared in the place of instinctual satisfaction and were, in essence, a symbolic solution to an unconscious conflict and not a reaction to frustration [1]. It is evident that the "somatic" symptoms of conversion hysteria are symbolic in that they refer to a *fantastic* body in the literal sense of the word, a body functioning as a small child might imagine, or a fantasy body such as might be contrived by primary process thinking. Then, Freud came to consider hysterical conversion and hysterical identification as *ego defenses*. In this way, the well-known list of hysterical symptoms was incremented with those which use the body to translate inhibition of id [1] impulses as a reaction to the repressive forces of ego [2], and superego. Thus, inhibitions of bodily functioning, such as constipation, impotence, frigidity, insomnia, and so on, have come to be considered as closely allied to classical conversion symptoms.

In every case, *the symptom tells a story*. Once decoded, the story always reveals the hero to be a guilty victim of forbidden wishes who has met setbacks along the pathways of desire. The subject's symptoms might be said to result from the combined effect of his unconscious fantasy life and the structure of his ego defenses. These symptoms, undoubtedly of psychogenic origin, do not form part of what is denoted by the term *psychosomatic*. We might say that in hysteria, the body lends itself and its functions to the mind to use as the mind wills, whereas in psychosomatic illness the body does its own "thinking." The drama which is being expressed is a more "archaic" one and its elements have been stored differently. The symptoms are signs, not symbols, and follow somatic rather than psychic laws. Unlike the hysterical dramatizations, the thinking of the soma is carried out with, sometimes literally, deadly precision. The recurring character of science fiction, the mechanized robot who takes over, without even a pale shadow of emotion or identification with the common human wishes and conflicts, is a pristine image of the workings of the psychosomatic symptom. The soma is no longer concerned with translating the wishes of the psyche, as in neurotic illness. If we attempt to define the area covered in today's terminology by the word *psychosomatic*, we might say that this term is reserved for *organic disorders of demonstrable physiological (of physiology) dysfunction* (and then pathological or physiological nature), *but although they have no apparent symbolic significance, they appear nevertheless to be linked with the patient's personality structure, life circumstances, and history*, i. e., they declare themselves in connection with situations of stress arising either from within the individual or from his immediate environment. The psychosomatic subject, however, is rarely aware of any such connections and is frequently *unaware* of being under any particular stress. This definition, though extremely vague, serves to distinguish such disorders from hysterical manifestations, in which there is no physiopathological lesion, and also from organic illness, in which no links with the personality or environmental stress appear to be involved.

At this point, we would like to come back to the fact that the mental and the physical are indissolubly linked, yet at the same time essentially different. The psyche-soma functions as an entity. There is little doubt that every psychological event has its effect on the physiological body, just as every somatic event has repercussions on the mind, even when these are not consciously registered.

Freud's position regarding the psyche-soma should be recalled. He grounded the psychoanalytic theory of mind on firm biological territory and constantly emphasized the tendency of the human organism to function as a whole. Nevertheless, he chose to concern himself solely with the psychological aspects of the psyche-soma, and showed a distinct disinclination to cross the frontier between the psychological and the physiological, even in areas where he recognized organic illness as being of psychosomatic origin. At the same time, he was constantly preoccupied with the relations between body and mind, and the fact that psychic processes grow out of organic ones.

We must also remember the theoretical model of the more recent Parisian psychosomatic school which comprises an economic theory of psychosomatic transformation, and the concept of psychosomatic transformation as opposed to neurotic, psychotic, perverse, etc., structures. The economic concept is closely allied to the early theory of real neurosis, emphasis being laid on urgent instinctual discharge, which escapes psychic elaboration because of deficient representation and diminished affective response: in short, an impoverishment of the capacity to symbolize instinctual demands and their conflict with reality, and to elaborate fantasy. Instinctual energy, bypassing the psyche, thus affects the soma directly, with catastrophic results. This particular theoretical approach to psychosomatic formations is in complete contrast with the theory of hysterical formation: the latter being the result of repressed fantasy elaborations, while the former would result precisely from the lack of such psychic activity. The failure to represent instinctual conflict symbolically leads to a specific mode of mental functioning and this may in turn lead to a "psychosomatic character pattern" [3]. On the basis of several years of research (interviews and psychotherapy), these investigators have delineated certain characteristics observed in seriously ill psychosomatic patients. We can summarize as follows:

1. Unusual object relationship, notably lacking in libidinal affect. This is also manifest in the interviews insofar as these patients show little interest in the investigation and practically none in the investigator.
2. An impoverished use of language marked in particular by what the authors call operant thinking ("*la pensée opératoire*"). This refers to thoughts that are pragmatic in the extreme. For example, "What kind of woman is your mother?" Reply: "Well, she's tall and blonde." "What was your reaction when you learned of the death of your fiancé?" "Well, I thought I'd have to pull myself together." In these interviews, one is struck by the flat response and an impression of unusual detachment. These have a psychotic resonance, yet there is no resemblance to a psychotic ego functioning in other aspects of these patients' lives, nor to any form of psychotic thought disorders. Indeed, "operant thinking" may be highly intellectual and abstract. De M'Uzan [4, 5] has pointed out that the outstanding feature of such thinking is its detachment "from any truly alive internal object representations."
3. A marked lack of neurotic symptoms and neurotic character adaptations.
4. Facial movements, bodily gestures, sensorimotor manifestations, and physical pain will appear where one might expect neurotic manifestations.
5. Preliminary interviews with psychosomatic patients are usually characterized by a type of inertia which threatens to bring discussion to an end, unless the investigator makes vigorous efforts to stimulate associative material concerning the patient's relationships, life experience, and illness. Dramatic or painful events are recounted with little emotional overtone or are omitted if not directly solicited.

Along similar lines, Sifneos [6] sees in psychosomatic patients a sort of agenesis of symbolic thought which he calls "*alexithymia*". Alexithymic patients are distinguished as primary, those in whom alexithymic traits are due principally to genetic or neurophysiologic causes (lack of connection between the limbic lobe – seat of the emotions – and the neocortical regions – neurophysiologic base for a critical evaluation of feelings), and secondary, those in whom the structural role of cultural and psychodynamic factors prevail. The characteristic features of alexithymic patients are, according to Sifneos, an impoverished fantasy life, poor dream recall, an inability to express feelings with words ("*no words for moods*"), and a utilitarian mode of thinking which is concerned with conscious psychic processes and has no appreciable relationship with unconscious fantasies. Sifneos concludes that since alexithymic patients are unable to produce fantasies or to establish an emotional interaction with others (including their therapist), psychodynamic psychotherapy is contraindicated [6].

Nevertheless, Engel [7] and Musaph [8] have independently claimed that many of their psychosomatic patients express themselves freely and have rich creative fantasy lives. Without disputing the presence of alexithymia in many psychosomatic and other physically ill patients, we question some of the conclusions which have resulted from its identification, in particular the implications for psychotherapy.

Now let us examine transactions within the doctor-patient relationship, with particular attention to *counter-transference* phenomena. Heimann [9, 10] suggested that the prefix "counter" implies additional factors and she used the term counter-transference to cover "all feelings which the analyst experiences towards the patient." She stressed the positive value of counter-transference and viewed it as "an instrument of research into the patient's unconscious." Heimann assumed "that the analyst's unconscious understands that of his patient. This rapport on the deep level comes to the surface in the form of feelings which the analyst notices in response to his patient, in his counter-transference." She stated "this is the most dynamic way in which his patient's voice reaches him." Heimann's contribution was to show clearly that the reaction of the analyst may be the first useful clue to what is going on in the patient. During the analytic work, the emotions aroused in the therapist are often "much nearer to the heart of the matter than his reasoning, or, to put it in other words, his unconscious perception of the patient's unconscious is more acute and in advance of his conscious perception of the situation... The counter-transference is not only part and parcel of the analytic relationship, but it is the patient's *creation*, it is part of the patient's personality" [9, 10].

Similar views are expressed by Bion [11] and Money-Kirle [12], who consider that by way of a pre-verbal or archaic kind of communication, some patients succeed in imposing a fantasy and its corresponding affect upon their analyst in order to deny it in themselves. At first sight, the therapist experiences these as being his own response to something, not recognizing that they have been made by the patient. The effort involved is in differentiating the patient's contribution from one's own. By using the theory of projective identification, the therapist can analyze his counter-transference and then develop appropriate interventions and interpretations. Various negative counter-responses to projective identification have been described by Money-Kirle [12]: for example, "the analyst may reproject the patient as something not understood, or foreign, in the external world." Projective identifications from the alexithymic patient may therefore be reprojected as statements that he is a mechanical kind of being with a neurophysiological defect. The affects of dullness, boredom, and frustration which the patient evokes appear to facilitate this reprojection and serve as rationalizations for the conclusions that he is blocked up inside an impregnable wall, and is unsuitable for psychodynamic psychotherapy. We believe that access may be gained to the patient's inner life by considering the feelings of dullness, boredom, and frustration as counter-transference experiences.

Grotjahn [13] and Fliess [14] discussed the affects of dullness and boredom, which they indicate may evoke a stage of ego disintegration and ego reconstruction. "Dullness is an ego danger because it is a stage of ego starvation. The dull situation offers no opportunity to apply the cognitive or motor abilities of the ego so that the ego is put into a desperate situation of unemployment, faces a mental death and the result is a certain disintegration" [13]. With the alexithymic patient, the therapist enters into a relationship expecting to be fed interesting fantasies and feelings, only to encounter increasing frustration, dullness, and boredom. If the therapist relaxes ego control, he may experience *oral-sadistic and oral-erotic fantasies which, as Fliess [14] indicates, parallel the infant's response to the trauma of weaning. Fliess has also referred to an implied "sucking-biting conflict" in the situation of boredom.* These feelings and fantasies may be regarded as counter-transference phenomena which are evoked by the patient's projective identifications. Analysis of the counter-transference therefore provides "secret access" into the patient's inner world which the patient is still unable to perceive consciously. According to Grinberg [15], Hanna Segal suggested that violent projective identifications made by patients presumably result from infantile experiences during which the child was subject to violent projective identifications on the part of the parents [16]. As the doctor-patient relationship parallels the mother-infant relationship, there is an unconscious re-creation of early feelings and fantasies associated with introjective and projective maneuvers. By sustaining and analyzing the counter-transference, the therapist can develop appropriate therapeutic strategies and interpretations which render the relationship with the alexithymic patient anything but sterile.

A paper by Fain and David [17] deals with the cardinal importance of dreaming and of unconscious fantasy in the maintenance of psychic equilibrium. In their conclusions, the authors state that the psychosomatic patient reveals a damaged capacity for creating fantasy to deal with infantile and present-day anxieties. Comparisons are drawn with psychotic patients who, in circumstances similar to those which precipitate psychosomatic illness, suffer hallucinatory episodes. Unlike the psychotic, "the psychosomatic patient remains closely attached to facts and things in external reality." The ego may show impoverishment but there is no distortion. However, in both cases pathological problems arise in proportion to the inability to use regression or dream functioning. This comparison calls to mind the clinical findings of Sperling [18]. Although she adduces quite different theoretical conclusions, she noted alternations between psychotic states and psychosomatic illness in the same individuals. Thus, if psychosomatic personalities may be said to be "antineurotics" due to their inability to create neurotic defenses, from another standpoint they may also be considered as "antipsychotics," in that they are "over-adapted" to reality and the difficulties of existence. Although the ego differences are striking from a phenomenological point of view, both states would appear to derive from some breakdown in symbolic functioning and we might expect similarities at some point. We have already mentioned two similarities, a certain quality of object relationship and a tendency to stifle or to lack affectivity.

In Bahnson's pathogenetic model of "psychophysiological complementarity," stress provokes a regression that can be either behavioral or somatic according to the way in which the subject's defenses are utilized: in one case, defenses of protection and removal which involve interpersonal relationships prevail, and the result is neurosis, or even psychosis; in the other case, there is a prevalence of repression/denial defenses which discharge the regression inside the body and result in hysteria, hypochondria, "psychosomatosis," organic illnesses, and even cancer [19].

Yahalom [20] reports Ekstein's work with psychotic children: this can give us an insight into certain features which call to mind aspects of psychosomatic patients. The study of the preoccupation of psychotic children with monsters and its connection with their inability to contain and to elaborate internal excitement offers several points of reflection. Yahalom writes: "The pressure of what the psychotic child wants yet fears, gives ground before his inward drive. He tries to cling to something concrete, reachable by his immediate senses, so that he can escape being overwhelmed by a flood of archaic matter. He then calls upon some creature, a delusionary introject, as a kind of substitute superego." This mechanism is closely allied to the tendency of the psychosomatic personality to cling to the concrete and factual aspects of living and to pursue them with intensity. Yahalom says: "In order to release an impulse with relief there must be a representation of an 'object' that absorbs the release. This can be called a safety element. The original safety element is the 'satiating mother' and the safety explains the insistent search for a mothering echo." The "satiating mother" recalls in striking fashion the "addictive mother" of infants suffering from psychosomatic illnesses (see below). In either case, satiating or addictive mother, the children run the risk of not being genuinely object-related.

In trying to come to terms with the substructure of all "action disorders" including psychosomatic "acts," we are in the area of transitional phenomena and are witnesses to the *attempt to make substitute objects in the external world do duty for symbolic ones which are absent or damaged in the inner psychic world.* Such attempts are ineluctably doomed to failure and the victim of this kind of lack is equally doomed to endless repetition and addictive attachment to the outer world and external objects. To come back then to the striking *differences* between psychosomatic and psychotic creations, we might say that, whereas the psychotic child clutches onto the delusional "monster" to palliate the lack of the internal object brutally projected outwards, the psychosomatic sufferer has precociously laid his monsters to rest. He has lost them. We agree with McDougall [19] that there are deeply buried archaic fantasy elements encapsulated somewhere in the unconscious or conscious thought. Stored at a pre-symbolic level, they do not find expression even in dreams. With a psychic substratum in which the "monsters" have been neither allowed to grow up nor projected in a hallucinatory fashion, but simply neglected through lack of psychic nourishment, what is missing is something much more subtle. Perhaps a concept such as *negative hallucination* might be invoked here. Such a mode of mental functioning would lead to an arrest in ego development, markedly different from that found in psychosis. The split is drawn in differently. In psychotic states, the ego is overwhelmed by the imaginary world once it slips out of its traces and is then no longer able to perform its initial function of inhibiting hallucinatory fulfilments [1]. The psychosomatic ego chokes the archaic elements of fantasy in their very beginnings and thus becomes split off from its instinctual roots, leaving few elements available for the creation of psychotic delusions.

Fain [21] has done studies on the earliest beginnings of fantasy life and their role in the predisposition to psychosomatic illness. This includes findings on babies suffering from serious psychosomatic disturbances in the 1st month of life. One group comprised infants who were only able to sleep if rocked continually in their mothers' arms, and otherwise suffered from almost total insomnia. The studies suggest that these mothers have failed in their function as a protective shield against exciting stimuli, precisely through overindulging the exercise of this function. Instead of the development of a primitive form of psychic activity akin to dreaming, which permits most babies to sleep peacefully after feeding, these babies require the mother herself to be the guardian of sleep. The author links this breakdown of the capacity to re-create symbolically a good internal state of being, to an allied failure to develop autoerotic activity. Fain's observations lead him to the conclusion that these babies do not have a satisfying mother ("*mère satisfaisante*") but a tranquilizing mother ("*mère calmante*"). The latter, because of her own problems, cannot permit her baby to create a primary identification which will enable him to sleep without continual contact with her. Cases of infantile asthma show a similarly disturbed mother-nursling relationship. Analogous observations have been made concerning the mother of "allergic" children: these mothers appear to allow no satisfactions which are not obtained in direct contact with themselves. Autoerotic activity and the capacity for psychic development is blocked in these children. "We have postulated that these mothers unconsciously wish to bring their children back to foetal bliss inside their own bodies," writes Fain [21]. This represents a pathological exaggeration of what is fundamentally a normal instinctual attitude on the mother's part, namely, to create a sheltering womb-like world for her newborn until he is able to provide this for himself. But, because of her own unconscious needs, she does not create conditions in which the baby can take over this function. If her libidinal interest in the other aspects of her life, particularly her love-life, does not lead her to *disinvest* her baby sufficiently (e. g., wishing it to go peacefully off to sleep leaving her free for other occupations), she may overdo her protective role, thus keeping her baby tied to her bodily presence. Here we point out that also Ammon [22] paid particular attention to the psychodynamic implications in dermatologic patients. In his exemplary interpretation of a case of atopic dermatitis, the skin disease was considered "related to a disturbed archaic mother-child relationship in which a dominating and rejecting mother on the one hand took possession of her child as to body and psyche, but on the other was not capable of any spontaneous tender body contact and thus exposed him to serious abandonment anxieties." This example belongs to Ammon's original ego-structural view, according to which the symptoms of the psychosomatic disease try to fill in the "hole in the ego," that is the deficiency in the ego-structure caused by the disturbed mother-child relationship (*psychosomatogenous mother*): the final aim is to impede disintegration of the personality. With this point of view we look to Winnicott [23] for support and start out from the relationship between the child and the *"not good enough mother"*, only to arrive through the action of the affective conflict at a schism of self, a division between the psyche and soma, which creates the "psychosomatic" disease to avoid anguish [23].

Fain describes three types of baby sleep-patterns related to early psychic functioning: the first infant makes small sucking movements while sleeping, the second sleeps with his thumb firmly planted in his mouth; the third sucks frenetically and does not sleep. We have here three modes of autoerotism which manifest qualitative differences in the balance between motricity and the capacity for psychic representation. This in turn implies a difference in the distribution of narcissistic libido and that part of the libido which remains attached to the object [21].

The first baby reinforces his capacity to maintain sleep through some form of hallucinatory discharge of excitation, the second requires a real object for a much longer period of time; babies of the third category are thrown into a perilous cycle of endless discharge. Fain concludes from his observation of the mothers that "the continual investment of the baby by the mother impedes the development of primary autoerotism and this automatically leads to a most dangerous vicissitude – the exclusion of libidinal activity from the symbolic chain... This type of maternal failure is frequently accompanied by a corresponding failure in the father's role as a figure of authority" [21].

This reference to parental attitudes indicates that the groundwork for eventual reactions to the oedipal crisis is already being laid down.

At the opposite end of the scale of infantile psychosomatic disorders is the strange disease known as "*merycism*" in which the baby constantly regurgitates and then swallows his stomach contents until dehydration and exhaustion set in. Here, the baby has created *prematurely* an autoerotic object which enables him to dispense with his mother. Observations of the mothers reveal that, among other unusual restrictions, they impose severe prohibitions on all normal autoerotic activity. "They react to thumb-sucking as though it were a truly Oedipal masturbation to be suppressed at all costs" [21]. In comparison with the tiny insomniacs, the merycist babies show a significant contrast: they sleep well. The author points out that in order to sleep, a baby must develop the capacity for adequate autoerotic activity, as well as the autonomous ability to maintain a protective barrier against stimuli both from within and without. These children succeed in decathecting the sensorium, but there is nevertheless a serious symbolic gap in that the mother's absence is in no way compensated *psychically*; it is totally disavowed through the baby's having precociously created its own protective barrier against her absence, and one which continues to isolate him from her even in her presence. She is the helpless witness of his autoerotic activity. "The external object is first 'perceived' in that part of the body formed by the mouth-esophagus-stomach area. For these children there is a total separation between the instinctual world and the somatic area where the oral impulses make themselves felt, and, on the other hand, the sensorium where the stimuli from the outer world are captured." Instinctual aims and autoerotic activity then run the risk of becoming literally *autonomous*, detached from any *mental representation of an object*. According to McDougall, this may be here the foundation for a subsequent separation between psyche and soma in adult life.

From a historic-genetic viewpoint, Fain's research suggests that there are at least two predominant trends in disturbed baby-mother relationships which are apt to create a predisposition to *psychosomatic pathology*. The first is unusually severe prohibition of every attempt on the baby's part to create autoerotic substitutes for the maternal relationship, thus vitiating the nodal point for the creation of inner object representations and the nascent elements of fantasy life. The second trend is the antithesis of this, namely, the mother's continual offering of herself as the only object of satisfaction and psychic viability. Fain's observations agree with Spitz's findings [24] on mother-child relationships and their importance in creating or hindering the development of autoerotism. One might consider it a question of leaving the baby too much or too little psychic space in which to be mentally creative on his own.

With the expansion of psychodynamic knowledge and the ever increasing accumulation of clinical experience and research findings, it was inevitable that psychoanalysis would concern itself with psychosomatic symptoms arising in patients, and would try to decode their meaning. It was equally inevitable that psychoanalysts would at first try to reconstruct the underlying fantasy formations which the somatic symptoms might symbolize, following the well-known pattern of hysterias. However, this proved to be more difficult than expected: Freud, in fact, had already made the discovery that such symptoms, unlike hysterical ones, yielded no answers under hypnosis. Other analysts observed that with psychosomatic patients presenting few neurotic symptoms, the analytical process did not by any means reveal the clear oedipal and preoedipal structures, with their contingent of fantasy, sexual symbolism, and object-relation patterns, which were the fruit of analytical work with patients suffering from hysterical and obsessional neuroses and sexual perversions. In fact, most of the patients whose reactions to anxiety were almost exclusively psychosomatic were quite refractory to analytical therapy. Nevertheless, many correlations were found between specific emotional conflicts and specific personality traits on the one hand, and specific psychosomatic afflictions on the other. These were studied by psychiatrists using both physiological and psychological techniques. At the same time, analysts using only their therapeutic skills and intuitions drawn from classical psychoanalysis, attempted to reconstruct the unconscious fantasies which might underlie somatic symptoms. One of the best known of these is the hypothesis suggested by Garma (cited by McDougall [19]): in speaking of patients with gastric ulcers, he described the ulcer as a vengeful "bite" which the patient was obliged to give himself as a punishment for his babyhood wishes to bite his mother's breast. Thus, out of unconscious guilt, the future ulcer patient might select food harmful to himself, and procure for himself an introjected bite simultaneously into his stomach and psyche. In addition, ulcers were ultimately found to carry miscellaneous symbolic meanings related to the castration complex.

It is worth noting that since the interaction of psyche and soma are so intricate and so inevitable, we may easily lose sight of their fundamental difference. A cartesian metaphor like "body is black and mind is white" might yield the idea that *psychosomatic manifestations could be considered as an infinite series of grays*. However, such a simplified model would overlook the essential difference between psychic and somatic functions. It would be better to compare the psyche-soma to a fusional substance like seawater. In spite of its unity, saltwater can be transformed on the one hand into a heap of dried salts and on the other into a cloud of watery vapor. We might consider the salts as the somatic elements, whereas the psychic dimension is represented by the watery cloud. This metaphor allows us to conceive the two components as different in substance and subject to different laws. The fact that they combine should not allow us to obliterate their dissimilarity. Taking the analogy a little further, one might also emphasize that neither substance quite adds up to a piece of living ocean. Thus, we can readily sympathize with those who find that a somatic approach to the problem resembles a pile of dried dust, drained of its psychic fluid. And we understand equally well that the somaticians and the psychobiological experimenters, when faced with the archaic fantasy constructions and hypotheses which a less rigid psychological approach allows, feel they are called upon to take arms against a sea of suppositions: a cloud of watery vapor with no solid matter left. In fact, neither tells us much of what is going on in the stormy ocean. Nevertheless, theoretical confusion will result if we overlook the fact that somatic processes and psychic processes are governed by different laws of functioning. We cannot apply the laws which structure psychological functions to those which govern physiological functioning. There is not a causal but an analogical relationship between the two orders. This concords with the observations and reflections of Konrad Lorenz, who concluded that the movement from soma to psyche will remain forever mysterious. From a psychoanalytical viewpoint, we are constantly made aware of the intricate and ineluctable interdependence of psyche and soma, while being confronted with their ineradicable difference.

Thus, in concluding this section, it is opportune to point out some of the elementary concepts which form the basis of our idea of psychosomatics.

1. The body (soma) and the mind (psyche), treated separately for too long, at least in Western medicine, constitute a single unit. Separating the two and treating them individually should be considered a reductive necessity or abusive operative simplification for the investigator and/or the doctor; this method of proceeding has hypertrophied, accentuated by the use of different methods for studying and intervening on the one hand on the body and on the other on the mind. Psychosomatic medicine proposes the examination of psyche and soma as a unit "in sickness and in health" and, in the former case, useful intervention in the attempt to re-establish equilibriums that have been altered.
2. A long series of observations suggest, with certainty for some, inconclusively for others, that certain somatic functions and certain diseases, even cutaneous, are influenced, triggered, or caused by factors which belong to the psychic sphere and which we could define generically as "emotional". We note that H.I. Kaplan and B.J. Sadock, in their *Pocket Handbook of Clinical Psychiatry* [25], point out that "the psychosomatic disorder refers to physical conditions caused or aggravated by psychological factors. Although most physical disorders are influenced by stress, conflict, or generalized anxiety, some disorders are more affected than others" [25].
   A very ample series of observations signal the influence which many diseases (especially cutaneous ones, because of their unaesthetic consequences) exercise on psychic homeostasis. In such cases, we prefer to speak of somatopsychics. A vicious circle may be established by the superimposition of psychosomatic and somatopsychic influences.
3. We would suggest that in so-called alexithymic patients, feelings are neither denied nor absent, but are, rather, deeply buried and experienced as highly dangerous and ego-disruptive. Through his counter-transference responses, the therapist gathers information about the primitive internalized object relationships of the patient. The doctor-patient transactions may then be conceptualized in terms of introjective-projective relatedness and in fostering the development of psychotic transference, intense feelings, fantasies, and dreams are released.
4. The patient must be considered in a unitary way (holistic) as an inseparable mind-body relationship [26].

The "psychosomatic idea" may oscillate between the ambitious assumption of interpreting a disease as determined by a psychic disturbance and the necessity of suggesting that the doctor use a better psychological approach in managing his patient. Psychosomatic interpretation of certain diseases, including cutaneous ones, has always come up against the quantitative terms (the "scientific method" of Newton and Galileo, so respected by the majority of the biological and medical sciences), in opposition to "indeterminate" methods, like those of the "sciences of man" (those related to psychology and psychiatry). Psychosomatics uses both routes, excludes no fields, and looks for clinical confirmation of relationships (supposed or glimpsed) between psyche and soma, which have marvelous, sophisticated, and continually better-identified anatomo-physiologic ties. Winnicott says, significantly, that the hyphen uniting the two terms of the expression (psyche-soma) is the most important part of the word (psychosomatic), because it defines the area that needs to be studied: "the hyphen at the same time unites and divides the two aspects of medical practice." This hyphen is the area in which those who deal with psychosomatic illnesses work, and it is here that we find the fundamental disturbance of the patient; that is, his "dissociation" that tends to separate the two terms and thus to make space for the hyphen [26, 24].

17.2 Orality and Oro-alimentary Behavior

Sigmund Freud, the father of psychoanalysis, died in London in 1939 at the age of 83 from cancer of the jaw. In 1917, Freud suffered from swelling of the palate, and from then on thought he might have a carcinoma. Since the swelling appeared in a period when he was forced to give up smoking, because cigars were not available, and it disappeared when he started smoking again, he thought perhaps the symptom was psychogenic. In February 1923, he became aware of a tumor on the right side of his palate. This was removed in the first of 33 operations which Freud underwent for this affliction. Then, 6 months later, the famous Viennese mouth surgeon Hans Pichler performed a radical operation, removing the diseased areas from Freud's jaw and palate, which irremediably compromised the quality of life for Freud from then on. He had to wear an uncomfortable prothesis, which he called "the monster," necessary to close up the cavity resulting from the surgery, but insertion and removal were very painful, and when in place it caused sores and severe pain. The specialists consulted were unable to improve the situation, and Freud's life was practically unbearable from that time on: talking and eating were difficult, as was smoking cigars, which was presumably the origin of the disease.

The face presents three organs which exercise different basic functions: the eyes to see, the mouth to eat, breathe, and talk, and the nose to smell and breathe. We can presume that when investigated under a psychosomatic profile, many of the complex behavioral patterns studied in the psychology of mimical expressions, and in a broader sense also the pathological aspects involving that part of the body, are merely elaborations and further developments of these more simple functions.

The basic activity of "seeing," for example, involves not only perceptual-visual activity, but also a more elaborate activity of a cognitive character – from seeing we pass on to observing, recognizing, identifying, and so on – and these psychological operations are closely related, in turn, to attention. Thus, also so-called emotional behavior acquires in this area a particular meaning with a perceptive-cognitive character. The orientation reflex of aspecific attention can become alarm, fear, fright, etc., all responses close to the operation of identification of a stimulus. A stimulus identified as threatening, for example, provokes responses in the alarm-fright axis which are functional to the development of survival behavior (attack, flight, etc.).

The fundamental function of the mouth is, instead, strictly related to oral alimentary behavior. One must remember that the mimetic muscles of this area indicate first of all the relationship with ingestion of food in the simplest forms of sucking, chewing and biting (the latter is included also in the aggressive responses). Through the oral district, therefore, the environment is concretely taken in by the organism. Thus, while the ocular organ observes, the oral one gives absolute prevalence to taking in, expelling, etc. In any case, the relationship is one that involves active, peculiar manipulation of part of the environment, although different from manual activity. In children, the oral region also has the important function of knowledge and cognitive decodification of the environment.

Furthermore, oral alimentary behavior is closely connected with the internal conditions of the organism. Hunger, in fact, arises following alteration in homeostasis (specifically related to hypoglycemia), and satiation means that the homeostasis has been reestablished. Thus, the perioral muscles may, through contraction and relaxation, represent a complex system of "signals" which refer to internal conditions, indicating states of discomfort or satisfaction, both physical and/or psychological. For example, the hunger cry of an infant involves a particular positioning of the lips (the mouth assumes a quadrangular form due to the contraction of the quadrate muscles of the upper and lower lips and the contraction of the depressor anguli oris), which manifests an internal discomfort of alimentary origin. Obviously, these signals indicate originally to the mother the well-being or discomfort of the child. In fact, Charlesworth and Kreutzer [27] distinguish between the smile, explicitly of relational significance, which appears at the 3rd month, from the smile of the first few weeks of life, which appears prevalently in phases of sleepiness and irregular sleep, and which indicates internal states of the organism specifically related to glycemia levels.

The difference between the newborn infant and the 3-month-old is that of more punctual "means of communication" of positive and negative internal conditions and states, which become more and more differentiated in time. The infant's first experiences regard fairly general internal states, such as hunger, pain, satisfaction, and dissatisfaction. More differentiated emotions appear later [28], but make use of the schemes and expressive signs of preceding phases, for example smiling and crying. The infant goes from indicating hunger-satiation to indicating internal emotional conditions of pleasure-suffering. Even refusal and disgust, operations originally related to food [29], are extended to non-alimentary classes of behavior and psychological judgement. Thus, for example, disgust goes beyond the original physiological horizon: its use is extended to the definition of objects and persons; it acquires a psychological quality, increasing its metaphoric psychological capacity for reference.

The nasal region (the Schneiderian membrane) is closely connected with the oral region (the oral mucosae: inside the cheek, the palate, and the tongue, even allowing for specific differences among the three). Taste and smell interact in analyzing pleasant-unpleasant alimentary stimuli. Thus, even semantic transfer to classes of psychological events, such as disdain-refusal, involves the muscles of both regions.

The oral region is, together with the nasal one, a basis of both respiratory activity and language. It is important at this point to emphasize the possibility that also language represents a "pulling out," "expression," and therefore can be the object of favoring and inhibiting systems. One can imagine the possibilities for superimposition, of behavioral schemes aimed at withholding not only foodstuffs, but also "sonoric material," which always has a strong interactive, relational component. Themes of "not saying," "not expressing," "not communicating," are extremely important psychologically, and thus *psychosomatically*, and can be read and traced in the mimical movements of the face (including those which indicate endo-oral motions such as sucking, gritting the teeth, pushing the tongue, etc.).

It is important to note that there are two fundamental oral alimentary behaviors, sucking and chewing. Sucking is the typical behavior of the newborn, and consists mainly in aspirating the mother's milk. Chewing, instead, is possible only after the teeth have appeared, and it consists in breaking up food into small pieces to favor digestion. These two summary descriptions evidence the psychophysiological differences between these two behaviors. In sucking, the infant aspirates the mother's milk, that primordial food that comes from the outside world (in close contact with that privileged and privileging organ, the maternal skin), without exercising any evident active transformation (except for the addition of that secret component that comes from the salivary glands). In chewing, instead, the predominant factor is the transformation-decomposition that the individual operates on the material introduced from outside. This transformation consists in decomposing-fragmenting-grinding the material introduced in various ways, using the hand's (touching) and/or an instrument (spoon, etc.); in other words, this is a substantially destructive operation. Psychoanalysis attributes great importance to this, maintaining that issues regarding orality can involve various psychological components that may represent unresolved problems specific to neurotic conditions in adults. In fact, psychoanalysts tend to identify two periods in the oral phase corresponding to the two periods of sucking (the so-called passive-receptive stage) and chewing [30].

One must remember that the oral experience with its impulses of destruction (death instinct) and desire (life instinct), as they are defined by psychoanalysts, is at the base of a series of more general processes involving the individual and which go beyond the simple problem of food intake. The famous psychoanalyst Melanie Klein [31–33] studied individual orality [in her patient(s)] by examining the development of the relationship between the infant-subject who eats and the mother-object. Dr. Klein individuates a primary oral phase, which she defines as schizo-paranoid, in which the child learns to distinguish between food and bad objects. This process involves going beyond the mere problem of edibility, through operations that develop on a more general "semantic" level. The child learns to separate the bad object from the good one, to refuse it, expel it, to attribute characteristics of badness to external (outside) elements. Badness, moreover, although attributed to the outside, is in reality a part of the Self (of the subject himself). The operation arises from the necessity to control anxiety. Thus, in the same phase, the subject projects outwards onto the object also positive components of his own self, establishing in this way some control over the object. This schizo-paranoid phase, according to Klein, is followed by a so-called "depressive" one, characterized by a new complex relational method in which the subject no longer relates to a partial object (the breast), but to an entire object (the mother), towards whom ambivalent feelings of destruction and love emerge.

These "Kleinian phases", initially related to the interaction-conflict of the two apparently simple processes of sucking and chewing, could account for the death instinct which Klein evidences in these early phases, and which is presumably related to the emotionally negative experience of so-called chewing *sine materia*, which may happen with early activation of chewing, with or without tooth development. The "breast" object, although it excites a possible mastication reflex, is not usually subjected to being chewed for various reasons (lack of teeth, withdrawal of the breast), and thus frustration ensues. Furthermore, we know that mastication blocks a hypothalamic hyperexcitation by a feedback mechanism. In this case, since chewing cannot be effected, there is no stop signal, for the state of excitation related to the partially executed program (of chewing and biting), a program whose activation tends to destroy the object. It is precisely this negative emotional experience, which also interferes with sucking behavior, which the infant uses as a preferential scheme and with which he must confront. If the child's confrontation involves the entire object, the mother, one passes beyond the oral modality through the sense-motor experience, with the meeting of eyes, i. e., through one or more new modalities (Piaget's sense-motor phase) [34]. This passage is not always automatic or easy. The mother has a guiding role in teaching and facilitating new relational and sense-motor patterns. If this does not occur, the child may perceive, precisely because of the lack of new modalities, an inadequacy of normal oral paths, which tend to destroy the object and not to establish "contact" with it. The new relational scheme involving confrontation with the entire object tends, instead, to conserve such constructive contact. Moreover, the oral apparatus, with its very important role in the child's experiences, has a precise function in the child's learning about analyzing the object.

For psychoanalysts, orality is not only a basic element of personality structure, but is also at the base of processes defined as cognitive in experimental psychology. In Bion's development of Kleinian thought, the significant organization of meanings deriving from oral experiences are defined as fantasies or "first thoughts." These are the first intellectual operations, which Bion calls "protomental" [35, 36]. The first order of intellectual operations would include meanings of experiences related to "inside-outside," inside-outside the mouth, inside or outside the self, in other words the distinction between one's own self and something else. Thus, the child places attention on the breast as "something that enters in." Slowly, inside and outside become organized according to modalities more apt to reality through recognition of the existence of a breast that is outside the mouth. The first relationship experienced by the human mind is, therefore, an inside-outside relationship, one of entry and exit, of having inside and not having, between things that always have something else that can contain them. The authors cited maintain, thus, that the first inside-outside experience is of fundamental importance in the development of the human mind. Such compensating fantasies are at the base of the first operations of knowledge, and thus influence cognitive processes. Bion talks of container-content models situated abstractly in mental interaction which implies the genesis of thought.

We feel that this broad theme should not be underestimated in experimental psychophysiology. In fact, these psychodynamic interpretations related to such proto-experiences would be at the root of the organization of instinctive and emotional processes in the adult. Management of these processes leads to development of precise attitudes found in integrated processes, such as "withholding-expelling," that is, operations subsequent to those described above. These are not, however, merely cognitive acquisitions, but are also correlated with the experience of pleasure.

Adults have styles of oral behavior in which one particular phase is more important than others in the normal oral-alimentary sequence. Psychoanalysts express this concept with the term of "fixation" in the oral stage, to indicate the subject's lack of psychological evolution in managing his oral pulsions. For psychoanalysts, this process of non-maturation constitutes a personality trait. Abraham [37] individuates five types of oral personality: oral with inhibited desire, hyperprotected oral, frustrated oral, demanding oral, and productive oral. In synthesis, however, the characteristic of the oral trait is the need to be nourished, to be protected, to be loved, and form a unit with the love object. The individual fixed in this stage also appears passive, and being nourished not only has the alimentary significance of satiety, but also of possibility of consolation. Such is the case when the fixation refers to the first phase of the psychoanalytic scheme, called the *passive-receptive phase.*

The second oral stage, the *aggressive-possessive phase* [30], considered to appear in the second half of the 1st year of life, comports an attitude of "active taking," and, simultaneously, the tendency to develop a destructive aggressive behavior. This psychoanalytic model was the basis for Alexander's [38] psychosomatic model, which emphasizes how, in this "oral fixation," the parasympathetic and the trophotropic structures are activated simultaneously, with a tendency to hypersecretion of the various regions of the digestive tube. According to Alexander, an oral fixation, therefore, favors the onset of psychosomatic pathology in the gastric region by creating a condition of trophotropic hyperactivity. The sequence is more complex and passes through the following phases: hyperactivation of the oral systems, with subjective sensations of dependence (which, according to Alexander, would also provoke "guilt feelings"). Such activation would stimulate a compensatory countersystem of attack-escape which, however, once activated would accentuate the subjective needs of protection-nourishment, and, in other words, augment the problem of oral dependency with further hyperactivation of the attack-escape system.

The psychoanalytical system is more complex, however, because, in addition to talking about "oral fixation," in which case we expect to find the signs of hypertrophic oral behavior, it also talks about "removal" of the so-called oral pulsions.

The existence of a relationship between vegetative life (orality/oral phase) and relational life (environmental exploration behavior), which can influence the subject's subsequent behavior, has been demonstrated experimentally. In 1972, Hofer [39] showed that rats deprived of their mother's milk presented marked bradycardia and a tendency toward accentuated explorative behavior regarding their environment. When the animals were later given sufficient amounts of the right milk, the bradycardia disappeared, but the explorative behavior was maintained and became a stable personality trait. This finding confirmed that there is a relationship between orality and personality development.

While psychoanalysts tend to point out the components of oral fixation in the neurotic adult, emphasizing the oral phase that is undoubtedly a developmental stage, Bowlby [40] widens the view of the mother-child relationships in a wider category, called attachment. This means that while psychoanalysts evidence certain psychophysical problems, which are semantic transfers related to this phase (incorporation, oral aggressivity, etc.), such that they form a picture characterized by a more general passive-receptive attitude (oral typology), Bowlby's method evidences better the relational and psychological components (dependence, attachment) which are not necessarily triggered by oral problems. In this regard, other classic studies [41, 42] on monkeys have emphasized the heteroceptive tactile-sensorial-thermal component in the mother-child relationship. The monkeys who took their food from a metal "mother" presented autistic type behavior. Furthermore, in addition to the tactile receptive component, there is a motor component involving active manipulation of the environment. It appears, therefore, that orality, which without doubt involves specific problems, must be included in this wider, unified view of the situation.

Oral fixation, according to Alexander [38], accompanied by a prevalence of the parasympathetic sphere and infantile dependence pulsions, is not opposed to aggressive behavior, but rather the individual-environment relationship matures through the exercise and practice of relational life (motor and sensorial events, looks, acquisition of meaning, language) that do not necessarily pass through activation of aggressive behaviors. The dialectic becomes one of maturation, but not in the sense, or at least not only in the sense, that one passes from the oral phase to the anal phase, but in the sense that systems of interaction with the environment are developed. The merging of such systems means that the classic instinctive-pulsional components take second place, and less space, in the overall picture of individual experience.

Therapeutic strategies should consider also this dialectic-evolutional relationship between pulsional and relational moments, and should be able to arbitrarily transfer the "objects" specific to the so-called pulsional life to one's relational life. The existence of such processes of transformation are, therefore, not negated: fantastic objects or transfer of pulsional tendencies to symbolic objects. There is no doubt that the discovery of these processes has opened enormous horizons to psychology, but there are also paths of development that are modulated by needs which adapt to the individual's relationship with the environment and its rules and schemes, rather than by internal needs in the classic sense of pulsions.

The majority of cognitive processes arise from an immediate event in the decodification of the environment and which is, in fact, contemporaneous with the entire system of oral-alimentary behavior, rather than as transformations of signals of homeostatic re-equilibrium related to hunger. A banal example of this is the application of a burning stimulus to a newborn, in which situation orality seems to be absolutely extraneous. Withdrawal of the limb after "recognition" of the damaging stimulus is just as fundamental to survival as nourishment is. Therefore, it does not seem possible (in fact, even Freud worked with this viewpoint, after some delay) to follow along a path exclusively of the history of pulsions, for example the passage from the oral phase to the anal one, without understanding the evolutive and maturative role of the pulsion-organizational sphere in relational life, which not only is contemporary to the two pulsional moments (the oral and anal phases), but also occupies all the intermediate transitional space. It is therefore possible that an individual may not get over the oral phase, to use the psychoanalytic terminology, not only because of an inability to cope with pulsional components, but also because that individual may not learn (have learned) to grow in relational life.

Gestalt theory, instead, does not deal so much with the generalization and "transfer of oral pleasure" (a particular form of the libido, according to Freud) as with the problem of introjection. That is, Gestalt psychology places emphasis on the role of chewing in the breaking down of food into constituents that consent assimilation. Incomplete mastication, according to Perls, Hefferline, and Goodman [43], does not break down the material introduced and produces assumption of food that is inadequately transformed, such that the individual assumes but may not assimilate. A similar scheme can be applied in reference to assumption-assimilation of reality of a psychological character, because mastication has, in fact, a complex emotional meaning. The process of assimilation of "psychic" substances is, of course, fundamental to psychological development. Clearly, non-psychoanalytic and non-Gestalt psychology prefers to talk of behaviors that *imitate* models or symbolic figures, while the term introjection, although often used confusedly, does not refer to explicit paths specific to orality. Thus, it would appear preferable to talk of observation of behaviors to imitate, and thus of sensorial relational channels. However, insistence on the oral path indicates realization that the assimilative and imitative process may necessarily include a phase involving breaking down of material. According to Gestalt psychology, therefore, although the capacity to chew and break down food is correlated to mere digestive function, in actual fact it is the very expression of the capacity to break down, decompose, and destroy.

Framing the problem in these terms, it is no longer necessary to hypothesize transfer from concrete mastication to masticating as an abstract psychological operation. The capacity to masticate is only the strictly biological aspect of a more ample psychophysical operation. This hypothesis seems to be confirmed by Gestalt clinical experiences which point out the existence of material that has been "introjected" compared to "assimilated," i. e., not chewed in the symbolic sense and thus not digested, meaning that it cannot be harmoniously integrated in the individual personality. The introjected material ends up as a bag of parasitic behaviors that burden, rather than "nourish," the individual psychologically.

17.3 Disorders of the Oral Cavity Related to Psycho-emotional Factors

17.3.1 Psychosomatic Aspects

Psychosomatic dermatology (the term we prefer to the equivalents "psychocutaneous," used principally in the United States, and "psychodermatology," used especially in Holland), refers to affections of the skin and mucosae with more or less high incidence of reports of psychoemotional factors (based on the hypothesis, more or less supported by research, that they constitute pathogenetic factors) [25, 26]. As Table 17.1 shows, few of these affections involve the oral mucosae. However, as we discuss in the next section of this chapter, certain mouth lesions comport somatopsychic rebound (from the periphery, the oral mucosae in this case, to the mind).

Table 17.1. Affections of the skin and mucosae with higher incidence of reports of psychoemotional factors

- Acne
- Alopecia areata
- Atopic dermatitis
- Dyshidrosis
- Glossodynia
- Herpes simplex
- Hyperhidrosis
- Lichen planus
- Lichen simplex
- Pruritus sine materia
- Psoriasis
- Rosacea
- Seborrheic dermatitis
- Telogen effluvium
- Urticaria
- Vitiligo
- Warts

Only lichen planus and herpes are included in this list. We wish to make a few comments on these two clinical pictures in relation to psychosomatics and then treat glossodynia in a separate section.

Lichen Planus. This dermatosis has always been "suspected" of having a psychosomatic pathogenesis, and we investigated this aspect in 1984 [26]. This usually self-limiting eruption most commonly affects middle-aged adults. It can involve glabrous skin, mucous membranes, hair, and nails. After the cutaneous form, oral lichen planus (Fig. 17.1) is the most commonly reported form of this disorder and is the sole manifestation of the disease in 15 %–35 % of patients. Six different types of oral lesions have been described: reticular, plaque-like, atrophic, papular, erosive, and bullous. The reticular variety is usually considered to be the most prevalent form, although in one ample study of 570 patients with oral involvement, erosive lichen planus was found to be the most common [44]. Erosive lesions may provoke a painful or "burning" sensation. A metallic taste in the mouth has been described. Older patients tend more often to have erosive lesions at initial presentation.

The buccal and glossal mucosae are most commonly involved, whereas sublingual and palatal disease is unusual. Gingival involvement may potentially lead to a picture of desquamative gingivitis. Symmetric involvement is the rule. Oral disease may be precipitated by trauma: lesions have been noted to develop after periodontal surgery and after irradiation for lymphoma [45].

The typical histologic markers are thickening in the granular layer, liquefaction of the basal cells,

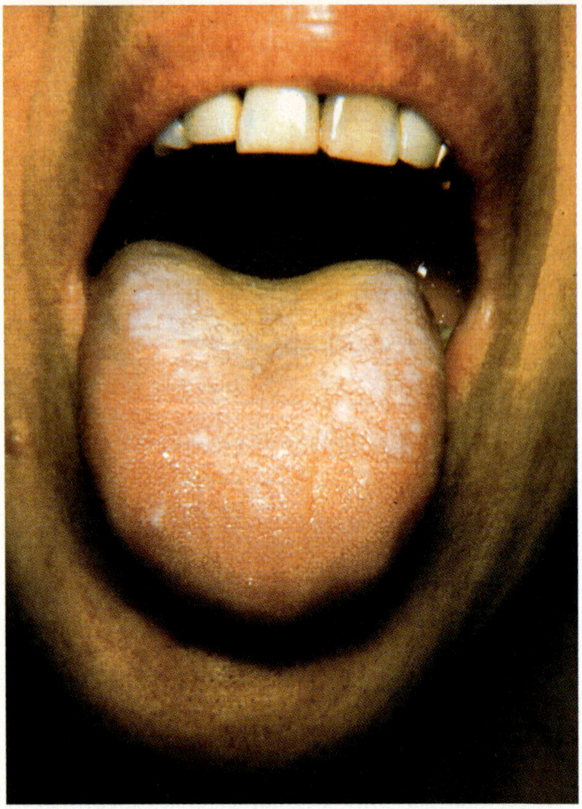

Fig. 17.1. Lichen planus with oral involvement: whitish papules on the tongue

and a band of infiltration in the superficial derma. The infiltrate is composed prevalently of T-lymphocytes with cytotoxic activity affecting the keratinocytes in the basal layer as part of a hypothesized mechanism related to cell-mediated immunity.

The etiology is unknown. Clinical forms identical to lichen planus are caused by ingestion of certain drugs (quinacrine, chlorochine, phenothiazine, etc.), contact with chemicals used in film developers (p-phenylenediamine salts), and during graft versus host reaction.

There are numerous bibliographic references to lichen as being a disease with "neuropsychiatric genesis." These reports were critically reviewed by Obermayer [46], and Cossidente [47]. In two patients with lichen planus, Obermayer evidenced by plethysmography "psychogenic" waves which were, according to him, influenced by unconscious emotional content and he proposed the idea of the cutaneous projection of a psychological conflict predisposed by an inorganic dysfunction in early infancy [46]. Many other observations of patients with lichen planus regard the significant incidence of emotional factors, the presence of states of tension and anxiety, psychological shock as a triggering event, pre-existing prolonged psychophysical stress (Arndt pointed out the increase in cases in certain parts of Europe during World War II) [46], fixation at the oral stage, and reduction of energies used in other spheres with probably abnormal organic localization. All this implies vital energy not directed at self-realization but withdrawing into bodily limits, increasing vulnerability to frustrating stimulations, with a tendency to self-accusation, etc.

The onset, exacerbation, diffusion, and relapses of lichen planus caused by emotional stress have been emphasized by Samman and Arndt and others [46]. Griesemer and Nadelson [48] noted a high incidence of emotional triggering (82 % of the cases observed), with a biologic incubation interval ranging from a few days to a couple of weeks. In their classification of "psycho-cutaneous alterations," Meluzzi and Zina [49] include lichen planus among the "specifically psychosomatic dermatoses with a latency that is prolonged with respect to the stressor."

We did a targeted study on 100 cases of lichen planus using formal psychiatric interviews in all the cases and psychodiagnostic reactive test in 14 [47, 50]. The tests used were the Rorschach, Cattel's form C 16 PF, Cattel Anxiety Scale, STAl X1, STAl X2 self-evaluation questionnaire, and Eysenck's Maudsley Personality Inventory (a psychophysiological questionnaire). These indicated a significant character base with noteworthy emotional instability and emergence of neurotic components, such as anxiety and mood depression, noticeable tendency to somatize psychic tension, modest presence of prolonged psychophysical stresses, and an irrelevant incidence of emotional-affective shock before the manifestation of the symptoms. In our clinical experiences with this disease in liaison consultation, we observed that while the neurotic factors found were of no particular significance for a specific etiopathogenesis (in that they are alterations in the psychic equilibrium with a notoriously high endemic incidence), the character bases of emotional hyperreactivity can be compared with those more generally found in other dermatological forms with possible psychosomatic pathogenesis, such as non-allergic chronic urticaria, rosacea, alopecia areata, etc. On such predisposed ground, the stressors have more effect even when they are relatively mild and not easily quantifiable by the patient; thus, a determinant mechanism of repeated or "creeping" emotional incitement becomes more important than the mechanism of (punctual) affective-emotional shock. Moreover, we observe that both of these mechanisms are important in modulating the course of the disease once it has manifested, conditioning the relapses. We have also noted that patients with lichen planus almost never have somatopsychic rebound of any practical importance.

Boyd and Neldner, in their review on lichen planus, observe that patients with lichen planus frequently report worsening of the disease during periods of stress, while others have noticed onset and exacerbation with fatigue [45]. The disease has been noted to erupt usually 1–2 weeks after severe emotional stress, or to be seen in "nervous, highly tense" subjects [51]. In a large questionnaire survey, Altman and Perry [52] found that although only 10 % of affected patients could recall a stressful situation at the onset of their disease, 60 % believed that chronic tension aggravated it.

Most studies investigating a link between mental health and lichen planus have involved oral disease. Lowenthal and Pisanti [53] evaluated 49 patients with oral disease and concluded that an association existed between emotional stress and erosive disease, without asymptomatic variants. A similar study involving 48 lichen planus patients and control subjects evidenced no significant link with stressful life events [54].

It is known that even diseases caused by specific biological noxae can be influenced by psychosocial factors. This has been reconfirmed recently by rigorously documented psychoneuroimmunological studies [55] in which the investigators give value to the meaning behind the words of the "typical mother" who says: "If you don't get some rest, you are going to get sick." Such factors are valid also, and especially, for viral infections, many of which have onset in or involve the oropharyngeal mucosae.

To date, the infectious disease with the most clinical evidence of dependence on emotional stress is *herpes simplex* (HSV), both type 1, which causes prevalently herpes simplex labialis, and type 2, which causes prevalently, but not exclusively, herpes genitalis; both types are usually recurrent. The latter form belongs to the sphere of sexually transmitted diseases and has become diffuse to the extent of being an epidemic disease of enormous proportions with evident, unjustified, psychosocial repercussions in part due to the old, never-spent feelings of guilt and sin connected with sexuality.

Everyone knows that the recurrent manifestations of these two forms (type 1 – with predominant localization on the mouth or nearby areas – and type 2 – primarily located on the mucosae of the genital organs, or in nearby areas) can be triggered by emotional stimuli. Some statistics, including also varicella zoster virus infections [48], report a 36 % incidence of emotional triggering with a very brief incubation interval, as well as triggering by physical trauma, fever, menstruation, foods, drugs, sunshine, etc.

HSV infection is a true puzzle: this double-stranded DNA virus is a mystery, with its icosahedral nucleocapsid which lives latent, hidden, and silent in the sanctuary of the dorsal root ganglia, and then descends via the peripheral nerves to attack the skin with its typical (the same features known from the time of Hippocrates) crop of clustered vesicles. It is ubiquitous and dependent on hygienic, environmental, social, and even economic situations (overcrowded conditions) with contagion by kissing and sexual relationships, as well as immunologic factors and stress in general, emotional in particular. Psychodependence is such a common observation that there is no need to cite the many reports, old and new. We will mention, however, Rasmussen's [56] experiment in which he observed that mice subjected to an avoidance-learning task by stimulation with mild electric shocks became more susceptible to herpes simplex virus. Regarding man, there are numerous reports dealing with recurrence under hypnotic suggestion [57, 58], specific character profiles and psychopathologic alterations [59], and new attacks in connection with episodes of extramarital intercourse with "feelings of guilt" [46] or as a "form of self punishment." According to Whitlock [60], however, such interpretations must be evaluated very cautiously or even refuted; instead, he very rightly points out that "one might consider the possibility that changes in immunity could well occur as a result of emotional stress." In fact, according to Whitlock, there is growing evidence that major life changes can influence the incidence and the course of illness through their impact on the immune response. In fact, it has been reported that natural killer (NK) cell activity declines significantly in medical-student blood samples taken before and during examinations [61]. NK cell activity is important in tumor surveillance, as well as in the control of virus infection. Two other factors are significantly related to NK activity, stressful life events and loneliness, with high scorers on both having significantly lower levels of NK activity.

As said above, considerable anecdoctal speculation has linked stress and the appearance, duration, and intensity of herpesvirus infections, with such effects presumably reflecting alterations in cellular immunity. There is an increased risk for infection by Epstein-Barr virus (EBV) in West Point cadets associated with certain psychosocial risk factors (high levels of motivation, poorer academic performance, and having a father who was an overachiever) [62]. Another study found that general unhappiness among student nurses was predictive of the frequency of herpes labialis lesions [63]. Such effects may be related to cellular immune competence. Glaser and coworkers [64] carried out a study using a prospective design to examine the influence of examination stress and loneliness on herpesvirus latency as measured by changes in antibody levels to three herpes viruses, Epstein-Barr virus (EBV), herpes simplex type 1 (HSV-1), and cytomegalovirus (CMV). Three blood samples were obtained from 49 1st-year medical students, with the first sample drawn 1 month before final examinations, the second on the 1st day of final examinations, and the third during the 1st week after their return from summer vacation. A median split on the UCLA Loneliness Scale divided subjects into high- and low-scoring loneliness groups. There were significant changes in the antibody titers to all three herpesviruses across the sample points, with the lowest levels found in the third (low stress) sample. High loneliness subjects had significantly higher EBV antibody titers than low-loneliness subjects.

Although it may be triggered by an emotional stressor, herpes labialis creates in turn, in more sensitive individuals, a great disturbance, instigating touching, picking, licking, etc. Herpes labialis is second perhaps only to herpes genitalis in its noteworthy somatopsychic rebound in many subjects. This fact reminds us of the idea of the old masters. Brocq, Wise, and Sulzberger et al., mentioned by Obermayer [46], maintained that all, or many, inflammatory diseases of the lips, and various types of cheilitis were "manifestations of emotional instability" and in some cases even of neuropsychiatric disturbances. In discussing the various types of cheilitis, Rook [65] proposed that the exfoliative and glandular forms might possibly be psycho-influenced. We believe, also on the basis of our experience, that any lesion on the lips can provoke in particularly sensitive persons a sort of tic of self-manipulation (licking, touching, picking, etc., even with various instruments), often perpetuating the cheilitis.

Bilisoly et al. [66] call attention to more strictly neural factors: they observed that 90 % of patients who undergo a resection of the trigeminal nerve had an attack of herpes labialis which could be avoided by denerving the involved area beforehand.

Numerous types of oral ulcerations have been described, independent of orally located herpes. In particular, the very bothersome recurrent aphthae, of unknown etiology but probably of immunoreactive origin, have been seen to be related to emotional stress and "significantly designated as ulcus neuroticus mucosae oris" [46].

17.3.2 Somato-psychic Aspects

Physicians in general, but especially dermatologists, frequently see patients alarmed by: (1) white lesions in the mouth (leukoplasia, lichen, candidosis), (2) ulcerated or other erosive lesions, especially of long duration (due to various causes, such as trauma, inflammatory, or tumoral affections), and (3) aspecific inflammatory factors, even of minimal importance. In many cases, the alarm is not justified, but is due to the current diffuse divulgation of medical and scientific knowledge aimed at stimulating preventive measures by informing the general public of the possibly cancerogenous nature of uncommon or suddenly manifested dark lesions on the skin or lesions, especially leukoplasia, on the oral mucosae. Silence on the part of the specialist, or his insistent request for laboratory tests, may serve to alarm the patient further. Doubts and diagnostic difficulties on the part of the physician often generate fear for the worse in the patient. In the most unfortunate cases, once the patient is alarmed, it is very difficult to convince him/her that there is no reason for alarm, notwithstanding sincere reassurances and the results of eventual histologic tests.

The patient may have severe oncophobia and may even believe that the histologic documentation has been falsified. Oncophobia is the fear of having a presumed cancer, which preventive medicine brings more often despite early diagnosis; the oncophobic patient will continue in his belief despite the negative results of all tests and examinations. Such patients often need psychiatric help, but often refuse it because they do not believe that their suffering is based on "mental" factors. Physicians must be extremely cautious in referring unwilling patients to a psychiatrist or psychologist: the patient who has chosen to present to a regular physician, a dermatologist, or other specialist, usually believes that is the kind of help he needs and there have been cases of suicide in patients forced to refer against their will to a psychiatrist or psychologist.

17.4 Glossodynia and Related Disorders

The term "*glossodynia*" (GD) is derived from the Greek *glossa* for tongue, and *odyne* for pain. The earliest references are attributed to Buisson (1854), Schwimmer (1886), and Magitot (1887) [67–69], but perhaps the best is the one presented by Oppenheim [70] in 1913: "paraesthesia, particularly a burning and prickling sensation on the tongue extending perhaps to adjacent membranes. It may be continuous, paroxysmal, and may even disturb the sleep… Nothing is found on examination."

Although investigators agree on the normal appearance of the tongue, opinions differ on what constitutes GD. Fox [71] restricts the term to those cases with a psychogenic or idiopathic cause, but others [72–75], like us, include cases with an identifiable cause. The International Association for the Study of Pain (IASP) definies GD as a "burning pain in the tongue, involving the tip and lateral borders of glossal mucosa, palate, lips, and other buccal mucosa often associated with odd taste, dry mouth, uncomfortable bite or denture intolerance" [75, 76]. We prefer to consider GD as a symptom, according to the definition of the IASP, without specifying the eventual presence of clinical signs, and, thus, the tongue may or may not present a normal appearance [75] (Figs. 17.2, 17.3). GD is not a disease *sui generis*, but a symptom. In the scientific literature, a variety of terms are used to describe similar symptoms, such as glossopyrosis, pain in the tongue, burning tongue, orodynia, burning mouth syndrome, glossalgia, stomatodynia, oral dysesthesia, and even "oral galvanism." Generally, these terms describe symptoms of an unexplained, prolonged sensation of pain and/or burning in the mouth. The so-called syndrome of oral galvanism describes a situation of chronic pain or atypical taste sensations in the mouth due to metal taste and galvanic currents caused by metal (mainly amalgam and nonprecious alloys) used in dental work. In spite of what appears to be an etiology, this syndrome has characteristics similar to those of GD and can often be considered as a variant [77–82].

The true incidence of GD is unknown: in fact, this is partly due to the lack of unanimity concerning the definition, and partly due to the fact that subjects with GD present to a variety of specialists (dentists, dermatologists, neurologists, psychiatrists, otorhinolaryngologists), with different patterns of presentation to each speciality. The age of initial onset is usually between 40 and 60 years; it appears only rarely before the age of 30 years, and never in children or adolescents.

The typical GD patient is a middle-aged woman. Nearly all investigators report a strikingly higher percentage of women suffering from the syndrome, up to 90 %. Symptoms usually occur in more than one site of the mouth, with the tongue as the most common site of sensation. Other areas include lips, palate, buccal mucosa, upper and lower denture-bearing tissues, throat, and pharyngeal cavity [75, 83–95]. The prevalence of oral sites at which a burning sensation occurs has been reported to be: tip of tongue (78 %), anterior two-thirds of tongue (58 %), ventral side of tongue (17 %), posterior third of tongue (11 %), floor of mouth (13 %), anterior third of hard palate (49 %), posterior two-thirds of hard palate (26 %), soft palate (6 %), oropharynx (13 %), mucosal portion of lower lip (24 %), mucosal portion of upper lip (18 %), lower alveolar ridges (25 %), upper alveolar ridges (24 %), and buccal mucosa (14 %) [94]. The patient may complain of pain despite the absence of any observable lesion on the

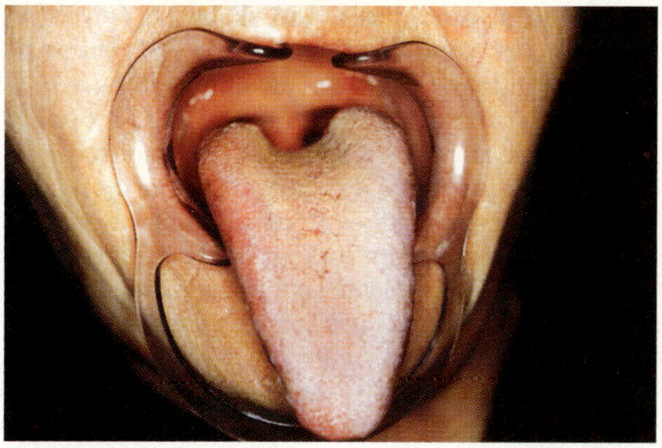

Fig. 17.2. Glossodynia: this is a typical case, with no evident pathological lesion on clinical examination

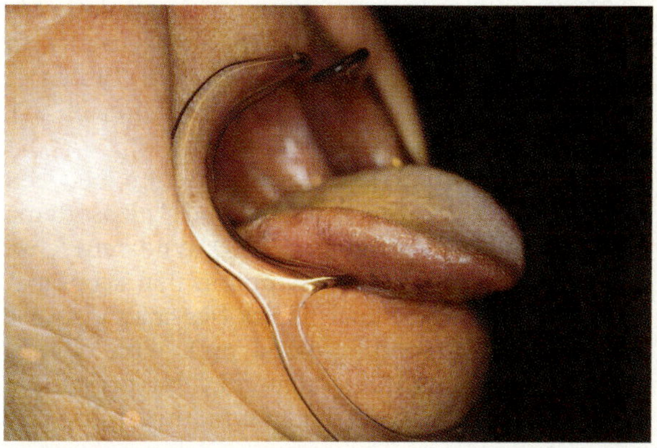

Fig. 17.3. For legend, see Fig. 17.2

tongue or elsewhere in the mouth. The surface of the tip of the tongue is often smooth and atrophic from constant rubbing against the front teeth. The symptoms are often poorly localized. Characteristically, the pain does not interfere with eating or sleeping, and usually occurs only during the day [75, 96]. A sour or bitter taste often accompanies the burning. Patients with chronic GD commonly describe all of the physicians and dentists consulted previously and the unsuccessful treatments prescribed [97].

Most patients suffer from the syndrome for a long time, reportedly ranging from months up to 18 years [75]. The onset was reported to be gradual for 63 % of the subjects and sudden for the others [94]. Although many patients tend to relate the onset of symptoms to previous dental procedures (up to 70 %) (e.g., extractions) or to a previous illness (up to 10 %), up to 57 % could not relate it to any prior event.

Several causes have been proposed as possible etiologic factors for GD, including local irritation by environmental factors, such as denture base, oral parafunction, deficiency states, hormonal changes occurring in menopause, change in salivary composition, candidiasis, and diabetes. Nevertheless, studies conducted comparing GD patients with age- and sex-matched control subjects have provided little support for some of the earlier proposed etiologic factors, such as dentures, oral habits, candidiasis, and nutritional deficiency. Furthermore, different sensory modalities (tests of touch, two-point discrimination, warmth scaling, and oral stereognostic ability) have showed no significant differences between the two groups [94]. Moreover, GD may be associated with a wide variety of clinical conditions which can be classified etiologically (Table 17.2). Although it is not uncommon for several conditions to be implicated (and consequently diagnosis and management can be complicated), we point out that the importance of systemic problems as a cause of GD (for example anemia or nutritional deficiencies) is, in view of all those authors concerned with such patients, almost always overrated. Table 17.2 presents a possible etiological classification of GD, and we will discuss each item below.

Our classification makes a distinction between "glossodynia syndrome" (GDS) and "glossodynia disease" (GDD). By the term "GD syndrome", we mean that glossodynia is a symptom that accompanies another well-defined illness (we may also use the term symptomatic glossodynia), with clinical and histological features that may be present at the onset of the glossodynic symptomatology or may present later. The term "GD-disease" refers to a picture that is characterized only by the subjective glossodynic symptom, without any other clinical manifestations for the entire duration of the disease. Obviously, this distinction between GD syndrome and GD disease is an attempt to clarify the possible etiopathogenesis of this still unclear symptom/disease. Very careful follow-up is necessary to verify whether the patient has GD syndrome or GD disease. In fact, as mentioned below, the clinical features of well-known diseases may present some years after the onset of the glossodynic symptom. So, we believe that in most cases, a follow-up of about 3 years must be done before establishing if the glossodynic symptom is a manifestation of GD disease (idiopathic GD), or a symptom of other disease (GD syndrome). Nevertheless, the suggested 3 years of follow-up were arbitrarily established by us [75].

Table 17.2. Proposed etiological classification of "glossodynia"

I. Glossodynia syndrome (symptomatic glossodynia)
Denture factors
Ill-fitting dentures
Dental plaque
Residual monomer irritant
Deficiency states
Iron
Vitamin B_{12}
Folate
Vitamin B_2 (riboflavin)
Vitamin B_6 (pyridoxine)
Zinc
Endocrine disorders
Diabetes
Myxedema
Sex steroid hormones
Menopause
Neurologically mediated disorders
Referred from tonsils/teeth
Neuropathy of the lingual nerve
Glossopharyngeal neuralgia
Esophageal reflux
Menopause
Xerostomia
Diabetes
Scleroderma
Sjögren's syndrome
Systemic lupus erythematosus
Radiation therapy
Chemotherapy
Pharmacologic agents
Over-the-counter products
Caffeine
Alcohol
Drugs
Iatrogenic
Mouthwash
Pharmacologic agents
Skin diseases with oral involvement and oral diseases
Lichen planus
Erythema multiforme
Candidiasis
Herpes virus infections
Aphthous stomatitis
Pemphigus vulgaris
Benign migratory glossitis
Squamous cell carcinoma
II. Glossodynia disease (idiopathic glossodynia)
Psychological
Cancerophobia
Debility-induced neurosis
Depression
Idiopathic

Recently, some authors suggested a possible *psychogenic etiology* for GD [75]. A thorough clinical work-up should be done initially to determine whether a local or systemic cause is involved (see Table 17.2). If local and systemic factors are ruled out and it is possible to exclude a GD syndrome (symptomatic GD), then inquiries need to be made to determine positive evidence of a psychogenic cause. Nevertheless, one must keep in mind that also a subject with symptomatic burning mouth syndrome may experience psychic discomfort due to possible somatopsychic rebound. In fact, the symptom of GD has long been a medical problem and has given rise to a wide range of differential diagnostic considerations. Despite this, the fact that it might also point to a disorder of psychiatric relevance is not well enough known, although Albert [98] speculated that psychiatric disturbance could be a possible contributory factor as long ago as 1885.

Although GD is a condition familiar to virtually all general practitioners, dentists, and medical specialists, there are very few publications considering the symptom of burning tongue on a general nonspecialist basis. Marxkors and Muller-Fahlbusch [99], who wrote a monograph dealing with psychogenic artificial denture intolerance (a symptom related to GD), were the first authors to go beyond the dental, internistic, and allergological aspects and give considerations to the important psychiatric aspects of the condition.

In their studies, they found that the diagnosis "psychogenic denture intolerance" masked depression in 57 % of cases, neurotic developments in 21 %, abnormal psychic reactions in 19 %, and schizophrenia in 3 %. True denture intolerance is only very rarely seen to be the cause of GD. However, the fitting of dentures, or some other dental or medical intervention, often triggers or exacerbates the condition [99].

Maier [100] published a report on eight patients with "vital disorders of the oral region (glossodynia)" which occurred within the framework of an endogenous depression. In these patients, the basic depressive syndrome faded into the background compared to the glossodynia. In one study of 150 cases of psychogenic GD, it was found that involvement most frequently implicates multiple locations, and involvement at a single location is rare [101, 102].

Baurle and Schoenberger [103] submitted 100 patients with GD to patch testing for suspected allergic stomatitis, with negative findings in all cases. For this reason, the authors drew attention to the lack of clinical relevance of allergens in the etiology of GD. Such patch testing, they maintained, could be considered superfluous, and denture replacement usually resulted in no decisive improvement in the symptomatology. They concluded that "the time spent on patch testing should rather be employed for a carefully conducted interview of the patient, or else an attempt should be made to convince the patient that the condition is possibly psychiatric in origin, thus preparing the ground for further psychiatric diagnostic evaluation" [103].

With respect to the premorbid personality of patients with GD, Haneke [104] reported that almost all appeared nervous or even tense, and many appeared to be anxious and introverted, depressed or even tearful. Almost half of the patients associated the onset of their complaints with medical or dental treatments.

Gottwald [105] noted that these subjects appear "psycho-vegetatively" labile and depressive in mood. In general, however, it should be noted that individuals with GD are usually not recognized immediately by non-psychiatrists as having psychiatric/psychological problems.

In 1984, in their review of "psychiatric syndromes with dermatologic expression", Cossidente and Sarti proposed that GD be included in the sphere of the hypochondrias and the so-called phobias [106]. They agree with Obermayer [46] that GD is a phobic syndrome similar to cancerophobia. Obermayer cites Ziskind and Moulton [107], who pointed out that the psychological basis of the syndrome is "sexual frustration and maladjustment prior to the menopause, with an increase in sexual anxiety at the approach of the menopause." Cossidente and Sarti point out that in general, sentiments of fear and guilt are present in patients with GD. In their opinion, the pain, therefore, represents at times the threat of danger or the means to make amends. For these authors, GD is sometimes a depressive equivalent, i. e., a somatic sign of masked depression [106].

Zaidens hypothesizes that GD symbolizes the fear of death (above all expressed as fear of cancer), localized in particular in the oral cavity which, as the site of food introduction, is directly connected with the preservation of life [46].

From a deep-psychological point of view, the mouth and tongue region is of considerable significance from the earliest age onwards. In the infant, apart from the skin, the mouth is the "primary site of social contact", and the tongue is the first mediator of infantile objectal relationship. In adulthood, too, this area plays a central role in the intake of food and beverages, in the use of tobacco, and also in the sexual sphere. Suppressed feelings and emotions, and buried conflicts find expression in oral symptoms, in particular during sleep, but also during the day, in such symptoms as "oral habits" (grinding of teeth or bruxism, movements of the mouth). According to Haneke [108], particular oral habits not infrequently lead to muscular tension, aches, and temporo-mandibular joint syndromes. These "pain dysfunction syndromes" may give rise to the sensation of burning of the tongue. The intimate relationship between the personality structure of patients with GD and the temporo-mandibular joint syndrome (Costen's syndrome), which often has a psychogenetic etiology, is well known. In 1984, Feinmann [109] described two facial pain syndromes, possibly psychogenic in origin, Costen's syndrome or "facial arthromyalgia" and atypical facial pain. There have been suggestions of an association with masked or atypical depression, and some investigators propose antidepressants as an effective treatment of such pain.

In one study, 160 GD patients were submitted to a psychodiagnostic questionnaire survey (only 10 % of subjects were male and the average age was

60 years) which showed state-of-anxiety and trait-anxiety scores clearly higher than the average scores of healthy subjects, but lower than the average recorded for psychiatric outpatients [109]. The corresponding depression scores (state and trait) were higher than those of inpatients suffering from somatic diseases, but much lower than those of depressed psychiatric patients. The scores for neuroticism and neurosomatic lability were considerably higher than the mean scores observed in the general population. Thus, subjects with GD have been found to score higher than the normal population on state and trait anxiety, depression, somatic reactions to stress, and neuroticism [91]. In another study, 39 % of the study population was found to suffer from clinically significant anxiety and 13 % from depression [88]. Another study evidenced psychiatric disorders in 44 % of GD patients compared with only 16 % in a control group [86], and in another series of ten treated GD patients, seven presented a pathologic personality disorder and three a mild psychiatric disorder [110].

The psychopathologic profile of subjects with GD basically resembles the psychological distress reported for other chronic pain populations [111–113]. For example, the psychopathologic profile of the GD patient shows elevations in scales of somatization and depression resembling the elevations reported for a general chronic pain population in the United States [111]. The relative elevation in the scales of somatization and depression is evident when GD patients are compared with other groups of dental patients, such as dental phobics who have been treated successfully for their dental fear (0.94 vs. 0.63 on the somatization scale, 0.93 vs. 0.70 on the depression scale) [114]; their psychopathological profile is higher for all parameters than that of a general, healthy population of dental patients.

Although such comparisons should be carried out with care (differences in population characteristics, sociocultural contexts, research design, etc.), it seems that the increased psychological distress of the GD patient is associated with the chronic pain condition. This situation concords with Grushka's study [84] pointing out some psychopathology in GD patients whose personality profiles show elevations in certain personality characteristics (e. g., depression, anger, anxiety), changes that tend to increase with pain.

The psychological findings in GD patients may be either the consequence of the chronic pain condition or its cause. Many of these patients often live alone, and their psychologic distress is significantly associated with their single status. A relatively high percentage report having had psychiatric or psychological treatment in the past and/or present. All of the patients who reported having had such treatment initiated it over 5 years before the study (conducted by Eli et al.), whereas the GD symptoms in most of the patients began 1–3 years before this study. Thus, it is possible that personal distress plays a role in the development of the syndrome. However, the possibility that some patients may have developed psychologic distress after the onset of symptoms and initiated treatment as a result, cannot be overlooked. Today, it is generally accepted that syndromes involving prolonged chronic pain, such as GD, are indeed closely associated with increased psychological distress in the individual. For example, a significant excess of adverse life events has been found before the onset of lower back pain [115]. In fact, chronic pain (like GD) and depression seem to be closely related. Ott [101] conducted a study on 131 GD patients, submitting them to a careful examination that included a neurological work-up, detailed psychiatric interview, and numerous psychological tests (Achievement test for endogenous depression, Multiple choice vocabulary test measuring verbal intelligence, Erlangen depression scale, Anxiety-aggression scale, Scale for general somatic symptoms, Scale for vegetative functional disorders, Abbreviated pain scale, Self-rating scale for state of well-being, Self-rating anxiety scale, Self-rating depression scale). Particular attention was paid to psychosomatic and psychopathologic disorders. The finding that 73 % of GD patients are female contrasts with earlier reports [111, 112] in which it is stated that about 90 % of the patients are women. The author concludes by saying that postmenopausal women, in particular, may develop the symptoms of GD. The probability that depression is the causal factor is high, so treatment with antidepressants would appear to make good sense. In Ott's study, 49.2 % of the patients were diagnosed as depressive (8.2 % major depression, 41 % minor depression). Such data may justify treatment with antidepressant drugs.

Finally, quite often, GD is a somatic manifestation of a psychological illness that may range from life stress reactions with anxiety or minor depression, or both, to major depression. Both organic and psychogenic factors may be obviously present; for example, a patient with candidiasis may also have major depression. Moreover, there may be a genuine *cancerophobia* [116, 117]. Cancerophobia is common in patients with GD and it is one of the hypochondriacal disorders. Patients with hypochondrias are preoccupied with the convinction that they are incurably ill with a specific disease. The physician should ask about fear of cancer, because many patients may not voluntarily express their intense fears and convinctions unless this information is elicited directly. Also, patients should be asked if a close

Table 17.3. Basic outline for a preliminary screening of the glossodynic subject

Pain directly associated with eating → local cause	
Pain with onset some time after eating → myogenic or neurologic cause	
Pain diminishing while eating → psychological cause	

friend or relative has had oral cancer, for obvious reasons. Thus, when a patient has an unusual complaint and there seem to be few objective physical findings, the physician is challenged to provide an appropriate differential diagnostic workup. Obviously, the examiner's bias can influence findings, especially when there is a major psychologic stressor like glossodynia. The simple process of giving a name to a symptom is often a major stress reliever; fear of the unknown can be worse than dealing with a chronic problem. The Greek word *odyne*, which means pain, has been used in medicine for many years to indicate localized discomfort [75].

The aim of assessment of GD is the identification of correctable causes. We believe that the first step is to try to evaluate whether the subject with GD presents a symptomatic GD or an idiopathic GD (i.e., GD syndrome versus GD disease). We realize that this distinction may be very difficult or dangerous, and in some cases it may be made only after many months (or even years) of follow-up. Table 17.3 presents a very basic outline for a preliminary screening of the glossodynic subject [75]. Obviously, a thorough history including psychological stress factors is essential (including history of anxiety or depression). The examiner should investigate kindly familial and social situations, possible cancerophobia, and whether the burning mouth syndrome interferes with sleep, and ask frankly about possible depression (for example: "Do you feel down-hearted and blue? Do you feel hopeful about the future? Are you restless and can't keep still? Do you get tired for no reason? Does your heart beat faster than usual? Do you have trouble sleeping at night?" etc.). Glossodynia is sometimes a symptom of a complex systemic disease rather than a pathologic entity; thus, a full otorhinolaryngological examination is required, with particular attention to any macroscopic changes in the mouth and oropharynx, and the state of the teeth. A general examination may reveal signs of systemic disorder.

Even in the presence of an identifiable cause, there may be contributing and aggravating factors (such as psychological implications or intrapsychic conflicts), and further investigation is advisable. A bacteriological swab is easily taken, and a full blood count and film. To establish iron, folate, or vitamin B_{12} deficiency, a hematologic screening that includes complete blood count, red-cell, serum-iron, vitamin B_{12}, folate levels, and serum zinc should be performed [118]. Although they are rarely required, specific tests for suspected niacin, pyridoxine, and riboflavin deficiency are available in specialized centers. Although GD related to nutritional deficiency is statistically uncommon, it is easily curable with replacement therapy. Identification of a vitamin deficiency through early oral symptoms can forestall development of serious and irreversible systemic and neurologic damage.

Random blood sugar and thyroid function tests are easy and should probably be performed in every case. If the GD is thought to be related to the onset of the menopause, the existence of ovarian failure can be confirmed by measuring serum follicle stimulating hormone (FSH). An orthopantomogram may reveal dental pathology, and a barium swallow will confirm or negate suspected esophageal reflux. Finally, when there are dentures, a dental opinion may reveal an ill-fitting prosthesis, dental plaque, or an irritant residual monomer [75].

As mentioned above, the importance of generalized medical diseases as a cause of GD, for example anemia or nutritional deficiencies, is almost always overrated. It is our opinion, in fact, that most subjects who report burning mouth syndrome present an idiopathic-psychogenic GD (GD disease), whereas few subjects present complaining of symptomatic GD. Nevertheless, we emphasize that the physician must not forget this possibility and should remember to prescribe specific tests and/or examinations. Table 17.4 presents a very short system for assessing GD syndrome [75].

Table 17.4. A short system for assessing glossodynia

Anamnesis

General physical examination

Laboratory tests
a) Bacteriological swab
b) Mycological tests
c) Hematological tests
  - Full blood count and film
  - Random blood sugar
  - Serum iron
  - Serum vitamin B_{12}
  - Serum folate
  - Serum zinc
  - Serum thyroxine
  - Serum follicle stimulating hormone (FSH)
  - Serum erythrocyte glutathione reductase activity (for assessment of riboflavin status)
  - Serum erythrocyte aminotransferase activity (for assessment of pyridoxine status)
d) Radiological tests
  - Orthopantomogram
  - Barium swallow

Dental examination

Table 17.5.5. Diagnostic-therapeutic flow chart of glossodynic patient

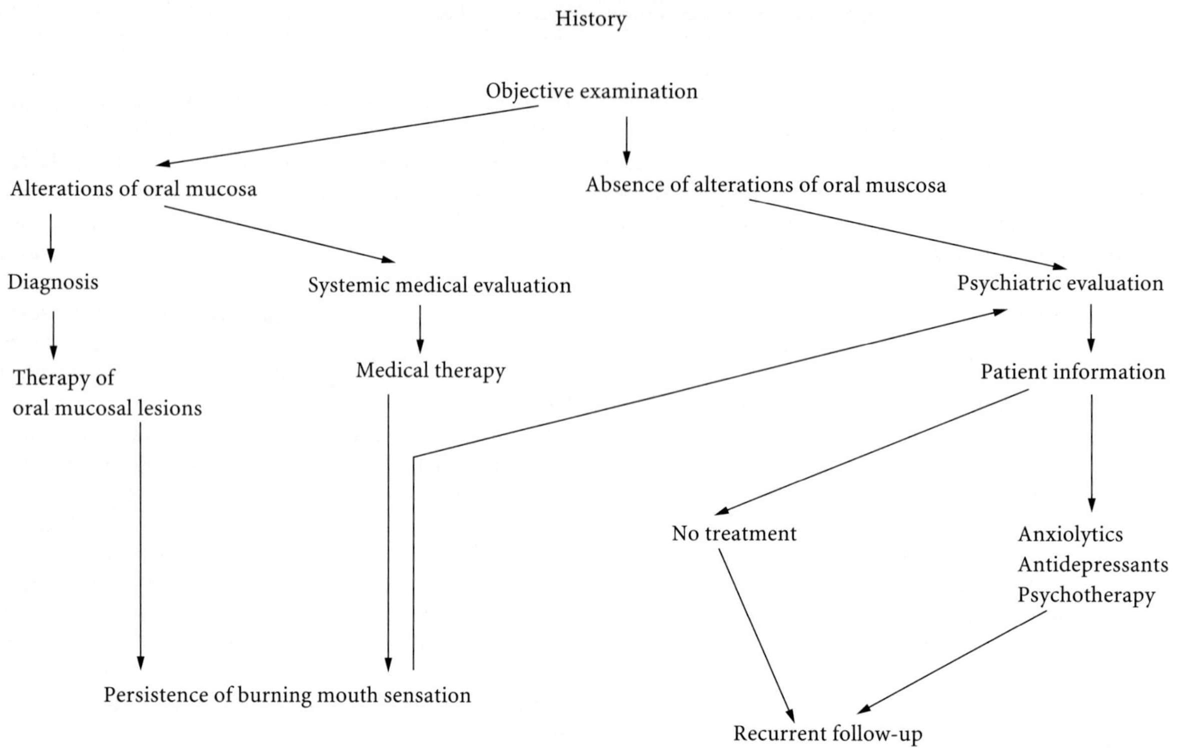

It may be useful to try to identify the causes of GD on the basis of the type of discomfort referred by the patients. In Table 17.5 we present a possible diagnostic-therapeutic flow chart for the management of the GD patient [75].

Finally, we note that the presence (or absence) of depression in chronic pain patients has been shown to affect treatment response [119]. Therefore, early identification of any possible psychological factors may contribute significantly to the understanding and treatment of GD patients. In fact, several recent studies suggest that GD patients can be divided into those responsive to treatment and those who resist it. When the psychological profiles of cured versus noncured patients are compared, the latter are found to be more unstable, apprehensive, and tense [120].

Management of the glossodynic patient should focus on correcting suspected causative factors. Thus, one should eliminate the medications known to provoke or aggravate xerostomia. In the cases of symptomatic GD (GD syndrome) treatment is based essentially on correct therapy of the underlying disease. Thus, for example, antimycotic agents in the case of candidiasis, nutritional supplements for deficiency states, estrogen, and hormonal replacement in endocrine disorders. Irritants, such as alcohol-based mouthwashes, should be avoided. The pain, itching, and stinging are appropriately treated with topical anesthetic agents (for example, diphenydramine hydrochloride 12.5 mg/5 ml mixed with one tablespoonful of water, before each meal). An elixir of equal parts of diphenydramine, kaolin, and pectin retained for 1–2 min and then expectorated, 30 min before meals [73], has been reported to give some relief.

In the cases of GD disease (idiopathic glossodynia) or psychogenic GD, as well as cases of GD syndrome which present an important somatopsychic rebound, psychoactive drugs may also be employed. First, however, we recommend that these subjects be reassured that there is no evidence of any important local or systemic disease, including malignancy. In their very recent comprehensive review of burning mouth syndrome, Huang et al. [73] suggest the use of amitryptiline (75–150 mg daily) and doxepin (75–150 mg daily), the most commonly prescribed tricyclic antidepressants. We emphasize, however, that, tricyclic antidepressants also have an anticholinergic effect and often induce xerostomia. Thus, we prefer to prescribe the newer serotonin uptake inhibitor antidepressants, such as fluoxetine or paroxetine, in patients presenting symptoms of depression of depression equivalents. Also, pimozide (a neuroleptic drug), alone or in combination with antidepressants, has been reported effective [75, 121].

However, no specific treatment recommendations, except for psychotherapy, are usually given. Unfortunately, patients with psychosomatic symptoms are most often resistant to, and may even be indignant about, referrals to a psychiatrist. Their intense preoccupation with their symptoms often overshadows the underlying depression. With some depressed patients, the same or other somatic symptoms reappear with each recurring depression. These patients are often unable to recognize the effects of the depressed mood, and they return to their doctors, expecting a physical cause for the symptoms. Such patients commonly deny a depressed mood, even though it is evident to their doctor. This is known as "masked" depression or "smiling" depression. Depressed patients with GD require a comprehensive diagnosis that leads to more specific treatment by the consulting doctor, or treatment recommendations for the referring doctor, or both. Fortunately, the recent literature on psychogenic glossodynia focuses on the diagnosis of treatable depressive disorders. The "burning" is a symptom of the depression. If the depression is adequately treated, the GD will subside. Kuffer [102] found that 60 % of cases of psychogenic GD were associated with depression that responded to treatment with antidepressant medication, often within 2–3 weeks after beginning treatment.

As with most medical problems, the patient expects a diagnosis and subsequent treatment for a physical, nonpsychogenic condition. From a medical point of view, it is usually in the patient's best interest that the psychologic cause be suggested by the clinician at the same time that physical causes are presented. However, too often this is not done, perhaps as the doctor is reluctant to offend or anger the patient. Nevertheless, it is desirable that the clinician tell the patient that tension and depression can indeed have a biologic basis that causes physical symptoms such as tension headaches or nervous diarrhea. The clinician should emphasize that effective treatment is available and that the symptoms are real and not being imagined. This approach is usually accepted by patients who are fervently searching for an explanation for, and relief from, their distress.

In evaluating patients, the referring physician should inquire directly about a history of depression in both the patient and the patient's parents and siblings, as well as whether the patient is presently depressed and/or being treated for depression. Some patients will not give a history of their emotional illnesses or treatments unless they are asked directly, because they believe it will bias the doctor unfairly in the diagnostic evaluation. Patients should also be asked if they have had other physical complaints that have been difficult to diagnose or treat. Patients with depression often have more than one "psychosomatic" symptom. Depression is commonly triggered by an actual or a threatened personal loss, such as the death of a spouse or serious disability, or the loss of a job or job status. The physician should ask specifically if such an event preceded the onset of the glossodynia. Also, as stated above, cancerophobia is sometimes present in patients with GD. If cancerophobia is a manifestation of major depression, it will usually respond to antidepressant medication. If the cancerophobia is a hypochondriacal symptom without considerable depression, it is often difficult to treat. In the latter situation, the physician should emphasize the lack of clinical findings and, with the assistance of the patient's family, try to get the patient to accept a psychiatric consultation. Finally, some patients with GD have anxiety disorders [102, 104, 108]. These are seen most commonly in patients with secondary guilt, especially in patients with emotional conflicts over sexual practices. Frank discussion may help elicit pertinent information from some of these patients. If warranted, anxiolytic medications can be given for a limited time so that psychological dependency on the medications is minimized. In such cases, benzodiazepine chlordiazepoxide has been reported to lead to complete remission in 15 % and some relief in 52 % of treated patients [73, 122].

17.5 Conclusions

As stated at the beginning of this chapter, the psychosomatic creations seem to be the most mysterious since they refer to the overall desire to live. While their psychological function is conspicuous by its absence, their biological meaning also eludes us. We believe that man's irrepressible psychic fertility, of whatever order, is coexistent with life itself. If we admit that something like psychic death may occur, then it is possible that when psychic creation faulters or comes to a halt, man may be threatened with biological death. The psychic processes that create and maintain psychic health, as well as those responsible for maintaining psychic ill-health, are nevertheless on the side of life. When the individual, for any reason, fails to create some form of mental management to deal with psychic pain, a psychosomatic process may take over.

Research into the meaning and treatment of psychosomatic illness (including the presence of certain parameters such as chronicity, involvement of a psychic stress, and characteristic and constant personality traits) is at the crossroads of various scientific disciplines. In the first part of this chapter, we have focused mainly on the psychosomatic features that can be evidenced through that very peculiar viewpoint, psychoanalytic interpretation.

Thus, we believe that it is inevitable that the skin (which continues in the mucosae) and its diseases become the object of medical observation and interpretation from a psychosomatic point of view. The structure that we notice first in a human being, the skin, the body's surface, constitutes the individual's enveloping shell and is, therefore, the liaison with everything that surrounds it and for everything which fundamentally defines the person. The skin and its mucosal prosecutions appear to be the most appropriate site for somatic transformation of subjective psychological content.

One of the most important functions of the mouth (and oral mucosa) is, instead, strictly related to oral alimentation behavior. One must remember that the mimetic muscles of this area indicate first of all the relationship with ingestion of food in the simplest forms of sucking, chewing, and biting (the latter is included also in the aggressive responses). Through the oral district, therefore, the environment is concretely taken in by the organism. Thus, the oral organ gives absolute prevalence to taking in, expelling, etc. In any case, the relationship is one that involves active, peculiar manipulation of part of the environment, although different from manual activity. As said above, in children, the oral region also has the important function of knowledge and cognitive decodification of the environment. Furthermore, oral-alimentary behavior is closely connected with the internal conditions of the organism. Thus, we focused particular attention on an enigmatic syndrome: glossodynia, or burning mouth syndrome. This disease is a condition characterized by burning and painful sensation in a mouth with generally normal mucosa. Oppenheim's words were: "nothing is found to examination". Five words say that objective examination usually does not reveal any coarse alterations in the oral cavity; but, if the physician pays attention to the psychosocial aspects and personality profile of the patient (and he should always do so), he may discover important, causative factors that may explain and justify the painful sensation of the mouth and tongue. Burning mouth syndrome is a multifactorial disease with varying somatic and psychological symptoms which, in many cases, can occur in other oral conditions. Therefore, when studying glossodynia it is important from a diagnostic point of view to separate this disease as a clinical entity from other oral conditions with similar symptoms. Furthermore, the dentist or physician must fully control the different clinical parameters that might influence the disease, including the many etiologic factors.

In order to establish a sound scientific basis for the future management of these patients, it is essential to perform clinical and psychological prospective studies. In fact, our personal opinion is that strict diagnostic criteria must be agreed upon if crucial research is to be done in this field. Sometimes, organic changes are found in these patients and basic science research is needed. We all see many of these patients and yet have no unified approach to their treatment as none is effective in all patients. Reassurance and support are essential if good quality of life is to be maintained.

References

1. Freud S. Opere. Torino: Bollati Boringhieri, 1967
2. Laplanche J, Pontalis JB. Vocabulaire de la psychoanalyse. Paris: Presses Univ. de Paris, 1967
3. Marty P, De M'Uzan M, David C. L'investigation psychosomatique. Paris, Presses Univ de Paris, 1963
4. Marty P, De M'Uzan M. La "pensee operatoire". Rev Fr Psychoanal 1963; 27:1345–1356
5. De M'Uzan M. Psychodynamic mechanisms in psychosomatic symptom formation. Psychother Psychosom 1974; 23:103–110
6. Sifneos PE. The prevalence of alexithymic characteristics in psychosomatic patients. Psychoter Psychosom 1973; 22:255–262
7. Engel G. Discussion in physiology, emotion and psychosomatic illness. Ciba Foundation Symposium, No 8. Amsterdam: Elsevier, 1972: 27
8. Musaph H. The role of aggression in somatic symptom formation. Int J Psychiat Med 1974; 449–460
9. Heimann P. On counter-transference. Int J Psychoanal 1950; 31:81–84
10. Heimann P. Counter-transference. Br J Med Psychol 1960; 33:9–15
11. Bion WR. Attacks on linking. In: Second thoughts. London: Heinemann, 1967
12. Money-Kyrle RE. Normal counter-transference and some of its deviations. Int J Psychoanal 1956; 37:360–366
13. Grotjahn M. The process of awakening. Psychoanal Rev 1942; 29
14. Fliess R. Boredom, in Ego and body ego. New York: Int. Univ Press, 1961; 191–194
15. Grinberg L. On a specific aspect of counter-transference due to the patient's projective identification. Int J Psychoanal 1962; 43:436–440
16. Taylor GJ. Alexithymia and the counter-transference. Psychother Psychosom 1977; 28:141–147
17. Fain M, David C. Aspects fonctionels de la vie onirique. Rev Fr Psychanal 1963; 27:241–343
18. Sperling M. Psychosis and psychosomatic illness. Int J Psychoanal 1955; 33:121–226
19. McDougall J. The psychesoma and the psychoanalytic process. Int Rev Psychoanal 1974; 1:437–459
20. Yahalom I. Sense, affect and image in the development of the symbolic process. Int J Psychoanal 1967; 48:373–383
21. Fain M. Prelude a la vie fantasmatique. Rev Fr Psychoanal 1971; 35:291–364
22. Ammon G, Schibalski-Ammon K, Herold J, Finke G. Psychodynamics and ego structure in skin disease. In: Panconesi E (Ed). Stress and skin diseases. Philadelphia, Lippincott, 1984: p.43
23. Winnicott DW. Psychosomatic illness in its positive and negative aspects. Int J Psychoanal, 1966; 47:510–516

24. Spitz R. Autoerotism. Psychoanal Study Child 1962; 17
25. Kaplan HI, Sadock BJ. Pocket handbook of clinical psychiatry. 2nd Ed. Baltimore: Williams and Wilkins, 1996
26. Panconesi E. Stress and skin diseases: psychosomatic dermatology. In: clinical in dermatology. Philadelphia: Lippincott, 1984
27. Charlesworth WR, Kreutzer MA. Facial expression of infant and children. In: Ekman P (Ed). Darwin and facial expression: a century of research in review. New York: Academic Press, 1973
28. Bridges KMB. Emotional development in early infancy. Child Dev 1932; 3:324–341
29. Anochin PK. Biologia e fisiologia del riflesso condizionato. Roma: Bulzoni, 1975.
30. Braetigam W, Christian P. Psychosomatische Medizin. Stuttgart: Thieme, 1975
31. Klein M. A contribution to the psychogenesis of manic-depressive states. In: Contributions to psychoanalysis. London: Hogarth Press, 1948
32. Klein M. Noes on some schizoid mechanisms. In: Klein M (Ed). Developments in psychoanalysis. London: Hogarth Press, 1952
33. Klein M. Individia e gratitudine. Firenze: Martinelli, 1969
34. Piaget J. La rappresentazione del mondo del fanciullo. Torino: Boringhieri, 1966
35. Bion WR. Trasformazioni. Roma: Armando, 1973
36. Bion WR. Apprendere dall'esperienza. Roma: Armando, 1972
37. Abraham K. The first pregenital stage of the libido. In: Selected papers on psychoanalysis. New York: Basic Books, 1953
38. Alexander F. Medicina psicosomatica. Firenze: Giunti-Barbera, 1972
39. Hofer MA. Physiological and behavioral processes in ealy maternal deprivation. In: Ciba Foundation Symposium, N 8. Amsterdam: Elsevier, 1972
40. Bowlby J. Attaccamento e perdita: attaccamento alla madre. Torino: Boringhieri, 1979
41. Harlow HF. The nature of love. Am Psychol 1958; 13:673–685
42. Harlow HF. The development of affectional patterns in infant monkeys. In: Foss B (Ed). Determinants of infant behavior. New York: Wiley, 1961
43. Perls K, Hefferline RF, Goodman P. Teoria e pratica della terapia della Gestalt. Roma: Astrolabio, 1971
44. Silverman S, Gorsky M, Lozada-Nur F. A prospective follow-up study of 570 patients with oral lichen planus: persistence, remission, and malignant association. Oral Surg Oral Med Oral Pathol 1985; 60:30–34
45. Boyd AS, Neldner KH. Lichen planus. J Am Acad Dermatol 1991; 25:593–619
46. Obermayer ME. Psychocutaneous medicine. Springfield: Charles C. Thomas, 1955
47. Cossidente A, Devoto G, Melli MC. Indagine psicologico-psichiatrica su cento casi di lichen planus. G Ital Dermatol Venereol, 1982; 6:337–340
48. Griesemer RD, Nadelson T. Emotional aspects of cutaneous disease. In: Fitzpatrick IM, Eisen AZ, Wolff K (Eds). Dermatology in general medicine. New York: McGraw Hill, 1979: 1353–1363
49. Meluzzi A, Zina G. Le malattie dermatologiche. In: Pancheri P (Ed). Trattato di medicina psicosomatica. Firenze: USES, 1984: 699–750
50. Devoto G, Cossidente A. Risultato di un'indagine con test psicodiagnostici in una casistica di pazienti affetti da lichen planus. Med Psicosom 1983; 28:277–286
51. Kaplan B, Barnes L. Lichen planus and squamous carcinoma. Arch Otolaryngol 1985; 111:543–547
52. Altman J, Perry HO. The variations and course of lichen planus. Arch Dermatol 1961; 84:179–191
53. Lowenthal U, Pisanti S. Oral lichen planus according to the modern medical model. J Oral Med 1984; 39:224–226
54. Allen CM, Beck FM, Rossie KM. Relation of stress and anxiety to oral lichen planus. Oral Surg Oral Med Oral Pathol 1985; 61:44–46
55. Ader R, Felten DL, Cohen N. Psychoneuroimmunology. 2nd Ed. San Diego: Academic Press, 1991
56. Rasmussen AF, March JT, Brill NQ. Increased susceptibility to herpes simplex virus in mice subjected to avoidance learning stress or restraint. Proc Soc Exp Biol Med 1957; 96:183–186
57. Helig R, Hoff H. Ueber psychogene Entstehung des Herpes labialis. Med Klin 1928; 24:1472
58. Ullman M. Herpes simplex and second degree burns induced by hypnosis. Am J Psychol 1947; 103:828–830
59. Blank H, Brody MW. Recurrent herpes simplex: a psychiatric and laboratory study. Psychosom Med 1950; 12:254–360
60. Whitlock FA. Psychophysiological aspects of skin disease. Philadelphia: WB Saunders, 1976
61. Kiecolt-Glaser JK, Garner W, Speiche CE. Psychosocial modifiers of immunocompetence in medical students. Psychosom Med 1984; 46:7–14
62. Kasl SV, Evans AS, Neiderman JC. Psychosocial risk factors in the development of infectious mononucleosis. Psychosom Med 1979; 41:445–466
63. Luborsky L, Mintz J, Brightman VJ. Herpes simplex and moods: a longitudinal study. J Psychosom Res 1976; 20:543–548
64. Glaser R, Kiecolt-Glaser JK, Speicher CE. Stress, loneliness and changes in herpesvirus latency. J Behav Med 1985; 8:249–260
65. Rook A. The lips. In: Rock A, Wilkinson DS (Eds). Textbook of dermatology. 3rd Ed. London: Blackwell Scientific Publication, 1979; 1803–1908
66. Bilisoly FN, Goodell H, Wolff HG. Vasodilation, lowered pain threshold and increased tissue vulnerability. Arch Intern Med 1954; 94:759–773
67. Buisson, quoted by Butlin HT and Spencer WG. Diseases of the tongue. New York: Cassell, 1900; 410
68. Schwimmer EL. Beiträge zur Glossopathologie. Wien Med Wochenschr 1886; 36:337–341
69. Magitot EJ. De la glossodynie: glossalgie (Breschat): rheumatisme musculaire de la langue; nevralgie linguale; ulcerations imaginaires de la langue (Verneuil). Gaz Hebd de Med 1887; 24:788–791
70. Oppenheim H. Lehrbuch der Nervenkrankheiten. Berlin: S Karger, 1913; 943
71. Fox H. Burning tongue glossodynia. NY State J Med 1935; 35:881–884
72. Zisken DE, Moulton R. Glossodynia: a study of idiopathic orolingual pain. JADA 1946; 33:1422–1432
73. Huang W, Rothe MJ, Grant-Kels JM. The burning mouth syndrome. J Am Acad Dermatol 1996; 34:91–98
74. Main DMG, Baker RM. Patients complaining of a burning mouth. Br Dent J 1983; 154:206–211
75. Hautmann G, Panconesi E. Glossodynia. J Eur Acad Dermatol Venereol 1996; 7:207–227
76. Merskey H (Ed). Classification of chronic pain: descriptions of chronic pain syndromes and definitions of pain terms. Pain 1986; 3(Suppl):1–226
77. Jontell M, Haraldson T, Persson L-O, et al. An oral and psychosocial examination of patients with presumed oral galvanism. Swed Dent J 1985; 9:175–185
78. Yontchev E, Hedegard B, Carlsson GE. Outcome of treatment of patients with orofacial discomfort complaints. Int J Oral Maxillofac Surg 1987; 16:312–318
79. Agerberg, G. Signs and symptoms of mandibular dysfunction in patients with suspected oral galvanism. Acta Odontol Scand 1987; 45:41–48
80. Hampf G, Ekholm A, Salo T, et al. Pain in oral galvanism. Pain 1987; 29:301–311
81. Hugoson A. Results obtained from patients referred for the investigation of complaints related to oral galvanism. Swed Dent J 1986; 10:15–28
82. Haraldson T. Oral galvanism and mandibular dysfunction. Swed Dent J 1985; 9:129–133
83. Zilli C, Brooke RI, Lau CL, et al. Screening for psychiatric illness in patients with oral dysesthesia by means of the General Health Questionnaire: twenty-eight item version (GHQ-28) and the Irritability, Depression and Anxiety Scale (IDA). Oral Surg Oral Med Oral Pathol 1989; 67:384–389
84. Grushka M, Sessle BJ, Miller R. Pain and personality profiles in burning mouth syndrome. Pain 1987; 28:155–167

85. Grushka M, Sessle BJ, Howley TP. Psychophysical evidence of taste dysfunction in burning mouth syndrome. Chem Senses 1986; 11:485–498
86. Browning S, Hislop S, Scully C, et al. The association between burning mouth syndrome and psychosocial disorders. Oral Surg Oral Med Oral Pathol 1987; 64:171–174
87. Lamey P-J, Lamb AB. Prospective study of etiological factors in burning mouth syndrome. Br Med J 1988; 296:1243–1246
88. Lamey P-J, Lamb AB. The usefulness of the HAD scale in assessing anxiety and depression in patients with burning mouth syndrome. Oral Surg Oral Med Oral Pathol 1989; 67:390–392
89. Basker RM, Sturdee DW, Davenport JC. Patients with burning mouths: a clinical investigation of causative factors, including the climacteric and diabetes. Br Dent J 1978; 145:9–16
90. Hammaren M, Hugoson A. Clinical psychiatric assessment of patients with burning mouth syndrome resisting oral treatment. Swed Dent J 1989; 13:77–88
91. van der Ploeg HM, van der Wal N, Eijkman MAJ, et al. Psychological aspects of patients with burning mouth syndrome. Oral Surg Oral Med Oral Pathol 1987; 63:661–668
92. Main DMG, Basker RM. Patients complaining of a burning mouth: further experience and clinical assessment and management. Br Dent J 1983; 154:206–211
93. Lamey P-J, Hammond A, Allam BF, et al. Vitamin status of patients with burning mouth syndrome and the response to replacement therapy. Br Dent J 1986; 160:81–84
94. Grushka M. Clinical features of burning mouth syndrome. Oral Surg Oral Med Oral Pathol 1987; 63:30–36
95. Grushka M, Sessle BI, Howley TP. Psychophysical assessment of tactile, pain and thermal sensory functions in burning mouth syndrome. Pain 1987; 28:169–184
96. Paparella MM, Shumrick DA (Eds). Otolaryngology, vol 3. Philadelphia: W. B. Saunders, 1980
97. Lynch MA. Burkett's oral medicine, 7th Ed. New York: Lippincott, 1977: 198–201, 357–359
98. Albert E. Einige seltenere Erkrankungen der Zunge. Med Presse 1885; 26:1–6
99. Marxkors R, Muller-Fahlbusch H. Psychogene Prothesenunverträglichkeit. Munich-Vienna: Hanser, 1976
100. Maier CH. Vitalstörungen des Mundbereichs (Glossodynie) bei depressiven Rückbildungspsychosen. Nervenarzt 1986; 57:113–115
101. Ott G, Ott, C. Glossodynia: psychodynamic basis and results of psychopathometric investigations. J Psychosom Res 1992; 36:677–686
102. Kuffer R. Les paresthesis buccales psychogenes. Ann Dermatol Venereol 1987; 114:1, 589–596
103. Baurle G, Schoenberger A. Glossodynie-Indikation zur Epikutantestung? Z Hautkr 1986; 61(16):1175–1184
104. Haneke E. Psychische Aspekte der Glossodynie. Dtsch Med Wochenschr 1978; 103:1302–1305
105. Gottwald W, Haneke E. Glossodynie – Ein Syndrom. Proc. V South-East-Europe Neuropsychiatr. Conf. Graz 1983; 110–120
106. Cossidente A, Sarti M. Psychiatric syndromes with dermatologic expression. In: Panconesi E (Ed). Stress and skin diseases. Psychosomatic dermatology. Philadelphia: Lippincott, 1984: 201–220
107. Ziskind DF, Moulton R. Glossodynia. A study of idiopathic oral-lingual pain. J Am Dent Assoc 1946; 33:1422–1432
108. Haneke E. Zungen- und Mundschleimhautbrennen. Munich: Hanser, 1980
109. Feinman CH, Harris M, Cawley R. Psychogenic facial pain. Presentation and treatment. Br Med J 1984; 288:436–438
110. Hampf G, Vikkula J, Ylipaavalniemi P, et al. Psychiatric disorders in orofacial dysaesthesia. Int J Oral Maxillofac Surg 1987; 16:402–407
111. Crisson JE, Keefe FJ. The relationship of locus of control of pain coping strategies and psychological distress in chronic pain patients. Pain 1988; 35:147–154
112. Jamison RN, Rock DL, Parris WCV. Empirically derived symptom check-list 90 subgroups of chronic pain patients: a cluster analysis. J Behav Med 1988; 11:147–158
113. Parker JC, Buckelew SP, Smarr KL, et al. Psychological screening in rheumatoid arthritis. J Rheumatol 1990; 17:1016–1021
114. Kleinhauz M, Eli I, Baht R, Shamay D. Correlates of success and failure in behavior therapy for dental fear. J Dent Rev 1992; 71:1831–1835
115. Craufurd DIO, Creed F, Jayson MIV. Life events and psychological disturbances in patients with low-back pain. Spine 1990; 15:490–494
116. Engman MF. Burning tongue. Arch Dermatol Syph 1920; 1:137–138
117. Marshall CJ. The papillae foliatae and carcinophobia. Br Med J 1928; 2:13
118. Domb GH, Chole RA. The burning mouth and tongue. Ear Nose Throat J 1981; 60(7):29–36
119. Dworkin RH, Richlin DM, Handlin DS, et al. Predicting treatment response in depressed and nondepressed chronic pain patients. Pain 1986; 24:343–353
120. Lamb AB, Lamey P-J, Reeve PE. Burning mouth syndrome: psychological aspects. Br Dent J 1988; 165:256–260
121. Koblenzer CS, Bostrom P. Chronic cutaneous dysesthesia syndrome: a psychotic phenomenon or a depressive symptom? J Am Acad Dermatol, 1994; 30:370–374
122. Gorsky M, Silverman S Jr, Chinn H. Clinical characteristics and management outcome in the burning mouth syndrome: an open study of 130 patients. Oral Surg Oral Med Oral Pathol 1991; 72:192–195

CHAPTER 18

Diseases of the Peripheral Nervous System

L. Bianchi, M. Argenta, and G. Nini

The oral cavity and the surrounding facial tissue may be part of the clinical spectrum of different neurological conditions. Most of these disorders involve the 7th, facial, and the 12th, hypoglossal, cranial nerves.

18.1 Facial Nerve Palsy

The facial nerve comprises motor, sensory, and secretomotor fibers. The motor component supplies all the muscles and expression on one side of the face. The sensory fibers carry the taste sensation from the anterior two-thirds of the tongue, whereas the secretomotor component acts on submaxillary, sublingual, and smaller salivary glands. Different clinical pictures are expressions of facial nerve disturbances resulting from defects at various sites [1, 2].

18.1.1 Bell's Palsy

Bell's Palsy represents the most common disease affecting the facial nerve; its etiology is still debated, an inflammatory reaction in or around the nerve at the stylomastoid foramen level being the common finding [3]. Sudden paralysis of upper and lower portions of the face, pain localized behind the ear, loss of taste in the anterior two-thirds of the tongue, and hyperacusis on the affected side are typical findings. Ballooning of the cheek with each respiration, drooping of the corner of the mouth, flattening of the nasolabial fold, with greatest weakness around the mouth, complete the clinical picture (Fig. 18.1). Secondary disturbances, such as food collection between the teeth and the lips, and dribbling of saliva from the corner of the mouth, may occur. The prognosis is benign in 80 % of patients without therapy, but if degeneration of facial nerve is total and denervation in the facial muscles occurs, recovery of function may be late and incomplete and may take a few months to a few years. This occurence may be observed in diabetic patients and when facial paresis

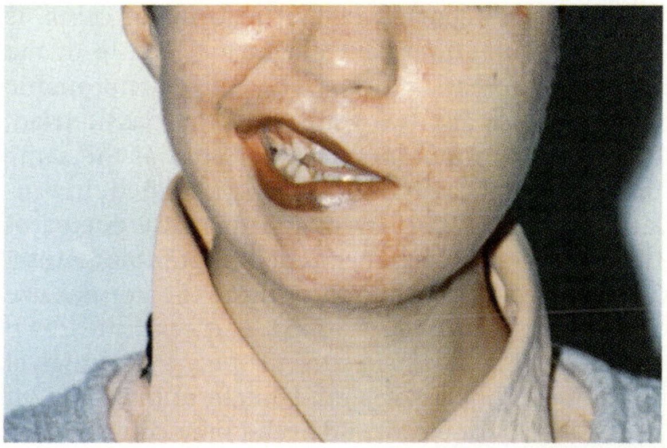

Fig. 18.1. Peripheral facial nerve palsy (Bell's palsy). The clinical picture includes paralysis of upper and lower portions of the face, flattening of the nasolabial fold and deviation and drooping of the corner of the mouth

is secondary to herpes zoster, featuring *Ramsay-Hunt syndrome*. This syndrome, due to viral involvement of the geniculate ganglion, includes either a cutaneous vesicular eruption localized on the tympanum, external auditory canal, between the ear and mastoid, in the oral cavity on the anterior pillar or fauces, or severe facial palsy, deep facial pain, or loss of taste over the anterior two-thirds of the tongue [4].

Among the other possible causes of peripheral facial palsy are Guillain-Barrè Strohl syndrome and Charcot-Marie Tooth disease, the former, a conduction block of the nerve, the latter, a slowly insidious neuropathy. Furthermore, cerebellopontine angle tumors, multiple sclerosis, and softening of the pons at the base may cause lesions of the intrapontine portion of the facial nerve; the former is generally associated with trigeminal, acoustic, and glossopharyngeal nerve damage and the latter, as in Millard-Gruber syndrome, with omolateral abducens nerve palsy and contralateral corticospinal lesion [5, 6]. Moreover, bilateral facial palsy (diplegia) may occur in idiopathic polyneuritis, sarcoidosis, and myasthenia gravis. Peripheral and nuclear facial palsy are distinguished from the supranuclear type since in the latter, the upper muscles of the face are less involved than those of the lower part, and aplasia and/or paralysis of the arm and leg are commonly found in conjunction.

18.1.2 Melkersson-Rosenthal Syndrome

Peripheral facial nerve palsy is one of the three signs of *Melkersson-Rosenthal syndrome* [7]. The complete disorder, uncommonly observed, includes recurrent orofacial swelling, lingua plicata, and intermittent facial palsy. The orofacial or oral mucosal involvement, reported in the majority of cases, is considered the dominant diagnostic feature of the monosymptomatic form. The oligosymptomatic form includes any two features of the classic triad, being all the symptoms rarely present at the same time. The oral cavity is affected by isolated, irregularly recurrent, short-lived, asymmetrical edema of the lip, known as Miescher's cheilitis granulomatosa. The affected lip is two to three times the normal size and appears fissured, chapped, and reddish-brown in color (Fig. 18.2). Recurrent polypoid gingival swelling may be associated. Unilateral involvement of the cheek, forehead, and eyelid may complete the facial clinical picture. The histological findings, when typical, reveal noncaseating epithelioid cell granuloma. The lingua plicata, reported in one-third of patients, seems the least important symptom. It appears as deep grooves and furrows on the dorsal surface, extending in all directions from the center line of the tongue. A dominant inheritance with incomplete penetrance is proposed for this disorder. Intermittent peripheral facial palsy, usually featuring the appearance of Bell's palsy, is reported in up to 90 % of cases. It may occur months to years before or after the diagnostic orofacial symptoms. The paralysis may be partial, complete, bilateral, or contralateral. Loss of taste along two-thirds of the tongue may also develop. Among the additional neurological manifestations, hyperhidrosis, hypogeusia, acroparesthesia, hyperacusia, and retrobulbar neuritis have been reported. The pathogenesis of the syndrome is unknown; it has been speculated that various factors, such as heredity, infective agents, and allergic reactions, could cause vasomotor disturbances of either the vasa nervorum or the small arterioles producing peripheral tissue damage.

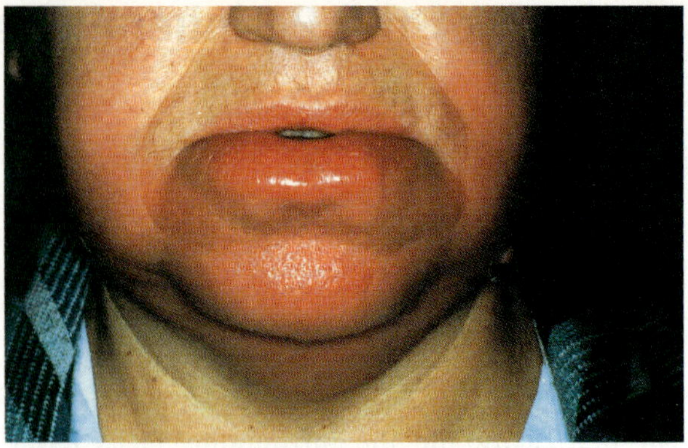

Fig. 18.2. Melkersson-Rosenthal syndrome. The monosymptomatic form is characterized by Miescher's cheilitis granulomatosa. The affected lip appears two to three times the normal size, edematous, chapped, and reddish-brown in color

18.2 Hypoglossal Nerve Palsy

The 12th cranial nerve is a purely motor nerve which supplies the ipsilateral intrinsic muscles of the tongue and the subglottic upper subpharyngeal muscles such as the hypoglossus, styloglossus, and genioglossus [8]. Unilateral lesions of the nerve affect the tongue, resulting in wrinkling, fasciculations (Fig. 18.3), fibrillations, atrophy, and weakness of protrusion of the tongue, with ipsilateral deviation of tongue and uvula (Fig. 18.4) due to of the action of the contralateral genioglossal muscle [9, 10]. Iso-

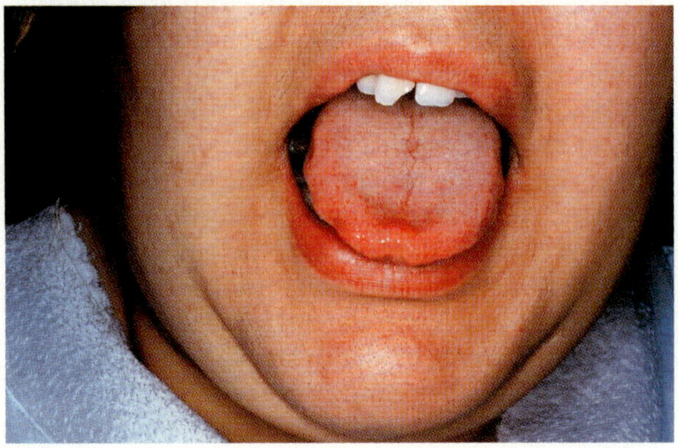

Fig. 18.3. Hypoglossal nerve palsy. Fasciculation of the border of the tongue

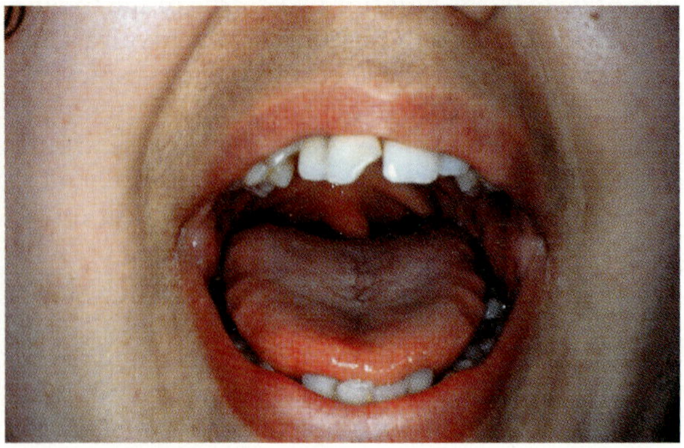

Fig. 18.4. Hypoglossal nerve palsy. Deviation of the uvula

lated involvement of the hypoglossal nerve is uncommon. Bilateral lesions can seriously affect the ability to protrude the tongue, with potential respiratory difficulties. Twelfth cranial nerve palsy is reported following surgical trauma, such as carotid endoarterectomy, cervical vascular anomalies, a penetrating mass or lesion of the neck, and radiation for head or neck tumors. The hypoglossal nerve can also be involved in extramedullary compressions or intramedullary tumors and softening, or as a complication of infectious mononucleosis. Furthermore, hypoglossal nuclei may be damaged in poliomyelitis and other motor system diseases [11].

References

1. Brodal A. The cranial nerves. III. Springfield: Charles C. Thomas, 1959
2. Mayo Clinic and Mayo Foundation. Clincial examinations in neurology. 4th Ed. Philadelphia: Saunders, 1976
3. Groves J. Bell's (idiopathic) facial palsy. In: Hinchcliffe R, Harrison D (Eds). Scientific foundations of otolaryngology. London: Heinemann, 1976: 446–459
4. Karnes WE. Diseases of the seventh cranial nerves. In: Dyck PJ, Thomas PK, Lambert EH (Eds). Peripheral neuropathy, vol. I (27). Philadelphia: Saunders, 1975: 570–573
5. Haymaker W, Kuhlenbeck H. Disorders of the brain system and its cranial nerves. In: AB Baker, LH Baker (Eds). Clinical neurology. RJ Joynt Editor. Philadelphia: JB Lippincott, 1990; vol 3(40)
6. Lapresle J, Lasjaunias P. Cranial nerve ischaemic arterial syndromes: a review. Brain 1986; 109:207–215
7. Greene RM, Rogers RS. Melkersson-Rosenthal syndrome. a review of 36 patients. J Am Acad Dermatol 1989; 21:1263–1270
8. Smoker WRK. The hypoglossal nerve. Neuroimag Clin 1993; 3:193–206
9. Afifi AK, Rifai ZH, Faris KB. Isolated, reversible, hypoglossal nerve palsy. Arch Neurology 1984; 41:1218–1224
10. Caparros-Lefebvre D, Girard-Buttaz I, Leclerc X, Hurtevent JF, Desaulty A, Pruvo JP, Francke JP, Petit H. Paralysie unilatérale des nerfs glossopharyngiens, vague et grand hypoglosse. Rev Neurol (Paris) 1994; 150(3):236–238
11. Keane JR. Twelfth-nerve palsy. Arch Neurology 1996; 53:561–566

CHAPTER 19

Precancerous Lesions and Benign Tumors of the Oral Mucosa

19.1 Oral Mucosa Changes Induced by Aging and Light

S. Humke and T. Ruzicka

19.1.1 Cheilitis Angularis (Perlèche, Angulus Infectiosus)

Definition. Cheilitis angularis is an acute or chronic inflammation of the angles of the mouth.

Etiology. Cheilitis angularis is a polyetiological clinical syndrome [1]. Several factors may be causative, alone or in combination; *Staphylococcus aureus* and *Candida albicans* are frequently found as infective agents [3].
Candida albicans is often isolated in patients who wear dentures, and may be an early manifestation of mucocutaneous candidosis due to an underlying immunological deficiency, which might be HIV, diabetes mellitus, or chronic granulomatous disease, for example [5]. Various mechanical factors can cause cheilitis angularis in elderly people, such as ill-fitting dentures and macerated skin of the angles due to overlying skin. Other mechanical factors are prognathism and hypersalivation (e.g., in Down's syndrome). In rare cases, the presence of sinuses of developmental origin may cause the condition [2]. Chronic inflammatory skin diseases, such as atopic eczema and seborrheic dermatitis, are also sometimes associated with inflamed anguli of the mouth. Nutritional deficiencies such as riboflavin, vitamin B12, and iron deficiencies, or general protein malnutrition are further possible causes.

Pathogenesis. Maceration due to various etiological factors leads to an impaired epidermal barrier and predisposes to infection with pathogenic organisms.

Oral Manifestations. Redness, superficial fissuring, and crusting occur at the angles of the mouth. The adjacent skin surface may also be involved, but the buccal mucosa is usually free [4] (Fig. 19.1).

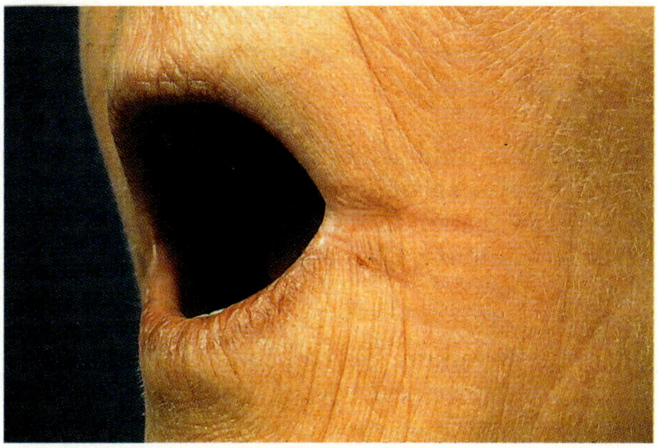

Fig. 19.1. Cheilitis angularis

Associated Findings. In *Candida albicans* infections, oral candidosis may also be present. Deficiency syndromes usually present with several clinical signs: in the case of riboflavin-deficiency cheilosis, tongue atrophy, blepharitis, and seborrheic dermatitis can occur. Patients with vitamin B12 deficiency often show hyperpigmentation on the extremities and Moeller-Hunter glossitis.
In patients with iron deficiency, atrophy and burning sensations of the tongue, gingivitis, parodontitis, koilonychia, and hair loss may be other clinical signs.

Diagnosis. Bacteriological and mycological examinations, including the parts covered by dentures, should be performed. To exclude deficiency syndromes, blood samples for serum iron and blood cell count should be obtained. Diagnostic gastric investigations may also be helpful. Mouth closure and teeth should be checked by a dentist.

Differential diagnosis. Papular syphilids (condylomata lata) in secondary syphilis present with a similar clinical picture.

Treatment. The treatment of cheilitis angularis consists mainly in the use of antiseptics, antibiotics, or antimycotics, depending on the cause. Topical 2%–

5 % silver nitrate, 0.5 % clioquinol in zinc lotion, or short-term glucocorticosteroids may be helpful [1]. In the case of vitamin or iron deficiencies, supplementation is essential to obtain cure. The occlusal vertical dimension should be corrected, if necessary.

19.1.2 Cheilitis Actinica Acuta

Definition. Cheilitis actinica acuta is an acute inflammation of the lips after exposure to sun. This sunburn of the lip occurs mainly on the lower lip.

Etiology. It occurs usually in summer, after intensive exposure to sunlight [3].

Pathogenesis. Sunburn is mainly a UVB effect. The release of prostaglandins leads to erythema by way of vascular dilation in the subepidermal connective tissue. In addition, UVB damages keratinocytes directly.

Oral Manifestations. Several hours after intensive UV exposure, painful edema, erythema, and, depending on the dose, vesicles and erosive lesions occur [1].

Associated Findings. Acute actinic dermatitis of other sun-exposed parts of the body is usually present.

Microscopic Findings. 12–72 h after sun exposure, sunburn cells (eosinophilic dyskeratotic cells with small nuclei and pale cytoplasm) are present in the upper and middle parts of the stratum spinosum. After intensive sun exposure, extensive epithelial necrosis can occur. There is a slight perivascular lymphohistiocytic infiltrate.

Diagnosis. The diagnosis is made from the clinical signs and the history.

Differential Diagnosis. As differential diagnoses of lupus erythematosus, lichen planus, contact cheilitis, angular cheilitis, glandular cheilitis, exfoliative cheilitis, factitious cheilitis, granulomatous cheilitis, and plasma cell cheilitis may be considered [2, 4].

Treatment. Avoidance of the sun is essential; the skin changes should then resolve within several days. Topical corticosteroids may be used if necessary [1].

19.1.3 Cheilitis Actinica Chronica (Cheilitis Exfoliativa, Solar Cheilosis, Actinic Keratosis of the Lip)

Definition. Cheilitis actinica chronica is a precancerous condition consisting of a chronic inflammation of the lip after excessive long-term sun exposure.

Etiology. Mostly older men with a lifelong history of chronic sun exposure, such as farmers or sailors, are affected. It occurs most frequently in fair-skinned individuals and is associated with squamous cell carcinoma of the lip [1].

Pathogenesis. The pathogenesis of the condition is analogous to that of actinic keratosis of the skin. UV irradiation leads to mutations in epidermal cells, which are transformed into atypical anaplastic cells [2].

Oral Manifestations. The lower lip is predominantly involved. The chronic changes include diffuse atrophy, a silver-gray color, and an ill-defined vermilion border. Poorly demarcated white keratotic plaques may be present. Dryness or erosions which heal slowly or are persistent are also common. Secondary infection of the lip may result in erosions and ulcers, which the clear with the disappearance of the infection.

If infiltrated regions can be felt or chronic ulcers appear, carcinomatous transformation is to be expected.

The lesions persist throughout the year [1, 2, 4] (Figs. 19.2–19.5). As a special form, cheilitis abrasiva praecancerosa Manganotti can be distinguished. It consists of chronic erosive lesions with crusts, with-

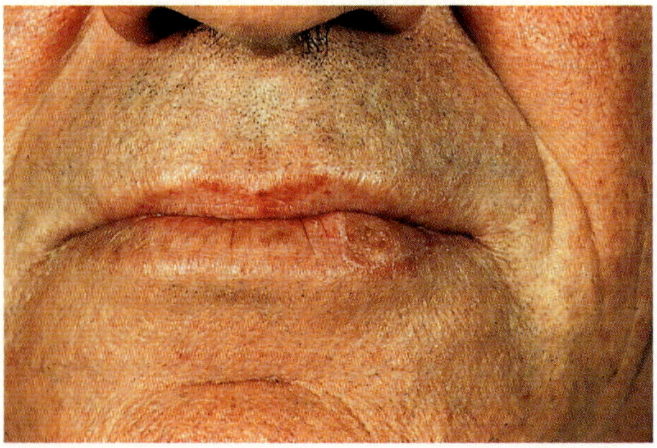

Fig. 19.2. Cheilitis actinica chronica, mild case

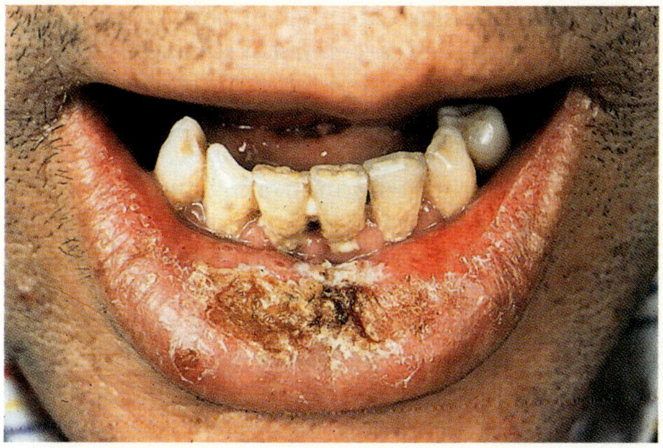

Fig. 19.3. Cheilitis actinica chronica, severe case

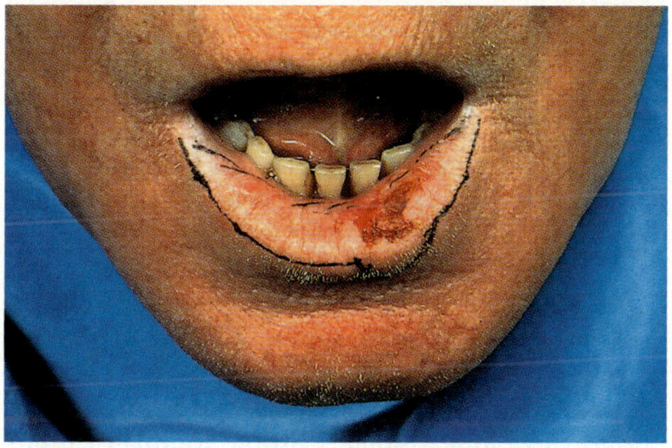

Fig. 19.4. Cheilitis actinica chronica, before vermilionectomy

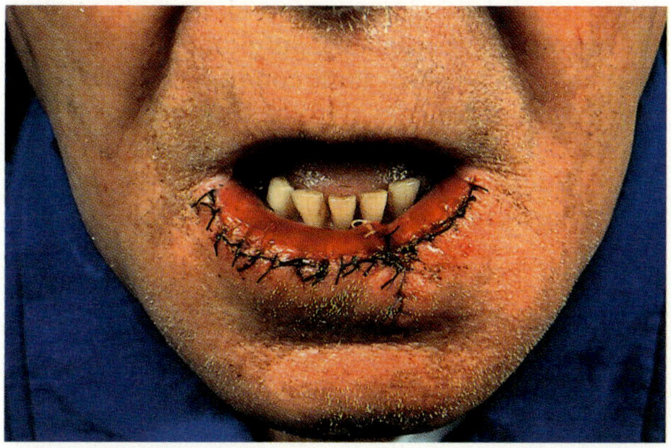

Fig. 19.5. Cheilitis actinica chronica, after vermilionectomy

out a sharp border, and has a higher risk of developing carcinoma [1].

Associated Findings. Other signs of chronic sun exposure and actinic keratoses on other sun-exposed parts of the body are common.

Microscopic Findings. Histopathologic examination shows ortho- and parakeratosis, with areas of hyperplasia, atrophy, dysplasia, and abnormal epithelial stratification with an inflammatory infiltrate [1].

Diagnosis. The diagnosis is made from the clinical signs and the history of chronic sun exposure. A biopsy is mandatory if carcinoma is suspected.

Differential Diagnosis. The differential diagnosis must take account of such skin diseases as lupus erythematosus and lichen planus. Contact cheilitis, leukoplakia, squamous cell carcinoma, angular cheilitis, glandular cheilitis, exfoliative cheilitis, factitious cheilitis, granulomatous cheilitis, plasma cell cheilitis, and cheilitis artefacta may present with a similar clinical picture [4].

Treatment. The treatment includes laser therapy, cryotherapy, topical 5-fluorouracil, and chemical peeling. In advanced cases, vermilionectomy or lip shaving may become necessary [7].
Protection from prolonged sun exposure is essential. If a carcinoma has already developed, excision with a sufficient safety margin must be performed, as squamous cell carcinoma of the lip metastasizes in up to 10 %–15 % of cases. In extensive carcinoma, neck dissection may be necessary [2].

19.1.4 Squamous Cell Carcinoma of the Lip

Definition. The squamous cell carcinoma is a malignant epithelial tumor.

Etiology. Lip carcinomas usually develop from precanceroses such as leukoplakia (often present in smokers, glass blowers, and tar workers), cheilitis actinica praecancerosa, or cheilitis abrasiva praecancerosa.
They occur after chronic UV exposure, including long-term phototherapy and photochemotherapy. Most people affected have skin types I and II. Other etiologic factors are ionizing radiation, chronic arsenic intoxication (e.g., drugs), and chronic skin damage. The latter may be due to chronic radiodermatitis, scars of lupus vulgaris or lupus erythematosus, or mechanically strained scars [8].

Pathogenesis. The squamous cell carcinoma is thought to arise from atypical epidermal keratinocytes.

Oral Manifestations. Squamous cell carcinoma usually starts as an adherent scale, nearly without infiltration. Later, ulceration and infiltration occur.

Other manifestations include small erosions with a firm base, primary painless ulcerations without exophytic growth and with a hard indolent base, and rapidly growing inflammatory nodules, which later show necrosis [9].

Metastases seen to develop after 1–2 years in 10%–15% of cases [10] (Figs. 19.6–19.8).

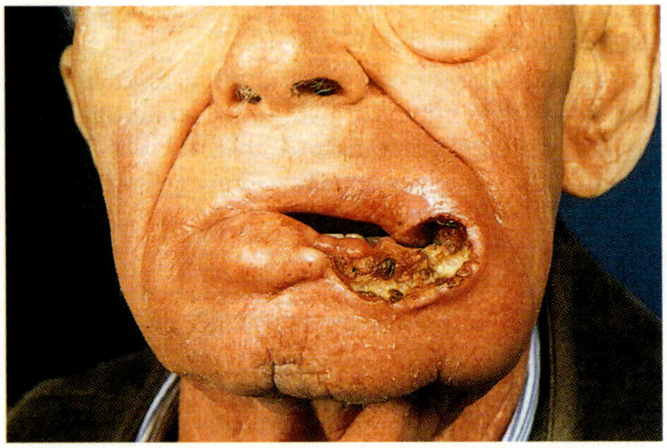

Fig. 19.6. Squamous cell carcinoma of the lip

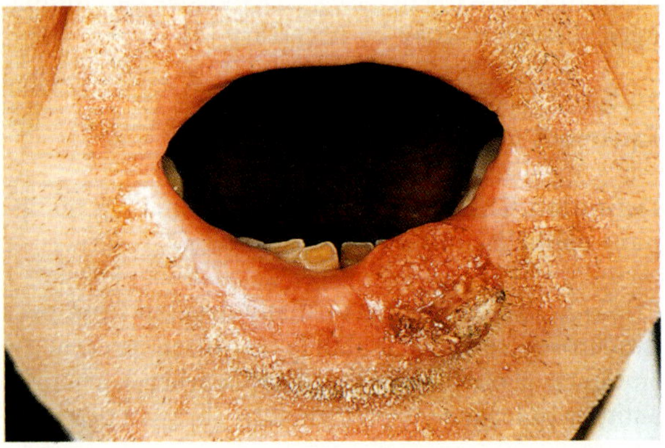

Fig. 19.7. Squamous cell carcinoma of the lip

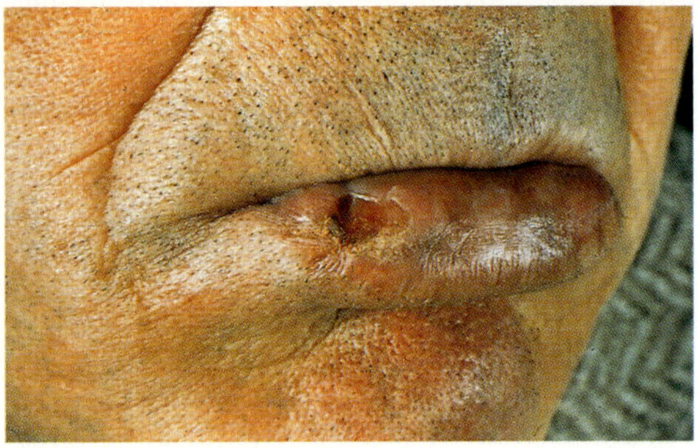

Fig. 19.8. Squamous cell carcinoma of the lip

Associated Findings. Other signs of chronic actinic damage, e. g., basal cell carcinoma or squamous cell carcinoma, may be present in other sun-exposed areas.

Microscopic Findings. Irregular tumor masses arise from the epidermis with infiltrating and destructive growth into the dermis.

Atypia of keratinocytes is present throughout the full thickness of the epidermis. The cells are large and rich in plasma. So-called horn cysts develop due to keratinization. There is a marked stromal reaction around the proliferating tumor masses, with aggregation of histiocytes and mast cells.

Diagnosis. The diagnosis is made from the typical clinical features. In cases of doubt, a biopsy should be performed if an excision in toto is not possible. The presence of a squamous cell carcinoma should always be confirmed by histological examination. The lesion may be sampled by shave, punch, or incisional biopsy, or by excision in toto. Palpation of the submandibular and the cervical lymph nodes is essential in every case of suspected squamous cell carcinoma.

Differential Diagnosis. Infectious conditions such as primary syphilis, syphilis gummosa, and tuberculous ulcer can be considered. Other tumors, e. g., keratoacanthoma, granuloma teleangiectaticum, or lymphoma, may look similar. Chronic trauma or lupus erythematosus might also be taken into consideration.

Treatment. The treatment is primarily surgical or destructive, depending on the size of the tumor and the age of the patient. Surgical excision is the treatment of choice. In some conditions, X-ray treatment offers advantages. Cytotoxic drugs can be used systemically (bleomycin) or locally (nitrogen mustard, 5-fluorouracil).

Follow-up is required for at least 5 years.

19.1.5 Basal Cell Carcinoma (Basalioma)

Definition. Basal cell carcinoma is a semimalignant tumor of the skin, with infiltrative and destructive growth, but very rare metastases.

Etiology. It occurs after chronic UV exposure, including long-term phototherapy and photochemotherapy. Most of those affected have skin types I and II. Other etiologic factors are ionizing radiation, chronic arsenic intoxication (e. g., drugs), and chronic skin damage. The latter may be due to chronic radiodermatitis, scars of lupus vulgaris or lupus erythematosus, or mechanically strained scars [8].

Pathogenesis. The tumor probably arises from immature pluripotent epithelial cells [13].

Oral Manifestations. Primary basal cell carcinoma occurs only on the lips. Manifestations in the oral cavity arise in continuity from facial primary lesions [11]. The most common appearance is a slightly translucent, waxy, or pearly papule or nodule, with surrounding or overlying telangiectasia. Secondary changes can include ulceration, crusting, scaling, pigmentation, erythema, cyst formation, and scarring. In the atypical rodent ulcer, the edge and the base of the tumor are indurated, but there is no thread-like margin.
Superficial basal cell carcinoma is a well demarcated and erythematous macule, with fine scaling and telangiectasia. A primary sclerosing basal cell carcinoma, also called morpheaform or infiltrating basal cell carcinoma, is relatively rare and appears as an ill-defined flat or depressed, yellowish, indurated plaque, sometimes with overlying telangiectasia [14] (Figs. 19.9, 19.10).

Associated Findings. Other signs of chronic actinic damage might be visible. The patient should be examined for basal cell carcinoma and squamous cell carcinoma on other sun-exposed areas.

Microscopic Findings. Pathologic changes that indicate the presence of a basal cell carcinoma include cytologically atypical cells with darkly staining, large, oval, elongated nuclei, and little cytoplasm collected in masses of various sizes. There is palisading of cells at the periphery of the tumor lobules and retraction artifacts from surrounding stroma. Stromal changes include mucin deposition and fibrosis of varying degrees [8, 9].

Diagnosis. The diagnosis is made mainly from the typical clinical appearance and confirmed by biopsy. The lesion may be sampled by shave biopsy, punch biopsy, incisional biopsy, or excision in toto. In cases of primary sclerosing basal cell carcinoma, photodynamic diagnosis may be performed.

Differential Diagnosis. As differential diagnoses, nevocellular or appendageal benign tumors, malignant melanoma, squamous cell carcinoma, keratoacanthoma, traumatic ulcers, and dermatitis artefacta can be considered [11].

Treatment. The treatment is primarily surgical or destructive, depending on the size of the tumor and the age of the patient. Surgical excision is the treatment of choice, with a minimum safety margin of 2–4 mm [15].

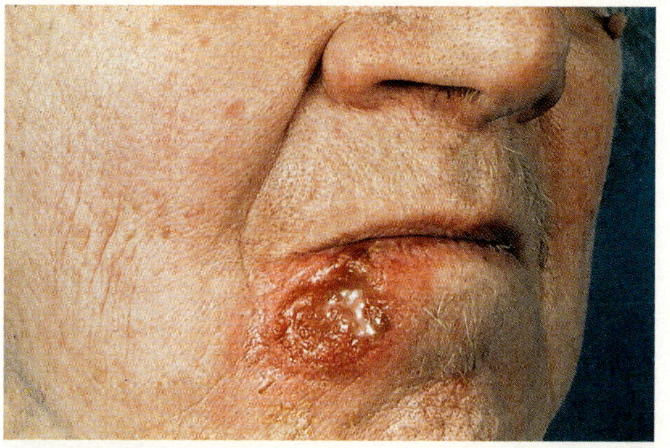

Fig. 19.9. Basal cell carcinoma

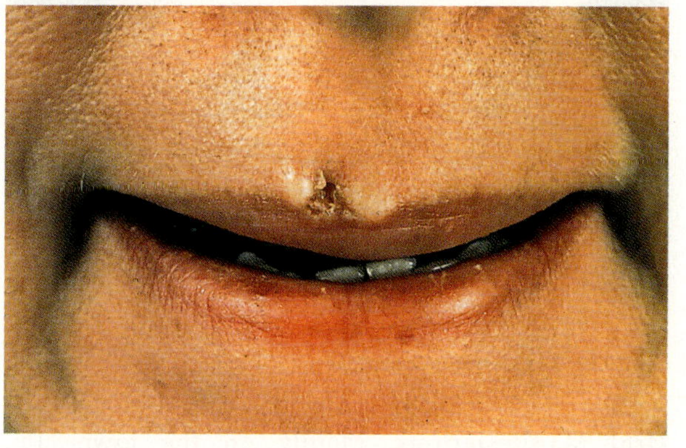

Fig. 19.10. Primary sclerosing basal cell carcinoma

Cryotherapy, radiation, laser surgery, photodynamic therapy, electrodesiccation and curettage, and Mohs micrographic surgery can also be performed. Follow-up is required for at least 5 years [12].

19.1.6 Xeroderma Pigmentosum

Definition. Xeroderma pigmentosum is a group of disorders with an autosomal recessive mode of inheritance associated with excessive sunburn reactions to minimal light, with early onset of freckling and severe actinic damage, leading to multiple malignant tumors.

Etiology. An abnormal reaction of the skin to UV irradiation, caused by DNA repair deficiency, leads to this condition.

Pathogenesis. Excision of UVB-induced pyrimidine dimers is impaired in genetic variants A-I; the so-called variant form consists of a defect of postreplication repair [18].

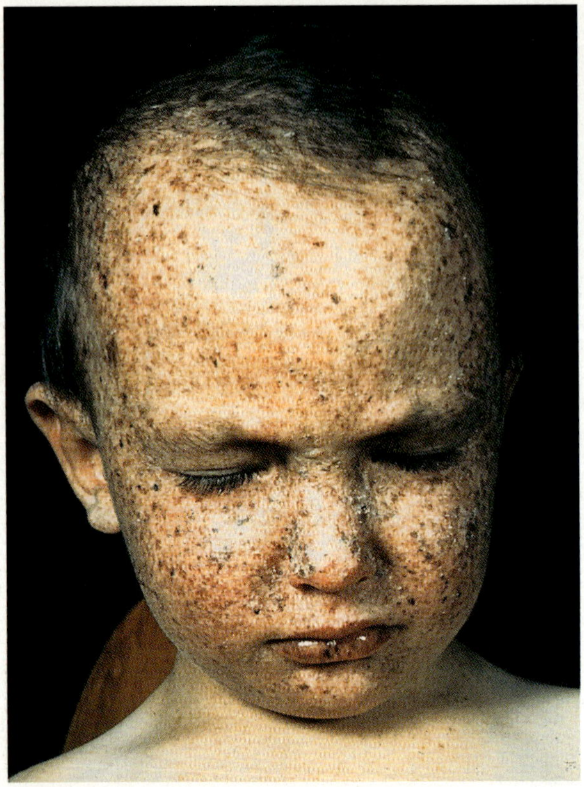

Fig. 19.11. Xeroderma pigmentosa

Oral Manifestations. Mainly on the lower lip, chronic light damage including various precancerous lesions occurs. Patients develop skin cancers in abundance, such as basal cell carcinomas and squamous cell carcinomas, but also malignant melanomas. Tumors arise even in childhood [16, 18] (Fig. 19.11).

Associated Findings. Severe actinic damage is found on all sun-exposed areas of the skin. Deafness, progressive mental deterioration, photophobia, conjunctivitis, and UV keratitis are sometimes associated with this [17].

Microscopic Findings. Poikiloderma-like and sun-damaged epithelial cells are found in combination with UV-induced tumors [16].

Diagnosis. The diagnosis is made from the clinical findings and by genetic complementation tests [18].

Treatment. The cornerstone of the therapy is early diagnosis and strict protection from any UV irradiation. This involves potent sun screens, restricted sun exposure, and protective clothes. Any premalignant or malignant tumor must be removed by excision, curettage, cryotherapy, etc. Regular checks are indicated so that the diagnosis of these lesions can be made at an early stage [16].

19.2 Precancerous Lesions of the Oral Mucosa

G. M. Palleschi, A. Giacomelli, and C. Vallecchi

The term precancerosis is a clinical expression defining various mucosal alterations that can each be the prelude to malignant neoplasms. The most frequent malignancy affecting the oral mucosa and lips is squamous cell carcinoma. On the lips, photoaging is the primary predisposing factor to precancerosis. On the oral mucosa, precanceroses are strictly related to tobacco and ethanol use. Other environmental factors are persistent trauma due to defective dental prostheses or sharp teeth, inflammatory disorders, and nutritional deficiency. These precanceroses are actinic cheilitis, leukoplakia, and erythroplasia. They do not resolve spontaneously and are defined as obligate precanceroses. Other diseases with possible spontaneous regression are considered precanceroses in a broad sense because they occasionally develop into cancer. These are oral deep fibrosis, leukokeratosis nicotina palati, erosive lichen planus, and atrophy caused by iron deficiency. Clinical diagnosis of a precancerous lesion of the oral mucosa should be confirmed by microscopic examination to evaluate the degree of dysplasia. Because of their potential for malignant evolution, these lesions should be treated in the early stage of onset.

19.2.1 Actinic Cheilitis (Cheilitis Exfoliativa, Solar Cheilosis, Actinic Keratosis of the Lip)

This disease is characterized by dryness, scaling, and fissuring with erosions of the lower lip related to sunlight exposure as discussed in Sect. 19.13. It is prevalent in outdoor workers. Sunlight exposure is the primary environmental factor, and wind and cold weather are important secondary environmental factors. The incidence is lower in blacks than whites and in females than males, probably because of the protection afforded by melanin pigment in blacks and use of lipstick in women. The pathogenesis of cellular damage is due to persistent UV radiation. The clinical manifestations are typical, generally involving the lower lip. Actinic cheilitis can be divided into acute and chronic forms. The former is characterized by initial edema, redness, congestion, and vesicles, followed by scaling, fissuring, superficial erosions, and even ulceration, and it resolves in some weeks. The latter is present in every season of the

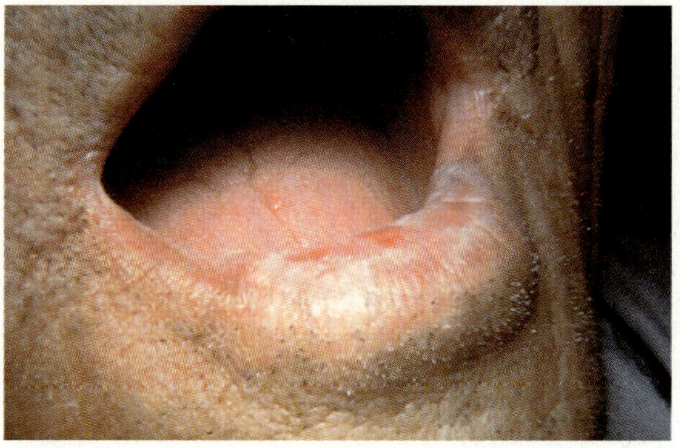

Fig. 19.12. Chronic actinic cheilitis of the lower lip: white-gray patches of marked hyperkeratosis with atrophic areas

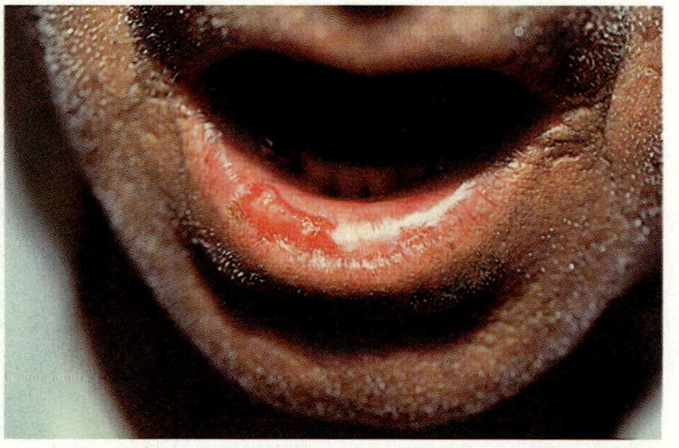

Fig. 19.13. Chronic actinic cheilitis of the lower lip with limited erosion

year and is characterized by patches of marked hyperkeratosis, which are whitish gray or light brown in color, with atrophic areas. Erosions and ulcerations are present. An association with squamous cell carcinoma is present in 50 % of chronic forms. The histopathological findings are: hyperkeratosis with parakeratosis, acanthosis, and superficial ulceration. The epithelial cells show dyskeratosis, abnormal mitoses, and nuclear atypia. There is reactive band-like infiltration of lymphocytes, plasma cells, histiocytes, and, occasionally, eosinophils and mast cells. The dermis shows ectasia of the capillaries and solar elastosis. The clinical diagnosis should be confirmed by histological examination to rule out squamous cell carcinoma. The differential diagnosis includes lichen planus, discoid lupus erythematosus, radiodermatitis, irritant or allergic (photoallergic) contact dermatitis, candidiasis, and factitial dermatitis. The treatment of acute forms is limited to photoprotection with sunscreens, topical antibiotics, and corticosteroids; in chronic forms, topical fluorouracil as 1 % or 5 % solution is useful, and, when needed, vermilionectomy or carbon dioxide laser vaporization can be employed (Figs. 19.12–19.14).

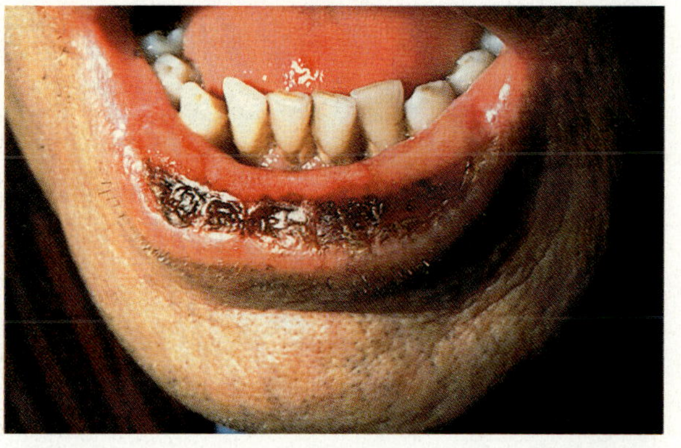

Fig. 19.14. Chronic actinic cheilitis of the lower lip with severe atrophy and extensive ulceration

19.2.2 Leukoplakia

The term leukoplakia is used for a white patch or plaque on the mucous membrane that cannot be rubbed off and is not recognized as a specific disease entity. The etiology is generally unknown, but some such patches are due to chronic physical (sharp edges of carious teeth or defective prosthesis), chemical (use of tobacco, oral snuff, or chewing) irritation, or chronic candidiasis. The pathogenesis is related to the progessive thickening of the epidermis, with various degrees of dysplasia. The clinical manifestations are usually represented by single lesions on the oral mucosa. Retroangular regions and the cheek mucosa are most frequently involved. Leukoplakia can be distinguished in four clinical forms: simplex, with a plane, homogeneous, sharply delimited lesion; speckled, with an irregular reddish-gray plaque; verrucosa, with an irregular, rough, warty surface; erosiva, with an erosive patch. Other diseases, such as candida infection and squamous cell carcinoma may be associated. Histopathology is characterized by hyperkeratotic or parakeratotic thickening of the horny layer, acanthosis, and chronic inflammatory infiltrate. The epithelial hyperplasia shows various degrees of dysplasia. The diagnosis is difficult on clinical examination. Incisional biopsy should be carried out and, for this, indurated red erosive or ulcerated areas should be selected rather than the more obvious whiter areas.

The differential diagnosis includes some congenital forms with different microscopic findings, such as white sponge nevus, dyskeratosis congenita (Zinsser-Engman-Cole), and dyskeratosis follicularis

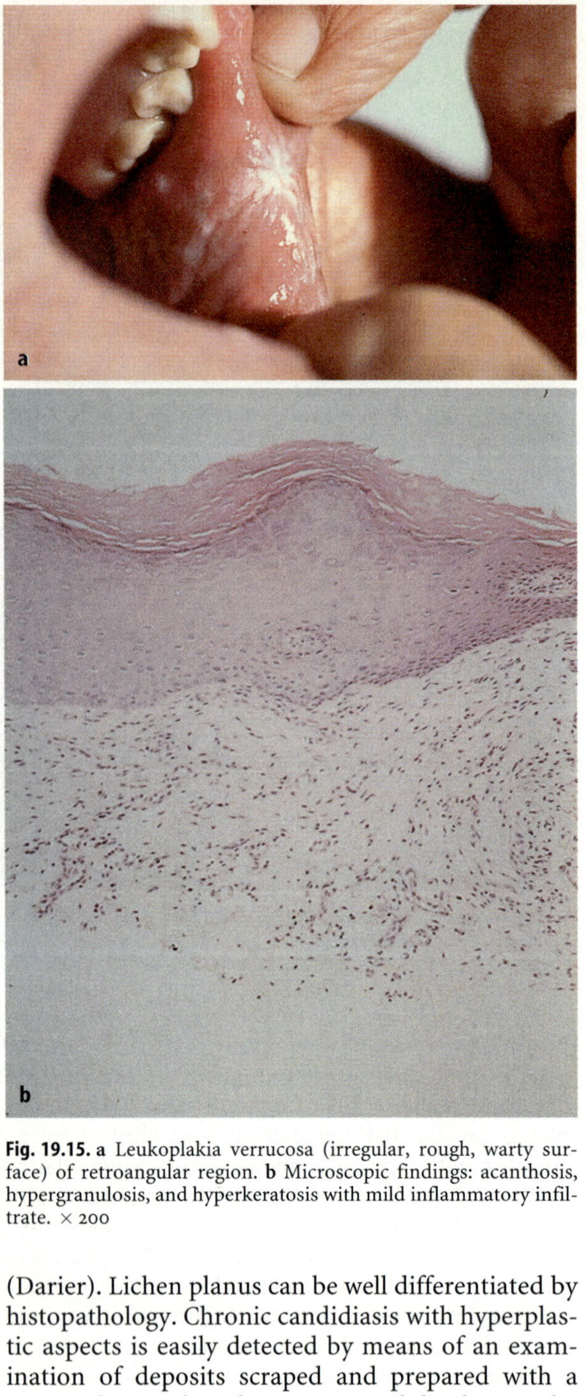

Fig. 19.15. a Leukoplakia verrucosa (irregular, rough, warty surface) of retroangular region. **b** Microscopic findings: acanthosis, hypergranulosis, and hyperkeratosis with mild inflammatory infiltrate. × 200

(Darier). Lichen planus can be well differentiated by histopathology. Chronic candidiasis with hyperplastic aspects is easily detected by means of an examination of deposits scraped and prepared with a KOH solution that shows up pseudohyphae, or by microscopic examination of a biopsy specimen. Hairy leukoplakia is characterized histologically by hair-like projections with parakeratosis.

Before treatment, any predisposing factors (sharp edges on teeth, alcohol consumption, smoking, or similar habits) must be reduced. Single, small lesions can be treated with topical tretinoin or topical bleomycin 0.5 %; systemic vitamin A derivatives can be used in larger and multiple manifestations. In the most severe cases, surgical excision or physical treatment with cryotherapy, electrocoagulation, or vaporization by CO_2 laser is necessary (Figs. 19.15–19.18).

19.2.3 Erythroplasia

Erythroplasia is a red, velvety lesion level with or depressed below the surrounding mucosa. It is far less common than leukoplakia in the mucosa of the oral cavity. Heavy alcohol consumption and tobacco smoking induce mucosal atrophy and may predispose to erythroplasia. Eryhtroplasia usually involves the floor of the mouth, the ventrum of the tongue, and the soft palate. It may appear as a velvety, reddish plaque, with or without patchy regions of leukoplakia, or as smooth, red areas with minimal or no leukoplakia.

In 90 % of cases an in situ or invasive carcinoma is demonstrable. Only 9 % of cases show moderate epithelial dysplasia with hypertrophy of the squamous cell layer, and lengthening and thickening of the rete ridges, often with superficial erosion. The acanthotic epidermis shows dysplastic changes. The dermis shows a pronounced stroma reaction with lymphocytes and plasma cells. The diagnosis, when suspected on the grounds of clinical examination, must be confirmed by histological examination. Differential diagnosis includes candidiasis, erosive lichen planus, and trauma. Incipient squamous cell carcinoma should be ruled out. Excision is the treatment of choice. Curettage and electrosurgery, cryosurgery, and 5-fluorouracil are also recommended.

19.2.4 Oral Submucous Fibrosis (Oral Deep Fibrosis)

Oral submucous fibrosis is a fibrosis of oral tissues with chronic course. It appears to be caused by exposure to constituents of areca nut. The fibrosis is reactive to the irritative stimulation caused by chewing areca nut with tobacco, betel leaf, and lime. Oral submucous fibrosis follows oral dysesthesia and vesicular stomatitis. It appears as symmetrical fibrosis of the cheeks, lips, or palate, developing in white, firm areas and causing restriction in opening of the mouth. Development of squamous cell carcinoma is possible in 2 % of cases over 10 years. Microscopic findings are characterized by subepithelial chronic inflammatory reaction, with fibrosis extending to the submucosa and muscle. Epithelial changes vary from atrophy to keratosis and there may be dysplasia. Anamnestic and clinical data allow the diagnosis. Surgery relieves the fibrosis. Jaw exercises and intralesional corticosteroids are useful.

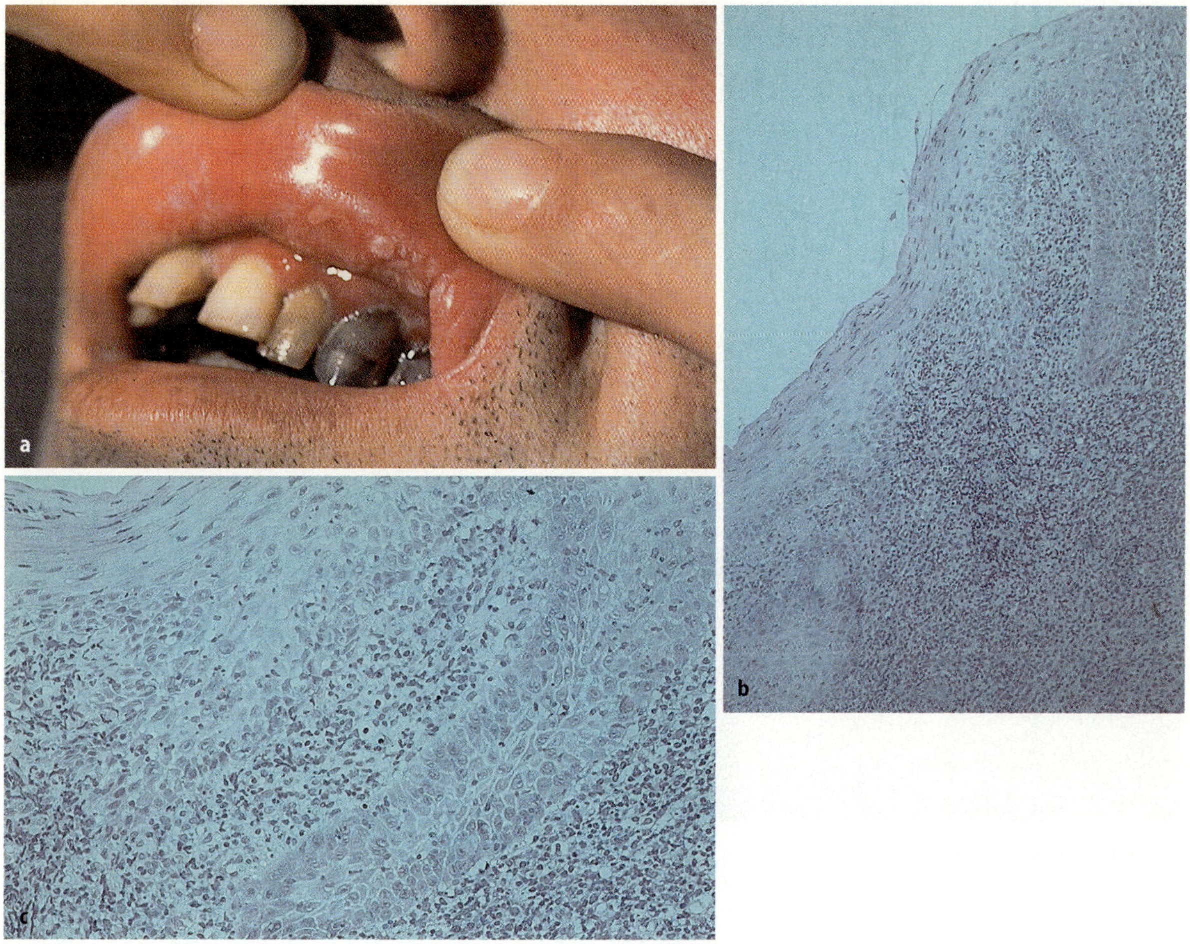

Fig. 19.16. **a** Leukoplakia of the upper lip mucosa, which has arisen from chronic irritation caused by a defective prosthesis. **b** Microscopic findings: parakeratotic thickening of the horny layer, acanthosis, and chronic inflammatory infiltrate. The epithelial hyperplasia shows various degrees of dysplasia. × 200. **c** Microscopic findings at a higher magnification: parakeratotic thickening of the horny layer, acanthosis, and chronic inflammatory infiltrate. The epithelial hyperplasia shows various degrees of dysplasia, × 400

19.2.5 Leukokeratosis Nicotina Palati (Stomatitis Nicotina – Smoker's Keratosis)

Leukokeratosis nicotina palati is a diffuse keratosis that develops in heavy smokers. The hyperplastic reaction of the epithelium of the palate to smoke is due to distillation products in the tobacco smoke, particularly in incompletely fermented tobaccos. Smoking cigarettes with the lit end held inside the mouth ("reverse" smoking) determines marked nicotina stomatitis, with an increased incidence of squamous cell carcinoma of the palate. Clinically, it appears as grayish-white, hard, flat papules 1–3 mm in diameter, isolated or clustered in a plastered appearance, located on the hard palate and occasionally spreading to the soft palate. Each papule is pointed with a red spot representing the opening of the inflamed palatal salivary gland. Typical microscopic findings are epithelial reactive hyperplasia with broadening of the rete ridges, accompanied by squamous metaplasia of the underlying ducts with a lymphocytic infiltrate. The diagnosis is supported by anamnestic and clinical findings. The treatment includes improved hygiene and discontinuation of smoking.

19.2.6 Erosive Lichen Planus

Erosive lichen planus is a clinical variant of lichen planus, characterized by bilateral white and erosive lesions involving the oral mucosa. Most cases of oral lichen planus are idiopathic, but the erosive and ulcerative forms are related to liver disease. Diabetes, hypertension, and immunodeficiency are also found in association with this condition. It com-

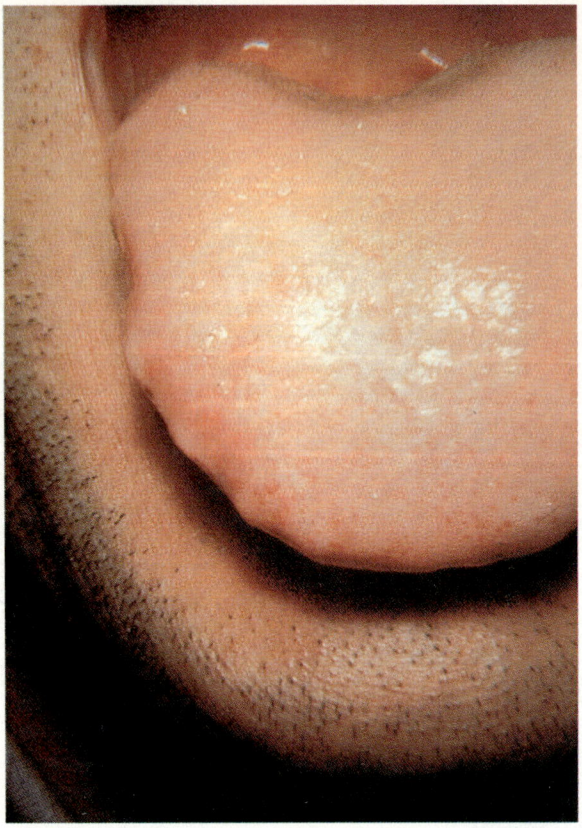

Fig. 19.17. Leukoplakia associated with macroglossia

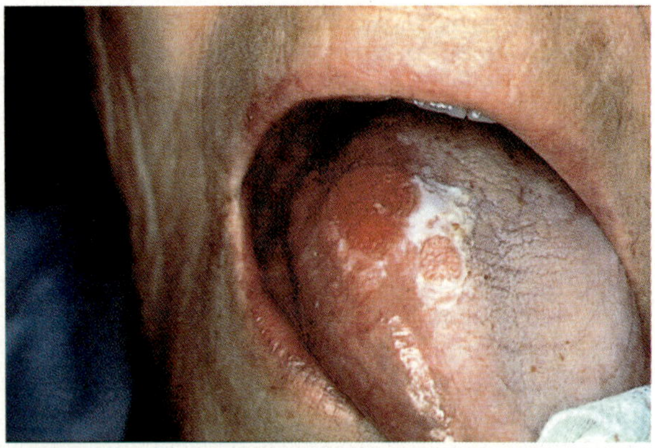

Fig. 19.18. Invasive squamous cell carcinoma, which has arisen on a patch of erythroleukoplakia of the tongue

monly appears as erosive or ulcerated areas, with irregular outline of buccal mucosa, lateral borders of the tongue, and, occasionally, gingiva. Typical reticular, papular, or plaque-like lesions of mucosal lichen planus are also present and can sometimes cause soreness. Microscopic examination reveals hyperkeratosis with or without parakeratosis. The

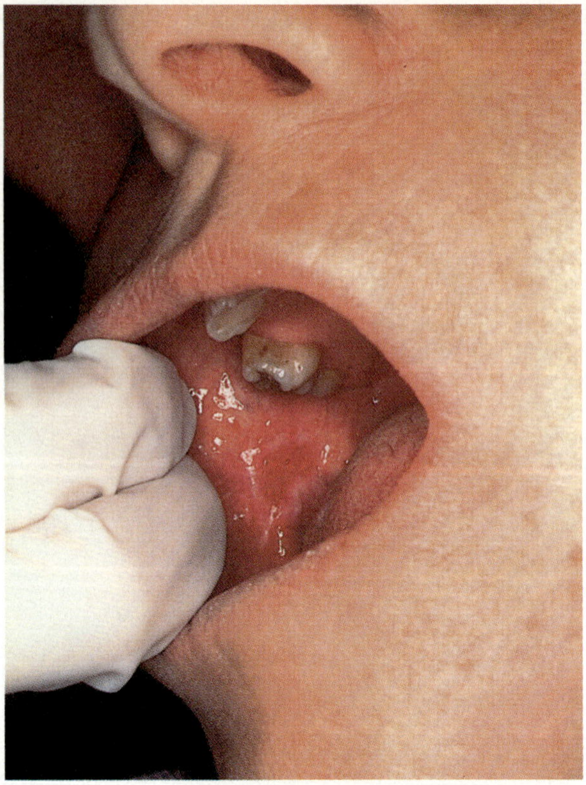

Fig. 19.19. Erosive lichen planus of the cheek mucosa: erosive lesion with irregular white border

epithelium may be atrophic and lack rete ridge formation, or acanthotic with the saw-toothed rete ridges. Individually keratinizing squamous cells (cytoid bodies) are found in the lower spinous cell layer. Degeneration of basal cells is characteristic. In the subjacent connective tissue, there is a band-like inflammatory infiltrate, sometimes obscuring the epithelial/connective tissue junction. It is made up of lymphocytes and some eosinophils and plasma cells. Erosive lesions develop either through the rupture of vesicles or as a result of necrosis of the epithelium. A clinical diagnosis must be supported by microscopic examination to exclude keratosis, lupus erythematosus, and malignancy. Treatment includes topical or intralesional corticosteroids. Topical retinoids and cyclosporin can be useful in the management of this chronic disease from which squamous cell carcinoma develops in less than 1% of cases (Figs. 19.19–19.21).

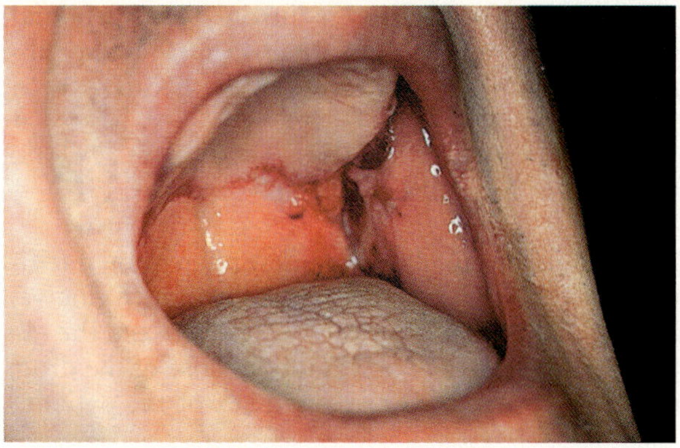

Fig. 19.20. Erosive lichen planus of buccal mucosa: multiple ulcerative lesions of cheek and palatal mucosa

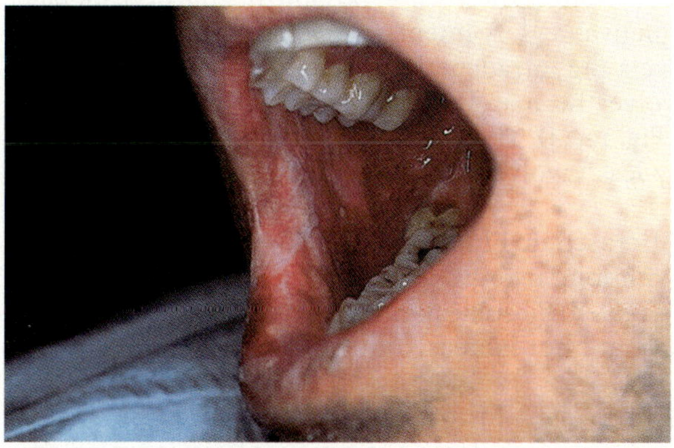

Fig. 19.21. Erosive lichen planus of the lower lip: the erosion is associated with the typical papular plaque-like lesions found in mucosal lichen planus

19.3 Benign Tumors of the Oral Mucosa, Muscle, Nervous System, Bone, and Cartilage

C. C. Zouboulis, P. G. Stavropoulos, and K. D. Wolff

19.3.1 Benign Tumors of the Oral Mucosa

19.3.1.1 *Epithelial Benign Tumors*

19.3.1.1.1 *Verrucous Hyperplasia*

Definition. Verrucous hyperplasia [19] is a precancerous lesion of the oral mucosa, which has some clinical and histological features in common with verrucous carcinoma. It is frequently associated with leukoplakia (54 %), verrucous carcinoma (31 %), and squamous cell carcinoma (8 %).

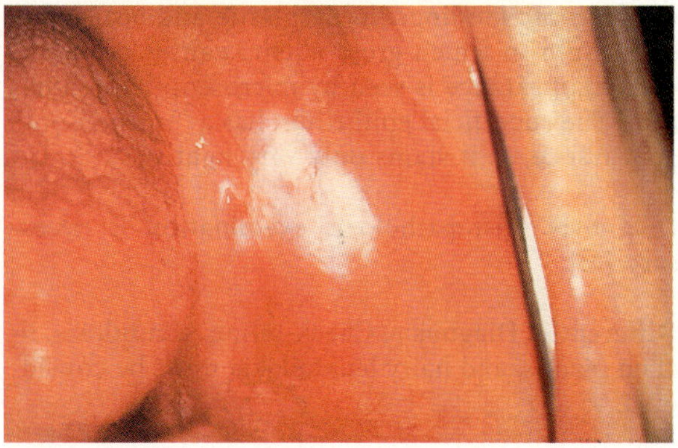

Fig. 19.22. Verrucous hyperplasia of the buccal mucosa

Etiology. Smoking and aging (patients older than 65 years) are the main causes.

Oral Manifestations. Two clinical types have been described: the "sharp" type, in which the verrucous process is narrow and white, and the "blunt" type, with the verrucous processes flat and broader. The lesions are located mostly in the gingiva and alveolar mucosa. The buccal mucosa and tongue can also be involved (Fig. 19.22).

Microscopic Findings. Histopathologic features are verrucous epithelial hyperplasia and, in nearly 60 % of cases, focal dysplasia confined to the suprabasal area.

Diagnosis. Histopathologic examination.

Differential diagnosis. Verrucous leukoplakia, verrucous carcinoma, squamous cell carcinoma.

Treatment. Surgical excision.

19.3.1.1.2 *White Sponge Nevus (Pachydermia Oralis, White Folded Gingivostomatitis)*

Definition. This is a rare familial disorder inherited as an autosomal dominant trait and having an excellent prognosis [20].

Etiology. Abnormal tonofilament aggregation.

Oral Manifestations. Painless, shaggy, folded white lesions typically affecting the buccal mucosa bilaterally. Other areas may also be involved, but rarely the gingival margins.

Microscopic Findings. Hyperplastic and acanthotic epithelium in which gross edema causes a basket-weave appearance is seen by microscopic examination. The superficial epithelium has a "washed-out" appearance, as it stains only very lightly.

Diagnosis. Histopathologic examination is necessary [21].

Differential Diagnosis. Cheek-biting, candidosis, lichen planus, and hairy leukoplakia must be considered.

Treatment. No treatment is required.

19.3.1.1.3
Papilloma

Definition. Papilloma is a cauliflower-like lesion with a whitish or pinkish color and may resemble a wart. It does not undergo malignant transformation [22].

Etiology. It is caused by human papillomaviruses (HPV).

Oral Manifestations. It can appear anywhere in the mouth (Fig. 19.23), but occurs most commonly at the junction of the hard and soft palate.

Microscopic Findings. Acanthotic and sometimes hyperkeratotic epithelium with occasional koilocytosis.

Diagnosis. Histopathologic examination is needed.

Differential Diagnosis. Fibroepithelial polyp (normal colored papilloma) must be excluded.

Treatment. Total excision is the only treatment and must be deep and wide enough to include any abnormal cells beyond the zone of the pedicle.

19.3.1.1.4
Drug-Induced Gingival Hyperplasia

Definition. Certain drugs, namely phenytoin, nifedipine, cyclosporin, and diltiazem, can induce gingival hyperplasia. There is no correlation between the extent of overgrowth [23–25] and the dose of the drug, its serum levels, or the age and sex of the patient.

Etiology. Presumably, the condition is an effect of the drug on fibroblast activity. The hyperplasia is aggravated by poor oral hygiene.

Oral Manifestations. A variable degree of firm, pale, gingival enlargement, which characteristically affects the intradental papillae first and may then involve the marginal and even the attached gingiva (Fig. 19.24). The lingual gingiva and palate are usually less involved.

Microscopic Findings. Marked epithelial thickening with long overgrowths into the connective tissue is revealed. Fibroblasts show increased mitotic activity but are not increased in number.

Diagnosis. A history of drug intake must be elicited, and histopathologic examination is also necessary.

Differential Diagnosis. Epulis, idiopathic gingival hyperplasia, and hypertrophic gingivitis (pregnancy) all need to be excluded.

Treatment. Improvement of oral hygiene is pivotal. It may be feasible for the physician to change the medication. Excision may be followed by recurrence.

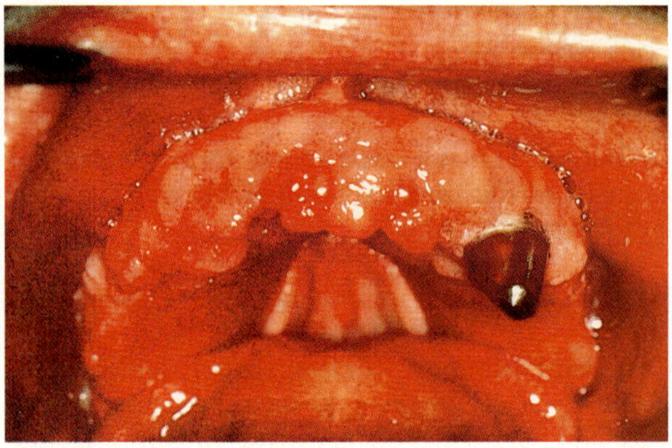

Fig. 19.23. Papilloma of the gingiva

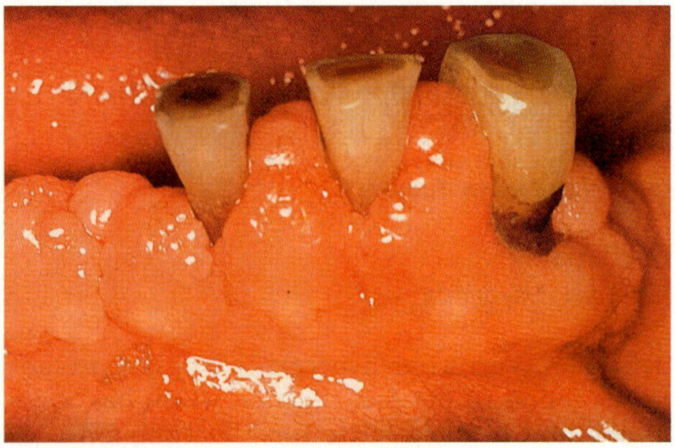

Fig. 19.24. Drug-induced gingival hyperplasia

19.3.1.1.5
Verruciform Xanthoma

Definition. This is an uncommon benign oral mucosal lesion and seems to have a predilection for women in the 5th and 7th decades of life. The size ranges between 0.2 and 2 cm. There is no association with hyperlipidemia [26, 27].

Etiology. It is not known how the lesion arises.

Oral Manifestations. It appears as a flat or slightly raised, well-circumscribed, papillary lesion, ranging in color from white to red and most frequently located on the alveolar ridge and the gingiva.

Microscopic Findings. There is symmetrical elongation of rete ridges, and numerous foam cells are present within the connective tissue papillae. Immunohistochemically, the lesion is characterized by the presence of Langerhans' cells [26].

Diagnosis. Histopathologic examination is necessary for the diagnosis.

Differential Diagnosis. Papilloma and oral verruca vulgaris must be excluded.

Treatment. Excision is the only treatment. Recurrences have not been reported.

19.3.2
Benign Tumors of the Epithelium-Lamina Propria Junction

19.3.2.1
Melanocytic Nevi of the Oral Mucosa

Definition. This lesion is defined as a collection of nevus cells in the epithelium or the lamina propria of the oral mucosa, or both. There are congenital and acquired melanocytic nevi. Acquired melanocytic nevi of the oral mucosa have their highest incidence in adults between 30 and 40 years of age (mean 35 years).

Etiology. These are developmental malformations from melanoblasts of the neural crest.

Oral Manifestations. Melanocytic nevi occur rarely in the oral cavity, in contrast to their common presence on the skin. Nevi of the oral mucosa are most frequently located in the hard palate (38 %; blue nevus 60 %) and the buccal mucosa (19 %). The majority of melanocytic nevi of the oral mucosa are pigmented (83 %). Clinically, they are asymptomatic, brown, brownish-black, or blue macules or papules (Fig. 19.25). The hard palate and the buccal mucosa can also be rare areas of involvement of the oculodermal melanocytosis of Ota, which mostly appears in mongoloid and female subjects (female-to-male ratio, 5 : 1).

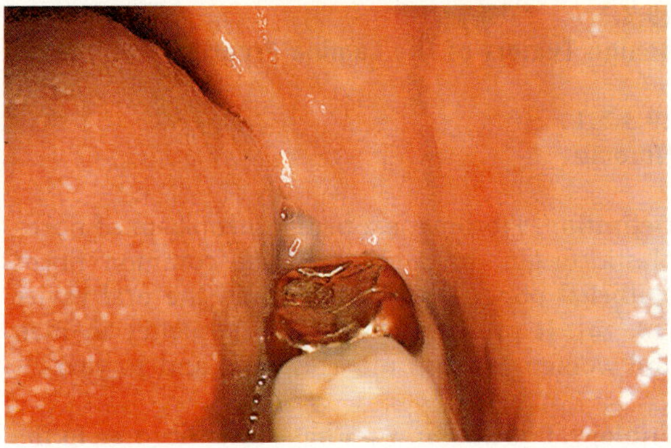

Fig. 19.25. Blue nevus of the oral mucosa located in the supramolar area

Microscopic Findings. Melanocytic nevi of the oral mucosa are classified into the following types, dependending on the location of nevus cells and the presence or absence of junctional activity: intramucosal nevus (nevus cells in the lamina propria, 55 %), junctional nevus (clusters of nevus cells at the epitheliomesenchymal junction, 2.8 %), compound nevus (rare), and blue nevus (spindle melanocytic cells in the lamina propria, 36 %). The nevus of Ota resembles blue nevus. Intramucosal and blue nevi can be S-100- and HMB-45-positive, in contrast to intradermal nevi. Therefore, these antibodies do not differentiate benign from malignant melanocytic lesions of the oral mucosa.

Diagnosis. Histopathologic examination is needed for diagnosis.

Differential Diagnosis. Amalgam tattoo, lentigo simplex/maligna, and malignant melanoma must be considered.

Treatment. With the exception of the rare junctional nevus (surgical excision), no treatment is required. Transformation of a mucosal nevus to melanoma is an extremely rare event (except in the case of junctional nevus).

19.3.3 Benign Tumors of the Lamina Propria

19.3.3.1 *Fibroma*

Definition. Fibroma is a benign neoplasm of fibroblastic origin. In contrast to the common fibroepithelial polyp, fibroma is rare in the oral cavity [28, 29]. It presents with equal frequency in men and women between the ages of 30 and 50 years.

Etiology. It is not known what causes fibroma in the oral cavity.

Oral Manifestations. Fibroma is an asymptomatic, continuously enlarging, single, firm, well-defined, sessile or pedunculated tumor with a smooth surface (Fig. 19.26). Its diameter usually ranges between 1 and 1.5 cm, and it appears on the gingiva, buccal mucosa, tongue, lips, and palate.

Microscopic Findings. Signs of marked proliferation of fibroblasts are seen. Cell nuclei are of uniform shape and size without any findings of atypia.

Diagnosis. Histopathologic examination is needed.

Differential Diagnosis. Fibroepithelial polyp, fibrous histiocytoma, neurofibroma, lipoma, myxoma, and pleomorphic adenoma must be excluded.

Treatment. Total, deep, and wide surgical excision is the only treatment.

19.3.3.2 *Pyogenic Granuloma*

Definition. Pyogenic granuloma is a common granulation tissue overgrowth [30, 31]. It occurs most frequently in persons between 10 and 40 years of age, and the female-to-male ratio is 2:1.

Etiology. Tissue reaction to mild irritation or trauma is known to cause this lesion.

Oral Manifestations. A pedunculated or sessile, reddish, painless, nodular, soft, exophytic mass (Figs. 19.27, 19.28). Its surface may be smooth or lobulated, or even ulcerated, and may be covered by a thin surface. The lesions grows rapidly, usually reaching a final size of 0.5–1 cm, and present a hemorrhagic tendency after irritation. The gingiva is the commonest site of involvement; tongue, lips, buccal mucosa, and palate can also be involved.

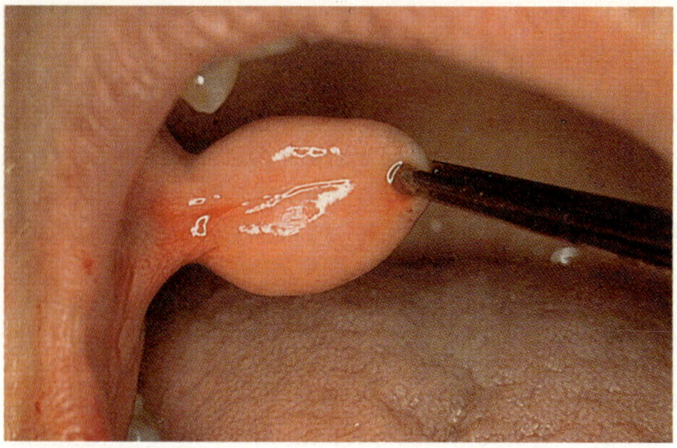

Fig. 19.26. Fibroma of the buccal mucosa

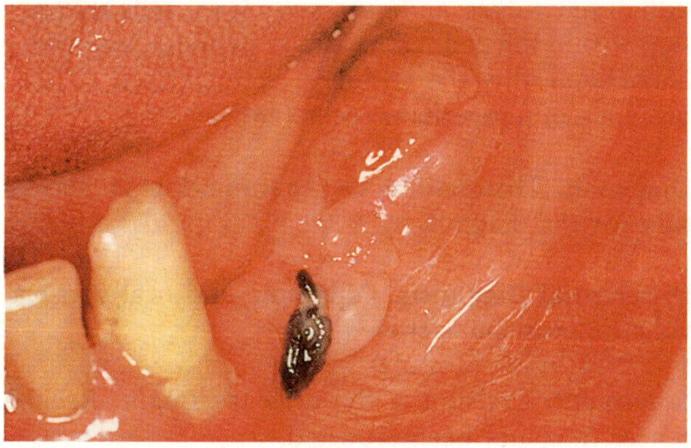

Fig. 19.27. Pyogenic granuloma of the oral mucosa

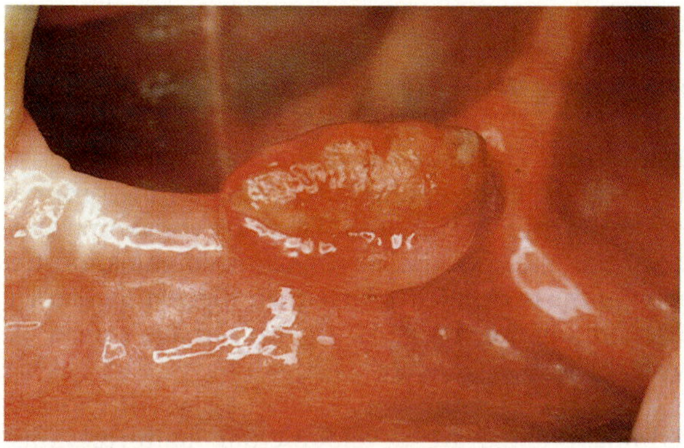

Fig. 19.28. Pyogenic granuloma of the oral mucosa

Microscopic Findings. There are signs of proliferating small blood vessels which erupt through a breach in the epithelium, to produce a globular pedunculated tumor. A thin layered epithelium forms a collarette at the base of the lesion and covers part, or all, of the tumor.

Diagnosis. Histopathologic examination is needed for diagnosis.

Differential Diagnosis. Epulis, hemangioma, leiomyoma, bacillary angiomatosis, Kaposi sarcoma, and metastatic tumors must be excluded.

Treatment. Surgical excision (classic, CO_2 laser, cryosurgery).

19.3.3.3
Epulis (Congenital Epulis, Granular Cell Myoblastoma, Giant-Cell Epulis, Peripheral Giant-Cell Granuloma, Fibroepithelial Polyp, Fibrous Epulis, Fibrous Lump, Epulis-Fissuratum, Denture-Induced Hyperplasia, Denture Granuloma)

Definition. An epulis is a granulation tissue overgrowth. Five types are mainly defined: congenital epulis, representing a rare benign swelling on the maxillary alveolus in infants (8:1 female predominance); giant-cell epulis, being a solitary tumor with characteristic clinical and histopathologic features (more common in males under 16 years of age; over 16 years; female:male ratio of 2:1); pregnancy epulis; fibroepithelial polyp; and epulis fissuratum, defined as a lesion caused by poorly fitting dentures.

Etiology. It represents a mesenchymal tissue reaction due to chronic irritation (except the fibroepithelial polyp, which also occurs after acute trauma). Chronic irritation or trauma trigger hyperplasia of mucoperiosteum and excessive production of granulation tissue. Occasionally, giant-cell epulis is a feature of hyperparathyroidism. Pregnancy epulis is assumed to be mediated by sex steroids and other products of the immune response.

Oral Manifestations. Congenital epulis is usually a pedunculated, firm, pink swelling, exclusively appearing on the alveolar ridges of the maxilla and mandible. Giant-cell epulis arises interdentally adjacent to permanent teeth that have had deciduous predecessors (Fig. 19.29). The size of the lesion ranges from 0.5 to 2 cm. Fresh lesions are deep red in color, hemorrhagic, and can ulcerate, becoming paler with time. Pregnancy epulis has the feature of a fresh giant-cell epulis, but tends to resolve at least partly on parturition. A fibroepithelial polyp is a solitary, red, shiny, and soft or pale, stippled, and firm nodule, depending on the acuity of inflammation (Figs. 19.30, 19.31). Initially, it grows rapidly, to stop at a maximum size of 2.5 cm. Epulis fissuratum resembles fibroepithelial polyp; it presents as single or multiple elongated fibroepithelial enlargements of the vestibular mucosa, with or without erosions among the single lesions (Fig. 19.32).

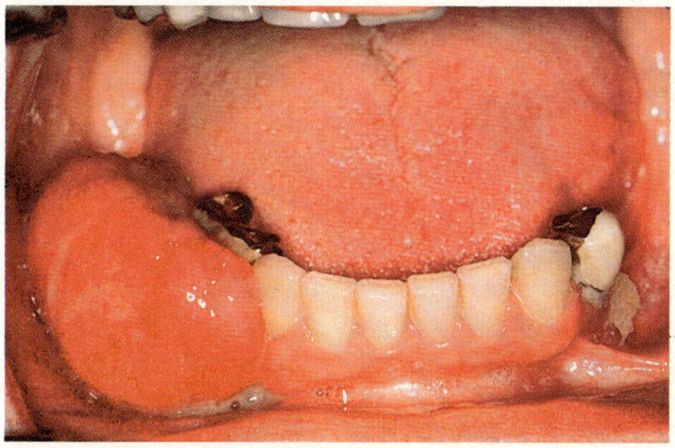

Fig. 19.29. Giant-cell epulis

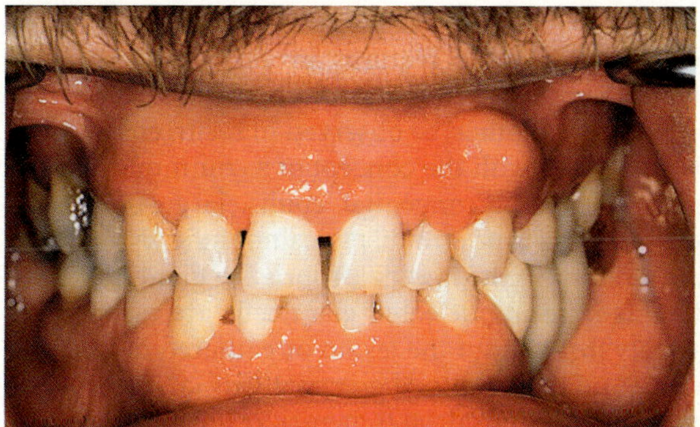

Fig. 19.30. Fibroepithelial polyp on the gingiva

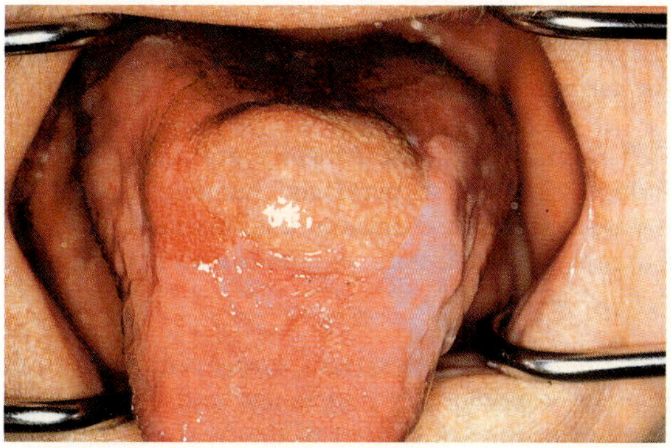

Fig. 19.31. Fibroepithelial polyp on the tongue

Microscopic Findings. Histologically, epulis resembles a pyogenic granuloma. It can be classified into giant-cell-, granulomatous- and fibromatous-type lesions. It represents self-limiting, reactive gingival overgrowth of granulation tissue, displaying com-

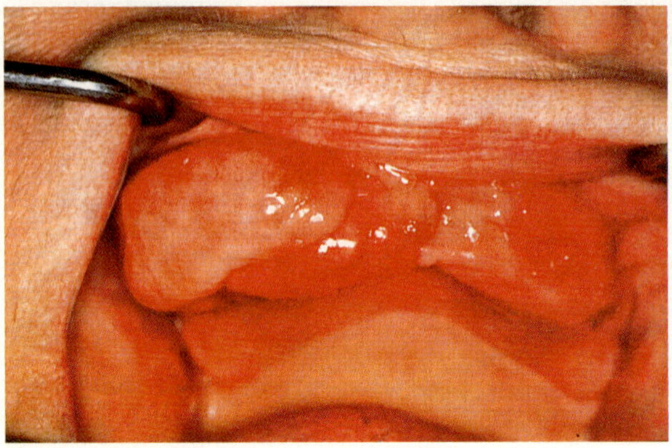

Fig. 19.32. Epulis fissuratum in a toothless patient who normally wears a denture

mon morphologic features in all three histologic types. The transition of a given histologic type of epulis into another, as observed in recurrent lesions, is consistent with the concept of a common histogenetic entity. In congenital epulis, large polygonal cells, with a fine granular eosinophilic cytoplasm, are present in the lamina propria. In giant-cell epulis, many multinucleated giant cells are distributed widely throughout the lesion or gathered in clumps. In pregnancy epulis, the immaturity of the vessels may lead to superficial ischemia, resulting in ulceration. In fibroepithelial polyp and epulis fissuratum, a well-keratinized, stratified epithelium overlies a connective tissue exhibiting thick collagenous bundles.

Diagnosis. Histopathologic examination is needed for diagnosis of epulis.

Differential Diagnosis. Pyogenic granuloma, drug-induced gingival hyperplasia, hemangioma, leiomyoma, fibroma, bacillary angiomatosis, Kaposi sarcoma, and metastatic tumors can all have similar appearances.

Treatment. Surgical excision, improvement of oral hygiene, especially in pregnancy, and appropriate denture fitting are all part of the treatment.

19.3.3.4
Myxoma

Definition. Myxoma is quite a rare benign tumor of the connective tissue. It appears in males more frequently than females and at any age. It is a slowly-growing, quiescent lesion that may suddenly enlarge.

Etiology. The etiology is unknown.

Oral Manifestations. A well-defined, mobile, soft tumor is located on the buccal mucosa, palate, or floor of the mouth.

Microscopic Findings. Myxoid degeneration of the connective tissue, resembling undifferentiated embryonal mesenchyme. Although benign, it has a tendency to infiltrate normal tissue [32].

Diagnosis. Histopathologic examination is needed for diagnosis of this lesion.

Differential Diagnosis. Lipoma, fibroma, focal mucinosis.

Treatment. Surgical excision with no reported recurrences

19.3.3.5
Hemangioma

Definition. Hemangioma is a common benign lesion of the oral cavity often present at birth.

Etiology. Hemangioma occurs due to overproliferation of blood vessels. It should not be considered as a true neoplasm but as an abnormality in development, which is strongly supported by its presence at birth.

Oral Manifestations. Hemangiomas are classified as capillary hemangiomas (red in color; Fig. 19.33) and

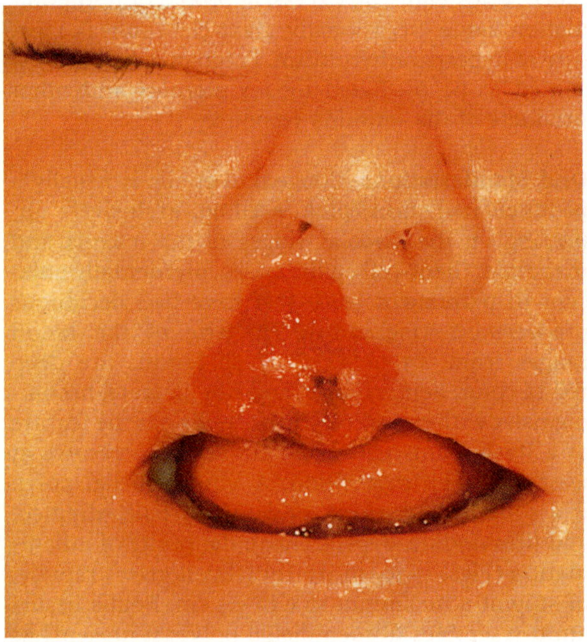

Fig. 19.33. Capillary hemangioma of the upper lip

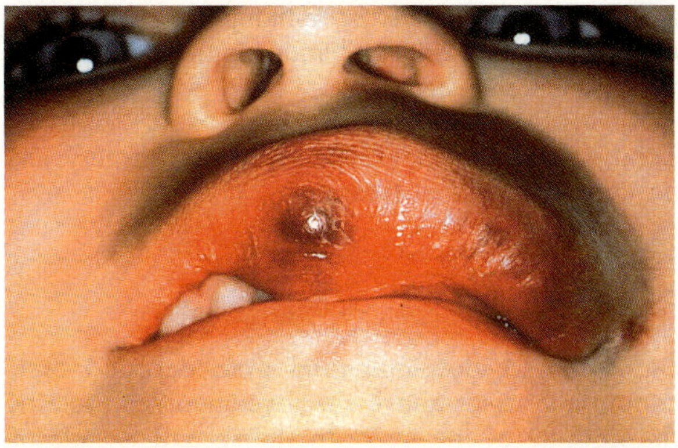

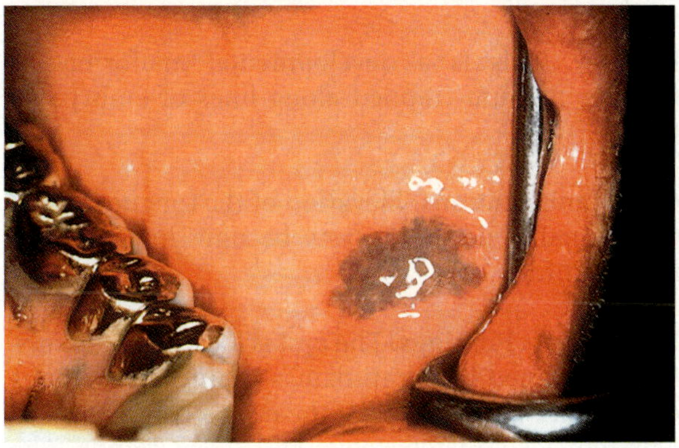

Fig. 19.34, 19.35. Cavernous hemangiomas of the upper lip (Fig. 19.34) and the buccal mucosa (Fig. 19.35)

cavernous hemangiomas (blue; Figs. 19.34, 19.35). They are located in the lip, tongue, and buccal mucosa. They range in size from millimetres to extensive lesions. Occasionally, they cause organ deformities (macroglossia, macrocheilia). On pressure, the red color characteristically disappears, returning when pressure is discontinued.

Microscopic Findings. Histology reveals two main types of hemangiomas: the capillary hemangioma, which consists of numerous small capillaries, and the cavernous type, whose main feature is the presence of large dilated sinuses filled with blood.

Diagnosis. Histopathologic examination allows the diagnosis.

Differential Diagnosis. Syndromes with oral vascular lesions (Sturge-Weber, Maffuci, Rendu-Osler-Weber, Klippel-Treauny-Weber), hemangioendothelioma, and Kaposi sarcoma must be excluded.

Treatment. Surgical excision, cryosurgery, and embolization or ligation of feeding vessels are effective. Some hemangiomas undergo spontaneous remission, especially in newborn children.

19.3.3.6
Lymphangioma

Definition. Lymphangioma is an uncommon tumor of the mouth, typically arising during the first years of life.

Etiology. Lymphangioma would probably be more correctly classified as hamartomatous malformation in most cases.

Oral Manifestations. Oral lymphangiomas are small, soft, slightly elevated, red-yellow nodules mimicking tiny cysts. They are located mostly on the tongue and sometimes on the lips, buccal mucosa, soft palate, and floor of the mouth (Fig. 19.36). Usually, they are asymptomatic, but as they enlarge in size, pain and discomfort may be felt during speaking, chewing, and swallowing. Recurrent infection and macroglossia cause considerable distress to the patient.

Microscopic Findings. Histology reveals dilated lymph channels of various sizes lined with normal lymphatic epithelium. These changes frequently extend into subcutaneous fat and even muscle.

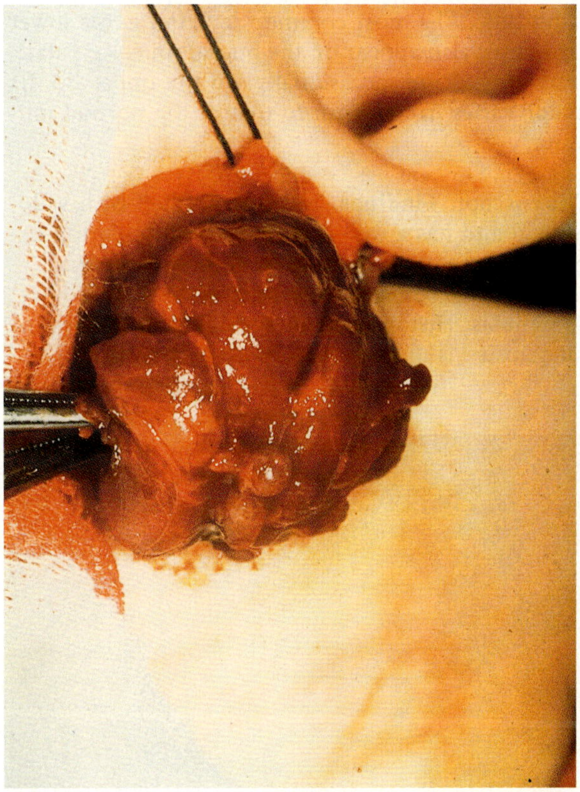

Fig. 19.36. Excision of a lymphangioma located on the floor of the mouth

Diagnosis. Histopathologic examination is needed for the diagnosis.

Differential Diagnosis. Hemangioma, epulis, lingual thyroid.

Treatment. Surgical excision is the only treatment.

19.3.3.7
Mucocele (Mucous Cyst)

Definition. Mucocele is the most common cyst of the oral soft tissue. It originates from minor salivary glands or their ducts. Two types are described: the more frequent extravasation mucocele (80 % of cases) and the rare retention mucocele. There is no sex predilection and it can occur at any age.

Etiology. Duct rupture from trauma due to biting seems to be the cause of extravasation mucocele. The pathogenesis of retention mucocele is related to partial obstruction of the duct due to infection or sialolithus.

Oral Manifestations. Examination of the mouth reveals a painless, spherical, single tumor, a few millimeters to some centimeters in size (Fig. 19.37). It appears suddenly, growing rapidly, and persisting for a long time. The most common location is the lower lip; it can also appear on the buccal mucosa, palate, and tongue and, occasionally, on the upper lip. Its color varies from bluish to that of the normal mucosa.

Microscopic Findings. The cyst is filled with sialomucin and has a wall composed of granulation tissue. Degeneration of connective tissue is found.

Diagnosis. Histopathologic examination allows the diagnosis [33].

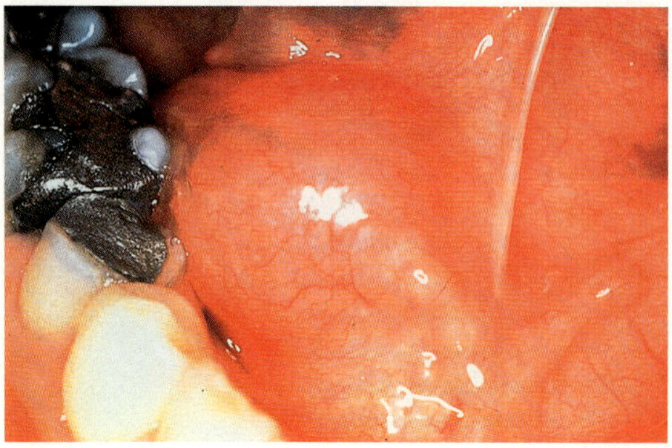

Fig. 19.37. Mucocele on the floor of the mouth

Differential Diagnosis. Lymphangioma, hemangioma, cystic neoplasm, and mucoepidermoid tumor must all be excluded.

Treatment. Surgical excision and cryosurgery are the only methods of treatment.

19.3.3.8
Dermoid Cyst

Definition. A developmental cyst, dermoid cyst, commonly arises above the myelohyoid muscle in the midline of the neck. In the second decade of life it becomes clinically obvious.

Etiology. This is a developmental malformation from epithelium trapped along lines of embryonic fusion [34].

Oral Manifestations. Elevation of the tongue is seen. Occasionally, dermoid cysts become infected and then painful.

Microscopic Findings. The cyst is located in the subcutis and lined by keratinizing, stratified squamous epithelium. In some cases, the cyst is complete with hair follicles and sebaceous and sweat glands. The lumen contains lipids, keratin, and hair.

Diagnosis. Histopathologic findings allow the diagnosis.

Differential Diagnosis. Thyroglossal cyst, ectopic thyroid gland, and intraoral abscess must be excluded.

Treatment. Surgical excision is the only treatment

19.3.3.9
Sebaceous Adenoma

Definition. Sebaceous adenoma is an extremely uncommon benign tumour of the oral mucosa [35].

Etiology. Sebaceous adenoma seems to originate from Fordyce's granules.

Oral Manifestations. The lesion appears as a yellowish, smooth or granular, single, firm, spherical mass (Fig. 19.38). Its diameter ranges between 0.5 and 1 cm.

Microscopic Findings. Sebaceous adenomas consist of hyperplastic blood vessels and sebaceous glands, with an increase in collagen synthesis.

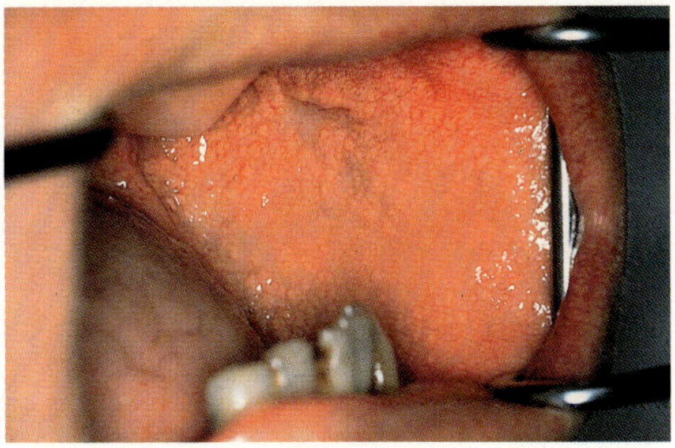

Fig. 19.38. Sebaceous hyperplasia (adenoma) caused by ectopic sebaceous glands in the oral mucosa

Diagnosis. Histopathologic examination is needed for diagnosis.

Differential Diagnosis. Verruciform xanthoma, lipoma, myxoma, and fibroma must be considered.

Treatment. Surgical excision is the only treatment.

19.3.3.10
Pleomorphic Adenoma

Definition. Pleomorphic adenoma is the commonest benign neoplasm of the major and minor salivary glands [36]. It represents 70 % of all tumors of the former and 60 % of tumors of the minor salivary glands. No sex predilection is reported, and the tumor occurs in subjects between 40 and 70 years of age.

Etiology. Major and minor salivary gland hyperplasia gives rise to this tumor.

Oral Manifestations. It is an asymptomatic, slow-growing, firm swelling, in most cases located in the parotid gland. Ulceration is uncommon, and the lesion is covered by normal epithelium (Fig. 19.39). Problems in chewing, speaking, and fitting a denture may arise in some patients.

Microscopic Findings. On histological examination, the major and minor salivary glands appear significantly hyperplastic.

Diagnosis. Histopathologic examination is needed for diagnosis.

Differential Diagnosis. Other salivary gland tumors and lipomas should be considered.

Treatment. Surgical excision is the only treatment.

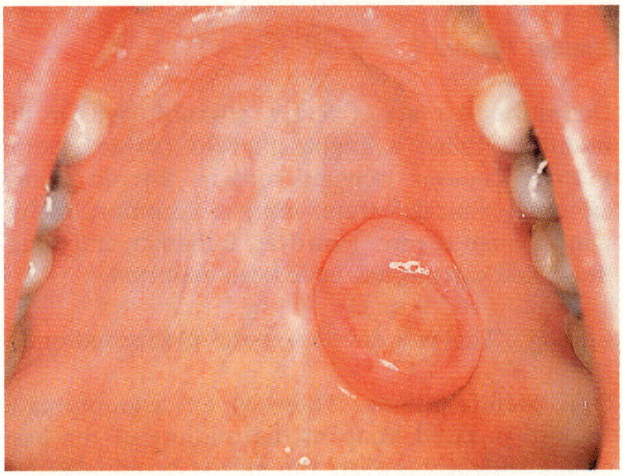

Fig. 19.39. Pleomorphic adenoma on the hard palate

19.3.3.11
Lingual Tonsil

Definition. Lingual tonsil is a mass of lymphoid tissue in the posterior third of the tongue.

Etiology. This is a developmental malformation.

Oral Manifestations. Lingual tonsil is localized between the epiglottis posteriorly and the cirumvallate papillae anteriorly. It is usually divided in the midline by a ligament. It may be small and asymptomatic, but in atopic patients, it may become enlarged. Sometimes, it is so prominent that it fills the vallecula and impinges on the epiglottis. A globus sensation, alteration of the voice, dyspnea, or obstructive sleep apnea may be caused. Lingual tonsilitis with a red, swollen, painful tongue, fever, and neutrophilia is not uncommon [37].

Microscopic Findings. Histopathologic examination reveals the ectopic lymphoid tissue.

Diagnosis. Histopathologic examination is necessary for the diagnosis.

Differential Diagnosis. Lingual thyroid and benign and malignant tumors of the tongue need to be excluded.

Treatment. Treatment may be required when the enlarged tonsil causes symptoms. Electrocautery and cryotherapy are regarded as quite safe procedures. Surgery can be hazardous because of the blood supply to the tongue base.

19.3.3.12
Lingual Thyroid

Definition. A mass of ectopic thyroid tissue in the mouth is called a lingual thyroid [38–40]. Some 10 % of cadaver tongues contain thyroid tissue, although clinical features are less common. Malignant change is rare. However, follicular and squamous cell carcinomas have been reported.

Etiology. This is a developmental malformation.

Oral Manifestations. There is an asymptomatic smooth-surfaced lump in the midline of the base of the tongue between the sulcus terminalis and the epiglottis, at the site of the foramen caecum. Occasionally, dysphagia, coughing, or pain may be present.

Microscopic Findings. Histopathologic examination reveals the ectopic thyroid tissue. Thyroid function should also be tested.

Diagnosis. Histopathologic examination is needed for the diagnosis.

Differential Diagnosis. Lingual tonsil and benign and malignant tumours of the tongue must all be excluded.

Treatment. Surgery is the basic treatment; thyroid hormone supplements should be administered when TSH levels are high.

19.3.3.13
Intraoral Abscess

Definition. An intraoral abscess is a localized collection of pus in the oral mucosa.

Etiology. Most intraoral abscesses are odontogenic in origin, as a final consequence of dental caries. Occasionally, they follow trauma or the presence of a foreign body, or are related to oral infections such as actinomycosis, nocardiosis, or botryomycosis.

Oral Manifestations. Firm, erythematous, painful nodules, occasionally associated with general illness and fever (Fig. 19.40). Abscesses may discharge into the mouth on the buccal gingiva. They can also discharge on the chin or in the submental region.

Treatment. Drainage and appropriate antimicrobial therapy must be instituted. Dental attention is helpful; dental abscesses are drained by tooth extraction, incision and drainage or through the root canal.

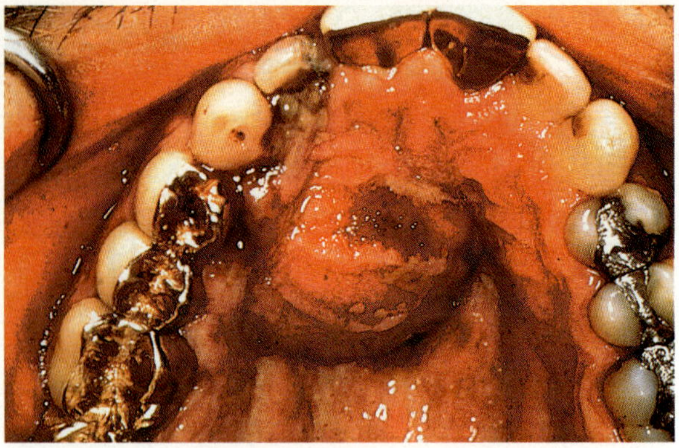

Fig. 19.40. Intraoral abscess

Suggested Further Reading

Lucker J. A case of lingual abscess. Br Dent J 1985; 159: 300–309

19.3.4
Benign Tumors of the Fatty Tissue

19.3.4.1
Lipoma

Definition. This benign neoplasm of the adipose tissue is relatively rare in the oral cavity [41]. While it appears in subjects of all ages, the average age at onset is 55 years, being somewhat higher in women than in men.

Oral Manifestations. It presents as an asymptomatic, sessile or pedunculated, slow-growing, solitary soft tissue tumor located mainly in the buccal mucosa, and then in the buccal sulcus, floor of the mouth, tongue, and lip (Fig. 19.41). It varies in adipose consistency and, depending on its localization, it can be yellowish in color. The covering epithelium is thin with visible blood vessels.

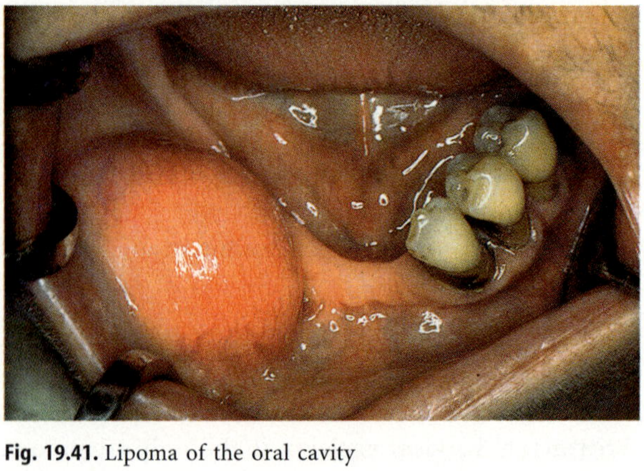

Fig. 19.41. Lipoma of the oral cavity

Microscopic Findings. The histological pattern varies according to the proportions of fibrous, vascular, and adipose elements present; thus, diagnoses vary: true lipoma, fibrolipoma, etc.

Diagnosis. Histopathologic examination is essential for the diagnosis.

Differential Diagnosis. Myxoma, fibroma, mucocele, and dermoid cyst must all be borne in mind.

Treatment. Surgical excision is the only treatment. The prognosis is excellent if the lesion is totally excised [38].

19.3.5 Benign Tumors of the Muscles

19.3.5.1 *Leiomyoma*

Definition. Leiomyoma is an uncommon benign tumor derived from smooth muscles [42]. Both sexes are equally affected during middle age.

Etiology. It derives from the smooth muscle of blood vessel wall and from the circumvallate papillae of the tongue.

Oral Manifestations. Leiomyoma is a slow-growing, usually painless, reddish, well-defined tumor. It is fairly soft and movable. It mainly occurs on the tongue, but also in the lower lip and palate (Fig. 19.42).

Microscopic Findings. There is smooth muscle cell proliferation, producing interweaving bundles of spindle-shaped cells, which are strongly eosinophilic.

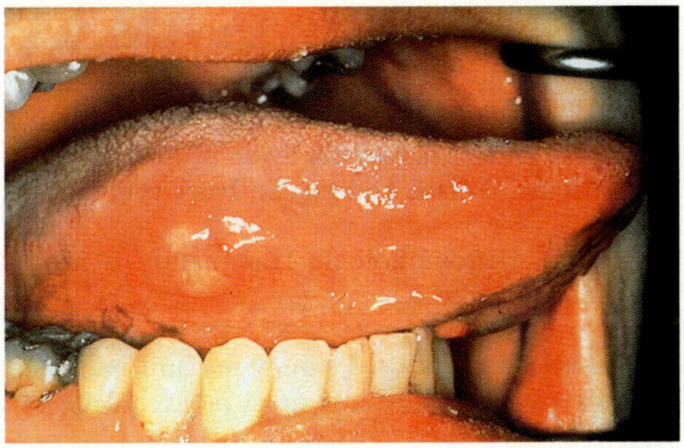

Fig. 19.42. Leiomyoma of the tongue

Diagnosis. Histopathologic examination is necessary for the diagnosis.

Differential Diagnosis. Glomus tumor must be excluded (when painful).

Treatment. Surgical excision is the only treatment.

19.3.5.2 *Rhabdomyoma*

Definition. Extracardiac rhabdomyomas [43] are subdivided into adult, fetal, and genital types. The adult type is seen mostly in men in the oral cavity, pharynx, and larynx. The age of patients is around 60 years, and the neoplastic nature of this rare tumor is doubtful.

Etiology. This is a hamartomatous malformation.

Oral Manifestations. Rhabdomyomas present in the oral cavity as lumps, especially on the floor of the mouth, tongue, and soft palate.

Microscopic Findings. Histologic examination reveals the presence of large cells with abundant, glycogen-rich cytoplasm. Cross-striations are variably developed.

Diagnosis. Histopathologic examination allows the diagnosis.

Treatment. Surgical excision is the only treatment.

19.3.6 Benign Tumors of the Nervous System

19.3.6.1 *Neuroma*

Definition. Spontaneous solitary neuroma has to be differentiated from the neuromas that are a symptom of the familial syndromes of multiple endocrine neoplasia (MEN) [44]. The latter present in at least three separate clinical patterns. The type 3 MEN syndrome is characterized by medullary carcinoma of the thyroid, and pheochromocytoma associated with multiple mucosal neuromas.

Etiology. Solitary neuroma usually occurs after trauma. Type 3 MEN syndrome has an autosomal dominant inheritance.

Oral Manifestations. Neuroma can occur on the buccal mucosa, gingivae, palate, and tongue.

Microscopic Findings. Histologic examination reveals classic findings of peripheral nerve tissue.

Diagnosis. Histopathologic examination is necessary for the diagnosis.

Differential Diagnosis. Neurofibroma and neurilemoma must be excluded.

Treatment. Surgical excision is the only treatment.

19.3.6.2
Neurilemoma (Schwannoma, Neurinoma)

Definition. This is a tumour of nerve sheaths, composed of cells resembling Schwann cells.

Etiology. It presents mostly as a symptom of neurofibromatosis generalisata (von Reckinghausen's disease).

Oral Manifestations. The tumor is a rounded or ovoid, circumscribed nodule varying size up to 5 cm. It usually occurs on the tongue, but other mucosal areas can be involved (Fig. 19.43).

Microscopic Findings. Histologic examination reveals a rounded, circumscribed, and usually encapsulated tumor of spindle-shaped cells, enclosed by a stringy meshwork of argyrophilic intercellular fibrils. Electron microscopy shows evidence of association with Schwann cells.

Differential Diagnosis. Neuroma (type 3 MEN syndrome) and neurofibroma must be excluded.

Diagnosis. Histological examination is necessary for the diagnosis.

Treatment. Surgical excision is the only treatment.

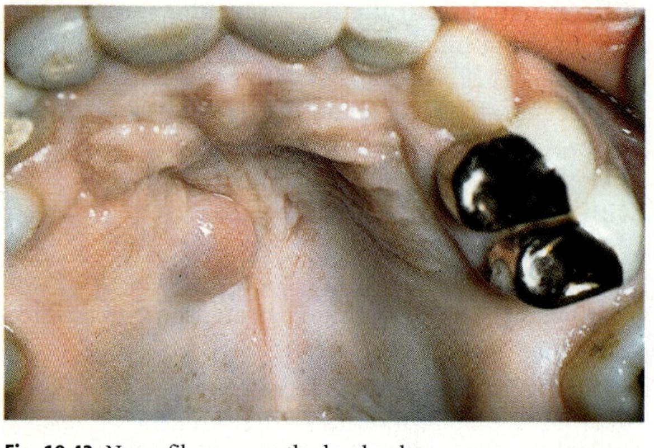

Fig. 19.43. Neurofibroma on the hard palate

19.3.6.3
Neurofibroma

Definition. This solitary tumor is considered to be a manifestation of abortive neurofibromatosis or, in the case of multiple lesions, a symptom of neurofibromatosis generalisata.

Etiology. Its etiology is unknown.

Oral Manifestations. Solitary, slowly-growing gray-white, rounded nodule varying in size.

Microscopic Findings. Histologic examination reveals a rounded, but not encapsulated, tumor composed of spindle-shaped cells with characteristically wavy nuclei. Cholinesterase is present and S-100 and neuron-specific enolase antibodies are positive.

Differential Diagnosis. Neuroma and neurilemoma must be excluded.

Diagnosis. Histological examination is necessary for the diagnosis.

Treatment. Surgical excision is the only treatment.

19.3.6.4
Granular Cell Myoblastoma (Abrikosoff's Tumor, Granular Cell Tumor)

Definition. This tumor is composed of cells with a characteristic granular cytoplasm.

Etiology. The etiology is unknown.

Oral Manifestations. The solitary tumor is flesh-colored to pink or grayish-brown and is situated beneath the epithelium of the tongue. It is firm and rounded but with rather indefinite margins and can be sessile or pedunculated; it is between 5 and 20 mm in size.

Microscopic Findings. Histologic examination reveals large polyhedral cells arranged in sheets, which infiltrate the dermal connective tissue and subcutaneous fat. The cells contain S-100 protein and neuron-specific enolase and myelin basic protein.

Diagnosis. Histopathologic examination is needed for the diagnosis.

Differential Diagnosis. Leiomyoma and malignant granular cell myoblastoma must be excluded.

Treatment. Surgical excision is the only treatment.

19.3.7
Benign Tumors of the Jawbones and the Cartilage

19.3.7.1
Benign Odontogenic Tumors

19.3.7.1.1
Ameloblastoma (Adamantoma, Multicystic Jaw Tumor, Epithelioma Adamantinum, Epithelial Odontoma, Odontogenic Epithelioma, Epithelioma Ameloblastoides, Basiloma)

Definition. Ameloblastoma is a unilocular, aggressively infiltrating tumor. Although it is basically not age-dependent, half of all cases are found in patients in the 3rd and 4th decades of life. Very rare cases of metastasizing ameloblastomas have been reported. Since these metastases have never been detected before treatment of the primary, but occurred only after tumor removal, it must be assumed that their spread is the result of aspiration in the lungs with subsequent lung metastasis. Generally, there is a marked tendency to tumor recurrence, so that long-term clinical follow-up is necessary.

Etiology. This tumor is a benign chondroma.

Pathogenesis. The tumor develops from the remains of the dental lamina or from the enamel organ itself, but also possibly from the Malassez rest. In rare cases, ameloblastoma can develop from follicular cysts.

Oral Manifestations. Ameloblastoma is most frequently localized in the mandible, especially the horizontal branch in the lateral dental region (Fig. 19.44 a). Macroscopically, the tumor appears grayish-white and predominantly solid, though also partly cystic. With the exception of swelling, an ameloblastoma rarely causes symptoms. Occasionally, pain and inflammation are observed in connection with cystic changes. In rare cases, there are surface ulcerations or loosening of the teeth in the tumor region. With severe broaching of the bone in the maxilla, nasal breathing impairment and nasal bleeding may occur.

Radiological Findings. There is mainly multilocular, cystic translucence varying in size, which can be designated as a soap bubble or honeycomb configuration. Unilocular cysts occur more frequently in the maxilla and more rarely in the mandible (Fig. 19.44 b). In adjacent teeth, especially the wisdom tooth, there are absorption signs at the root apex. If the tumor encloses an impacted tooth, it gives the impression of a follicular cyst.

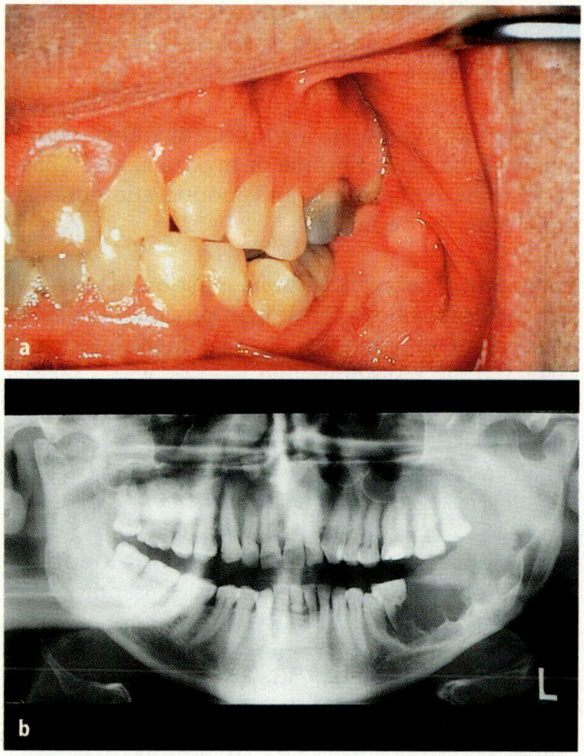

Fig. 19.44. **a** Ameloblastoma at the horizontal branch of the left mandible in the lateral dental region, and **b** its radiological appearance

Microscopic Findings. The terms ameloblastoma and adamantinoma are misnomers insofar as there is basically no amelogenesis, but rather histologically cylindrical cells are found, which only look like ameloblastomas. Four types are differentiated, according to the arrangement of the epithelial components: follicular, plexiform, acanthoid, and granular cell types of ameloblastoma. In the follicular type, there are round or elongated depositions of epithelial cell nests, which are not interconnected, while in plexiform ameloblastoma, these epithelial sections are interconnected and often pass through the tumor in long strands. In acanthoid ameloblastoma, squamous epithelium metastases develop in the interior of the epithelial island. In ameloblastoma containing granular cells, there are large round cells with PAS-positive and acidophilic granules in place of the reticular component in the interior of the epithelial island.

Diagnosis. The diagnosis can only be made histologically, and even then it is particularly dependent on assessment of the connective tissue component, since the ameloblastoma is considered to be an epithelial odontogenic tumor without any inductive effect on the surrounding stroma. Despite the amount of radiological signs, the diagnosis of an ameloblastoma cannot be established by radiological examination alone.

Differential Diagnosis. Giant cell reparative granuloma, odontogenic fibroma or myxoma, ameloblastic fibroma or myxoma, and monocystic bone tumors must be excluded.

Treatment. The involved bone must be resected far into the healthy bone. Treatment procedures such as enucleation or curettage involve high recurrence rates and are not admissible.

19.3.7.1.2
Odontogenic Myxoma
(Odontogenic Mixofibroma, Soft Odontoma)

Definition. The odontogenic myxoma is a rare benign tumor of the facial skeleton. It is not sealed off and can infiltrate the soft tissue without clear delineation. Malignant degeneration of a myxoma in the jaw has not yet been observed. It occurs primarily in patients in the 2nd and 3rd decades of life, rarely in children under the age of 10 years. There is no gender specificity.

Etiology. Since the tumor is found exclusively in the jaws, an odontogenic origin is probable.

Pathogenesis. It is suspected that the odontogenic myxoma develops from the connective tissue of the dental papilla.

Oral Manifestations. The tumor is found more frequently in the mandible than in the maxilla (Fig. 19.45a). Myxoma primarily causes painless swelling, which in extreme cases can lead to distortion of the face. Sensitivity disorders of the lower lip can occur when the mandible is involved. If it is localized in the maxilla, the entire maxillary sinus can be affected by the tumor, resulting in sensitivity disorders in the infraorbital nerve. Tilting and loosening of teeth have been observed with larger tumors.

Radiological Findings. There is rare but predominantly multiloculate osteolysis, with sharp differentiation from the healthy bone (Fig. 19.45b). Root absorption is seen in individual cases.

Microscopic Findings. There is grayish-white soft tissue, from which mucus can be swabbed off. The sections with predominantly collagen fibers are adjacent to those containing mucus. The tumor is poor in cells. Typical are round and stellar cells interconnected by cell branches. Mitoses are rarely seen. The term myxofibroma is derived from the histological finding of collagen-rich sections in which fibroblasts have settled. The rest of the odontogenic epithelium, which are confirmatory for the histological diagnosis, are rarely found.

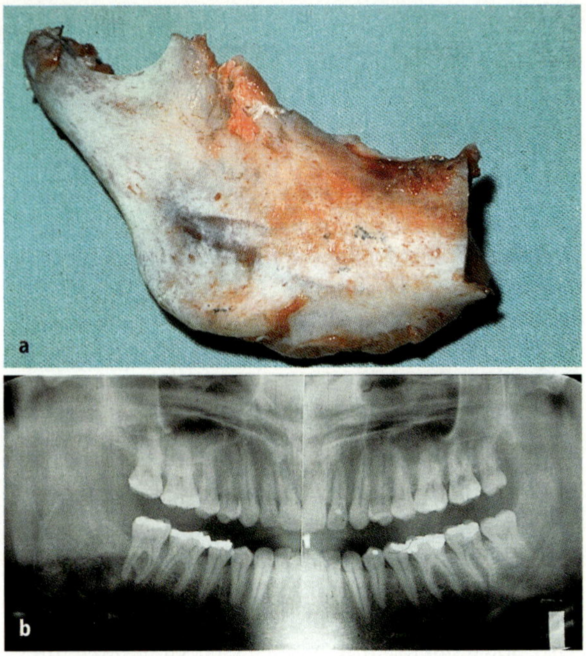

Fig. 19.45. **a** Surgical preparation of an odontogenic myxoma in the right mandible and **b** its radiological appearance

Diagnosis. Histopathologic examination is needed for the diagnoses.

Differential Diagnosis. Chondromyxofibromas, cysts, ameloblastoma, giant cell reparative granuloma, fibrous dysplasia, and aneurysmal bone cysts must be considered.

Treatment. Since myxofibroma has a high recurrence tendency and locally invasive growth, surgical removal with resection limits into healthy tissue are necessary. A recurrence rate of up to 25 % has been reported after curettage

19.3.7.1.3
Cementoma (Benign Cementoblastoma, Gigantiform Cementoma, Periapical Cement Dysplasia, Cementifying Fibroma)

Definition. Cementoma is a mesenchymal odontogenic tumor, which is mainly detected by chance on X-rays, as an opaque tumor surrounding the root apex of a tooth. Periapical cement dysplasia which develops reactively must be differentiated from cementomas. Cementoma occurs more frequently in men than in women, with a peak incidence in the 3rd decade of life.

Etiology. Since the tumor primarily spreads into the cement substance of the root, it is assumed that it originates from the cement of the tooth. However, cementoblastoma may be a variation of osteoblastoma, since uncalcified cementum in the tumor periphery has been described, which differs from osteoid only in the density of embedded cells.

Oral Manifestations. The typical localization is the molar or premolar region of the mandible. As an initial symptom, pain or asymmetry of the bones with increased size may lead to the diagnosis of cementoma. Swelling increases only slowly, but can reach a diameter of several centimeters. The tumor can push the roots apart, causing tilting of the teeth. However, the teeth remain vital in most cases.

Radiological Findings. The cementoma is characteristically seen on the X-ray as surrounding the apex of a molar or premolar root (Fig. 19.46). While the central tumor component is opaque, the periphery is radiolucent, so that the tumor can be differentiated from the surrounding bone. Despite the benign character of the tumor, absorption signs can be seen at the root.

Microscopic Findings. Extensive areas of calcified, very cell-poor, or even cell-free, ground substance are seen. There is cell- and vessel-rich stroma between the cement depositions or in the tumor periphery. The tumor usually spreads directly into the cement substance of the root and can also grow into the cavity of the tooth.

Diagnosis. Although the diagnosis can only be definitively made by histological examination, the typical localization of the tumor at the root apex facilitates the radiological diagnosis.

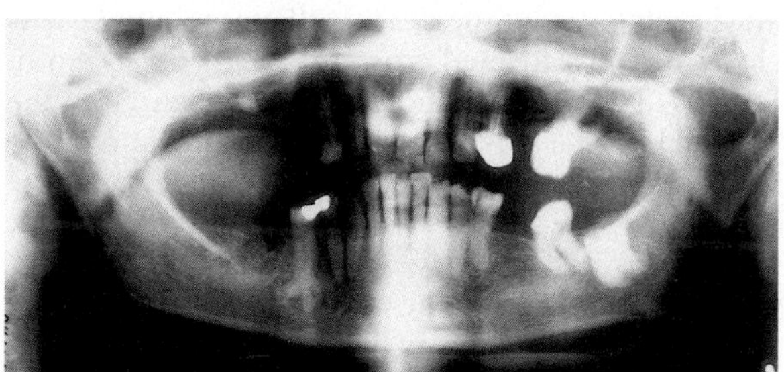

Fig. 19.46. Cementoma at the left manibular region

Differential Diagnosis. Osteoblastoma, osteoid osteoma, and osteosarcoma must be excluded.

Treatment. Enucleation of the tumor is the only treatment with or without extraction of the involved tooth. The affected tooth cannot be preserved if the tumor infiltrates the tooth cavity. Recurrences have not be reported.

19.3.7.1.4
Odontogenic Keratocyst (Primordial Cyst, Epidermoid Cyst of the Jaw, Cholesteatoma of the Jaw)

Definition. This is mostly a single, and occasionally a multichamber, cyst which is marked by a strong recurrence tendency. In rare cases, carcinoma can develop from an odontogenic keratocyst.

Etiology. This tumor originates in the undifferentiated cells of the dental lamina. The disease peaks in the 4th decade of life; men are more often affected than women. In a special form of Gorlin-Goltz syndrome, there is an accumulation of odontogenic keratocysts combined with multiple basaliomas.

Oral Manifestations. It is seen twice as often in the mandible as in the maxilla and is found predominantly in the region of the wisdom tooth of the mandible and in the canine region (Figs. 19.47, 19.48). Usually, keratocysts do not cause any pain, so that, despite swelling and rare fistulas in the oral cavity, no symptoms can be recognized. Occasionally, there is loosening, tilting, or displacement of the teeth. A yellowish, partly fetid, thin secretion flows out when the cyst lumen is opened.

Radiological Findings. On the X-ray image, mono- as well as multicystic keratocysts can be seen. They are sharply delineated and are frequently found in connection with an impacted tooth, mainly a wisdom tooth (Figs. 19.49, 19.50). Absorption at the root is possible.

Microscopic Findings. The odontogenic keratocyst is marked by a thin cyst wall, which is composed of 4–10 cell layers. One characteristic is that the basal cell layer is partly made up of cylindrical cells, which look like ameloblasts. Cellular atypias and mitoses are rare; there are horn rests in the cyst lumen.

Diagnosis. Histolopathological examination is needed for the diagnosis.

Differential Diagnosis. Ameloblastoma, odotogenic myxofibroma, and follicular cyst must be consid-

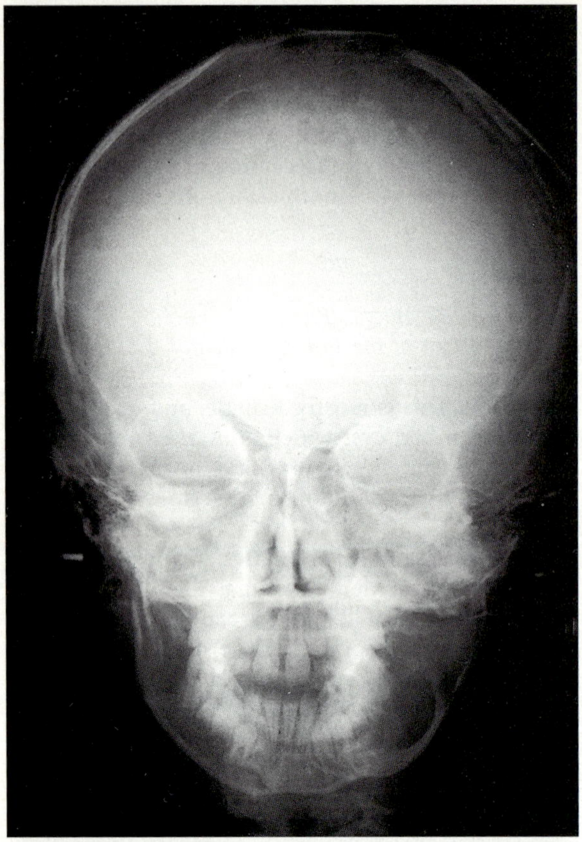

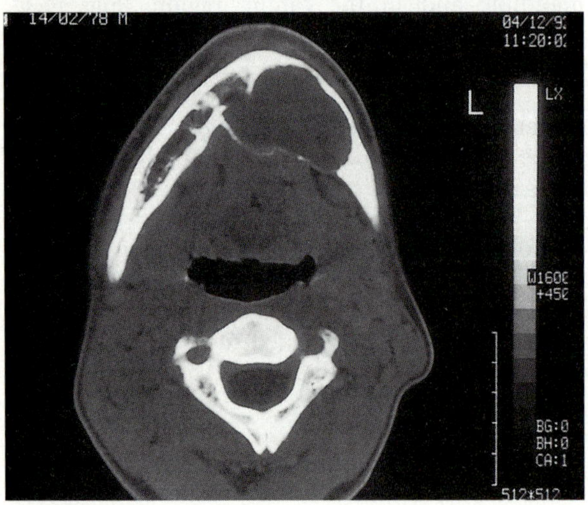

Fig. 19.47, 19.48. Odontogenic keratocyst on the left maxilla (Fig. 19.47) and the left mandible (Fig. 19.48)

ered, the last especially in combination with an impacted tooth.

Treatment. Treatment consists in complete removal of the cyst wall, which can also be performed after pretreatment with Karnoy's solution. Owing to the

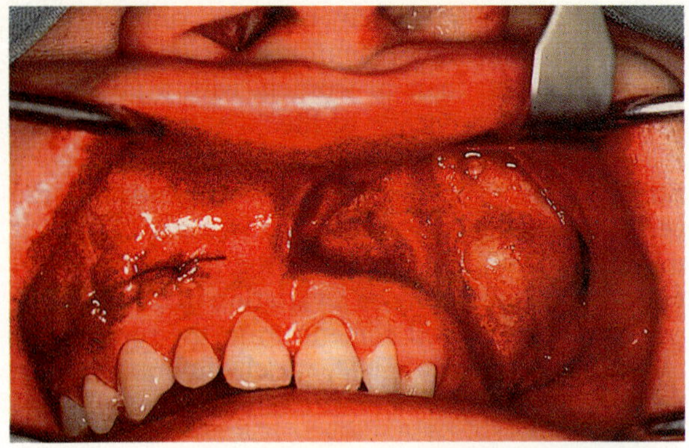

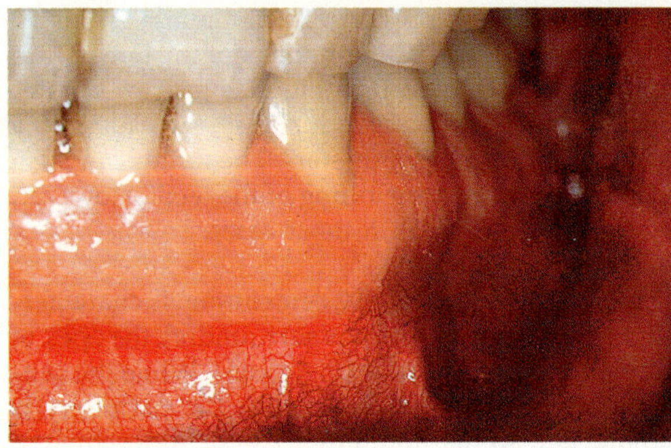

Fig. 19.49, 19.50. Odontogenic keratocyst (*arrows*) in the left facial area shown on X-ray (Fig. 19.49) and CT (Fig. 19.50)

high recurrence rate, close follow-up is needed in addition to careful removal of all cyst components.

19.3.7.1.5
Follicular Cyst (Coronary Cyst, Dentigenous Cyst)

Definition. This is a common benign odontogenic tumor, which in rare cases can be the origin of odontogenic tumors, carcinomas, and mucoepidermoid tumors. It occurs particularly often in the 3rd to 5th decades of life, with the same frequency in men and women.

Etiology. The follicular cyst develops from the enamel membrane of the dental follicle and mostly encloses the fully formed crown of an impacted tooth. In 75 % of cases, the follicular cyst is localized in the mandible, especially at the wisdom tooth, and in the remaining 25 %, in the maxillary wisdom and canine regions.

Oral Manifestations. The follicular cyst is primarily identified radiologically in the context of general dental check-ups, or after infection of the cyst lumen if there is a connection with the oral cavity. It can cause painless swelling by displacing the thinned bone wall.

Radiological Findings. The follicular cyst is seen on X-ray as a sharply delineated unilocular osteolysis infiltrating the crown of a tooth (Fig 19.51). It can be differentiated from a normal dental follicle by determining the distance seen on the X-ray between the cyst wall and the crown. If the distance is greater than 2.5 mm, it is a follicular cyst.

Microscopic Findings. The macroscopically hard, grayish-white tumor is histologically recognized by a thin epithelial layer of monomorphic cells of the same size. There are no rete ridges. Under the epithelial layer, loose connective tissue without any inflammatory signs is seen, in which there are occasional small odontogenic epithelial rests. In the case of infection, the epithelium is thickened and looks like that of a radicular cyst.

Diagnosis. Histopathological examination is needed for the diagnosis.

Differential Diagnosis. Odontogenic keratocyst and radicular cyst must be considered.

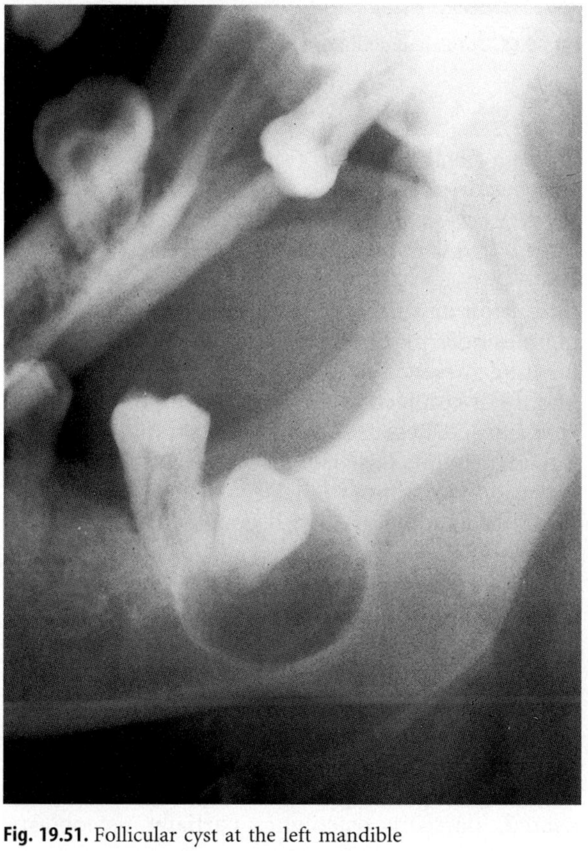

Fig. 19.51. Follicular cyst at the left mandible

Therapy. Cystectomy with removal of the impacted tooth; it is rarely possible to preserve the impacted tooth. In the cases of a large cyst, the defect can be filled with autologous spongiosa to accelerate bone healing or to prevent a spontaneous bone fracture. The follicle must be thoroughly removed, since odontogenic tumors can develop from odontothecal rests.

19.3.7.1.6
Radicular Cyst (Periapical Cyst, Apical Periodontal Cyst)

Definition and Etiology. This is a very frequent, benign cystic process, which develops from the roots of devitalized teeth. Radicular cyst occurs at any age and without any gender prevalence.

Oral Manifestations. Radicular cyst can develop under any devitalized teeth, but the root apices of the front teeth are especially affected. It is incidentally discovered on routine X-ray examinations. Clinical symptoms such as swelling or pain only occur when the cyst has reached a certain size or if the cyst lumen is superinfected. In cases of extensive spreading of the cyst, there is displacement or loosening of the teeth.

Radiological Findings. The radicular cyst is seen as an osteolytic change of more than 5 cm in diameter at the root apex of a devitalized tooth (Figs. 19.52, 19.53). Early forms are described as apical granulomas. The sharply delineated unilocular cyst lumen is mostly surrounded by a sclerotic halo. Occasionally, there is slight absorption of the root apex of the involved tooth.

Microscopic Findings. The cystic cavity is coated with uni- or multilayered, nonkeratinized squamous epithelium. In the loose connective tissue of the cyst wall, inflammatory cells may be present, which secondarily destroy the epithelium. There are sections of flagellated epithelial cells as well as beaker cells. The cyst cavity is filled with a cholesterol-containing liquid.

Diagnosis. Histopathological examination in connection with the relatively typical X-ray picture allows the diagnosis.

Differential Diagnosis. Odontogenic keratocyst and follicular cyst must be excluded.

Therapy. Removal of the causative devitalized tooth and cystectomy are necessary. With very large cysts, the cyst lumen must be kept open (cystostomy).

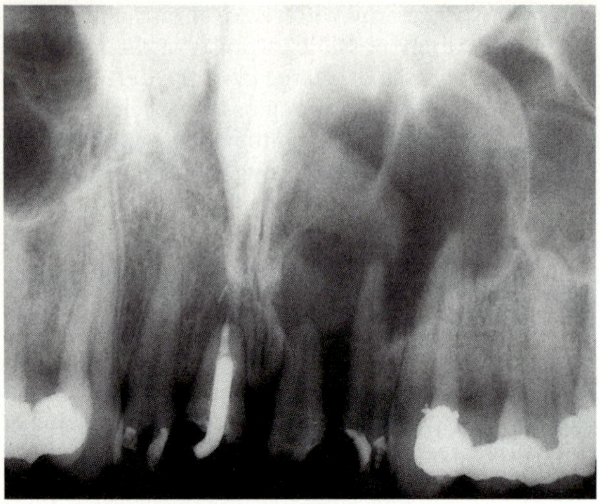

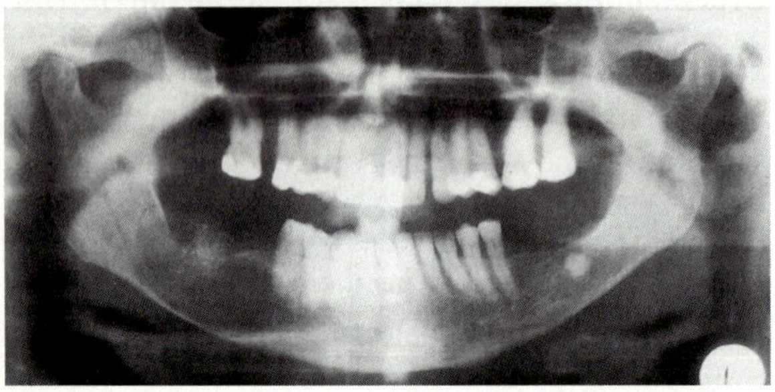

Fig. 19.52, 19.53. Radicular cysts in the central maxillary area and in the left mandible. An adenomatoid odontoma can be seen in the left part of the mandible

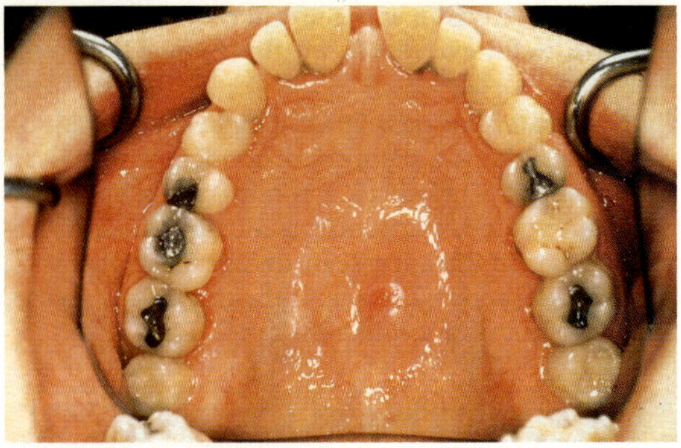

Fig. 19.54. Torus palatinus

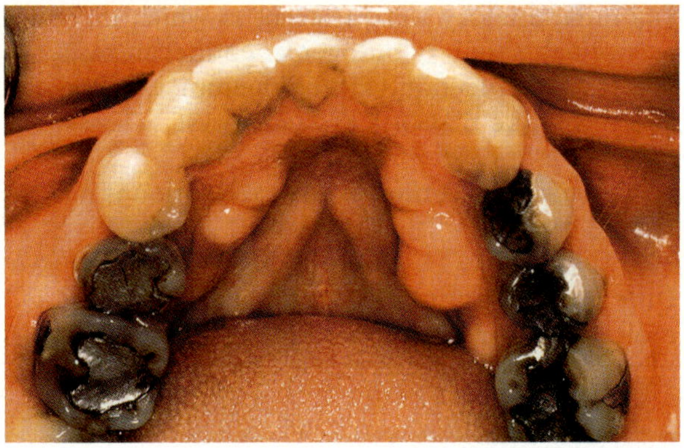

Fig. 19.55. Torus mandibularis

19.3.7.2
Benign Nonodontogenic Tumors of the Jawbones and Tumor-like Lesions

19.3.7.2.1
Torus Palatinus and Torus Mandibularis

Definition. These are common benign exostoses without consequence, apart from occasionally interfering with denture construction.

Etiology. They are developmental malformations.

Oral Manifestations. Torus palatinus occurs in the center of the hard palate as a painless nonenlarging bony, hard lump, with a normal overlying mucosa (Fig. 19.54). Its surface may be smooth or nodular. Torus mandibularis is found lingual to the premolar tooth, usually bilaterally (Fig. 19.55).

Diagnosis. Radiologic examination.

Treatment. Surgical excision is rarely indicated.

19.3.7.2.2
Ossifying Fibroma (Fibrous Osteoma, Fibro-osteoid, Osteoma, Sclerotic Fibroma, Osteodystrophia Fibrosa Localisata, Hypertrophic Localized Osteitis, Osteitis Fibrosa Localisata, Cement-Ossifying Fibroma)

Definition and Etiology. Ossifying fibroma is a benign tumor, probably originating from the bone-forming mesenchyme, which is initially composed mainly of connective tissue, ossifying only with increasing age. Because of this ossification, a transition into an osteoma has been discussed. It shows a manifestation maximum in the 3rd decade of life and later. Both genders are about equally affected.

Oral Manifestations. Slow invasive tumor growth, when localized in the maxilla, may lead to impairment of nasal breathing, or even exophthalmus or bulbar elevation. There is crowding and tilting of teeth. Typical are painless tumefactions that may persist unnoticed for a long time (Fig. 19.56a).

Radiological Findings. The X-ray shows well delineated, partially osteolytic, partially osteoblastic

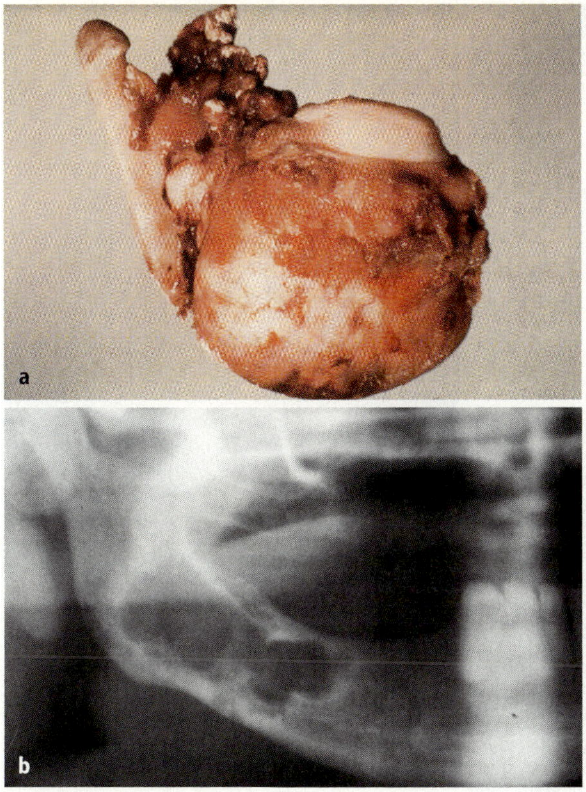

Fig. 19.56. **a** Surgical preparation of ossifying fibroma and **b** its radiological appearance in the right mandible

alterations (Fig. 19.56b). The mineralization of the trabecula formed by the tumor increases with age, making it more opaque. This produces frosted-glass-like shadows such as are seen in fibrous dysplasia, or more or less pronounced mineralization areas, giving rise to a spotted pattern in the X-ray image.

Histological Findings. Depending on the degree of mineralization, the coarse to bone-hard tumor has cell-rich, collagen fiber-containing connective tissue, with a large number of irregularly distributed trabeculae. These consist in part of fibrous and in part of lamellar bone. The fibrous portion exhibits isomorphous fusiform cells without mitoses or atypias. In most cases, the bony and the fibrous portion are of equal size.

Diagnosis. Histolopathological examination is needed for diagnosis.

Differential Diagnosis. Osteoblastoma, fibrous dysplasia, odontogenic cyst, and other tumors must be excluded.

Therapy. Since the tumor grows invasively, total removal with margins in the healthy bone is required. Primary irradiation is not recommended, because of poor irradiation sensitivity and danger of later transformation to osteosarcoma.

19.3.7.2.3

Fibrous Dysplasia (Focal Fibrosis of the Bone, Bone Cyst, Jaffé-Lichtenstein-Uehlinger Disease, Osteodystrophia Fibrosa, Osteofibroma, Osteitis Fibrosa, Unilateral Polyostotic Fibrous Osteitis, Cystofibromatosis)

Definition and Etiology. Fibrous dysplasia is usually viewed as a bone disease of adolescents, since it occurs mainly in the first three decades of life with a slight female preponderance. Owing to the different implications for treatment, differentiation from ossifying fibromas is important.

Oral Manifestations. Fibrous dysplasia occurs almost only localized in one bone. About one third of all monostotic fibrous dysplasias are localized in the region of the jawbone (Fig. 19.57a). The maxilla is more often affected than the mandible. Since fibrous dysplasia rarely causes symptoms, it is often detected incidentally, especially if there is only mild swelling or asymmetry. Displacement of the bulbus and tumefaction of the maxilla may also be observed. The tumor is pain-free even while growing and, if it is very large, can lead to pronounced facial asymmetries.

Radiological Findings. The X-ray image of fibrous dysplasia is nonspecific. Clearly delineated osteolytic foci are mainly observed, which are consistently opaque and honeycombed, with the corresponding radiotransparency (Fig. 19.57b,c). The well-defined corticalis may be displaced and thinned, reactively leading to periostal new bone formation, which may occasionally also be sclerotic. In the maxilla, protrusion into the maxillary sinus and involvement of the cheek bone is often observed.

Microscopic Findings. The macroscopically yellow-reddish coarse tissue shows histologically cell-rich connective tissue with fusiform cells and evenly distributed capillaries. In this stroma, a metaplastic bone formation of fibrous trabecula is found, the fibers of the stroma typically spreading directly into those of the trabecula.

Diagnosis. Histopathological examination is necessary; the history and local findings can only confirm a suspicion of fibrous dysplasia.

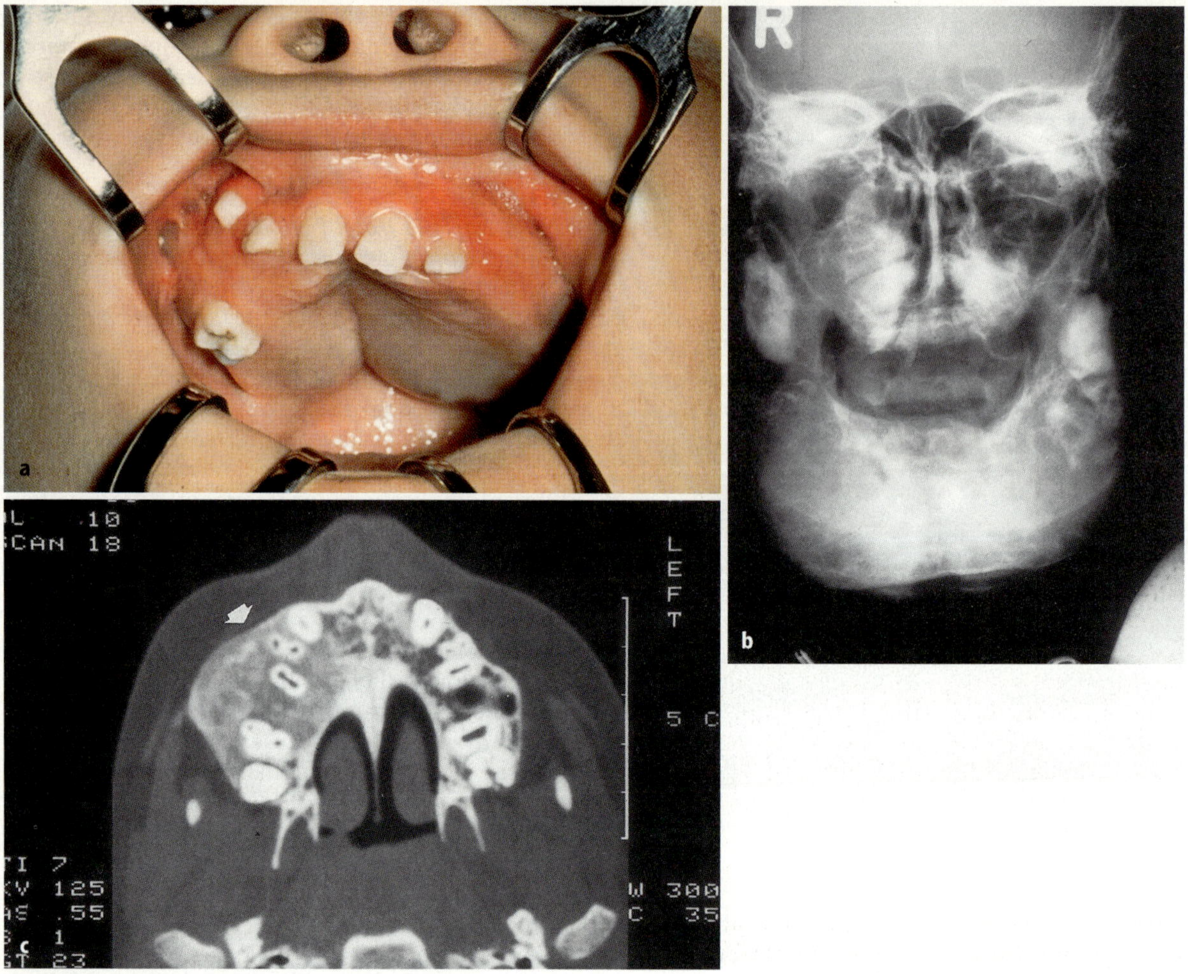

Fig. 19.57. a Fibrous dysplasia. The X-ray (**b**) and the CT (**c**) show the lesion as consistently opaque and honeycombed with the corresponding radiotransparency (*arrow*)

Differential Diagnosis. Cysts, giant cell reparative granuloma, ossifying fibroma, and ameloblastoma must be considered. Differentiation from ossifying fibroma is extremely difficult histologically. Differentiating characteristics are the fibrocartilaginous trabeculae metaplastically formed in the fibrous dysplasia and the missing secondary transformation.

Treatment. Modeling osteotomy is performed to remove disfiguring asymmetries. These interventions should only be carried out after the end of puberty. Owing to the possibility of occasional periods of renewed growth of malignant degeneration, careful clinical and radiological follow-up is necessary.

19.3.7.2.4
Osteoma Mucosae (Osseous Choristoma)

Definition. Osteoma mucosae is a rare primary benign tumor of bone, usually in the tongue. It occurs mostly in women in the 3rd or 4th decade of life.

Etiology. It may arise from thyroid anlages.

Oral Manifestations. It appears as a hard, pedunculated, painless lump on the dorsum of the tongue, immediately posterior to the foramen caecum.

Microscopic Findings. Spicules of bone of varying size may be found within the lamina propria or the subcutaneous tissue.

Diagnosis. Histopathological examination allows the diagnosis.

Differential Diagnosis. Osteoblastoma, chondroma, osteosarcoma, and chondrosarcoma must be excluded.

Treatment. Surgical excision is the only treatment.

19.3.7.2.5
Giant Cell Granuloma (Central Giant Cell Granuloma, Giant Cell-Containing Reparative Granuloma)

Definition and Etiology. The tumor is a reparative process characterized by local circulatory disorders and bleeding. Half of all cases occur in persons up to the age of 25 years. The mandible is more frequently affected than the maxilla, and there is a slight female predominance. Owing to the many morphological associations with aneurysmal bone cyst, which, in contrast to the giant cell granuloma, occurs mainly in the rest of the skeletal system and only rarely in the jaw, it is assumed that the two alterations are related processes. Transformation into a malignant tumor has not been observed thus far.

Oral Manifestations. Central giant cell granuloma occurs mainly in the tooth-bearing sections of the facial part of the skull. The tumor causes painless swelling that is only detected when facial asymmetries, impaired nasal breathing, and loosening and displacement of teeth are observed (Fig. 19.58a). The teeth, which are embedded almost only in granulation tissue, stay vital. Sensitivity disorders in the regional spread of the mental nerve have not been described. Penetration of the giant cell granuloma into the oral cavity is only observed in edentulous patients. In these cases there is a bluish-red protrusion in the gingiva. In a small number of patients, especially adolescents, multiple foci have been observed in the mandible and maxilla. The clinical picture of cherubism is seen if these cause symmetric swelling.

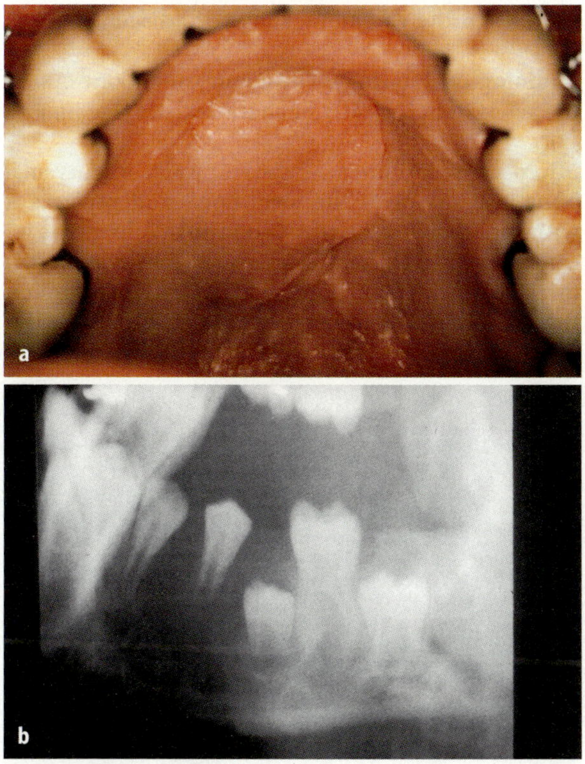

Fig. 19.58. **a** Giant-cell granuloma on the hard palate and **b** radiographic findings in another patient with a similar tumor

Radiological Findings. The X-ray shows single- or multichambered, sharply delineated osteolytic areas, which are occasionally only differentiated by a thin osseous cover (Fig. 19.58b). In some cases, absorption of the root apex of neighboring teeth is observed.

Microscopic Findings. Macroscopically, this is a grayish-red to brown tumor with granulation tissue that is histologically composed of fusiform fibroblast-like cells. Furthermore, there are irregularly distributed giant cells of the osteoblast type. Mitoses are rare and capillaries, numerous. A clear to pronounced fibrosis develops with increasing age of the alteration.

Diagnosis. Histolopathological examination is needed for diagnosis.

Differential Diagnosis. Odontogenic cyst, myxofibroma, ameloblastoma, giant cell tumor, aneurysmal bone cyst, brown tumor of hyperparathyroidism, and, especially with localization in the maxilla, fibrous dysplasia and ossifying fibroma must all be excluded. Histological differentiation is the most difficult.

Treatment. Curettage is the only treatment. The bone cavity is either primarily closed or, if the spread is very pronounced, filled with autologous spongiosa. Recurrences are observed in 13 % of cases and have to be treated in the same manner.

19.3.7.2.6
Solitary Bone Cyst (Simple Bone Cyst, Juvenile Bone Cyst, Traumatic Bone Cyst, Hemorrhagic Bone Cyst)

Definition and Etiology. The solitary bone cyst is a tumor-like or tumor-mimicking change of unclear etiology. As it was long thought to be of traumatic origin, it was often called 'traumatic bone cyst'. Solitary bone cysts are generally rare. They are predominantly observed in men.

Oral Manifestations. In 2 % of cases, solitary bone cysts are found in the jawbone. Two-thirds of these lesions are located in the mandible and one third in

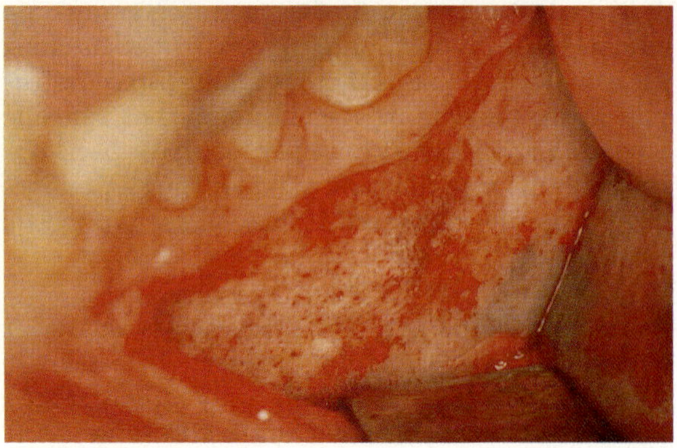

Fig. 19.59. Solitary bone cyst

the maxilla (Fig. 19.59). As a rule, solitary bone cysts are detected as incidental findings on plain radiographs. Swellings, pain, and supersensitivity of teeth are rare. Displacement of teeth or fractures of the jaw are only observed in rare cases, despite considerable volume of the change in some cases. Sensitivity disorders in the region of the mental nerve have not been described.

Radiological Findings. The cyst lumen is usually not clearly delineated in the X-ray image.

Microscopic Findings. Since empty cavities are the most frequent finding, it is difficult to obtain material for histological examination. A thin layer of connective tissue consisting of only a few cell rows is seen at the cyst lumen, in which hyaline masses are sometimes embedded.

Diagnosis. The diagnosis is made clinically, based on the empty cyst cavity and the macroscopically missing epithelium, as well as histologically. Five criteria are crucial for diagnosis of a solitary bone cyst: namely solitary cyst, absence of epithelial delineation, absence of any signs of acute or chronic inflammation, an empty cavity filled with clear liquid, and walls consisting of a mainly thin layer of connective tissue on an occasionally thin osseous lamella.

Differential Diagnosis. Aneurysmal bone cyst and giant cell reparative granuloma must be excluded.

Treatment. Dependent on the size and localization of the cavity, treatment of the solitary bone cyst consists either in merely removing an osseous lid or in curettage and filling with autologous spongiosa. The blood escaping into the cavity during surgery is collected here, thereby initiating healing.

19.3.7.2.7
Aneurysmal Bone Cyst (Expansive Hemangioma, Ossifying Hematoma, Periostal Hematoma, Benign Bone Aneurysm, Hemangiomatous Bone Cyst, Hemorrhagic Bone Cyst, Aneurysmal Giant Cell Tumor, Atypical Giant Cell Tumor, Pulsating or Benign Giant Cell Tumor, Subperiostal Giant Cell Tumor)

Definition. The aneurysmal bone cyst is a benign tumor-like alteration of the bone. The aneurysmal bone cyst is mostly located in the metaphyses of the large tubular bones and the vertebrae. Only 1%–3% of cases are found in the facial skeleton.

Etiology. The etiology of the aneurysmal bone cyst is controversial. A local circulation disorder with an increase of venous pressure resulting in an enlargement of the vascular space, a trauma with subsequent bleeding, and a reparative process that overshoots its mark are assumed. Aneurysmal bone cyst and giant cell reparative granuloma in the maxillofacial region are considered to be closely related.

Oral Manifestations. The aneurysmal bone cyst of the facial skeleton is predominantly localized in the mandible. The most frequent symptoms are swelling and pain. Expansion may lead to tilting and displacement of teeth, though the vitality of the teeth is preserved. There is no paresthesia or anesthesia in the spreading range of adjacent nerves.

Radiological Findings. The aneurysmal bone cyst of the jaw is radiologically uncharacteristic (Fig. 19.60).

Microscopic Findings. Macroscopically, aneurysmal bone cyst dissolves the local bone and replaces it with spongioid tissue with blood-filled chambers located under a thin cortical bone. The cyst wall is formed by collagen bundles. Close to the surface, there is often lamellar trabeculation from primitive

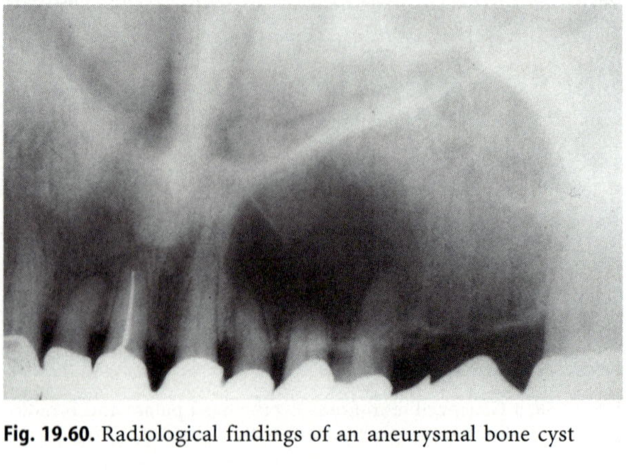

Fig. 19.60. Radiological findings of an aneurysmal bone cyst

fibrous bone. In the marginal sections, the connective tissue grows into the adjacent marrow spaces.

Diagnosis. Histopathological examination allows the diagnosis.

Differential Diagnosis. Giant cell reparative granuloma, odontogenic cyst, hemangioma, eosinophilic granuloma, myxofibroma, ameloblastoma, and tumor metastases must be excluded.

Treatment. Curettage is the only treatment. Depending on the size of the defect, the cyst must be filled with autologous spongiosa. Occasionally, spontaneous regression occurs. No recurrence has been observed of such a cyst localized in the facial skeleton.

19.3.8 Benign Tumors of Blood and Lymph Vessels

A. Patrizi and I. Neri

19.3.8.1 *Hemangioma (Angiomatous Nevus, Capillary and Cavernous Hemangioma, Strawberry Hemangioma)*

Definition. The term hemangioma is frequently used to encompass hamartomous vascular malformations and proliferative tumors, all of which appear during the first weeks of life or at birth [45]. In 1992, Mulliken and Glowacki differentiated this group of vascular birthmarks into two main groups: (1) hemangiomas due to abnormalities of endothelial cell proliferation and (2) vascular malformations resulting from developmental errors with normal endothelial turnover [46, 47].

Etiopathogenesis. Hemangioma, the most common benign tumor in infacy, is a vascular neoplasm characterized by a rapid proliferation phase followed by slow involution, leading to complete regression in most cases [48].

Clinically, well-developed hemangiomas can be differentiated into superficial, deep, and mixed on the basis of the size of the involved vessels [49]. The lesions may be present at birth as telangiectatic or pale macules [48]. After a few weeks, these lesions grow to present a strawberry-like appearance if they are the superficial type, and a bluish-red mass with poorly circumscribed borders in the deep lesions. A combination of strawberry and deep hemangioma is observed in the mixed type.

Oral Manifestations. Oral hemangiomas usually range in color from red to blue and blanch on pressure. The most commonly affected sites are the lips (Fig. 19.61) and tongue. In these sites, the lesions show a predominantly bosselated surface. The gingivae may also be affected with flat red macules (Fig. 19.62).

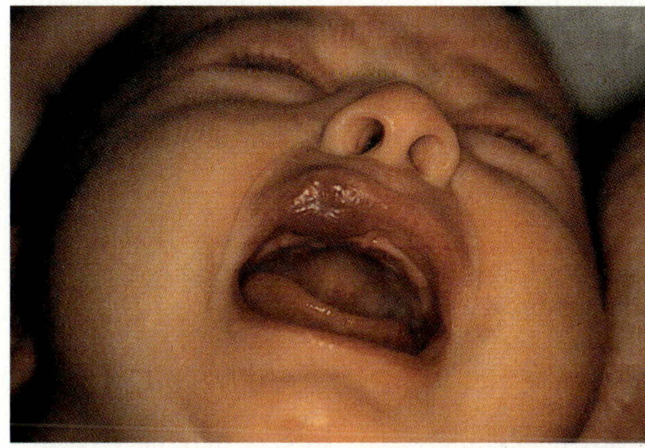

Fig. 19.61. Mixed hemangioma of the lip and oral mucosa

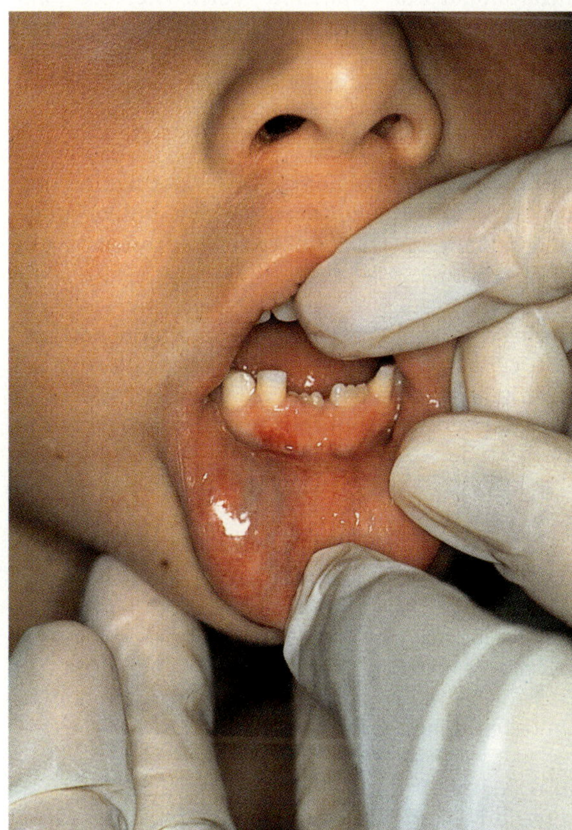

Fig. 19.62. Superficial hemangioma of the lower lip and gingiva

Oral hemangiomas are particularly at risk for complications such as ulceration and bleeding, especially caused by trauma [45, 48, 49].

Microscopic Findings. The well-organized hemangioma is microscopically characterized by vascular channels with different diameter lumina, which allow distinction between a capillary and a cavernous type. In the involutive phase [45], there is a progressive increase in intra- and interlobular fat and connective tissue [45].

Differential Diagnosis. In most cases, hemangioma is easily diagnosed clinically, but the differential diagnosis with vascular malformations or with lymphangiomas can sometimes be difficult. In these cases, magnetic resonance imaging (MRI), computed tomography (CT), and angiography should be performed [47].

Treatment. No treatment is normally required in most hemangiomas, owing to their frequent spontaneous resolution. Plastic surgery may be very successful for extensive lesions on the lips. Pulsed dye laser is a relatively useful modality for treating superficial hemangiomas.
Intralesional or systemic corticosteroids and cryotherapy are sometimes beneficial [47].

19.3.8.2
Lymphangioma

Definition. Lymphangioma is a developmental malformation of lymphatic vessels which, unlike congenital hemangioma, does not usually present involution over time.

Etiology. In some cases lymphangioma is probably best classified as a hamartomous malformation. Most lymphangiomas are present at birth or develop early in childhood, but they may also appear within the first 2 decades of life. They consist of dilated lymphatic vessels lined with normal lymphatic endothelium, varying in size from capillaries to large cystic cavities. Lymphangiomas can be classified into five main clinical types [50]: (1) simple lymphangioma, (2) L-circumscribed lymphangioma (LC), (3) cavernous or diffuse lymphangioma, (4) cystic hygroma or cystic lymphangioma [51], and (5) acquired progressive lymphangioma or benign lymphangioendothelioma.

Oral Manifestations. Simple lymphangiomas are blue-domed or skin-colored, solitary, insignificant lesions present in infancy. Levin et al. described multiple symmetrical simple lymphangiomas distributed in the posterior alveolar ridges of about 3 %–7 % of normal black newborns. These lesions often regressed spontaneously [52].
LC is the most common type. The tongue (Fig. 19.63) and the buccal mucous membrane are among the most frequently involved sites. On the tongue, LC may also be seen in conjunction with cavernous lymphangioma. They are usually asymptomatic and appear as grouped, translucent, small, deep vesicles with a "frog spawn" appearence (Fig. 19.64) [47].
LC [53] ranges in size from small plaques to very large lesions, sometimes involving the whole tongue. In these cases, a deeper component is almost always present and may be responsible for macroglossia. Lymphangioma of the lip can cause macrocheilia. Symmetrical involvement of the maxillary and mandibular gingiva has occasionally been reported [54, 55]. Rapid enlargement of a lymphangioma can suddenly occur as a result of infection and/or intralesional hemorrhage, particularly in childhood, in some cases causing obstruction of the airways, dysphagia, and rarely even death.

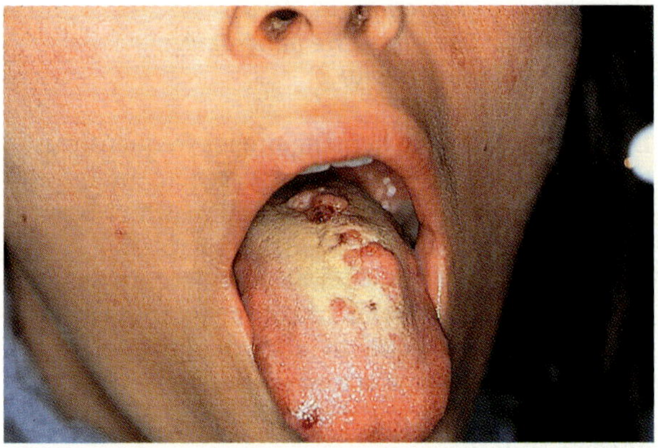

Fig. 19.63. Lymphangioma circumscriptum on the dorsal surface of the tongue

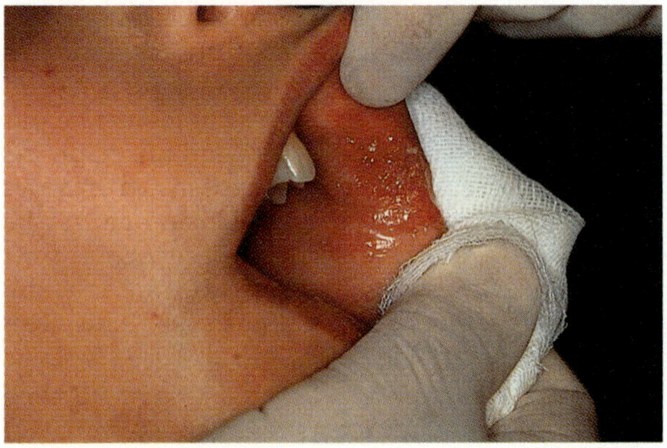

Fig. 19.64. Lymphangioma of the oral mucosa. Grouped, translucent, small vesicles with a "frog spawn" appearance

Microscopic Findings. In LC, numerous lymphatic vessels lined with flat endothelial cells are diffusely located in the submucosa immediately beneath the overlying epithelium. In deep lymphangiomas, there are diffuse, ill-defined masses of large dilated endothelium-lined, muscle-coated lymphatic spaces in the reticular dermis, subcutaneous tissue, and intermuscular septa.

Diagnosis. High-resolution ultrasonography is a diagnostic aid [56]. CT and MRI are sometimes indicated [47].

Differential Diagnosis. When there is only the deep component, lymphangioma can be confused with a lipoma or a cyst. Sometimes in LC, the vesicles contain blood: this conditions is called hemangiolymphangioma.

Treatment. Recurrent episodes of infection should be medically treated. Small superficial lesions may be treated with CO_2 and pulsed dye lasers [57], or with cryotherapy to obliterate the vesicular component [50]. A transfixation technique has also been used with good results [58]. Surgical excision is generally the treatment of choice, but recurrences are common, particularly in large lesions [47, 50]. In very large lesions, it is extremely difficult to obtain adequate excision, and often complete surgical excision is not practicable.

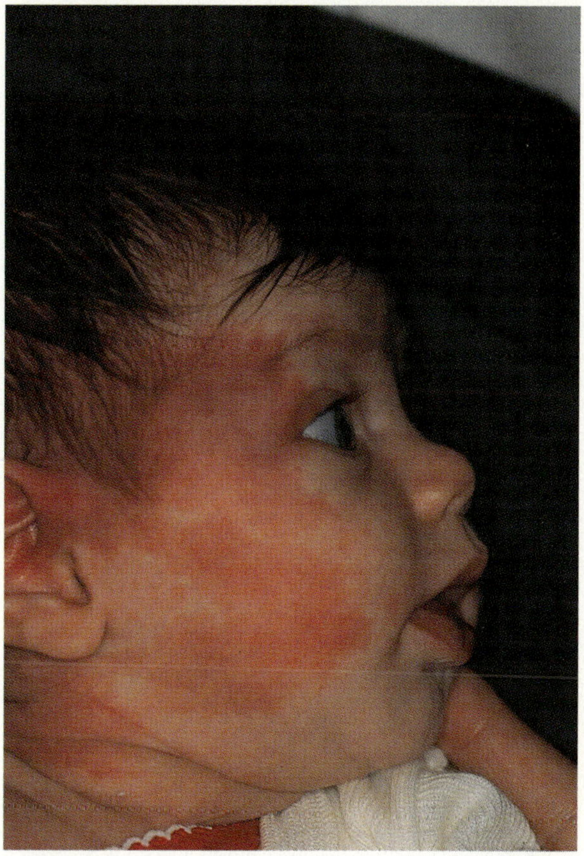

Fig. 19.65. Port-wine stain on the face of a 3-month-old child with Sturge-Weber syndrome

19.3.8.3 *Sturge-Weber Syndrome (Encephalofacial Angiomatosis, Encephalotrigeminal Angiomatosis, Cutaneous Angiomatosis with Cerebral Calcification, Sturge-Weber-Dimitri Disease)*

Definition. Sturge-Weber syndrome (SWS) is characterized by a facial port-wine stain associated with ipsilateral leptomeningeal vascular and cerebral cortex malformation. Ocular involvement is present in 30 %–50 % of cases. The port-wine stain in this syndrome is usually unilateral, involving the area of the first branch of the trigeminal nerve and sometimes also of the second (Fig. 19.65) [59]. The lesions may be small or large and can also have a bilateral extension [60]. Less than 10 % of patients with a port-wine stain over the first branch of the trigeminal nerve have SWS [61]. Complete involvement of the upper eyelid is not necessarily synonymous with SWS. The most common neurologic abnormalities include epilepsy, present in 75 %–90 % of patients, mental retardation and, more rarely, contralateral hemiparesis.

Etiopathogenesis. While etiology and pathogenesis remain unknown, a familial pattern has been observed in exceptional cases.

Oral Manifestations. The oral mucosae may show telangiectases. Sometimes, there is hypertrophy of the affected soft and/or skeletal tissue with swelling of the lips or gums [47]. The palate on the same side as the skin hemangioma may be involved.

Associated Findings. Port-wine stains in other cutaneous sites than the face have frequently been observed, and the association of SWS and Klippel-Trenaunay syndrome has sometimes been reported [62]. Other associations, such as SWS and oculocutaneous melanosis [63] and SWS and Wyburn-Mason syndrome [64] have occasionally been reported.

Microscopic Findings. Histology of the port-wine stain of SWS shows dilatation of mature superficial dermal capillaries.

Diagnosis. X-rays of the skull, electroencephalography (EEG), CT, and MRI of the brain help to establish the diagnosis. Repeated ophthalmologic examinations are also necessary.

Differential Diagnosis. Angio-osteohypertrophy syndrome is the main differential diagnosis [65].

Treatment. Port-wine stain can be treated with laser therapy. Medical and/or surgical treatments should be considered in every case with ocular and/or neurological symptoms. If phenytoin is used for control of seizures, generalized gingival hyperplasia may appear.

References

1. Braun-Falco O, Plewig G, Wolff HH (Eds). Disease of the lips and the oral cavity. Dermatology. 3rd Ed. Berlin Heidelberg New York: Springer Verlag, 1991: 800–821
2. Burton JL. The lips. In: Champion RH, Burton JL, Ebling FJG (Eds). Textbook of dermatology. 5th Ed. Oxford: Blackwell Scientific Publications, 1992: 2761–2774
3. Ohman SC, Dahlen G, Moller A. Angular cheilitis – a clinical and microbial study. J Oral Pathol 1986; 15: 213–217
4. Laskaris G. Diseases of the lips. In: Color atlas of oral diseases. Stuttgart: Thieme, 1988: 88–92
5. Pindborg JJ. Classification and oral lesions associated with HIV infection. Oral Surg Oral Med Oral Pathol 1989; 67: 292–295
6. Warnakulasuria KAAS, Samaranayake LP, Peiris JSM. Angular cheilitis in a group of Sri Lankan adults: a clinical and microbiologic study. J Oral Pathol Med 1991; 20: 172–175
7. Robinson JK. Actinic cheilitis: a prospective study comparing four treatment methods. Arch Otolaryngol Head Neck Surg 1989; 115: 848–852
8. Braun-Falco O, Plewig G, Wolff HH (Eds). Malignant epithelial tumors. Dermatology. 3rd Ed. Berlin Heidelberg New York: Springer Verlag, 1991: 918–1031
9. Burton JL. Epidermal skin tumors. In: Champion RH, Burton JL, Ebling FJG (Eds). Textbook of Dermatology. 5th Ed. Oxford: Blackwell Scientific Publications, 1488–1494
10. Dinehart SM, Pollack SV. Metastases from squamous cell carcinoma of the skin and lip. J Am Acad Dermatol 1989; 21: 241–248
11. Laskaris G. Malignant neoplasms. In: Color atlas of oral diseases. Stuttgart: Thieme Verlag, 1988: 230–251
12. Robinson JK. What are adequate treatment and follow-up care for nonmelanoma cutaneous cancer? Arch Dermatol 1987; 123(3): 331–333
13. Miller SJ. Biology of basal cell carcinoma. J Am Acad Dermatol 1991; 24: 1–13, 161–175
14. Wade TR, Ackerman AB. The many faces of basal-cell carcinoma. J dermatol Surg Oncol 1978; 4: 23–28
15. Wolf DJ, Zitelli JA. Surgical margins for basal cell carcinoma. Arch Dermatol 1987; 123: 340–344
16. Braun-Falco O, Plewig G, Wolff HH (Eds). Skin diseases due to physical and chemical causes. Dermatology. 3rd Ed. Berlin Heidelberg New York: Springer Verlag, 1991: 367–402
17. Kraemer KH, Slor H. Xeroderma pigmentosum. Clin Dermatol 1984; 2: 33–39
18. Thielmann HW, Popanda O, Edler L, Lung EG. Clinical symptoms and DNA repair characteristics of Xeroderma pigmentosum patients from Germany. Cancer Res 1991; 51: 3465–3467
19. Enzinger FM, Weiss SW. Soft tissue tumours. St Louis: Mosby 1995
20. Jorgenson RJ, Levin S. White sponge nevus. Arch Dermatol 1981; 117: 73–76
21. Terrier F, Bayle-Lebey P, Basex J. Cas pour diagnostic: white sponge naevus. Ann Der Venereol (Paris) 1993; 120: 397–398
22. Cida B. White sponge nevus of the oral mucosa. J Conn State Dent Assoc 1976; 51: 122–126
23. Hassell TM, Hefti AF. Drug-induced gingival overgrowth: old problem, new problem. Crit Rev Oral Biol Med 1991; 2: 103–137
24. Slavin J, Taylor S. Cyclosporin, nifedipine and gingival hyperplasia. Lancet 1987; II: 739
25. Stinnet E, Robn B, Grizzle WE. New developments in understanding phenyntoin-induced gingival hyperplasia. J Am Dent Assoc 1987; 114: 814–816
26. Helm KF, Hopfl RM, Kreider JW, Lookingbill DP. Verruciform xanthoma: a case report and immunohistochemical study. J Cutan Pathol 1993; 20: 84–86
27. Neville B. The verruciform xanthoma: a report of eight new cases. Am J Dermatopathol 1986; 8: 247–253
28. Christopoulos P, Sklavounou A, Patrikiou A. True fibroma of the oral mucosa. Int J Oral Maxillofac Surgery 1994; 23: 98–99
29. Weathers DR, Callihan MD. Oral fibroma. Oral Surg Med Pathol 1977; 37: 374–384
30. Buttler EJ, Macyntire DR. Oral pyogenic granulomas. Dent Update 1991; 18: 194–195
31. Vilmann A, Vilmann P, Vilmann H. Pyogenic granuloma: evaluation of oral conditions. Br J Oral Surg 1986; 24: 376–382
32. Elzay RP, Dutz W, Myxomas of the paraoral-oral soft tissues. Oral Surg 1978; 45: 246–251
33. Everson SW. Superficial mucoceles: pitfall in clinical and microscopic diagnosis. Oral Surg 1988, 66: 318–323
34. McAvoy JM. Dermoid cyst in the neck and head in children. Arch Otolaryngol 1976; 102: 529–533
35. Miller AS, Mc Crea MW. Sebaceous gland adenoma of the buccal mucosa. J Oral Surg 1968; 26: 593–595
36. Luna MA, Stimson PG, Bardwill JM. Minor salivary glands tumours of the oral cavity. Oral Surg 1988; 25: 71–75
37. Golding-Wood DG, Whittet HB. The lingual tonsil. A neglected symptomatic structure? J Laryngol Otol 1989; 103:922–925
38. Joseph M, Reardon E, Goodman M. Lingual tonsillectomy. Larynoscope 1984; 94:179–184
39. Jones JAM. Lingual thyroid. Br J Oral Surg 1986; 24: 58–62
40. Morgan NJ, Emberton P, Barton RP. The importance of thyroid scanning in neck limps. J Laryngol Otol 1995; 109:83–94
41. Rapidis AD. Lipoma of the oral cavity. Int J Oral Surg 1982; 11: 30–37
42. Merill RG, Downs JR. Oral leiomyomas: report of two cases. Oral Surg 1967; 23: 438–440.
43. Reid CO, Smith CJ. Rhabdomyoma of the floor at the mouth: a new case and review of recently reported intraoral rhabdomyomas. Br J Oral Surg 1985; 23: 284–291
44. Altmeyer P, Merkel KH. Multiple systematisierte Neurome der Haut und der Schleimhäute. Hautarzt 1982; 32: 240–244
45. Mulliken JB, Young A. Vascular birthmarks, hemangiomas and vascular malformations. Philadelphia: WB Saunders, 1988
46. Mulliken JB, Glowacki J. Hemangiomas and vascular malformations in infants and children: a classification based on endothelial characteristics. Plast Reconstr Surg 1982; 69: 412–20
47. Enjorlas O, Mulliken JB. The current management of vascular birthmarks. Pediatr Dermatol 1993; 10: 311–33
48. Patrizi A, Neri I, Voltolini, V et al. Nevi angiomatosi. Studio epidemiologico di 255 casi. G Ital Dermatol Venereol 1994; 129: 545–51
49. Esterly NB. Cutaneous hemangiomas, vascular stains and associated syndromes. Curr Probl Pediatr 1987; 17: 1–69
50. Rabinowitz LG, Esterly NB. Vascular birthmarks and other abnormalities of blood vessels and lymphatics. In: Schachner LA, Hansen RC (Eds). Pediatric dermatology. 2nd Ed. New York: Churchill Livingstone, 1996: 953–89
51. Seashore JH, Gardiner LJ, Ariyian S. Management of giant cystic higromas in infants. Am J Surg 1985; 149: 459–65
52. Levin LS, Jorgenson RJ, Jarvey BA. Lymphangiomas of the alveolar ridges in neonates. Pediatrics 1976; 58: 881–4
53. Brandrup F. Lymphangioma circumscriptum of the tongue. Dermatologica 1976; 153: 191–5
54. Josephson P, Van Wyk WC. Bilateral symmetrical lymphangiomas of the gingiva. J Periodontol 1984; 19: 47–48

55. McDaniel RK, Adcock JE. Bilateral symmetrical lymphangiomas of the gingiva. Oral Surg Oral Med Pathol 1987; 63: 224–7
56. Betti R, Nessi R, Blanc M et al. Ultrasonography of proliferative vascular lesions of the skin. J Dermatol 1990; 17: 247–51
57. Bailin PL, Kantor GR, Wheeland RG. Carbon dioxide laser vaporization of lymphangioma circumscriptum. J Acad Dermatol 1986; 14: 257–62
58. Vilalta MD, Mascaro JM. Hemangiolymphangioma of the tongue treated by transfixion technique. J Dermatol Surg Oncol 1985; 11: 2–5
59. Enjorlas J, Riché MC, Merland JJ. Facial portwine stains and Sturge-Weber syndrome. Pediatrics 1985; 76: 48–51
60. Uram M, Zubillaga C. The cutaneous manifestations of Sturge-Weber syndrome. J Clin Neuroophthalmol 1982; 2: 145–8
61. Lorette G, Abou Mrad J, Khallouf R, et al. A Port-wine stain angioma of the face and convulsion. Abstract Vth Congress ESPD, Rotterdam, September 4–8, 1996: 173
62. Schofield D, Zaatari GS, Gay BB. Klippel-Trenaunay and Sturge-Weber syndromes with renal hemangioma and double inferior vena cava. J Urol 1986; 136: 442–45
63. Noriega-Sanchez A, Markand ON, Herndon JH. Oculocutaneous melanosis associated with the Sturge-Weber syndrome: Neurology 1972; 22: 256–62
64. Ward JB, Katz NNK. Combined phakomatoses: a case report of Sturge-Weber and Wyburn-Mason syndrome occurring in the same individual. Ann Ophthalmol 1983; 15: 1112–16
65. Regezi JA, Sciubba J (Eds). Red blue lesions. In: Oral pathology. 2nd Ed. Philadelphia, WB Saunders, 1993

Suggested Further Reading

Alappat JP, Pillai AM, Prasanna D, Sambasivan M. Giant cell reparative granuloma of the craniofacial complex: case report and review of the literature. Br J Neurosurg 1992; 6: 71–74

Allen CM, Pellegrini A. Probable congenital melanocytic nevus of the oral mucosa: case report. Pediatr Dermatol 1995; 12: 145–148

Amling M, Werner M, Posl M, Maas R, Korn U, Delling G. Calcifying solitary bone cyst: morphological aspects and differential diagnosis of sclerotic bone tumours. Virchows Arch 1995; 426: 235–242

Anand VK, Arrowwood JP Jr, Krolls SO. Malignant potential of the odontogenic keratocyst. Otolaryngol Head Neck Surg 1994; 111: 124–129

Apisarnthanarax P. Granular cell tumor (review). J Am Acad Dermatol 1981; 5: 171–182

Awange DO. Fibrous dysplasia of the jaws: a review of the literature. East Afr Med J 1992; 205–209

Bochlogyros GN, Markopoulos A, Kanakis P. Intrakutaner Naevus auf der Mundschleimhaut. Quintessenz 1983; 8: 1487–1489

Boisnic S, Branchet MC, Pascal F, et al. Tretinoine topique dans le traitment des lichens planus et des leucoplasies de la muqueuse buccale. Evaluation clinique. Ann Dermatol Venereol 1994; 121: 459–463

Brannon RB. The odontogenic keratocyst. A clinicopathological study of 312 cases, part I. Oral Surg 1976; 42: 54–72

Brannon RB. The odontogenic keratocyst. A clinicopathological study of 312 cases, part II. Oral Surg 1977; 43: 233–255

Buchner A, Hansen LS. Pigmented nevi of the oral mucosa: a clinicopathologic study of 32 new cases and review of 75 cases from the literature. I. A clinicopathologic study of 32 new cases. Oral Surg 1979; 48: 131–142

Buchner A, Hansen LS. Pigmented nevi of the oral mucosa: a clinicopathologic study of 32 new cases and review of 75 cases from the literature. II. Analysis of 107 cases. Oral Surg 1980; 49: 55–62

Budtz-Jorgensen E. Oral mucosal lesions associated with wearing of removal dentures. J Oral Pathol 1981; 10: 65–80

Burton JL. The lips. In: Champion RH, Burton JL, Ebling FJG (eds) Textbook of dermatology. Oxford: Blackwell, 1992; 2761–2774

Chiodo GT, Rosenstein DI (1985) Dental treatment during pregnancy: a preventive approach. J Am Dent Assoc 110; 365–368

Colella G, De Luca F, Lanza A, et al. Transformazione maligna della leucoplachia del cavo orale. Revisione della letteratura e casistica clinica. Minerva Stomatol 1995; 44: 291–300

Colella G, Lanza A, Tartaro GP. Terapia della leucoplachia del cavo orale. Revisione della letteratura. Minerva Stomatol 1995; 44: 301–310

Daly BD, Chow CC, Cockram CS. Unusual manifestations of craniofacial fibrous dysplasia: clinical, endocrinological and computer tomographic features. Postgrad Med J 1994; 70: 10–16

Duffey DC, Bailet JW, Newman A. Ameloblastoma of the mandible with cervical lymph node metastasis. Am J Otolaryngol 1995; 16: 66–73

Duffey DC, Eversole LR, Abemayor E. Oral lichen planus and its association with squamous cell carcinoma: an update on pathogenesis and treatment implications. Laryngoscope 1996; 106: 357–62

Franklin CD, Pindborg JJ. The calcifying epithelial odontogenic tumor. Oral Surg 1976; 42: 753–765

Gazit D, Daniels TE. Oral melanocytic lesions: differences in expression of HMB-45 and S-100 antigens in round and spindle cells of malignant and benign lesions. J Oral Pathol Med 1994; 23: 60–64

Giansanti JS, Waldrom CA. Peripheral giant cell granuloma: review of 720 cases. J Oral Surg 1969; 27: 787–791

Gupta PC, Murti PR, Bhonsle RB, et al. Effect of cessation of tobacco use on the incidence of oral mucosal lesions in a 10-yr follow-up study of 12,212 users. Oral Dis 1995; 1(1): 54–58

Hahn SB, Kang ES, Jahng JS, Park BM, Choi JC. Ossifying fibroma. Yonsei Med J 1991; 32: 347–355

Harris MB, Toller P. The pathogenesis of dental cysts. Br Med Bull 1975; 31: 159–163

Huang X, Berthold H, Laeng RH. Epulis: a clinicopathological study of 120 patients with emphasis on recurrent lesions. ORL J Otorhinolaryngol Relat Spec 1994; 56: 230–235

Karmody CS, Forston JK, Calcaterra VE. Lymphangiomas of the head and neck in adults. Otolaryngol Head Neck Surg 1982; 90: 283–290

Kearns D, McGill T, Potsic W. Fibrous dysplasia. Head Neck 1992; 14: 510–512

Laskaris G. Colour atlas of oral diseases. Stuttgart: Thieme, 1988: 284

Lee KW. The fibrous epulis and related lesions. Periodontics 1986; 6: 277–299

Lever WF, Schaumburg-Lever G. Tumors and cysts of the epidermis. In: Lever WF, Schaumburg-Lever G (Eds). Histopathology of the skin: 7th Ed. Philadelphia: Lippincott, 1990: 523–577

Levin SL. Disorders of the mucous membrane. In: Farmer ER, Hood AF (Eds). Pathology of the skin USA: Prentice-Hall, 1990: 899–926

MacKie RM. Soft tissue tumours. In: Champion RH, Burton JL, Ebling FJG (eds) Textbook of dermatology. Oxford: Blackwell, 1992; 2073–2100

Manus DA, Sherbert D, Jackson IT. Management considerations for the granuloma of pregnancy. Plast Reconstr Surg 1995; 95: 1045–1050

Markaki S, Gearty J, Markakis P. Osteoma of the tongue. Br J Oral Surg 1987; 25: 79–82

Matt BH. Aneurysmal bone cyst of the maxilla: case report and review of the literature. Int J Pediatr Otorhinolaryngol 1993; 25: 217–226

Meiselman F. Surgical management of the odontogenic keratocyst: conservative approach. J Oral Maxillofac Surg 1994; 52: 960–963

Meyer JS, Davidson RS, Hubbard AM, Conard KA. MRI of focal fibrocartilaginous dysplasia. J Pediatr Orthop 1995; 15: 304–306

Motamedi MH, Yarzi E. Aneurysmal bone cyst of the jaws: analysis of 11 cases. J Oral Maxillofac Surg 1994; 52: 471–425

Murti PR, Bhonsle RB, Gupta PC et al. Etiology of oral submucous fibrosis with special reference to the role of areca nut chewing. J Oral Pathol Med 1995; 24(4): 145–52

Nair PN, Sjögren U, Schumacher E, Sundqvist G. Radicular cyst affecting a root-filled human tooth. Int Endod J 1993; 26: 225–22

Nastri AL, Wiesenfeld D, Radden BG, Eveson J, Scully C. Maxillary ameloblastoma: a retrospective study of 13 cases. Br J Oral Maxillofac Surg 1995; 33: 28–32

Peltola J, Magnusson B, Happonen RP, Borrman H. Odontogenic myxoma. A radiographic study of 21 tumours. Br J Oral Maxillofac Surg 1994; 32: 298–302

Piatelli A, Scarano A, Antinori A, Trisi P (1994) Odontogenic myxoma of the mandible. Report of a case and review of the literature. Acta Stomatol Belg 91: 101–110
Picascia DD, Robinson JK. Actinic cheilitis: a review of the etiology, differential diagnosis, and treatment. J Am Acad Dermatol 1987; 17: 255–64
Pindborg JJ, Hjoerting-Hansen E. Atlas of diseases of the jaws. Munksgaard: Copenhagen, 1974
Prein J, Remagen W, Spiessl B, Uehlinger E. Tumoren des Gesichtsschädels. Berlin Heidelberg New York: Springer, 1985
Reychler H. Neavus naevocellulaire buccal. Rev Stomatol Chir Maxillofac 1988; 89: 97–101
Rezaj RF. Torus palatinus, an exostosis of unknown etiology: review of the literature. Compend Contin Educ Dent 1985; 6: 149–152
Sakoda S, Shiba R, Irino S. Immediate reconstruction of the mandible in a patient with ossifying fibroma by replantation of the resected segment after freezing. J Oral Maxillofac Surg 1992; 50: 521–524
Schneider MS, Bise RN. Cementoma. Presentation predicates approach. J Craniofac Surg 1990; 1: 143–146
Sidoni A, Monico S, d'Errico P, Simoncell C. Giant cell reparative granuloma of the maxillary bone: case report and review of diagnostic criteria. Pathologica 1994; 86: 552–556
Slootweg PJ, Panders AK, Koopmans R, Nikkels PG. Juvenile ossifying fibroma. An analysis of 33 cases with emphasis on histopathological aspects. J Oral Pathol Med 1994; 23: 385–388
Stal S, Hamilton P, Spira M. Hemangioma, lymphangioma and vascular malformations of the head and neck. Otolaryngol Clin North Am 1986; 19: 769–796
Summerlin DJ. Precancerous and cancerous lesions of the oral cavity. Dermatol Clin 1996; 14: 205–23
Toller PA. Origin and growth of cysts in the jaw. Ann R Coll Surg Engl 1967; 40: 306–336
Webb JD, Wescott WB, Corell RW. Firm swelling on the anterior maxillary gingiva in an infant. J Am Dent Assoc 1984; 109: 307–308
Weissman JL, Snyderman CH, Yousem SA, Curtin HD. Ameloblastoma of the maxilla. CT and MR appearance. AJNR Am J Neuroradiol 1993; 14: 223–226
Williams TP. Management of ameloblastoma: a changing perspective. J Oral Maxillofac Surg 1993; 51: 1064–1070
Williams TP, Connor FA Jr. Surgical management of the odontogenic keratocyst: aggressive approach. J Oral Maxillofac Surg 1994; 52: 964–966
Young AE. Lymphatic malformations. In: Malliken JB, Young AE (eds) Vascular birth-mark – hemangiomas and malformations. Philadelphia: Saunders, 1988

CHAPTER 20

Malignant Tumors

20.1 Squamous Cell Carcinoma

J. M. Hall and R. S. Rogers, III

20.1.1 Squamous Cell Carcinoma of the Lip

Definition. Squamous cell carcinoma of the lip comprises 19 % of all oral carcinomas in the white population. In 90 % of the cases, it is seen on the vermilion border of the lower lip, just outside the line of contact with the upper lip or the junction of the wet and dry mucosa.

Etiology. The major known risk factors for carcinoma of the lip are rural residence and an outdoor occupation. Prolonged exposure to solar radiation is the suggested primary etiologic determinant. One of the strongest arguments for an actinic cause is the almost complete lack of mortality among dark-skinned populations. The disease is almost always in men, with incidence increasing in older age. Squamous carcinomas of the lip have also been noted to frequently arise at the site where a cigar, cigarette, or pipe is held. Carcinoma of the lip is a vanishing disease that has gone from the most common "oral" cancer to one that is only a quarter as likely to be diagnosed as any other intraoral carcinoma. The decrease in the United States in the formerly large numbers of outdoor white laborers probably contributes to the 4 % annual decline.

Pathogenesis. The pathogenesis is similar to that seen in the cutaneous development of actinic keratoses and squamous cell carcinomas of the sun-exposed skin.

Oral Manifestations. Approximately 90 % of premalignant and malignant lip lesions involve the lower lip vermilion. Early changes include atrophy, smoothing of the surface with blotchy pale areas, blurring of the demarcation between the lip vermilion and the cutaneous lip, and formation of rough scaly patches that may appear as leukoplakia. Leukoplakia is a sign on the lower lip that signifies malignancy or dysplasia in 14 %–23 % of patients. Crusted, oozing, nontender masses less than 1 cm across are also suggestive of early squamous cancer. Exophytic or indurated lesions are the result of long-standing malignancy.

Associated Findings. Submental lymphadenopathy associated with metastatic spread is seen in less than 10 % of the patients at the time of diagnosis.

Microscopic Findings. Most squamous cell carcinomas of the lip are well-differentiated, low-grade tumors and share the same characteristics as cutaneous squamous carcinomas. Actinic or solar cheilitis displays areas of orthokeratosis and parakeratosis, with degrees of atrophy, hyperplasia, and dysplasia similar to actinic keratoses.

Diagnosis. Biopsy is the only method that allows differentiation between solar cheilitis and early squamous cell carcinoma.

Differential Diagnosis. Dermatoses of the lip, such as lupus erythematosus and lichen planus, can produce scaly or erosive lesions that may bear a resemblance to squamous cell carcinoma. Their transient nature and multifocal distribution should provide clues to their nature. Similarly, recurrent herpes simplex labialis can produce crusted, oozing lesions that are short-lived. Chronic moderate to heavy keratinization, ulcerations, and erythroplasia should be viewed with concern.

Treatment. Surgery or radiotherapy have almost equal efficacy. Surgical management is preferred for most patients because of the advantage of tumor margin evaluation, avoidance of radiation complications, and rapid recovery. Lesions less than 3 cm across that involve the lower lip have an excellent prognosis, with 5-year survival rates in the range of 95 %–100 %. The rare squamous cancers of the upper lip seem to have a different biologic potential, with 25 % recurring and a 5-year survival of only 58 %. Worldwide variations in mortality of this disease may be due to differences in data collection, differences in age distribution, and failure to comply with the latest International Classification of Diseases. Management of solar cheilitis can be handled surgically, with antineoplastic medications such as 5-fluorouracil, cryotherpy, electrocautery, or laser ablation.

Suggested Further Reading

Kleinman DV, et al.. Cancers of the oral cavity and pharynx: a statistics review monograph 1973–1987. U.S. Atlanta: Department of Health and Human Services Public Health Service, 1991

Baker SR, Krause CJ. Carcinoma of the lip. Laryngoscope 1980; 90: 19–27

Neville BW, Damm DD, Allen CM, Bouquot JE. Oral and maxillofacial pathology. Philadelphia: WB Saunders, 1995: 259–321

Bouquot JE. Epidemiology. Pathology of the head and neck. Edited by Gnepp DR. New, Churchill Livingstone, 1988: 263–314

Douglas CW, Gammon MD. Reassessing the epidemiology of lip cancer. Oral Surg Oral Med Oral Pathol 1984; 57: 631–642

Shafer WG, Hine MK, Levy BM. A textbook of oral pathology. 4th Ed. Philadelphia: WB Saunders, 1983

Mincer HH, Coleman SA, Hopkins KP. Observations on the clinical characteristics of oral lesions showing histologic epithelial dysplasia. Oral Surg 1972; 33: 389–399

Bouquot JE, Gorlin RJ. Leukoplakia, lichen planus, and other oral keratoses in 23,616 white Americans over the age of 35 years. Oral Surg Oral Med Oral Pathol 1986; 61: 373–381

Waldron CA, Shafer WG. Leukoplakia revisited; a clinicopathologic study of 3256 oral leukoplakias. Cancer 1975; 36: 1386–1392

Cataldo E, Doku HC. Solar cheilitis. J Dermatol Surg Oncol 1981; 7: 989–993

Stanley RS, Roenigk RK. Actinic cheilitis: treatment with the carbon dioxide laser. Mayo Clinic Proc 1988; 63: 230–235

20.1.2 Squamous Cell Carcinoma of the Oral Cavity

Definition. Squamous cell carcinoma comprises over 90 % of all oral malignancies and about 4 % of the total malignancies in the United States. Pronounced geographical differences can be seen, however, with oral cancer constituting upwards of 20 % of all carcinomas in India.

Etiology. The precise etiology of oral carcinoma is unknown, but it is probably multifactorial with no single accepted agent. The most prominent factor is age, with the great majority of oral cancer patients being over the age of 45 years and prevalence increasing rapidly thereafter. Cigarette smoking and alcohol use are the other two most widely accepted correlates that figure in the etiology of oral cancer. India's high incidence is tied to the habitual use of betel quid. The relationship with smokeless tobacco is less compelling, but some report the risk of oral squamous cell carcinoma development in users is four times that in nonusers. These cancers usually form at the site of habitual placement of the tobacco and are often of the verrucous or exophytic type. Because of the higher-than-expected occurrence of oral carcinomas that behave more aggressively and appear at a younger age in AIDS patients, immunodeficiency may be relevant. Human papillomavirus has also been implicated as an etiologic factor, because of its presence in some oral cancers; however, these same viral types have also been found in normal oral epithelium. Other, previously suspected factors, such as vitamin deficiency, syphilis, and chronic irritation from dentures or irregular dentition, probably are not of consequence in the formation of oral squamous cell carcinoma.

Oral Manifestations. Early carcinoma of the oral cavity is most often seen as a white (leukoplakia) (Fig. 20.1) or red (erythroplakia Fig. 20.2) lesion. Leukoplakia is far more common than erythroplakia; however, a finding of erythroplakia is more ominous, with over 90 % of red lesions showing severe

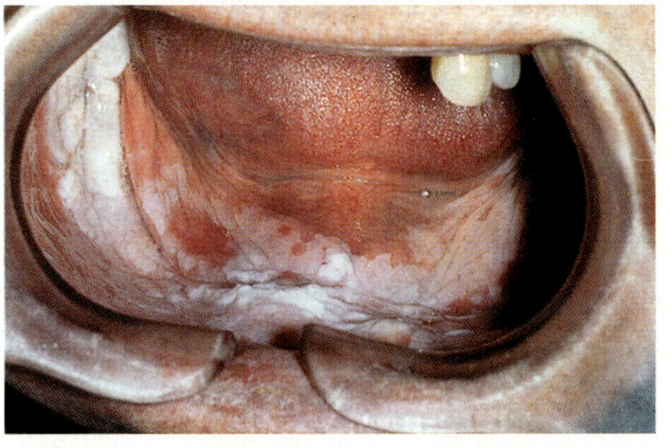

Fig. 20.1. Oral squamous cell carcinoma. Leukoplakia of the mandibular alveolus and floor of mouth. Biopsy revealed hyperkeratosis without dysplasia; however, verrucous carcinoma developed in the posterior component 2 years later

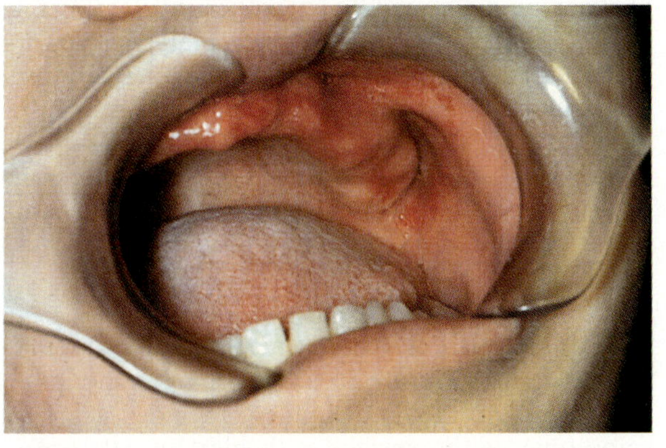

Fig. 20.2. Oral squamous cell carcinoma. Multifocal on the maxillary gingiva. Carcinoma in situ was found in several of the biopsy sites

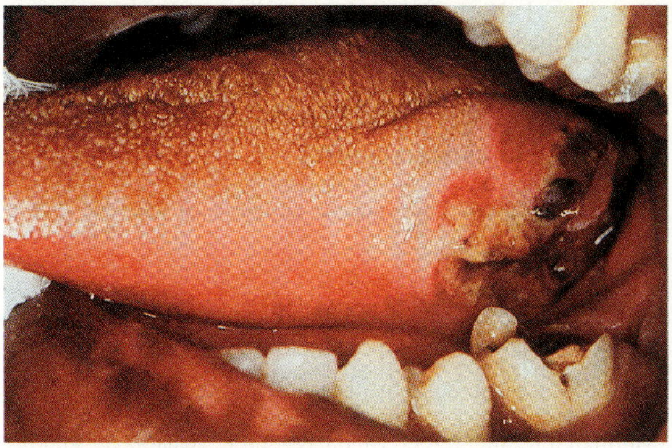

Fig. 20.3. Oral squamous cell carcinoma. Carcinoma on the posterior lateral tongue; one of the most common sites for development of oral squamous cell carcinoma

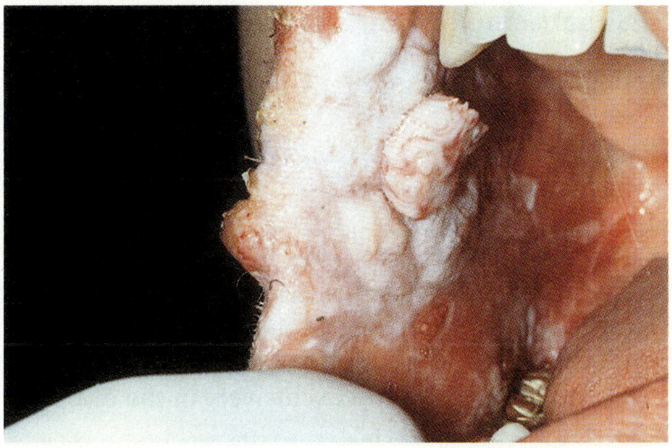

Fig. 20.4. Oral squamous cell carcinoma. Well-differentiated squamous cell carcinoma in areas of erythroplakia and leukoplakia

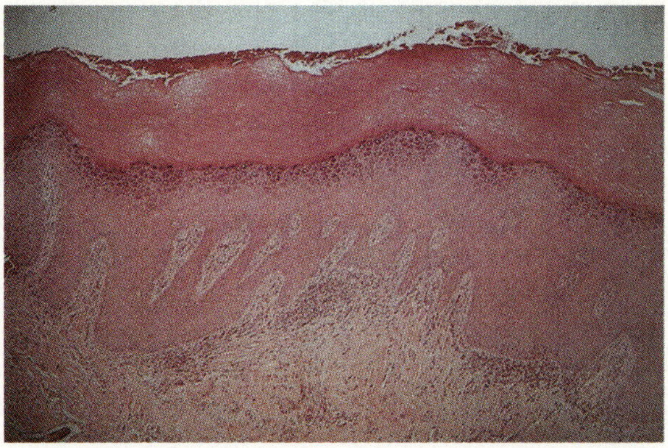

Fig. 20.5. Oral squamous cell carcinoma. Hyperkeratosis and acanthosis. Histologic findings from one of the biopsy sites of same patient as in Fig. 20.4

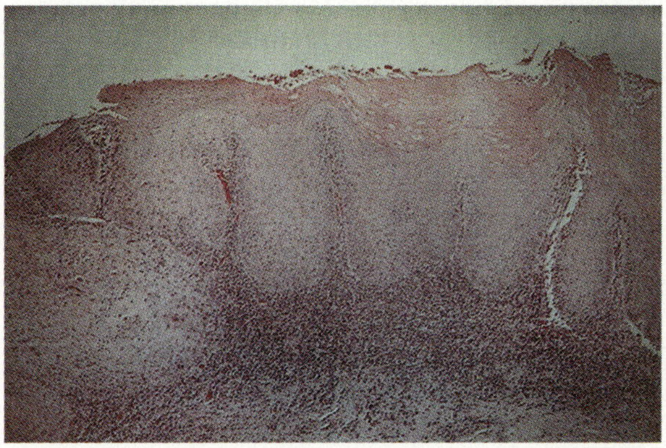

Fig. 20.6. Oral squamous cell carcinoma. Well-differentiated squamous cell carcinoma from one of the biopsy sites of same patient as in Fig. 20.4. The dense band of chronic inflammatory cells hugging the basement membrane should not be mistaken for a lichenoid process

dysplasia or invasive carcinoma on biopsy. Leukoplakias, on the other hand, are usually idiopathic benign hyperkeratoses, with only 4 %–8 % exhibiting significant dysplasia or malignancy and an eventual malignant transformation rate ranging from 5.9 % to 17.5 %, depending on the study. It should be noted that these studies included leukoplakias with a red erosive component. Approximately 90 % of the leukoplakias with malignant changes contained areas of erythroplasia. This underscores the prognostic importance of erythroplakia even when interspersed with leukoplakia. Another point of prognostic importance is that the great majority of oral squamous carcinomas develop on the ventrolateral tongue and the floor of the mouth (Fig. 20.3). Any lesion found in these areas should be viewed with heightened suspicion. Carcinoma of the gingiva, palate, and buccal mucosa follow in incidence (Fig. 20.4). Gingival cancers are most common on the posterior mandible, where they can closely mimic benign inflammatory changes such as periodontal disease or inflammatory hyperplasia associated with a denture flange. Ulceration, bleeding, pain, induration, and dysphagia are not seen until later stages, and at that point should not present a diagnostic challenge.

Associated Findings. Cervical lymphadenopathy may be seen as a late event in the progression of oral squamous carcinomas. Almost 21 % of patients present with cervical metastases at the time of diagnosis owing to delay in presentation. The relationship of *Candida albicans* to tumor formation is controversial, but a connection can be made because of the high rate of positive cultures in oral carcinomas, ranging from 53 % to 65 %. It is not known if the yeast produces dysplasia or is a secondary infection. Mutagenicity and carcinogenicity have not been proven.

Microscopic Findings. Leukoplakias are the result of hyperkeratoses with or without underlying malignancy or dysplasia (Figs. 20.5, 20.6). Erythroplakias almost always represent dysplasia or carcinoma. The lack of keratin formation, an atrophic epithelial layer, and a submucosal vascular proliferation associated with chronic inflammation impart the red color. Grades of dysplasia or carcinoma are similar to the cutaneous equivalents.

Diagnosis. Biopsy is the only valid method for diagnosis. No reliable clinical signs distinguish a reactive lesion from one that is neoplastic. A lesion that does not resolve 14 days after elimination of a suspected chemical, physical, thermal, or biologic stimulus is probably not reactive or inflammatory and needs further evaluation. A leukoplakia that persists for several years, occurs in a female, occurs in a smoker, is found on the floor of the mouth or ventrolateral tongue, or develops a granular or verruciform appearance is more likely to be malignant. All red lesions should be presumed malignant until proven otherwise.

Differential Diagnosis. Early squamous cell carcinomas of the oral cavity may bear a resemblance to tissue response from candidal infections, lichen planus, or injury of a physical, chemical, or thermal nature. An ulcer with a rolled border may be the result of a granulomatous process from a deep fungal infection, tuberculosis, tertiary syphilis, oral Crohn's disease, or chronic traumatic ulcers. Malignancies are usually seen as discrete lesions in high risk areas that persist despite the removal of local factors.

Treatment. Mild dysplasia is often the result of inflammation and resolves without treatment. It is not indicative of early malignancy. Lesions exhibiting moderate dysplasia, or worse, require removal or destruction by surgery, electrocautery, cryosurgery, or laser. Leukoplakias without dysplasia, if not removed, should be re-evaluated every 6 months because of the significant malignant transformation in as many as 17.5 %.

Carcinomatous change usually occurs between 2 and 4 years after the onset of a white plaque. Some white lesions have been successfully treated with systemic retinoids or topical applications of 0.05 % retinoic acid solution. Curative treatment for intraoral carcinoma consists of surgery and/or radiation. Chemotherapy is considered only as a palliative option. Surgery is favored for accessible tumors because of the long-term sequelae associated with radiation; xerostomia, osteoradionecrosis, and dental caries. Neck dissection and/or adjuvant radiation are indicated in tumors with histologically positive margins, perineural or vascular invasion, positive nodes, or a primary tumor site with a high rate of micrometastasis. The frequency of metastasis increases with the depth of invasion, the further posterior the tumor, and the lack of differentiation. Patients with one carcinoma of the throat or mouth are also at an increased risk for an additional malignancy. The tendency to develop multiple mucosal cancers has been termed "field cancerization".

Acknowledgement. Photographs courtesy of Michael Kahn, M.D.

Suggested Further Reading

Bouquot JE. Epidemiology. Pathology of the head and neck. Edited by Gnepp DR. New, Churchill Livingstone, 1988; 263–314

Silverman S Jr, Shillitoe EJ, Dillon WP, Fu K, Gallante M, Phillips TL, Silverberg IJ. Oral cancer. 3rd Ed. Edited by Silverman S Jr. American Cancer Society, Atlanta, 1990

20.2 Histopathology of Squamous Cell Carcinoma

A. Poiares Baptista and L. A. Born

Histopathology of squamous cell carcinomas (SCC) from the oral mucosa and from the skin is usually identical.

The main differences lie in the frequency of certain varieties. Whilst dyskeratotic, acantholytic, and spindle-cell forms are rare in the mucosa, florid oral papillomatosis, considered to be a variety of verrucous carcinoma, is found exclusively in the oral mucosa [1–3].

Squamous cell carcinomas are characterized by a proliferation of malpighian cells forming trabeculae or lobules with various shapes and sizes, arranged in different groupings. This proliferation, which continues more or less extensively with the mucosa of origin, may develop endophytically or exophytically. The limits of the proliferation may be clear or, as in most cases, imprecise and diffuse, with small groups of tumor cells dispersed in the surrounding stroma. The surface is usually ulcerated, and when it grows in depth it may reach underlying structures such as muscles, bone, and cartilage. Perineural infiltration, considered a marker of poor prognosis, is relatively rare.

There may be a variable inflammatory infiltrate on the peritumoral stroma, irrespective of the type and degree of tumor differentiation. It consists mainly of lymphomononuclear and plasma cells and, in tumors of the lip, also eosinophils.

Exocytosis is common, especially in lip carcinomas, sometimes forming intratumoral microabscesses.

The diversity of histopathological aspects results mainly from the cytological polymorphism and the type and degree of keratinization (Fig. 20.7): in well-differentiated forms, keratinization is fairly marked,

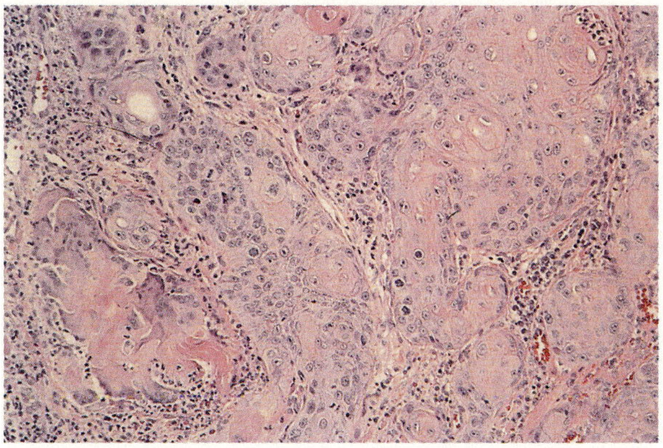

Fig. 20.7. Proliferation of malpighian cells in trabeculae with poorly defined limits, with some foci of keratinization, mitosis, and nuclear atypia

forming numerous horn pearls, and nuclear atypia and mitosis are rare and occur mainly at the periphery and in the deepest layers; in poorly differentiated and undifferentiated tumors, horn pearls are absent (the rare ones are incompletely formed) and there is nuclear atypia and frequent mitosis.

This is the basis for the classic classification of Broders: grade I (over 75 % keratinized cells); grade II (50 %–75 %); grade III (25 %–50 %), and grade IV (less than 25 % keratinized cells). Generally, there is some correspondence between the anatomical and clinical forms: exophytic keratotic papillomatous carcinomas are well differentiated (grades I and II), whilst the ulcerated endophytic forms are pooly differentiated and more aggressive (grades III and IV). However, there are many exceptions.

Among the different histopathological varieties of squamous cell carcinoma (dyskeratotic and acantholytic, spindle cell, verrucous, bowenoid), the following sections deal with the most relevant for oral mucosa.

20.2.1 Florid Oral Papillomatosis

The most striking feature of florid oral papillomatosis, a variety of verrucous carcinoma, is the contrast between its clinical aspect - papillomatous, expansive and aggressive - and its apparently benign histopathology.

The malpighian proliferation is characterized by accentuated hyperplasia, forming thick trabeculae with well-defined limits, hyperkeratosis and parakeratosis, conserved cellular stratification, no horn pearls, and infrequent nuclear atypia, which occurs only in the peripheral and deepest layers. In the papillary dermis, narrowed within the acanthotic proliferation, there is vasodilation and a scanty lymphomononuclear inflammatory reaction, sometimes with diffuse exocytosis of polymorphonuclear neutrophils (Fig. 20.8).

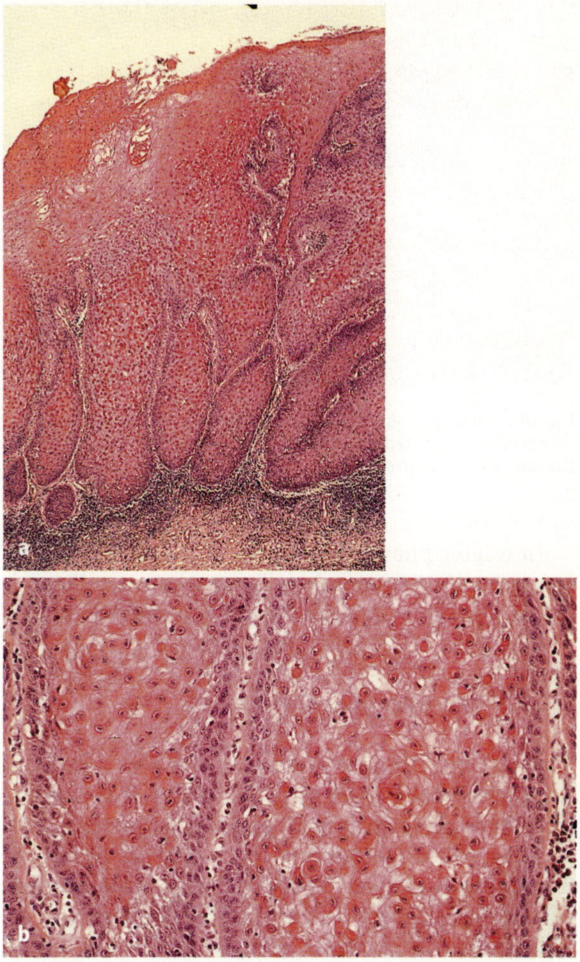

Fig. 20.8 a, b. Florid oral papillomatosis. **a** Hyperplasia with thick trabeculae with well-defined limits; **b** relative conservation of cellular stratification, intra- and extracellular edema, rare mitosis, and nuclear atypia at the periphery

In the most invasive lesions, there are areas of cellular atypia and abnormal mitosis and small groups of epithelial cells isolated in the dermis, suggesting evolution towards the more usual form of squamous cell carcinoma.

20.2.2 Bowenoid Squamous Cell Carcinoma

This is characterized by the relative thickness of the trabecular proliferation, its clear delimitation conserving the basement membrane, and, particularly, by loss of cellular stratification, great variability in size and shape of the nuclei, presence of numerous multinucleated cells, at all levels, frequency of dyskeratotic cells, and absence of horn pearls (Fig. 20.9).

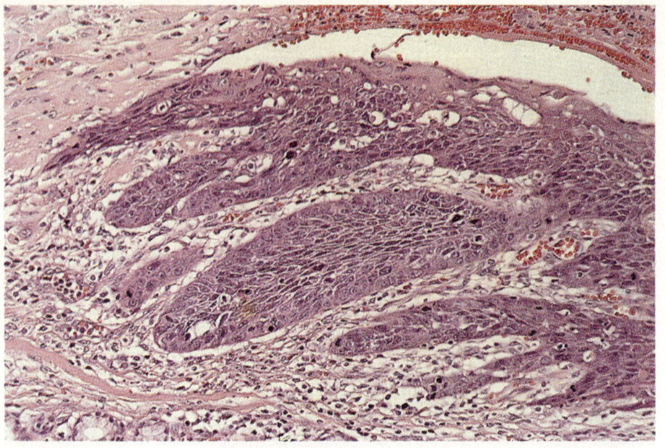

Fig. 20.9. Bowenoid squamous cell carcinoma: trabecular proliferation with well-defined limits, with complete loss of cellular stratification and widespread nuclear atypia

In a later phase, they can acquire the characteristics of an invasive trabecular squamous cell carcinoma, usually with a poor degree of differentiation.

20.2.3 Spindle Cell Squamous Carcinoma

This is quite rare in the mucosa, being usually localized at the free border of the lip, and it is characterized by a proliferation of spindle malpighian cells forming round (sometimes fasciculated), ill-defined masses, with nuclear atypia and a variable number of mitoses; corneal differentiation is absent or restricted to small cellular groups (Fig. 20.10).

Differential Diagnosis. The diagnosis of squamous cell carcinoma has to be discussed separately for each of its histopathological varieties.

Keratinizing and Trabecular Squamous Cell Carcinoma. This should be distinguished from pseudo-epitheliomatous hyperplasia which is associated with the benign lesions now listed.

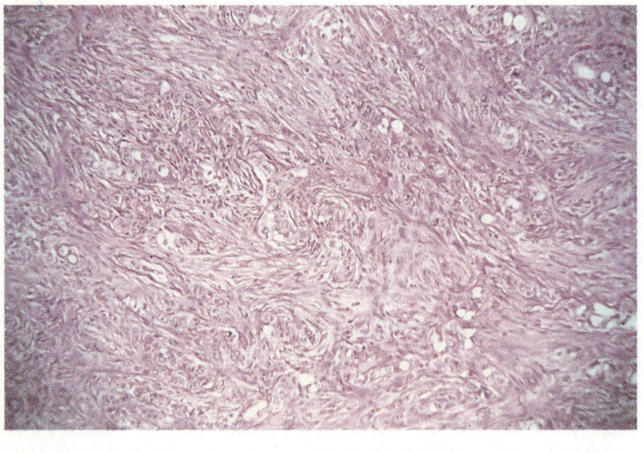

Fig. 20.10. Spindle-cell carcinoma: proliferation of malpighian spindle cells, scattered or in fasciculated strips

Granular cell myoblastoma (Abrikossov's tumor), a poorly keratinized papillomatous epidermal hyperplasia, is associated with the underlying proliferation formed by large polyhedral cells with clear cytoplasm containing acidophylic granules, arranged in strips that infiltrate the dermis.

In median rhomboid glossitis, malpighian hyperplasia is formed by thick and deep digitiform elongations, without nuclear atypia or mitosis, with well-defined limits, and there is an inflammatory infiltrate with lymphocytes, plasma cells, and polymorphonuclear neutrophils with exocytosis; at the surface there is parakeratosis and, particularly with a PAS stain, frequent mycelia can be seen.

Necrotizing sialometaplasia is characterized by one or two ulcerations about 1–2 cm in diameter on the palate, which regress spontaneously; it consists of foci of necrosis of the salivary glands associated with squamous metaplasia of the adnexa and salivary ducts.

Focal epithelial hyperplasia (Heck's disease) is of viral origin and consists of focal epithelial hyperplasia, acanthosis, and elongated rete ridges, with a ballooning type of nuclear degeneration.

Oral papillomatosis and warts are caused by human papillomavirus and characterized especially by acanthosis and sometimes hyperkeratosis, with occasional koilocytosis without nuclear atypia or mitosis.

Florid Oral Papillomatosis. Differential diagnosis is discussed mainly with the white sponge nevus: the proliferative type is identical, being also acanthotic, although less papillomatous and exophytic, and there is a characteristic intense vacuolization of the malpighian cells. The differential diagnosis is mainly clinical; this is familial, with an autosomic dominant mode of inheritance, begins in childhood, and may involve other mucosa (vagina, anus).

Spindle Cell Squamous Cell Carcinoma. Differential diagnosis is discussed with other spindle cell tumors, particularly amelanotic malignant melanoma and fibrosarcoma.

In favor of the spindle cell squamous carcinoma is the presence of areas of continuity with the epidermis, dyskeratotic cells, and intercellular bridges. However, in most cases, the differentiation is based on immunocytochemistry (keratins, S100 protein, HMB 45, etc.) and sometimes on electron microscopy.

20.3
Basal Cell Carcinoma (Basal Cell Epithelioma, Basalioma)

G. Landi and S. Feletti

Definition. Basal cell carcinoma (BCC) is a malignant epithelial neoplasm of the skin composed of basaloid cells similar to basal cells of the epidermis and its adnexa. It is a slow-growing tumor that extremely rarely metastasizes, although it can be strikingly destructive locally if neglected or inadequately treated.

Etiology and Pathogenesis. BCC is the most common cancer occurring in white races. Its prevalence increases with long-standing exposure to sunlight. Most people with fair skin, especially those who sunburn easily but tan poorly, are at increased risk [4]. However, many BCC develop on relatively sun-protected areas, such as the scalp, the inner canthus, and behind the ear, whereas the tumor is uncommon on the back of the hand and forearm. Thus, it has been suggested that besides the known effects of UV exposure, other regional factors, probably related to the density of pilosebaceous follicles, are capable of conditioning the distribution of BCC [5]. Indeed, BCC are seen almost exclusively on hair-bearing skin. They arise in the epithelium of pilosebaceous follicles, then spread over the adjacent surface epidermis. Furthermore, at least for the tumors located in the central panel of the face, a link with embryonic fusion planes may exist [6, 7].

The neoplastic epithelial cells take their origin from pluripotential primordial cells in the basal cell layers of the skin, and from the outer root sheath of the hair follicle or sebaceous gland or other cutaneous appendages [8].

Oral Manifestations. BCC are virtually unknown on the oral mucosa or the anogenital mucosa, due to the absence of follicular units on these mucous membranes. The vermilion of the lips is also nearly always spared. Even in the rare instances when BCC involves the vermilion, it does so from adjacent skin. BCC is most common on the upper lip, whereas squamous cell carcinoma is far more common on the lower lip.

Typically, the early lesions are small, smooth, skin-colored, roundish papules with a pearly, translucent appearance and overlying telangiectasia (Fig. 20.11). More advanced tumors, by a slow progressive course of peripheral extension, come to have a raised, rolled border, and at times central ulceration will develop (nodulo-ulcerative BCC) (Fig. 20.12).

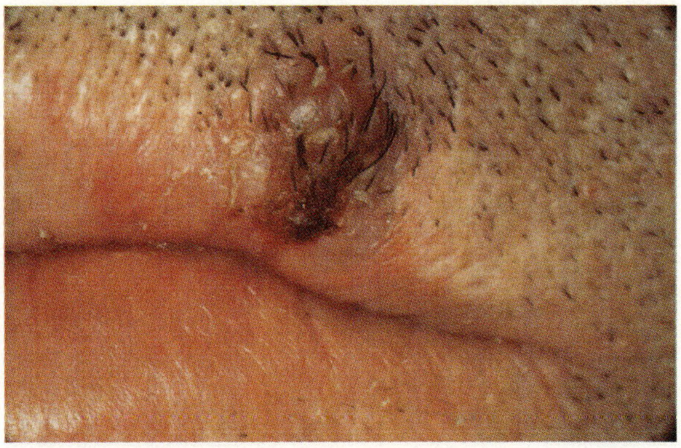

Fig. 20.11. Typical nodular basal cell carcinoma with exophytic growth and sharp delineation from normal skin

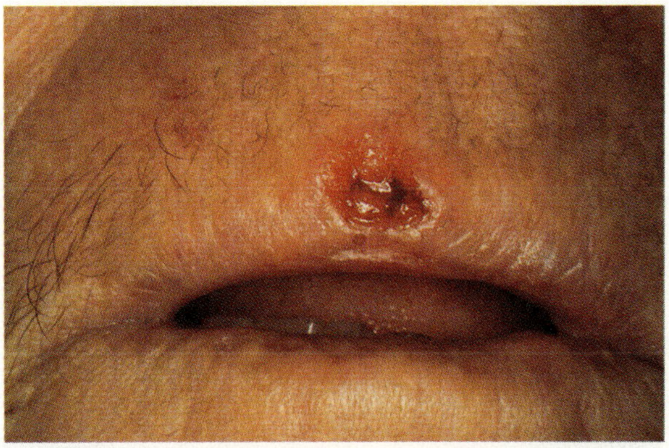

Fig. 20.12. Nodulo-ulcerative basal cell carcinoma in mild-portion of the upper lip. This lesion is characterized by a sharply circumscribed elevated border and a central ulcer covered by blood and crusts

Melanin pigment may be present to a variable extent, so that either only tiny flecks of brown pigment are apparent or a blue-black hue may involve the entire tumor, which may then be confused with a melanocytic lesion (pigmented BCC).

On the lips, less commonly than on covered portions of the trunk, BCC may spread only superficially, giving rise to large, plaque-like lesions. They have a slightly elevated thread-like border and an atrophic center. Discrete papules may occur within the plaque and slowly enlarge (superficial BCC; Fig. 20.13).

On occasion, BCC may present as a firm, thickened, scar-like plaque. The surface is smooth and ivory-colored (morpheaform BCC; Fig. 20.14). This lesion tends to develop in the nasolabial fold and is noted for its subclinical spread and high recurrence rate after treatment (Figs. 20.15, 20.16).

Associated Findings. BCC may arise in sebaceous nevi and other adnexal hamartomas. In some herita-

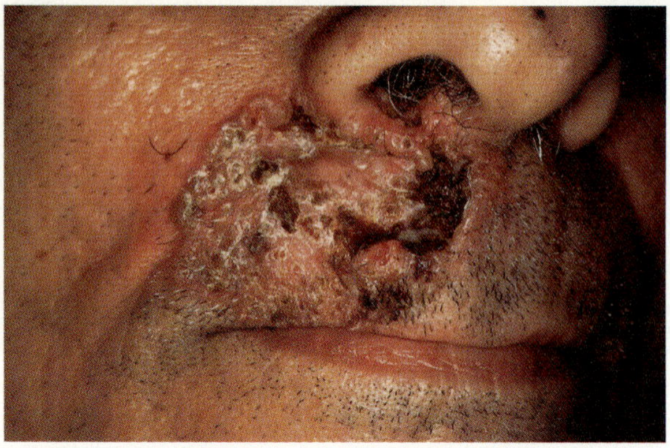

Fig. 20.13. Extensive neglected basal cell carcinoma on the whole right half of the upper lip. This lesion consists of a large, irregularly-shaped plaque with an elevated thread-like border. The surface is partially covered by scales and crusts, and tiny discrete papules are present

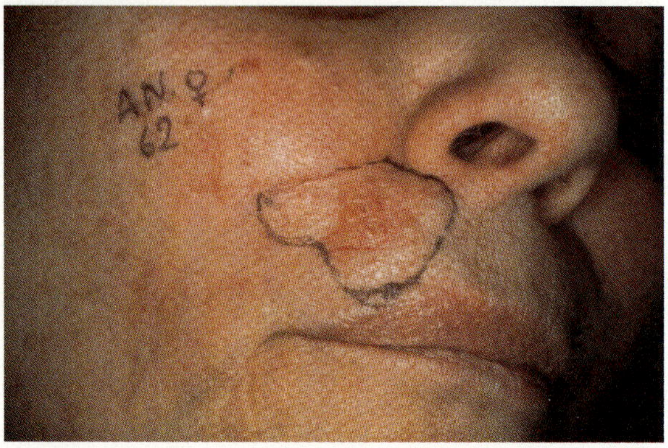

Fig. 20.14. Morpheaform basal cell carcinoma at a typical site in the nasolabial fold. Centrally translucent papules with telangiectases are present, and clinically ill-defined borders have been outlined by hand

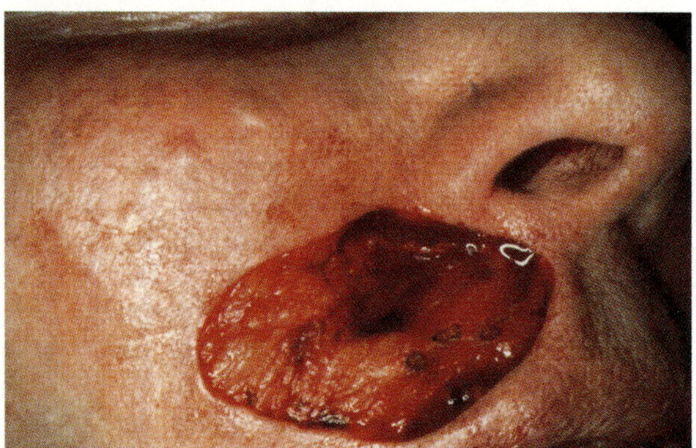

Fig. 20.15. Surgical defect following Mohs surgery for lesion in Fig. 20.14. Note extensive subclinical spread

ble syndromes, BCC develop more frequently and at a younger age than in the general population. Examples of these disorders include xeroderma pigmentosum and the nevoid basal cell carcinoma syndrome.

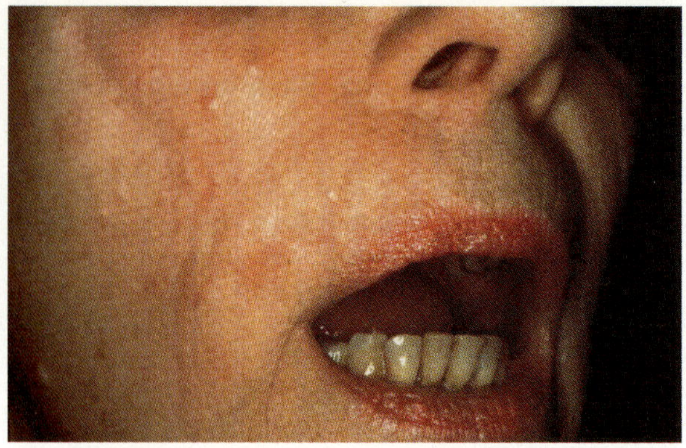

Fig. 20.16. Excellent cosmetic outcome after the surgical wound in Fig. 20.15 has been repaired with a transposition flap from the nasolabial fold

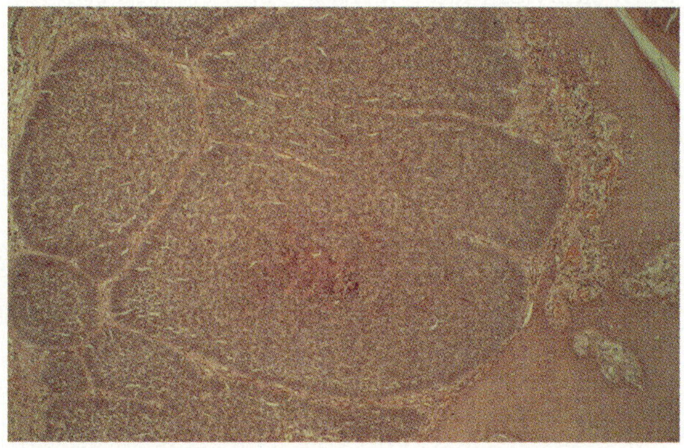

Fig. 20.17. Nodular basal cell carcinoma. It consists of large islands of uniform basaloid cells. At the periphery of each aggregation, the neoplastic cells are arranged in a palisade

Microscopic Findings. BCC are composed of irregularly sized and shaped masses of basaloid cells resembling those of the basal layer of the epidermis and the matrix cells of the appendages, embedded in a connective tissue stroma. Cells at the periphery of tumor islands tend to be arranged in palisades (Fig. 20.17). Characteristically, during tissue fixation, the stroma often shrinks close to edges of the tumor islands, producing artifactual clefts.

While most BCC grow as roundish expansile masses, some tumors are composed mainly of invasive strands penetrating the deeper structures [9] (Fig. 20.18).

Clinical Differential Diagnosis. BCC, especially in the initial stages, must be differentiated on occasion from trichoepithelioma, fibrous papule of the face (nose), melanocytic nevus, molluscum contagiosum, or senile sebaceous hyperplasia.

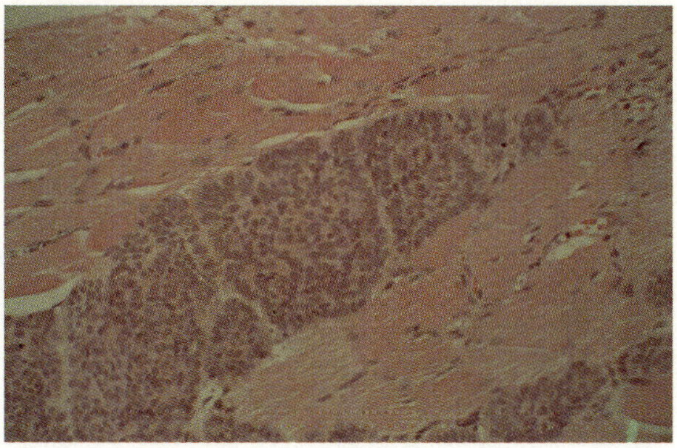

Fig. 20.18. Angulated strands of neoplastic basaloid cells without palisading penetrate the muscular tissue of the lip

Trichoepitheliomas, usually situated on the central panel of the face, lack the rolled borders and telangiectases of BCC. Fibrous papules of the face are usually solitary, firm, skin-colored, or pinkish papules without telangiectases or opalescent borders. Melanocytic nevi can be differentiated if hairs grow from the surface. In molluscum contagiosum and sebaceous hyperplasia, there is a central keratin-filled pit. It may be hard to distinguish BCC from keratoacanthoma and squamous cell carcinoma if scaling or crusting overlay the surface. On occasion, malignant melanoma may resemble darkly pigmented BCC. The borders of BCC are usually rolled with telangiectases and lack pigmented halo.

Treatment. Several therapeutic methods, surgical and nonsurgical, are currently available. The selection of the most appropriate modality depends on the tumor and on patient variables.

Tumor variables include whether the neoplasm is primary or recurrent, size and number of lesions, distinctness of the tumor borders, histologic growth pattern, and certain anatomic locations. The lips, like the nose, eyelids, ears, medial canthus, nasolabial fold, and scalp, are high-risk sites.

Patient variables such as age, medical status, and attendant medications must also be considered.

Nonsurgical Techniques. Radiation therapy is useful for definitive treatment of primary tumors and for palliation of inoperable cancers. This modality is usually reserved for elderly patients, particularly with rather extensive lesions, because the cosmetic results worsen with time, because of its potential carcinogenic effect, and because the chances of late radiation necrosis increase as time passes [10].

Topical chemotherapy with 5-fluorouracil has been widely used in recent years for managing small and superficial BCC. Topical 5 % should be applied twice a day for at least 6 weeks if not occluded or combined with curettage. Recurrence rates are greater than with other forms of treatment, so this method should be reserved for patients with superficial BCC for which no other therapeutic modality is feasible [11].

Surgical Techniques. Curettage and electrosurgery appear best suited for primary, well-defined, exophytic, nodular BCC as large as 1 cm in diameter, which are confined to the upper dermis and not situated in a high-risk area [12]. This method is less effective in the cure of recurrent lesions that are in scar tissue. Cryosurgery with liquid nitrogen has been advocated for primary small nodular BCC. In order to produce an adequate tumor kill, a double freeze-thaw cycle with a tissue temperature of $-50\,^{\circ}$C must be performed. However, because it is a blind treatment procedure, great care needs to be used in dealing with high-risk lesions [13].

Surgical excision is useful for both primary and recurrent BCC and has the advantages of histologic control, rapid healing, and optimal cosmetic result. Potentially, it can be employed for all types of BCC in all locations. The wound defects can be repaired primarily with side-to-side closures, grafts or flaps (Fig. 20.16), or allowed to heal by secondary intention [14, 15].

Mohs micrographic surgery is the treatment of choice for recurrent BCC, morpheaform BCC, extensively invading tumors, those in high-risk areas, and those that are ill-defined. With microscopic control of the completeness of removal at the entire perimeter and undersurface of the tumor, the procedure is capable of removing all neoplastic cells with minimal destruction to surrounding normal tissue [16] (Fig. 20.15).

20.4 Malignant Melanoma of the Oral Mucosa

A. Gollnick

Definition. Malignant melanoma of the oral mucosa is a rare, aggressive, highly malignant neoplasm of atypical melanocytes with a low survival rate, which was first described by Weber in 1859 [30]. Of all malignant melanomas, 0.2 %–8 % are located in the oral cavity, which represents an astonishing range of variance. Men are preferentially affected, with a sex ratio of 1.5–2 : 1, and mostly between the 40th and 60th years of life [22, 27, 30]. Oral mucosa malignant melanomas are more frequently observed in whites than in blacks [30].

Etiology. The etiology is unknown. In comparison with melanoma of the skin, there is no relation to

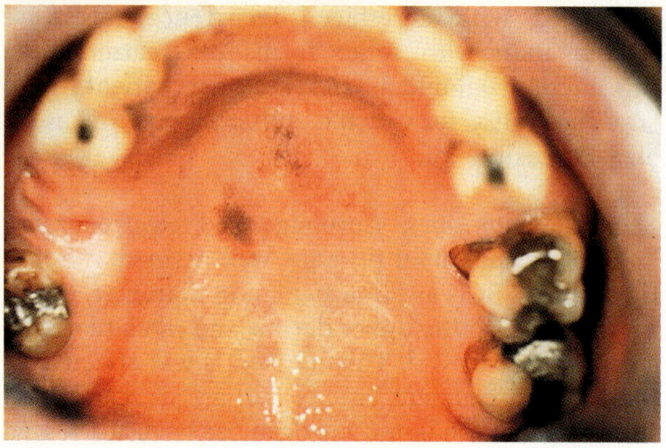

Fig. 20.19. Acrolentiginous melanoma of the oral mucosa

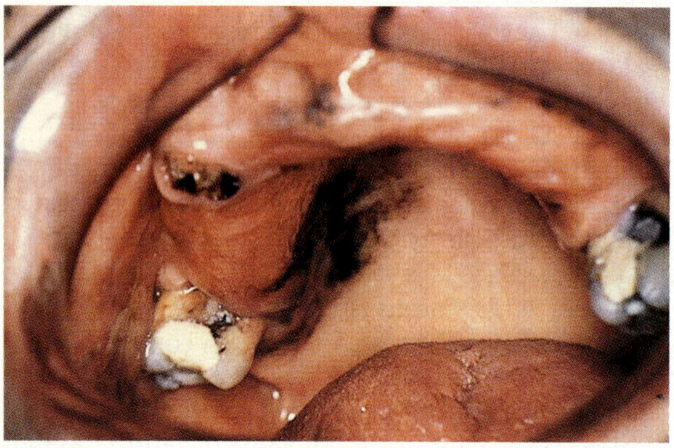

Fig. 20.20. Superficial spreading melanoma of the oral mucosa

sun exposure [24, 25, 33]. Whether local trauma predisposes to the condition, as in the case of lentigo maligna melanoma of the plantar skin in blacks, has to be further elucidated.

The origin of melanocytes is the neural crest cells. In the early fetal period, they migrate through cellular spaces enlarged by hydrated glycosaminoglycan and fibronectin of the basal cell layer to any localization of the organism. Generally, mucosal melanocytes are metabolically inactive and do not produce melanin. It is presumed that endogenic, exogenic, or local factors can disturb this chemical balance. The activation of a tyrosinase containing copper can initiate the production of melanin by polymerization of transformed products of dihydroxyphenylalanine (DOPA). The potential for oral nevi to undergo malignant transformation is unknown. Review of the literature revealed that in about 30 % of the patients with oral melanoma, pre-existing macular pigmentation was present for a variable period of time [20, 23].

Oral Manifestations. Four types of oral mucosal malignant melanoma are distinguished: acrolentiginous melanoma (ALM; mucosal malignant melanoma; Fig. 20.19); superficial spreading melanoma (SSM; pagetoid melanoma; Fig. 20.20); lentigo maligna melanoma (LMM); and nodular melanoma (NM).

The border of the almost indolent tumor is usually irregular and indistinct. The pigmentation is dark brown to bluish black, often accompanied by variations in color. Parts of the tumor may be free of pigment. Sometimes, the whole primary tumor is free of melanin (amelanotic melanoma). More than 50 % of oral mucosa malignant melanomas are located in the area of the hard palate, and about 20 % at the maxillary gingiva. It is rare for them to be found on the buccal gingiva, the tongue, or on the floor of the mouth. The cardinal symptoms are bleeding, pain during eating, recurring inflammation due to superinfections, removed prosthetic material, or perceptible resistance.

Associated Findings. In an advanced stage, the typical symptoms of late metastatic malignant melanoma occur, e.g., loss of weight, deterioration in general condition, metastases in lymph nodes - especially cervical lymph nodes - or visceral metastases - especially in brain, lungs, and liver, but also in any other organ, followed by corresponding visceral dysfunction.

Microscopic Findings. LMM is characterized by reticular aggregation of atypical, darkly pigmented melanocytic cells invading the basal cell layer and infiltrating the upper lamina propria as vertically growing masses. ALM has acanthotic squamous epithelium with atypical proliferating melanocytes penetrating into the lamina propria. In SSM, the acanthotic squamous epithelium is invaded by large, rounded, atypical melanocytes having abundant pale cytoplasm, similar to the that of cells in Paget's disease (pagetoid melanoma). In the lamina propria,

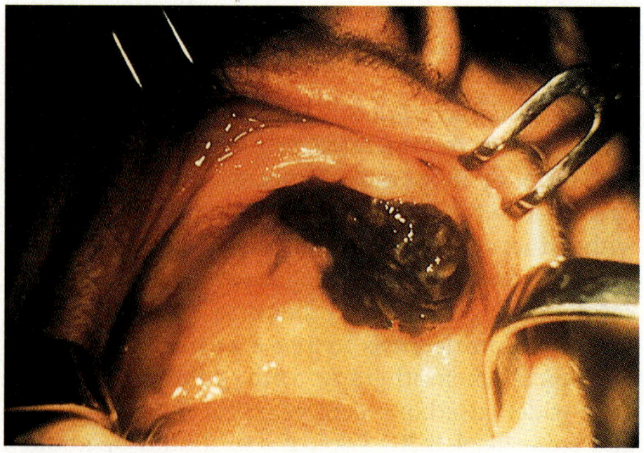

Fig. 20.21. Nodular melanoma of the oral mucosa

Table 20.1. Classification of mucosal malignant melanoma according to the invasion level [19, 20]

• Level I	Tumor limited to squamous epithelium and lamina propria
• Level II	Tumor has invaded submucosa to a depth of 1 mm
• Level III	Tumor has invaded submucosa to a depth of 1–2 mm
• Level IV	Tumor has invaded submucosa to a depth of more than 2 mm, but submucosal adipose tissue is not affected
• Level V	Tumor has invaded submucosal adipose tissue

there is usually a cellular inflammation. In the case of NM, melanoma cells (spindle-type, epitheloid, polymorphic, or nonmelanized cells) occur in the squamous epithelium, lamina propria, and (sometimes) in the submucosa. The stromal inflammatory reaction is pronounced.

The tumor volume and the depth of penetration are the determining parameters with substantial prognostic significance (Fig. 20.21, Table 20.1). Immunohistochemistry and melanin bleaching are used to assess the expression of antigens identified by anti-S-100, anti-HMB-45, or, for example, NKi-C3 antibodies on melanomas [21, 28]. Owing to the minimal cohesion of the melanocytes, cytologic investigations of oral smears seem to be possible. In the literature, the results of smear cytologies are controversially discussed [32].

Diagnosis. The symptoms and the clinical picture can point to the tentative diagnosis of an oral mucosal malignant melanoma, but histologic confirmation is required in each case. The definitive diagnosis of malignant melanoma requires a detailed examination, including computerized tomography of the cranium, abdomen, and, if necessary, the thorax. Sono-

Table 20.2. Oral mucosal malignant melanoma and differential diagnosis (+++ strong, ++ moderate, + low, – not present)

Diagnosis	Symptoms		Dermatological findings					
	Bleeding	Pain	Pigmentation		Border		Resistance	
			Color	Irregular	Irregular	Indistinct	Firm	Soft
Primary mucosal malignant melanoma	++	–/++	Dark brown to bluish black	+++	+++	+++	++	–
Mucosal metastatis of malignant melanoma	+	–	Gray to black, erythematous	+++/–	+++	+/–	+	+
Benign melanocytic nevi (junctional, intramucosal, compound nevi, lentiginous)	–	–	Light brown to dark brown to black	–/+	–/+	–/+	+	–
N. Blue nevus	–/+	–	Dark blue to bluish black	–	–	–/+	++	–
Foreign material (amalgam tattoo)	–/++	–/++	Gray to black	–	++	+	+++	–
Hemangioma varix	+/+++	+/++	Livid to dark blue, teleangiectatic	++	+/–	++	–	++
Hemosiderin	–	–	Yellow-brown	–	++	+	–	–
Papilloma fibroma	–	–	Mucosa-like to erythematous	–	–	–/+	–	++
Mucous cyst	–	–/+	Mucosa-like to anemic	–	–	–	Elast.	–
Granuloma	++	++	Erythematous to livid	–	+	+	+	–
Eruption cysts	–	–	Mucosa-like to bluish	+	–	–	+	–
Exostosis/tori	–	–	Mucosa-like	–	–/+	–	+++	–
Bone or cartilaginous neoplasm	–	–/+	Mucosa-like to erythematous	–	–/+	–/+	++	–
Lipoma/liposarcoma	–	–/+	Yellow-erythematous to mucosa-like	–	–	–	–	++
Carcinoma	++	–/++	Erosive-necrotic erythematous	+	++	++	+	–
Kaposi's sarcoma	+	–/+	Livid-erythematous to mucosa-like	+	++	++	++	–
Tertiary yaws	++	++	Necrotic-erythematous, ulcerous	–	–	–	+	–
Mucocutanous leishmaniasis	+++	++	Necrotic-erythematous, ulcerous	–	–	–	+	–

graphy of the lymph nodes, X-ray of the lung, and bone scan scintigram are also useful to detect metastases.

Differential Diagnosis. The differential diagnosis includes melanotic tumors as well as amelanotic tumors (Table 20.2). Sometimes, pigmented melanocytic lesions can point to several syndromes such as Peutz-Jeghers syndrome or Addison's disease. Hyperestrogenemia, for example during pregnancy, can also cause lentigines in the oral cavity. Following petechial bleedings, particularly in Wiskott-Aldrich syndrome, Bernard-Soulier syndrome, or idiopathic thrombocytopenic purpura, deposition of hemosiderin can occur. Frequently, following local trauma, postinflammatory hyperpigmentations, granulomas, or melanoacanthomas as mixed tumors made up of keratinocytes and melanocytes can occur. Particularly, the primary nodular malignant melanoma can be confused with metal impregnations, especially by amalgam. In the case of AIDS patients, macular or nodular Kaposi's sarcoma should be included in the differential diagnosis considerations [17, 18, 29, 30].

Treatment. Malignant melanoma of the oral cavity is a high-risk melanoma and should be classified as an advanced stage III–IV melanoma. In most cases, the diagnosis is made in advanced stages. The primary tumor should be treated by surgery whenever possible and as soon as possible. In conformity with general recommendations, cutaneous melanomas should be excised with safety margins of 3 cm all round. In the oral cavity, the excision has to be a function of the anatomy. If there is no evidence of distant metastases, the regional lymph nodes should be excised, even if they are not clinically palpable or detectable by sonography. Following surgical treatment, an adjuvant immunochemotherapy is indicated with various preparations, particularly dacarbazine, interferon alpha or beta, and vindesine (Table 20.3) [25, 31]. The surgical treatment of metastatic malignant melanoma, as defined by reduction of tumor, is indicated if there are solitary metastases. If there are distant metastases, a cytostatic treatment, combined in special cases with radiotherapy, can achieve reduction of the tumor mass (Table 20.4). In several studies, the response rates of immunochemotherapy with dacarbazine and interferon alpha are up to 20 %; the response rates to polychemotherapy with cisplatinum, vindesine and dacarbazine are up to 20 %–40 % [31]. Hematogenous metastasis spreads mainly to the lung, the liver, the bones, and – in view of the topography – to the brain. In the past, the treatment of cerebral metastases was a domain of neurosurgery and radiotherapy because most cytostatic agents are unable to pass the blood-brain barrier. Fotemustine, a nitrosurea derivative, can pass this barrier, being lipophilic, and can achieve a therapeutic level in liquor. In combination with telecobalt radiation, response rates of 40 %–50 % have been observed [34]. Radiotherapy of primary melanoma has only very low response rates and is only a palliative procedure in advanced cases of large ulcerated melanoma. The regression of irradiated metastases depends on the diameter of the metastasis and the individual dose. If the diameter is larger than 4 cm, the response rate is lower than 50 %. A total dose of 30–60 Gy should be applied [31, 34]. Experimental therapeutic procedures with cryoapplication and carbon dioxide laser are of some value in the oral cavity with regard to the functional anatomy, but determination of the prognosis is only possible if there is a complete histological review of the melanoma.

Table 20.3. Adjuvant chemotherapy

Scheme	Mode of administration
DTIC	200–250 mg/m^2 IV on days 1–5, repeated every 4 weeks (12–24 cycles)
DTIC + IFN alpha	20–250 mg/m^2 IV on day 1, repeated every 3 weeks (9–18 cycles) 9 million IU 3 times a week (1–2 years)
BHD	BCNU 150 mg/m^2 IV on day 1, every 2nd cycle Hydroxurea 1500 mg/m^2 PO on days 1–5 DITC 150 mg/m^2 IV on days 1–5, repeated every 4 weeks (6 cycles)

Table 20.4. Selection of chemotherapies for treatment of metastatic malignant melanoma

Author/year	Mode of administration
Garbe et al. (1993) [70]	Vindesine 3 mg/m^2 IV repeated every 2 weeks IFN alpha 3–9 million IU SC 3 times a week (1 year)
Dummer et al. (1990) [71]	DTIC 250 mg/m^2 CI on days 1–5 IL-2 18 million IU IV on days 21–24, 28–31, repeated every 7 weeks
Gunderson et al. (1987)	DTIC 200 mg/m^2 IV on days 1–5 Vindesine 3 mg/m^2 IV on day 1 Cisplatin 100 mg/m^2 IV on day 1, repeated every 4 weeks
Richards et al. (1992)	DTIC 220 mg/m^2 IV on days 1–3 BCNU 150 mg/m^2 IV on day 1 of every 2nd cycle Cisplatin 25 mg/m^2 IV on days 1–3 Tamoxiphen 2 × 10 mg/day. PO, repeated every 3 weeks
Falkson et al. (1991) [72]	DTIC 200 mg/m^2 IV on days 22–26 every 4 weeks IFN alpha 15 million IU SC on days 1–5 (3 weeks) then 10 million IU SC 3 times a week (2 years)
Ulrich et al. (1995) [34][a]	Fotemustine 100 mg/m^2 IV on days 1, 7, 14, then 100 mg/m IV every 3 weeks Telecobalt radiation to a dose of 60 Gy

[a] Cerebral metastases.

In advanced stages with extensive metastases, an improvement of the quality of life could be achieved with low expenditure by means of such methods. The prognosis is very poor. Compared with mucosal malignant melanomas in other localizations, such as the vulva, vagina, or rectum, the 5-year survival rate of this high-risk tumor is lower than 10 % [19].

20.5 Malignant Mesenchymal Tumors

20.5.1 Lymphomas and the Oral Cavity

G. Hautmann, M. Benci, and T.M. Lotti

20.5.1.1 *Mucosal and Cutaneous Lymphomas*

20.5.1.1.1 *Introduction*

Definition. Mucosal and cutaneous lymphoma (CL) is a monoclonal proliferation of lymphoid cells, presenting primarily in the skin and mucosa in the absence of any detectable extracutaneous lesion (despite careful and complete staging procedures) for at least 6 months from diagnosis.
Thus, it should be now accepted that involvement of the skin secondary to nodal lymphomas is something completely different from cutaneous lymphomas.

Classification. According to histoimmunologic and genotypic features, CL are divided into two main groups: cutaneous T-cell lymphoma (CTCL) and cutaneous B-cell lymphoma (CBCL). This distinction reflects some basic clinical and biologic differences: the long-term behavior and prognosis of CTCL are, as a rule, more aggressive and less favorable than those of CBCL. Moreover, therapy of CTCL creates great problems in terms of either complete remission rate or possibility of maintaining sustained complete remission. CL can be classified as reported in Table 20.5 [35–39].

Table 20.5. Mucosal and cutaneous lymphomas: a classification

1) Cutaneous B-cell lymphomas (CBCL)
   a) Chronic course
      SALT-related CBCL
      Follicular center cell lymphoma
      Immunocytoma
   b) Rare and/or unclassifiable CBCL
2) Cutaneous T-cell lymphomas (CTCL)
   a) Chronic course
      Mycosis fungoides (MF)
      CD30+ CTCL non-MF
      CD30− small to medium-sized, pleomorphic cells
   b) Aggressive course
      CD30− large-sized cells
   c) Rare and/or unclassifiable CTCL

Diagnosis. The diagnosis of CL and its differentiation from reactive lympho-proliferative disorders are actually supported by immunophenotyping and genotyping. In fact, the key criterion for the diagnosis of CL and its differentiation from pseudolymphoma is the demonstation of monoclonality.

20.5.1.1.2 *Mycosis Fungoides*

Definition, Epidemiology, Etiology. Mycosis fungoides is a cutaneous T-cell lymphoma; it is a chronic disease, usually with slow progression, of unknown etiology, which starts from the skin and remains a skin disease, but which in its later phases can also affect the lymph nodes and internal organs, and take a lethal course. It usually develops after the age of 40 years; there is no hereditary element, but there is male predominance of unestablished cause.

Clinical Features. The clinical course progresses in three stages: the premycotic, erythematous stage (an intensely pruritic eruption that may resemble psoriasis, so that it also used to be called parapsoriasis en plaque); the plaque stage, which is characterized by the presence of irregularly shaped, well-demarcated, slightly elevated, and indurated plaques; the tumor stage which usually occurs within the the flat infiltrated patches or on erythroderma. The tomato-type, hemispherical, mushroom-type, or indented tumors, are raised above the skin and are mostly soft, fungoid, and blue to brownish-red in color; these tend to ulcerating necrosis.

Oral Manifestations. Mycosis fungoides rarely involves the oral cavity. Less than 35 cases of oral CTCL had been reported in detail up to 1996. It usually develops after cutaneous lesions, in the plaque and tumor stages of the disease. Clinically, the most common presentation is an extensive erythema, which later progresses into indurated plaque (Fig. 20.22), ulcerated plaque, or tumor of the gingiva (Fig. 20.23), palate, or tongue, although any intraoral site can be involved.

Microscopic Findings. Histologic examinations of the oral lesions of mycosis fungoides usually show

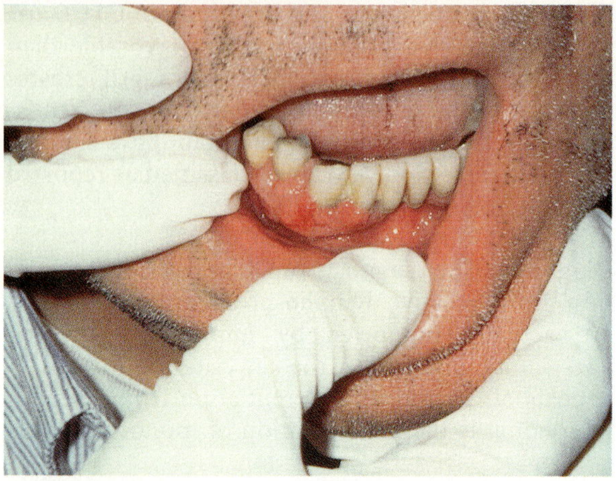

Fig. 20.22. Indurated plaque of the gingiva in a patient with mycosis fungoides

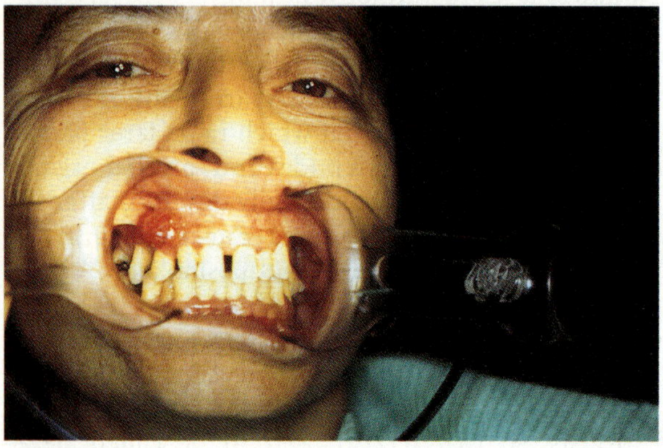

Fig. 20.23. Nodular lesion of the gingiva

a lichenoid lymphocytic infiltration of lamina propria; these cells are sometimes also present in the epithelium, forming microabscesses. These cells are small and atypical, with little cytoplasm and large nuclei.

Differential Diagnosis. It must be differentiated from oral lesions of dermatomyositis, lupus erythematosus, and other lymphomas.

Treatment. The choice of treatment depends on the staging of the disease, the size and site of the lesions, and whether involvement of the lymph nodes and/or visceral organs is present. Mycosis fungoides may be treated in the early stages with topical corticosteroids and/or carmustine, perhaps in association with UVB. PUVA therapy is also an option. In the plaque and tumor stages, the chemotherapeutic approach is largely used. Monochemotherapy (with bleomycin, cyclophosphamide, metothrexate, etc.) may be tried, or polychemotherapy, which is indicated in the tumor stages.

20.5.1.2
Systemic Lymphomas

20.5.1.2.1
Hodgkin's Disease

Definition and Epidemiology. This is a systemic malignant lymphoma, and skin lesions occur in about 30 %–50 % of patients. It can occur at any age, but incidence peaks between 15 and 35, and also after 50 years. There is a male predominance.

General Clinical Features. General symptoms are anorexia, weight loss, fever, night sweats. The lymphoma is classified into four stages and further characterized as A or B, depending on the absence or presence of systemic manifestations. The staging (along with the hystologic types) of disease influences the therapy.

Skin Lesions. The skin manifestations must be differentiated into specific and nonspecific skin changes. The nonspecific ones are relatively common, and polymorphous: pruritus, hyperpigmentation ichtyosis-type skin changes, herpes zoster, and, more rarely, alopecia diffusa, erythema nodosum, eczematoid reactions (Fig. 20.24), mucinosis follicularis, erythroderma, and nail growth disorders. The specific skin manifestations of Hodgkin's disease are very rare and are identified histologically by the specific criteria for this disease (demonstration of cells positive for the monoclonal antibody Ki-1). They comprise a heterotopic infiltration that appears as flat, infiltrated patches with diffuse margins or cutanous-subcutaneous brownish or livid-red firm nodules, as in other malignant lymphomas [35, 36]. These lesions may be single or multiple, and the preferred sites are the front and sides of the trunk, the lower abdomen, the inguinal region and thigh, and the scalp. The nodules can grow and develop ulcerating necrosis.

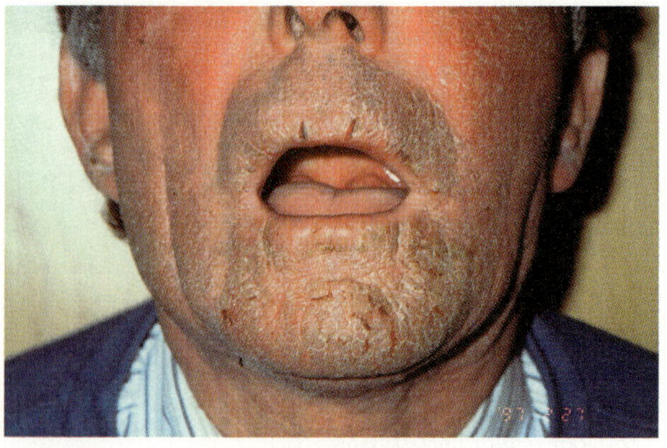

Fig. 20.24. Eczematoid reaction involves lips

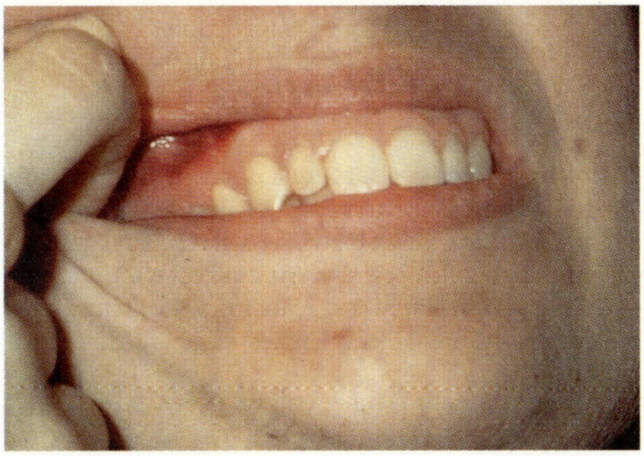

Fig. 20.25. A red, swollen area of the gingiva in a patient with Hodgkin's disease

Oral Manifestations. Sometimes, the initial signs of this lymphoma consist of specific infiltration of the lymphatic tonsillar ring, which can ulcerate. Moreover, the onset of the disease is often in a submandibular node or in a cervical lymph node with painless enlargement. Oral symptoms of Hodgkin's disease are rare and appear as ulcers or red, swollen areas (Fig. 20.25). The gingiva is usually not involved, in contrast to myeloid leukemia and agranulocytosis.

Diagnosis. For diagnosis, laboratory tests are essential, especially histologic examination and immunologic markers of infiltrating cells [35, 36].

20.5.1.2.2
Non-Hodgkin's Lymphomas

Definition and Epidemiology. Non-Hodgkin's lymphomas are a heterogeneous group of neoplastic diseases that originate from lymphocytic cell lines. They represent about 70 % of all lymphomas; they occur at any age and affect both sexes equally.

General Clinical Features. The onset can be fulminant or quiet, and the presenting symptom is usually represented by a painless lymphadenopathy. There may be weight loss and fever. The nodes most frequently involved are the cervical, axillary, and inguinal lymph nodes.

Oral Manifestations. Oral manifestations may be part of disseminated disease or the only manifestation. The lymphoma appears as a painless swelling, and in the advanced phases of the disease it may ulcerate; the ulcer presents an irregular surface; its base is inflamed and indurated. The most frequent sites involved are the tonsillar area, the palate, the tongue, the posterior gingiva, and the floor of the mouth.

Differential Diagnosis. The ulcer must be differentiated from Hodgkin's disease, Wegener's granulomatosis, lethal midline granuloma, eosinophilic ulcer, and squamous cell carcinoma.

Diagnosis. Diagnosis requires histologic examination and immunotyping of the infiltrating cells.

Treatment. The ulcer is usually treated by radiotherapy or chemotherapy [35, 36].

20.5.1.2.3
Burkitt's Lymphoma

Definition. Burkitt's lymphoma (African lymphoma, lymphoblastic lymphoma) rarely involves the skin; it is a high-grade malignant B-cell lymphoma that develops with great rapidity and affects mainly African children.

Epidemiology and Etiology. The distribution of this tumor depends largely on temperature and humidity, and it has been suggested that an infective agent might be incriminated, possibly with an insect vector. The infective agent is thought to be the Epstein-Barr virus (which is also the cause of mononucleosis).

General Clinical Features. This lymphoma is often bilateral and affects both maxillae and mandibles. Other organs frequently involved are the ovaries, kidneys, and adrenals, again often bilaterally. The celiac lymph nodes, liver, stomach, intestines, testes, spleen, and retroperitoneal tissues are often involved. The lungs, long bones, and brain are usually spared.

Oral Manifestations. The jaw involvement is most frequent in young children, occurring in 100 % of African cases below the age of 3 and then falling. This may provoke bone destruction and tooth loss, so that large ulcerating masses may be seen in the mouth.

Microscopic Findings. The histopathologic findings usually confirm the diagnosis: the histology is in fact characteristic: sheets of small, darkly staining round cells occupy the bulk of the soft tumor masses, which often contain areas of hemorrhage and necrosis. There are many clear spaces, which often contain one or more pale cells with a vesicular nucleus and large nucleoli: these give the characteristic "starry sky" appearance. The cells are small, non-cleaved, follicular center cells.

Differential Diagnosis. These oral manifestations have to be differentiated from other cancers of childhood and other types of lymphomas, and from central giant cell granuloma, ossifying fibroma, and odontogenic tumors.

Treatment. Treatment consists in radio- and/or chemotherapy [35, 36, 39].

20.5.1.2.4
Multiple Myeloma

Definition. In the course of multiple myeloma, extra-osseous lesions in association with multiple myeloma are not uncommon, and the skin is infiltrated in a fair number of cases.

General Manifestations. Primary involvement of the skin without evidence of bone marrow involvement is, however, extremely rare. The lesions present as small tumors of a red color, which enlarge and may metastasize. Histologically, they consist of a mass of plasma cells, mainly normal but with some abnormal forms. This disease is more common in men over 50 years of age. The most frequent sites of involvement are the skull, sternum, pelvis, ribs and clavicles.

Oral Manifestations. The jaws (particularly the mandible) are also frequently affected, and jaw involvement may be the presenting manifestation. The oral symptoms usually present are pain, paresthesia, bone swelling, and mobility of teeth; a painless, soft, nonspecific swelling on the gingiva and alveolar mucosa may complete the spectrum of the oral involvement.

Differential Diagnosis. It must be differentiated from the plasmocytoma of the oral mucosa. This is an unusual neoplasm that consists of plasma cells. It is considered to be a solitary extramedullary form of multiple myeloma that most often affects men over 50 years of age. The primary plasmocytoma of soft tissues generally arises in submucous tissues of the upper respiratory tract or oral cavity. It is localized on the palate, the gingiva, and, more rarely, on the buccal mucosa, the floor of the mouth, and the tongue. It appears as a painless soft swelling with a smooth normal surface, which may ulcerate in the advanced phases. It ranges from 1 to several centimeters in diameter. The subject with this disease can develop generalized multiple myeloma or can die as a result of local invasion [35, 36, 39].

20.5.2
Kaposi's Sarcoma

D. Cerimele and F. Cottoni

Definition. Kaposi's sarcoma is a multicentric angiogenic tumor. Four types of Kaposi's sarcoma (KS) have been described: (1) Classic or sporadic KS, (2) iatrogenic KS, (3) African or endemic KS, and (4) AIDS-related or epidemic KS. There is a male predominance in all types of KS [40].

Etiology. A viral etiology of KS has been suspected since 1972 [41], but only with the discovery of KSHV (HHV-8) was a sound candidate detected for the etiology of Kaposi's sarcoma [42].

Pathogenesis. Three factors appear to be at work in the pathogenis of KS: (1) genetic predisposition, (2) immunosuppression, and (3) a virus or viruses (KSHV/HHV-8) [43–46].
The relative relevance of these factors is different in the four types: immunosuppression is important in AIDS-related and in iatrogenic KS, while genetic predisposition is important in classic KS.

Oral Manifestations. Nodular or vegetating, usually ulcerated lesions, preferentially located on the hard palate (Fig. 20.26) are frequently observed in AIDS-related KS; violaceous patches (Fig. 20.27), or nodules (Fig. 20.28) may be observed on the oral mucosa in classic or iatrogenic KS.

Associated Findings. These also vary with the type of KS. In classic KS, violaceous macules or patches on the feet and scattered blue nodules, particularly on the legs, are characteristic features. In iatrogenic KS, which is observed mainly in renal transplant recipients, the lesions are nodules in most cases, with a

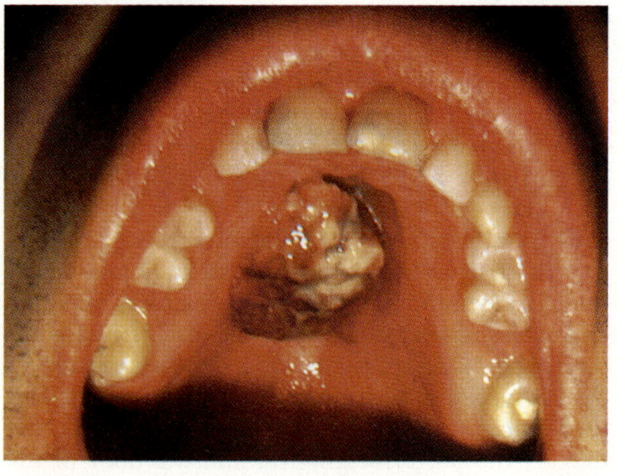

Fig. 20.26. Vegetating lesion of Kaposi's sarcoma on the hard palate

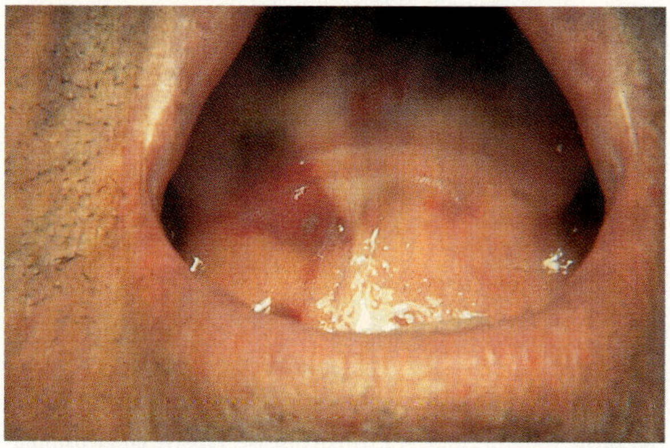

Fig. 20.27. Violaceous patch of Kaposi's sarcoma of the oral mucosa

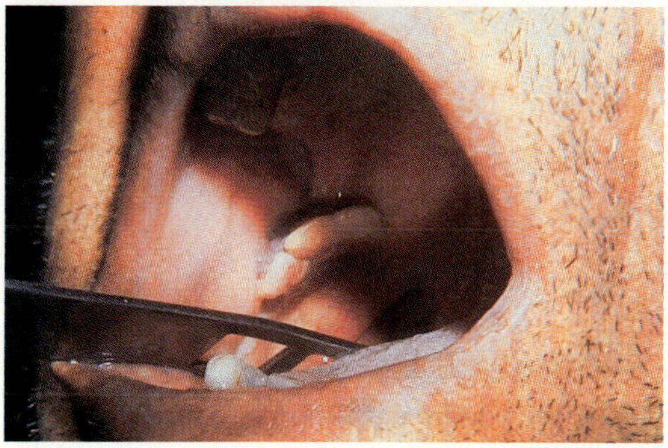

Fig. 20.28. Nodular lesion of Kaposi's sarcoma of the oral mucosa

quicker evolution and relatively more frequent involvement of gastric mucosa and lung. African KS is characterized by infiltrating and vegetating lesions on the feet and lower legs, with a very aggressive behavior. Sometimes, lymphadenopathic involvement is observed in young people. In AIDS-related KS, disseminated and rapidly spreading nodular or patch lesions on the skin are observed. On the trunk, the lesions sometimes assume a pityriasis rosea-like aspect; other times, a purpuric hue may be observed. Involvement of the oral mucosa is frequent: on the hard palate, vegetating, ulcerated, and bleeding lesions are characteristic.

Microscopic Findings. Two histological features are characteristics of KS: bundles of interweaving spindle cells and irregular vascular spaces, sometimes filled with erythrocytes. Extravasated erythrocytes are often present (Fig. 20.29). Bizarre, thin-walled blood vessels and scattered infiltrates of lymphocytes may be observed in initial lesions.

Diagnosis. The association of typical lesions on the skin, either disseminated or restricted to the feet or

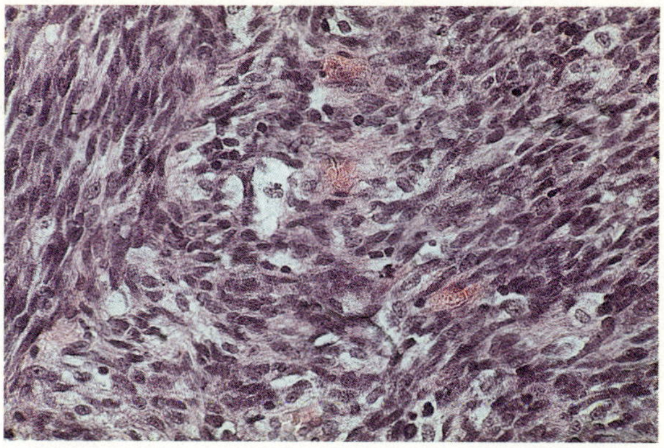

Fig. 20.29. Spindle cells, irregular vascular spaces, and extravasated erythrocytes seen on histopathological examination in a case of Kaposi's sarcoma

to the lower legs, is sufficient to justify suspicion of the diagnosis. Histological examination is necessary to confirm the clinical diagnosis.

Differential Diagnosis. Angiomas and benign lymphangioendothelioma must be taken into consideration in differential diagnosis.
Cavernous hemangiomas may develop on the cheek or on the tongue during the first months of life and, in many cases, these undergo at least partial spontaneous regression during subsequent years.
Senile angiomas may appear after the age of 50, particularly on the border of the lip: they appear as black or violaceous patches or nodules, and remain stationary or only slightly enlarging.
Benign lymphangioendothelioma, also termed acquired progressive lymphangioma, is characterized by the appearance of slowly extending, erythematous macules and plaques.

Treatment. Radiotherapy or intralesional infiltration with recombinant interferon (1–3 million units once a week) are the treatment of choice for isolated oral lesions. If disseminated skin lesions are present, general chemotherapy with bleomycin (15 mg IV twice a week up to 180–200 mg) or interferon-alpha (3–6 M every other day) is advisable.

20.5.3 Histiocytosis X

R. Caputo

Definition. Histiocytosis X (HX), now also termed Langerhans-cell (LC) histiocytosis [47], is characterized by a proliferation of a distinct histiocytic cell type; these cells are S100- and CD1a-positive and contain Birbeck granules in the cytoplasm. HX includes four clinical forms [48]: Letterer-Siwe disease (LSD), Hand-Schüller-Christian disease (HSC), eosinophilic granuloma (EG), and self-healing reticulohistiocytosis of Hashimoto-Pritzker (SHR). These four forms may best be regarded as being, respectively, the acute disseminated, the chronic progressive, the benign localized, and the purely cutaneous self-healing forms of HX. They range from a lethal multisystem disorder to easily curable or self-limiting single-system lesions (skin, mucous membranes, or bones). When the disorder involves at least two tissues or organs, the term disseminated HX has been used [2].

Etiology and Pathogenesis. HX has been variously regarded as a reactive disorder, an aberrant immune response, and a neoplastic process [49]. The detection of clonal histiocytes in all forms of HX suggests that this disease is probably a clonal neoplastic disorder with highly variable biologic behavior [50]. HX may arise from somatic mutations that cause the clonal expansion of LC [50], or it could result from a virally (Epstein-Barr virus, human herpes virus type 6) induced clonal proliferation of LC [51].

Oral Manifestations. Mucosal lesions may be sought in every patient with HX, except for neonates with SHR. The incidence of oral involvement varies from 10% [52] to 40% [53, 54] of cases. Of 114 patients with oral mucous membrane involvement collected by Hartman [52], 12% had HSC, 10% LSD, and 78% EG, and the majority were boys and men. In our 17 adult cases [54], oral manifestations were present in 6 cases of HSC and 1 case of EG.
Oral lesions are the initial sign of the disease in about 13% of all patients [53, 55], and 5% had only oral lesions at the time of presentation. Oral manifestations include soft tissue and bone involvement [52–56]. In LSD the lesions consist mainly of petechiae, purpura, vesicles, erosions, or ulcerations; in HSC and EG, the manifestations are usually noduloulcerative (Figs. 20.30–20.32). Gingival tissue is easily accessible and is the correct site from which to obtain biopsy material for diagnosis. Bone lesions may be present in the mandible and maxilla, with tender and swollen areas [55, 57–59]. The posterior mandible is the most commonly involved site. The lytic bone lesions [59] induce loss of permanent teeth and non-healing of extraction sites [59]. On radiographs, the teeth appear to be "floating" in the mouth as a consequence of the destruction of alveolar bone, with displacement of normal teeth. These "floating teeth" are pathognomonic of HX [58, 59]. Particularly in children, a dental evaluation should be suggested in every patient with HX. Oral lesions are frequently painful, may induce "foetor oris", and may result in gum retraction that makes fitting prosthetic dentures difficult [59].

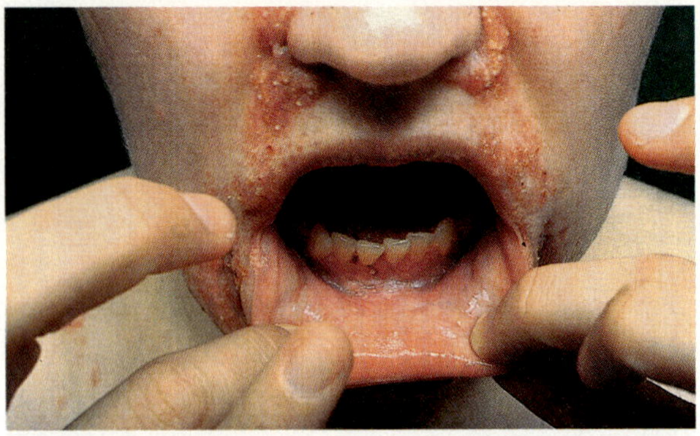

Fig. 20.30. Hand-Schüller-Christian disease. Erosive gingivostomatitis. Note the impressive perioral papulopostular lesions

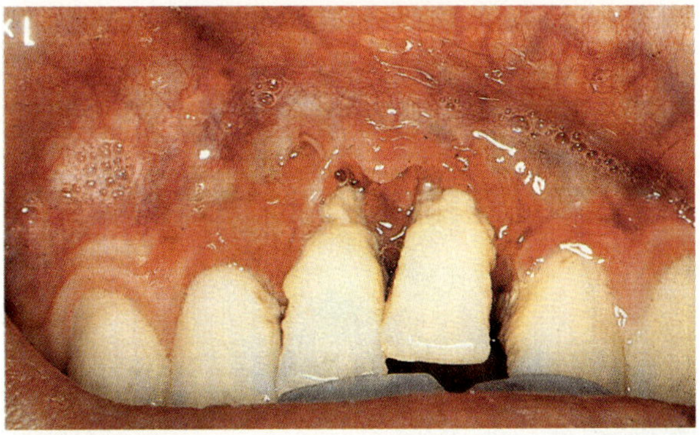

Fig. 20.31. Hand-Schüller-Christian disease. Swelling and ulceration of the gingiva

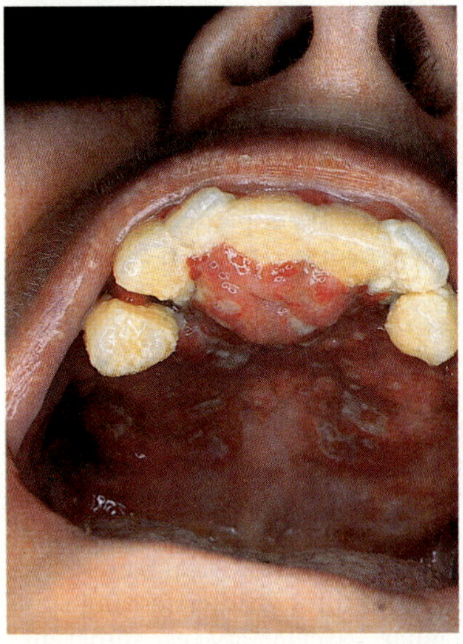

Fig. 20.32. Eosinophilic granuloma. Noduloulcerative lesions of the gingiva and palate

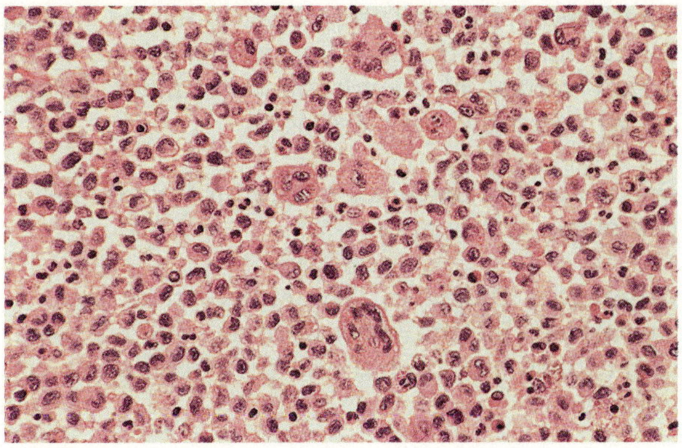

Fig. 20.33. Eosmophilic granuloma. Oral biopsy shows extensive aggregation of HX cells and inflammatory cells with some multinucleated histiocytes (granulomatous stage)

Associated Findings. In the presence of oral manifestations of HX, detailed screening of skin, bones, and viscera is appropiate.

Microscopic Findings. In contrast to the clinical heterogeneity of HX, the pathologic features of all forms are more uniform. The lesions consist predominantly of LC, with an accompanying inflammatory infiltrate [48]. LC have an irregular and vesiculated nucleus, often reniform, and an abundant, slightly eosinophilic cytoplasm (Fig. 20.33). In oral lesions, the histopathologic pattern is mainly proliferative or granulomatous [48, 60]. LC are S100- and CD1a-positive, and are ultrastructurally characterized by the presence of Birbeck granules within the cytoplasm [48].

Diagnosis. The diagnosis of HX is confirmed by the typical histopathological, ultrastructural, and immunohistochemical findings. A complete study of possible organ dysfunction (liver, bones, blood, bone marrow, and lungs) is mandatory.

Differential Diagnosis. Among the non-X histiocytoses, oral manifestations have been described in xanthoma disseminatum and in multicentric reticulohistiocytosis. In xanthoma disseminatum, oral lesions are papular and xanthomatous; in multicentric reticulohistiocytosis, the lesions are nodular, not ulcerated, and associated with severe polyarthritis, and show a characteristic histologic feature, i.e., the presence of numerous large, mono- or multinucleated histiocytes with an abundance of eosinophilic cytoplasm having a ground-glass appearance.

Aphthous and herpetic stomatitis can easily be ruled out because of their acute and episodic course. Chronic periodontitis and other inflammatory conditions may be clinically difficult to distinguish; histopathologic examination is necessary.

Treatment. Management of the manifestations of HX with local treatments, such as curettage or injections of corticosteroids, is usually unsatisfactory.

Monochemotherapy with vinblastine [48, 54] (0.1/0.2 mg/kg once a week intravenously for 1–3 months) [48, 54] or with etoposide (200 mg/m^2 orally on days 1–4, repeating every 28 days for four courses) [61, 62], has given excellent responses in both mucous and bone lesions in many cases. Recently, thalidomide (100 mg/day for 1 month) [63, 64] has been used successfully in a few patients with mucous membrane lesions.

20.5.4 Fibrosarcoma

G. Hautmann, G.L. Campanile, and T.M. Lotti

Definition. Fibrosarcoma is a malignant tumor of connective tissue, composed of cells that resemble fibroblasts. It is uncommon in humans, whereas it is frequently seen in rodents painted with carcinogens or exposed to UV radiation. Males are affected more frequently than females. Onset can be at any age, from birth onwards, with two peaks of incidence: in infancy and in old age.

It may occur, after a long interval, following intensive irradiation, in scars of lupus vulgaris, tertiary syphilis, and burns, and in xeroderma pigmentosum. The cells making up the tumor are anaplastic, spindle, usually large, and often pleomorphic, and they have frequent mitotic figures. The cells are disposed in a disorderly fashion, but tend to stream and eddy in bands in a herring-bone fashion [65].

Oral Manifestations. Fibrosarcoma may be located on the gingiva, buccal mucosa, palate, tongue, and lips. It consists of a relatively slow-growing, smooth-surfaced, firm, reddish or purple nodule. The more anaplastic examples grow faster and feel softer. Ulceration usually occurs sooner or later, and the more superficially placed lesions sometimes become pedunculated. Hemorrhage or necrosis within the mass provokes it to feel fluctuant. The more invasive lesions can produce extensive local destruction and metastasize by way of the blood stream.

Diagnosis. The diagnosis is based mainly on histopathologic examination.

Differential Diagnosis. Fibrosarcoma must be differentiated from histiocytoma, but fibrosarcoma exhibits progressive growth and becomes more vascular as it enlarges; it should also be differentiated from fibroma, dermatofibrosarcoma protuberans, amelanotic malignant melanoma, and squamous cell carcinoma.

Treatment. Surgical excision with a wide margin laterally and beneath the tumor is the treatment of choice.

20.5.5 Hemangiopericytoma

Definition. Hemangiopericytoma is a rare tumour with malignant potential, composed of vascular channels and proliferating pericyte-like spindle cells. It has been reported in all age groups including childhood. The sexes are equally affected. The usual situation is in the subcutaneous or intramuscular tissues. The cells may exhibit pleomorphism and mitotic activity. A proportion of 12 %–57 % metastasize to the lung and elsewhere [66].

Oral Manifestations. This tumor is extremely rare in the oral mucosa. It presents as a firm, often circumscribed, and nodular mass varying in size. In most cases, it is flesh-coloured and is not painful. The growth rate may be slow or quite fast.

Diagnosis. The diagnosis is based mainly on histopathologic examination.

Differential Diagnosis. Hemangioendothelioma, Kaposi's sarcoma, and benign tumors of blood vessel origin must all be considered in the differential diagnosis.

Treatment. Complete surgical removal is the treatment of choice.

20.5.6 Chondrosarcoma

Definition. Chondrosarcoma is a malignant neoplasm that is more common in men than women, especially between 30 and 60 years of age. It is characterized by the formation of aberrant cartilage tissue. Chondrosarcoma is subclassified as primary when it arises de novo, and secondary when it arises from a preexisting benign cartilage tumor. It is mainly found in the ribs, pelvis, femur, shoulder girdle, and jaws [67].

Oral Manifestations. Chondrosarcoma of the jaws is rare and presents as a painless, hard swelling that progressively enlarges, causing extensive bone destruction with loosening of the teeth. Occasionally, chondrosarcoma may present as a lobulated and ulcerated mass. In the maxillofacial area, a rare histological variant of chondrosarcoma, mesenchymal chondrosarcoma, may also occur.

Diagnosis. The diagnosis is based mainly on histopathologic examination.

Differential Diagnosis. The entities that must be considered include osteosarcoma, fibrosarcoma, chondroma, and central and peripheral giant cell granuloma.

Treatment. Surgical removal and radiotherapy are necessary.

20.5.7 Osteosarcoma

Definition. This is the most common malignant neoplasm of bone that affects males more than females, occurring at between 10 and 20 years of age. The tumor usually appears about 10 years later than a primary tumor elsewhere in the skeleton.

Oral Manifestations. The jaws are affected in 6 %–7 % of cases. The lesion presents as a hard swelling of the jaw bone, which grows rapidly, producing facial deformity and loose teeth. Pain, paresthesia, and bleeding may occur [68].

Diagnosis. The diagnosis is based mainly on histopathologic examination and X-ray examination.

Differential Diagnosis. Chondrosarcoma and fibrosarcoma are among the entities that must be excluded.

Treatment. The treatment consists in surgical removal, radiotherapy, and chemotherapy.

20.5.8 Leiomyosarcoma

Definition. Primary leiomyosarcomas are rare. Men are predominantly affected. The tumor is more or less circumscribed and the degree of differentiation can vary within different parts.

Oral Manifestations. The tumor is usually a solitary, firm, sometimes painful, nodule [69].

Diagnosis. Leiomyosarcoma can only be diagnosed by histopathologic examination.

Treatment. Surgical removal is the only treatment.

References

1. Andrade R, Gumport S, Popkin G, Rees H (Eds). Cancer of the skin. Biology, diagnosis, management. Philadelphia: Saunders, 1976: 101–111
2. Bearhs OH, Henson DE, Hutter RVP, Myers MH. Staging of lip and oral vacity. In: American Joint Committee on Cancer. Manual for staging cancer. American Joint Committee on Cancer 1988; 27
3. Stein AL, Tahan SR. Histologic correlates of metastasis in primary invasive squamous cell carcinoma of the lip. J Cutan Pathol 1991; 21: 16–21
4. Giles GG, Marks F, Foley P. The incidence of non-melanocytic skin cancer in Australia. Br Med J 1988; 296: 13–17
5. Moll R, Franke WW, Volc-Platzer B, et al. Different keratin polypeptides in epidermis and other epithelia of human skin: a specific cytokeratin of molecular weight 46,000 in epithelia of the pilosebaceous tract and basal cell epitheliomas. J Cell Biol 1982; 95: 285–95
6. Mora RG, Robins P. Basal-cell carcinomas in the center of the face: special diagnostic, prognostic and therapeutic considerations. J Dermatol Surg Oncol 1978; 4: 315–21
7. Panje WR, Ceilly RI. The influence of embryology of the mid face in the spread of epithelial malignancies. Laringoscope 1979; 89: 1914–20
8. Flaxman BA. Growth in vitro and induction of differentiation in cells of basal cell cancer. Cancer Res 1972; 32: 462–9
9. Jacobs GH, Rippey JJ, Altini M. Prediction of aggressive behavior in basal cell carcinoma. Cancer 1982; 49: 533–7
10. Chahbazian CM, Brown GS. Radiation therapy for carcinoma of the skin of the face and neck. Special considerations. JAMA 1980; 244: 1135–7
11. Epstein E. Fluorouracil paste treatment of basal cell carcinoma. Arch Dermatol 1985; 121: 207–13
12. Spiller WF, Spiller RF. Treatment of basal cell carcinoma by curettage and electrodesiccation. J Am Acad Dermatol 1984; 11: 808–14
13. Kuflik EG, Gage AA. Cryosurgical treatment for skin cancer. New York-Tokio: Igaku-Shoin, 1990; 143–153
14. Zitelli JA, Brodland DG. A regional approach to reconstruction of the lip. J Dermatol Surg Oncol 1991; 17: 143–8
15. Summers BK, Siegle RJ. Facial cutaneous reconstructive surgery: facial flaps. J Am Acad Dermatol 1993; 29: 917–41
16. Larson PO, Snow SN, Mohs FE. Mohs micrographic surgery – In: Lask GP, Moy RL (Eds). Principles and techniques of cutaneous surgery. New York: McGraw Hill, 1996; 561–78
17. Buchner A, Hansen LS. Pigmented nevi of the oral mucosa: a clinicopathologic study of 36 new cases and review of 155 cases from the literature. Oral Surg Oral Med Oral Pathol 1987; 63: 676–682
18. Buchner A, Merrell PW, Hansen LS, Leider AS. Melanocytic hyperplasia of the oral mucosa. Oral Surg Oral Med Oral Pathol 1991; 71: 58–62
19. Chung AF, Woodruff JM, Lewis L. Malignant melanoma of the vulva. Obstet Gynecol 1975; 45: 638
20. Clark WH Jr, Ainswoth AM, Bernadio EA, Yang CH, Mihm MC Jr, Reed RJ. The developmental biology of primary human malignant melanomas. Semin Oncol 1975; 2: 83–103
21. Gazit D, Daniels TE. Oral melanocytic lesions: differences in expression of HMB-45 and S-100 antigens in round and spindle cells of malignant and benign lesions. J Oral Pathol Med 1994; 23: 60–64
22. Haas N, Ernst TM, Finke C. Zum Konzept oberflächlicher Melanome an der Mundschleimhaut. Dtsch Z Mund Kiefer Gesichtschir 1988; 12: 97–102
23. Hinrichsen KV. Embryologie. 6th Ed. Stuttgart: Thieme, 1990: Suppl. 126–127
24. Horiuchi N, Tsunoda T, Suetake T, Kato T. Oral mucosa malignant melanoma in situ with involvement of the perioral skin. Dermatology 1994; 188: 66–68
25. Iversen K, Robins E. Mucosal malignant melanomas. Am J Surg 1980; 130: 660–664
26. Kato T, Takematsu H, Tmita Y, Takahashi M, Abe R. Malignant melanoma of mucous membranes. Arch Dermatol 1987; 123: 216–220
27. Kindermann D, Pape HD, Osborn JF, Krüger E. Primäre maligne Melanome der Mundschleimhaut. Fortschr Kiefer Gesichtschir 1988; 33: 122–127
28. Korabiowska M, Brinck U, Hoenig JF, Bartkowski SB, Mirecka J, Schauer A. An application of MIB antibody to the retrospective study of melanomas of oral mucosa and facial skin. J Cancer Res Clin Oncol 1994; 120: 365–368
29. Krüger N, Sanchez E. Tropenkrankheiten. Diagnostik, Therapie, Prävention. Darmstadt: Wiss. Buchgesellschaft, 1995: 107, 253
30. Nehse G, Mensing H, Maerker R. Differentialdiagnose und Therapie maligner Melanome der Mundhöhle. Fortschr Kiefer Gesichtschir 1988; 33: 127–130
31. Orfanos CE, Garbe C. Therapie der Hautkrankheiten. Berlin Heidelberg New York: Springer, 1995: Suppl. 857–881
32. Pfitzer P, Pape HD, Herzog M: Zur zytologischen, zytophotometrischen und klinischen Diagnostik des malignen Melanoms der Mundschleimhaut. Dtsch Zahnärztl Z 1982; 37: 517–520
33. Steidler NE, Reade PC, Radden BG. Malignant melanoma of the oral mucosa. J Oral Maxillofac Surg 1984; 42: 333–336
34. Ulrich J, Rosin C, Michael G, Gademann G, Gollnick H. Kombinierte Radio-Chemo-Therapie zerebraler Metastasen beim malignen Melanom. In: Tilgen W, Petzold D (Eds). Operative und konservative Dermatoonkologie. Berlin Heidelberg New York: Springer, 1995: 298–304
35. Laskaris G. Color atlas of oral disease. Stuttgart: Thieme, 1994
36. Braun-Falco O, Plewig G, Wolff HH, Winkelmann RK. Dermatology. Berlin Heidelberg New York: Springer, 1991
37. Giannotti B, Santucci M. Skin associated lymphoid tissue (SALT) related B-cell lymphoma. Arch Dermatol 1993; 129: 353–355
38. Pimpinelli N, Santucci M, Giannotti B. Cutaneous lymphoma: a clinically relevant classification. Int J Dermatol 1993; 32: 695–700
39. Willemze R, Beljaards RC, Rijlaarsdam JU. Classification of primary cutaneous large cell lymphomas. Dermatol Clin 1994; 12: 361–373
40. Piette WW. The incidence of second malignancies in subsets of Kaposi's sarcoma. J Am Acad Dermatol 1987; 16:855–861
41. Templeton AC. Kaposi's sarcoma. In: Andrade R (Ed). Cancer of the skin. Biology diagnosis management vol 2. Philadelphia: WB Saunders, 1976:1183–1225
42. Tedder RS, Shanson DC, Jeffries DJ. Prevalance in the UK of HTL V-1 and HTL V-2 infection in subjects with AIDS. Lancet 1984; ii: 125–127
43. Wit RDE, Boucher CAB, Veenhof KHN. Anti-retroviral effects of interferon in AIDS associated Kaposi's sarcoma. Lancet 1988; ii: 1218–1222
44. Chang Y, Cesarman E, Pessin MS, et al. Identification of herpesvirus-like sequences in AIDS-associated Kaposi's sarcoma. Science 1994; 266: 1865–9
45. Boshoff C, Whitby D, Hatziioannou T, et al. Kaposi's sarcoma-associated herpesvirus in HIV-negative Kaposi's sarcoma. Lancet 1995; 345: 1043–4
46. Decker L, Shanker P, Khan G et al. The Kaposi's sarcoma associated herpesvirus is present as an intact latent genome in KS tissue but replicated in the peripheral blood mononuclear cells of KS patients. J Exp Med 1996; 184: 283–8
47. Writing Group of the Histiocyte Society. Hystiocytosis syndromes in childhood. Lancet 1975: 208–209
48. Gianotti F, Caputo R. Histiocytic syndromes: a review. J Am Acad Dermatol 1985; 13: 183–404
49. Favara BE. Langerhan's cell histiocytosis: pathobiology and pathogenesis. Semin Oncol 1991; 18: 3–7
50. Willman CL, Busque L, Griffith BB, et al. Langerhan's cell histiocytosis (histiocytosis X). A clonal proliferative disease. N Engl J Med 1994; 331: 145–160
51. Leahy MA, Krejci SM, Friednash M, et al. Human herpesvirus 6 is present in lesions of Langerhans cell histiocytosis. J Invest Dermatol 1993; 101: 642–645

52. Hartman KS. Review of 114 cases with oral involvement in LCH. Oral Surg 1980; 49: 38–53
53. Fitzpatrick R, Rapaport MJ, Silva DG. Histiocytosis X. Arch Dermatol 1981; 117: 253–257
54. Caputo R, Grimalt R, Laterza A, et al. Mucocutaneous expressions of Langerhans cell histiocytosis in adults. Eur J Dermatol 1994; 4: 528–531
55. Sandor GK, McShane DP, Tharsis LM. Histiocytosis X its oral manifestations. Oral Health 1987; 77: 21–25
56. Esterly NB, Mauser HS, Gonzalez-Crussi F. Histiocytosis X. a seven-year experience at a children's hospital. J Am Acad Dermatol 1985; 13: 481–496
57. Blerius C, Dahlin DC, Lovestadt SH, et al. Oral and dental manifestations of histiocytosis X. Oral Surg 1959; 12: 473–483
58. Sigala JL, Silverman S, Brody HA, et al. Dental involvement in histiocytosis X. Oral Surg 1972; 33: 42–48
59. Komp DM. Long term sequelae of histiocytosis X. Am J Ped Hemat Oncol 1983; 3: 165–168
60. Belaich S. Langerhans cell histiocytosis. Dermatology 1994; 189 (Suppl 2): 2–7
61. Mayou SC, Chu AC, Munro DD, et al. Langerhans – cell histiocytosis. Excellent response to etoposide. Clin Exp Dermatol 1991; 16: 292–294
62. Sheehan MP, Chu AC. Oral, skin and bone multisystem Langerhans cell histiocytosis and its response to etoposide – a case report. Clin Exp Dermatol 1991; 16: 463–466
63. Gnassia AM, Gnassia RT, Bonvalet D, et al. Histiocytosis X avec granulome eosinophil vulvaire. Effet spectaculaire de la thalidomide. Ann Dermatol Venereol 1987; 114: 1387–1389
64. Thomas L, Ducros B, Secchi T, et al. Successful treatment of adult's Langerhans cell histiocytosis with thalidomide. Report of two cases and literature review. Arch Dermatol 1993; 129: 1261–1264
65. Dahl I, Angervall L. Pseudosarcomatous proliferative lesions of soft tissue with or without bone formation. Acta Pathol Microbiol Scand 1977; 85: 577–589
66. Enzinger FM, Smith BH. Haemangiopericytoma. An analysis of 106 cases. Hum Pathol 1976; 7: 61–82
67. Ajagbe HA, Daramola JO, Junaid TA. Chondrosarcoma of the jaws: review of fourteen cases. J Oral maxillofac Surg 1985; 43: 763–769
68. Clark L, Unni KK, Dahlin DC. Osteosarcoma of the jaws. Cancer 1983; 51: 2311–2315
69. Braun-Falco O, Kind P, Meister P. Kutanes Leiomyosarkom. Hautarzt 1984; 35: 428–429
70. Garbe C. Chemotherapy and chemoimmunotherapy in disseminated malignant melanoma. Melanoma Res 1993; 3(4): 291–9
71. Dummer R. et al. [Interleukin 2: immunologic background and clinical use in tumor therapy]. Hautarzt 1990; 41(2):53–5
72. Falkson CL et al. Improved results with the addition of interferon alfa-2b to dacarbazine in the treatment of patients with metastatic malignant melanoma. J Clin Oncol 1991; 9(8): 1403–8

Suggested Further Reading

Baker SR, Krause CJ. Carcinoma of the lip. Laryngoscope 1980; 90: 19–27

Banoczy J, Csiba A. Occurrence of epithelial dysplasia in oral leukoplakia. Oral Surg 1976; 42: 766–774

Bancozy J, Sugar L. Longitudinal studies in oral leukoplakia. J Oral Pathol 1972; 1: 265–272

Blot WJ, et al. Smoking and drinking in relation to oral and pharyngeal cancer. Cancer Res 1988; 48: 3282–3287

Bouquot JE. Epidemiology. Pathology of the head and neck. Gnepp DR (Ed). Edinburgh: New Churchill Livingstone, 1988; 263–314

Bouquot JE, Gorlin RJ. Leukoplakia, lichen planus, and other oral keratoses in 23,616 white Americans over the age of 35 years. Oral Surg Oral Med Oral Pathol 1986; 61: 373–381

Brugere J, et al. Differential effects of tobacco and alcohol in cancer of the larynx, pharynx, and mouth. Cancer 1986; 57: 391–395

Cataldo E, Doku HC. Solar cheilitis. J Dermatol Surg Oncol 1981; 7: 989–993

Douglas CW, Gammon MD. Reassessing the epidemiology of lip cancer. Oral Surg Oral Med Oral Pathol 1984; 57: 631–642

Kaugers GE, Burns JC, Gunsolly JC. Epithelial dysplasia of the oral cavity and lips. Cancer 1988; 62: 2166–2170

Kleinman DV, et al. Cancers of the oral cavity and pharynx. A statistics review monograph 1973–1987. US Department of Health and Human Services Public Health Service, Atlanta, 1991

Mashberg A, Samit A. Early diagnosis of asymptomatic oral and oropharyngeal squamous cancers. CA Cancer J Clin 1995; 45: 338–351

Miller CS, White DK. Human Papillomavirus expression in oral mucosa, premalignant conditions and squamous cell carcinoma. Oral Surg Oral Med Oral Pathol 1996; 82: 57–68

Mincer HH, Coleman SA, Hopkins KP. Observations on the clinical characteristics of oral lesions showing histologic epithelial dysplasia. Oral Surg 1972; 33: 389–399

Neville BW, Damm DD, Allen CM, Bouquot JE. Oral and Maxillofacial pathology. Philadelphia: WB Saunders, 1995: 259–321

Sankaranarayanan R. Oral cancer in India. an epidemiologic and clinical review. Oral Surg Oral Med Oral Pathol 1990; 69: 325–330

Shah JP, Lydiatt W. Treatment of cancer of the head and neck. CA Cancer J Clinic 1995; 45: 352–368

Shafer WG, Waldron CA. Erythroplakia of the oral cavity. Cancer 1975; 36: 1021–1028

Shafer WG, Hine MK, Levy BM. A textbook of oral pathology. 4th Ed. Philadelphia: WB Saunders, 1983

Silverman S Jr, Gorsky M, Lozada F. Oral leukoplakia and malignant transformation; a follow-up study of 257 patients. Cancer 1984; 53: 563–568

Silverman S Jr, Shillitoe EJ, Dillon WP, Fu K, Gallante M, Phillips TL, Silverberg IJ. Oral Cancer. 3rd Ed. Edited by Silverman S Jr. American Cancer Society, Atlanta, 1990

Silverman S Jr, Gorsky M, Kaugers GE. Leukoplakia, dysplasia, and malignant transformation. Oral Surg Oral Med Oral Pathol 1996; 82: 117

Sundstrom B, Bornstadt H, Axell T. Oral carcinomas associated with snuff dipping. J Oral Pathol 1982; 11: 245–251

Stanley RS, Roenigk RK. Actinic cheilitis. treatment with the carbon dioxide laser. Mayo Clinic Proc 1988; 63: 230–235

Waldron CA, Shafer WG. Leukoplakia revisited; a clinicopathologic study of 3256 oral leukoplakias. Cancer 1975; 36: 13886–1392

Orofacial Features of Leukaemia and Non-neoplastic Haematological Disorders with Involvement of the Oral Mucosa

21.1 Introduction

S.R. Flint

The leukaemias are a group of diseases characterised by malignant proliferation of leucocyte precursors in the bone marrow. Leukaemic cells then enter the peripheral blood and may be found in very high numbers. Infiltration of various tissues follows, but there is a predilection for the lymph nodes, liver and spleen, giving rise to lymph node enlargement and hepatosplenomegaly. The diffuse nature of the malignancy distinguishes it from local, solid tumours, such as carcinomas or lymphomas, and has important therapeutic implications, since practically all tissues will be infiltrated by leukaemic cells. Local leukaemic deposits may occasionally occur, typically in the skin, and may be difficult to distinguish histopathologically from lymphomas. As the malignant clone expands, the normal bone marrow becomes replaced by abnormal cells, leading to anaemia and thrombocytopenia. Although the leukaemic cells are present in large numbers their function is abnormal, and this leads to susceptibility to infections. The disease is fatal if untreated, usually as a direct result of overwhelming infection.

The leukaemias are classified according to the precursor cell line from which they originate. Thus, the malignant cells may derive from the lymphocyte, granulocyte or monocyte series. Acute and chronic forms are described. In acute leukaemias, primitive, non-functional blast cells appear in the peripheral blood, leading to their designation as acute lymphoblastic (ALL) and acute myeloblastic leukaemias (AML). The AML group can be further subdivided into acute promyelocytic, myelomonocytic and monocytic forms. A rare variant, acute erythroleukaemia, is also described (di Guglielmo's disease). Although it can occur at any age, ALL is generally seen in childhood, accounting for 50 % of childhood malignancies, with a peak incidence between 2 and 10 years. AML, on the other hand, affects adults in 80 % of all cases.

In chronic leukaemias the cells are much more highly differentiated and retain many phenotypic characteristics and some functions of their normal counterparts. As a consequence, chronic leukaemias run a more insidious and less aggressive clinical course. Chronic lymphocytic leukaemia (CLL) is the most common form of chronic leukaemia, and in a minority of elderly patients the disease may be asymptomatic and not affect life expectancy. Like AML, chronic myeloid leukaemia is also heterogeneous. Chronic granulocytic leukaemia (CGL) is the most common form, but a number of rarer variants are described, depending on the cell of origin. Chronic leukaemias may transform into their acute counterparts as the disease progresses – the so-called blast crisis.

The diagnosis of leukaemia depends on detection of abnormal cells in a peripheral blood film, along with histopathological analysis of the bone marrow. The cell of origin may be identified by demonstration of an array of cell-type-specific markers by immunohistochemistry.

Because of the diffuse nature of the disease, the mainstay of treatment of leukaemias is chemotherapy using cytotoxic drugs with or without radiotherapy. Of the acute leukaemias, AML requires much more aggressive therapy to induce remission. Bone marrow transplantation following total-body irradiation to ablate the host marrow offers hope for cure of those who relapse following the induction of a remission. Oral lesions may occur as a result of these treatments (see below).

21.2 Orofacial Manifestations of Leukaemia

21.2.1 Acute Leukaemias

Acute leukaemias typically present with features of bone marrow failure. In one study oral features were present in 38 % at the time of diagnosis. The mouth may be an important source of septicaemia. Orofacial features include mucosal petechial haemor-

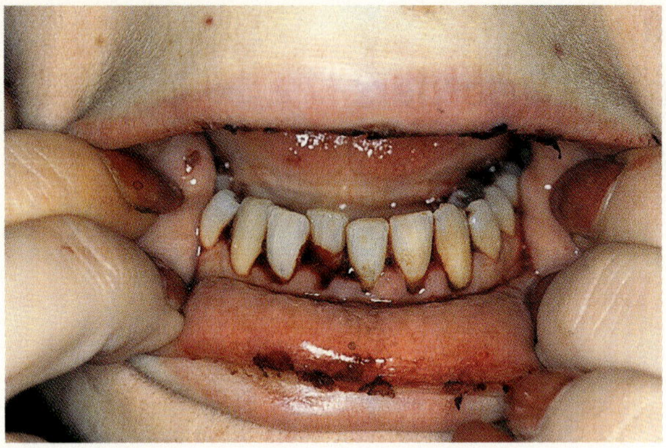

Fig. 21.1. Spontaneous gingival bleeding due to thrombocytopenia and mucosal pallor in acute myeloblastic leukaemia

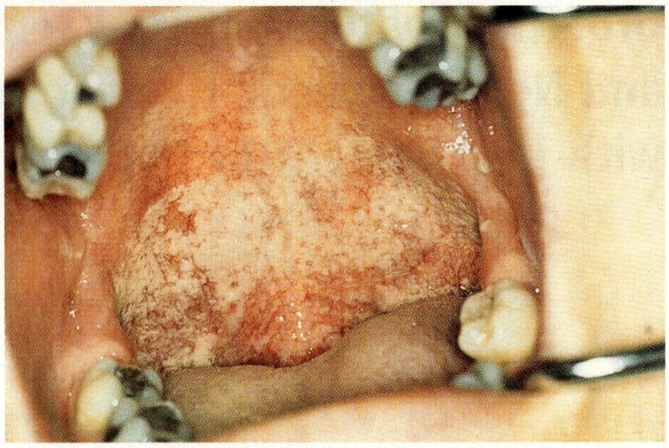

Fig. 21.3. Acute pseudomembranous candidosis affecting the soft palate in acute myeloblastic leukaemia

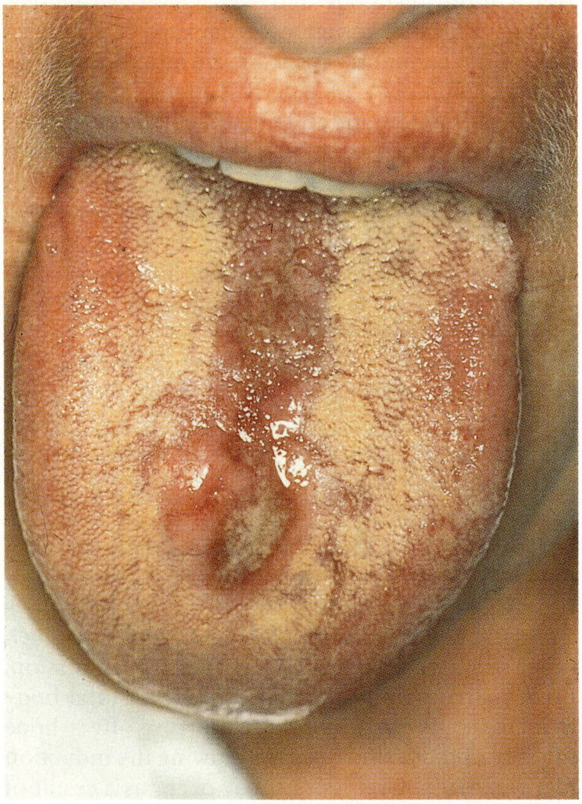

Fig. 21.2. Ulceration of the tongue caused by herpes simplex virus reactivation in acute lymphoblastic leukaemia

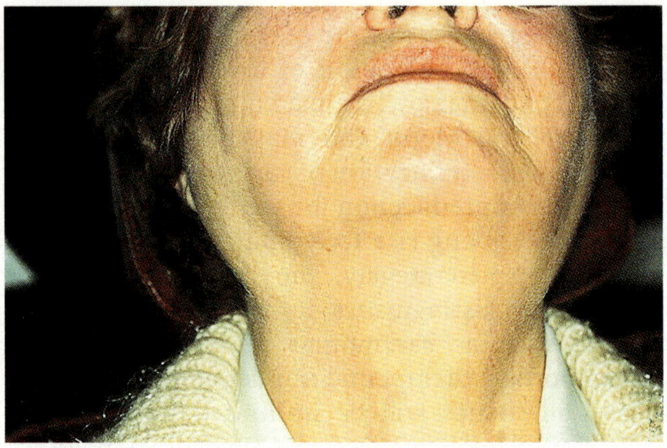

Fig. 21.4. Mikulicz syndrome in chronic lymphocytic leukaemia

rhages, ecchymoses, postextraction bleeding or spontaneous gingival bleeding due to thrombocytopenia (Fig. 21.1), mucosal pallor due to anaemia, and infections. Herpetic viral infections, particularly due to herpes simplex and zoster may cause typical or atypical mucosal ulceration (Fig. 21.2). Candidosis of the oral cavity is common (Fig. 21.3), and aspergillosis or mucormycosis of the paranasal sinuses may be highly invasive owing to the secondary immunosuppression. Odontogenic infections may be severe, spread rapidly and be difficult to control. Unusual bacterial species, particularly gram-negative bacilli such as Pseudomonas, may cause oral lesions such as ulceration, pericoronitis or sepsis. There may also be hepatosplenomegaly, and generalised persistent lymphadenopathy, which commonly affects the cervical lymph nodes. Swelling of the palatine tonsils may occur. Bone pain is also a feature, which may present as toothache or deep-seated jaw pain. Paradoxically, paraesthesia and numbness, particularly of the mental nerve, may also be a feature, possibly due to direct infiltration of the nerve or vasa nervorum. Leukaemic infiltration of the parotid and lacrimal glands with pain and diffuse swelling constitutes Mikulicz syndrome (Fig. 21.4).

Aggressive and rapidly progressive periodontal disease with bone resorption, apical pathology in the absence of caries, loosening of teeth and destruction of the crypts of developing teeth in the young may be presenting signs and prompt the diagnosis. Localised or generalised gingival enlargement may

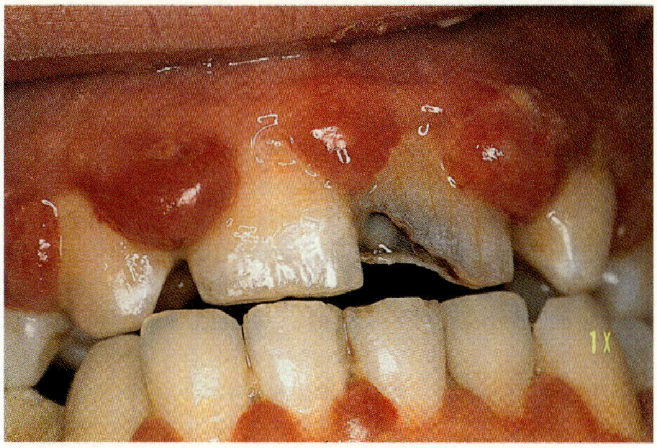

Fig. 21.5. Gingival swelling, ulceration and mucosal atrophy in acute myeloblastic leukaemia (Barret category 4)

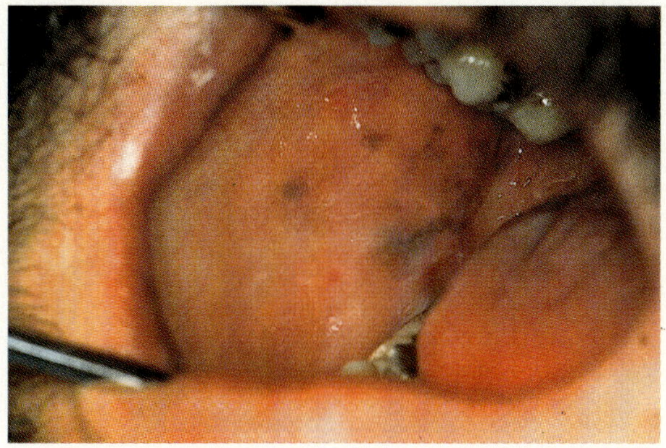

Fig. 21.6. Oral pigmentation in a patient treated with busulphan

be a feature of acute leukaemia, but is most commonly seen in AML (Fig. 21.5). Gingival swelling due to direct infiltration of the gingival tissues is seen, almost exclusively, in acute myelomonocytic leukaemia (and rarely in CLL). An aetiological classification has been proposed by Barret.

Category 1: gingival swelling due to direct infiltration of the tissues by leukaemic cells (unresponsive to strict oral hygiene and antimicrobial therapy).

Category 2: drug toxicity by chemotherapeutic agents, presenting as gingival swelling (cyclosporin), erosions and ulceration (cytotoxic drugs).

Category 3: graft-versus-host disease (lichenoid lesions, erosions, desquamative gingivitis).

Category 4: secondary effects of bone marrow suppression including haemorrhage, neutropenic ulceration, microbial infections such as acute necrotising ulcerative gingivitis or other mixed infections and mucosal atrophy, which respond, at least in part, to strict oral hygiene and antimicrobial therapy.

21.2.2 Chronic Leukaemias

The clinical course of chronic leukaemias tends to be much more insidious. In CLL, which generally affects the elderly, enlargement of the lymphoid tissue in Waldeyer's ring and cervical lymphadenopathy are orofacial manifestations. Patients with CLL seem to be particularly prone to herpes zoster which can affect the trigminal nerve. Gingival swelling due to infiltration is rare, but it does occur; gingival bleeding due to thrombocytopenia and mucosal pallor due to anaemia are more common. Neutropenic ulceration may be a presenting feature. Nodular leukaemic infiltration of the skin or soft palate may be seen.

In CML the hepatosplenomegaly may be massive, but orofacial manifestations are less common. Oral bleeding and Mikulicz syndrome have been reported. A rare manifestation is the "chloroma" (granulocytic sarcoma, leucotic sarcoma or myelosarcoma), a tumour-like deposit of leukaemic myeloid cells, which has been reported in the jaws. The name derives from the green appearance of the mass caused by myeloperoxidase in the leukaemic cells.

21.2.3 Orofacial Manifestations of the Treatment of Leukaemia

Cytotoxic chemotherapeutic agents cause cell death of rapidly dividing cells. During the neutropenic phase oral mucositis is common. Alopecia may also occur. Methotrexate may cause oral ulceration due to a direct toxic effect. The ulcers rapidly become secondarily infected. During this phase, septicaemia from the mouth may occur. The source of the infection may be from mucosal disruption, exacerbation of chronic dental abscesses or other foci of infection. Dry mouth has been reported as a complication of Adriamycin therapy, and oral pigmentation may be seen with busulphan therapy (Fig. 21.6).

Corticosteroid treatment, often at high doses, of lymphatic leukaemias will lead to a cushingoid facial appearance. Long-term cyclosporin-A therapy following bone marrow transplantation also causes a typical facies, with coarsening of the features and hirsuitism. Intraorally, non-inflammatory gingival hypertrophy is common. Once the gingival enlargement becomes gross, inflammation may be seen due to inadequate plaque control (Fig. 21.7). In graft-versus-host disease, where the donor graft attempts to reject the host, lichenoid lesions are seen in the oral mucosa (Fig. 21.8) and desquamative gingivitis has been reported. Late complications include a predis-

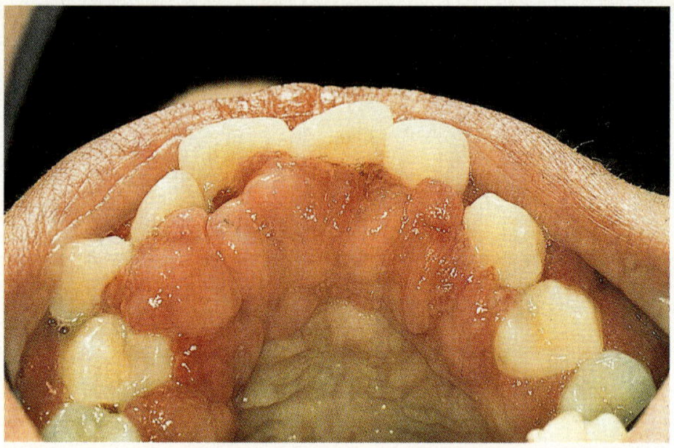

Fig. 21.7. Cyclosporin-A-induced gingival hyperplasia with superimposed inflammation due to poor plaque control

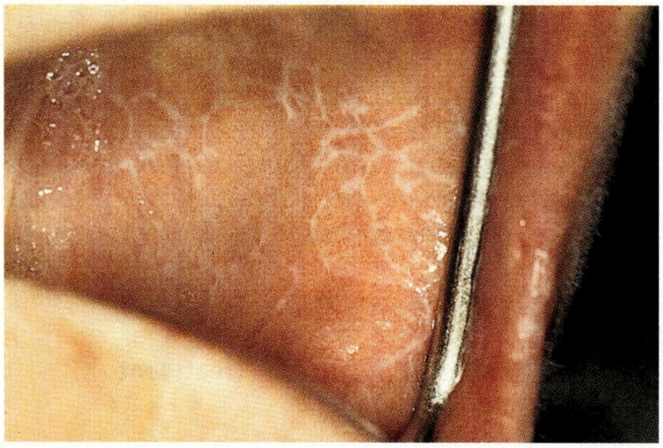

Fig. 21.8. Lichenoid lesion due to graft-versus-host disease

position to solid tumours, such as squamous cell carcinomas and lymphoma.

21.2.4 Dental Treatment Aspects of Leukaemias

The mouth is an important site of presentation of leukaemias, and leukaemia should be excluded if the clinician encounters cases of opportunistic infection, atypical ulceration, unresponsive or severe periodontal disease or odontogenic infections, spontaneous haemorrhage or postextraction bleeding without local cause. Dental treatment may be complicated by the bleeding tendency or susceptibility to infection and should be carried out in collaboration with the oncologist.

Patients who are to undergo chemotherapy or bone marrow transplantation should have a thorough dental examination to exclude any potential oral septic foci, and any discovered should be eradicated before chemotherapy is undertaken, since these may lead to septicaemia in the neutropenic phase before engraftment occurs. Oral sepsis eradication should be radical and may require haemostatic support. Oral hygiene should be optimised and its importance stressed to the patient. Patients who have central lines inserted in preparation for chemotherapy should have antibiotic prophylaxis before dental procedures are undertaken that could cause a bacteraemia, since the line may become infected. During chemotherapy, potential infective oral complications may be prevented by antibacterial (antibiotic cocktails), antiviral (acyclovir) and antifungal (nystatin, fluconazole) prophylaxis. Antiseptic mouthwashes are useful adjuncts. If specific infectious complications occur, appropriate antimicrobial therapy should be prescribed.

Following treatment for leukaemia, dental management may be complicated by drugs such as corticosteroids or cyclosporin-A. Mucocutaneous manifestations of graft-versus-host disease may be a marker of disease severity.

21.3 Non-neoplastic Hematological Disorders with Involvement of the Oral Mucosa

G. Hautmann, G.L. Campanile, and T.M. Lotti

21.3.1 Plummer-Vinson Syndrome

Definition. This syndrome is characterized by a combination of iron deficiency, dysphagia and oral lesions. It usually appears in middle-aged women.

Oral Manifestations. The oral signs include a characteristic smooth, atrophic and red tongue, identical to the appearance in iron deficiency anemia. Angular cheilitis and xerostomia are also common. Leukoplakia and oral and oropharyngeal squamous cell carcinoma may develop.

21.3.2 Thalassemias

Definition. These are a group of disorders characterized by an inherited abnormality of globin synthesis and are classified in several types: α, β, $\delta\beta$, δ, and $\gamma\delta\beta$, according to which globin chains are affected.

Thalassemia major, homozygous type, the severe form of the disease, usually develops during the first months of life and becomes progressively severe depending on an adequate transfusion program. The typical clinical features are skin pallor, low fever, malaise, weakness, and hepatosplenomegaly.

Oral Manifestations. The oral mucosa is pale. Glossodynia, loss of tongue papillae, and swelling of parotic glands may occur [1]. There is protrusion of the upper anterior teeth and malocclusion.

Diagnosis. The diagnosis is based on specialized hematologic tests.

Treatment. The treatment involves blood transfusion.

21.3.3 Congenital Neutropenia

Definition. This rare disorder is also known as infantile genetic agranulocytosis. It is characterized by a severe persistent decrease in circulating neutrophils, associated with life-threatening infections. The neutropenia is present at birth, probably due to an autosomal recessive genetic defect. Multiple bacterial infections involving the skin, lungs, middle ear, and urinary tract characterize the clinical picture of the disease [2].

Oral Manifestations. These include persistent and recurrent ulcerations, candidosis, and bacterial infections. Periodontal disease is very common, with severe gingival inflammation, tooth mobility, and extensive bone loss. The marginal and attached gingiva is red and edematous, and usually the interdental papillae are hyperplastic [3].

Diagnosis. Hematologic examination is the clue to the diagnosis. Radiographic examination of the oral cavity shows severe alveolar bone loss.

Differential Diagnosis. The differential diagnosis includes agranulocytosis, cyclic neutropenia, aplastic anemia, leukemia, acatalasia, hypophosphatasia, juvenile diabetes mellitus, Papillon-Lefevre syndrome, and glycogen storage disease type 1b.

Treatment. Local and systemic prophylaxis are suggested. Antibiotics and supportive treatment are to be provided.

21.3.4 Agranulocytosis

Definition. Agranulocytosis is a severe disorder characterized by a marked reduction of neutrophils or complete absence of all granulocytes. It may be a primary process of unknown cause or secondary due to a definite cause, such as drugs or infections. The most common drugs that may induce neutropenia are anti-inflammatory agents, analgesics, antibiotics, antihistamines, anticonvulsants, antithyroid drugs, etc. The onset of neutropenia is sudden with chills, fever, malaise, and dysphagia. Within 12–24 h, evidence of oral, pharyngeal, respiratory, or gastrointestinal infections appear.

Oral Manifestations. The presence of oral manifestations is an early sign; these consist of necrotic ulcers covered by grayish white or dark pseudomembranes without a red halo. The ulcers are usually multiple and measure up to several centimeters in diameter, involving palate, gingiva, tongue, and tonsils. The oral lesions are frequently accompained by increased salivation, painful mastication, difficulty in swallowing [4].

Diagnosis. Bone marrow aspiration and white blood counts in peripheral blood establish the diagnosis.

Differential Diagnosis. Conditions that must be considered include cyclic neutropenia, congenital neutropenia, aplastic anemia, acute leukemia, infectious mononucleosis, and Wegener's granulomatosis.

Treatment. Antibiotics, and in selected cases, white blood cell transfusions, should be prescribed.

21.3.5 Aplastic Anemia

Definition. Aplastic anemia is a stem cell disorder characterized by pancytopenia. It may be a primary process of unknown cause (constitutional or acquired) or a secondary process caused by drugs, radiation, chemicals, infections, and metabolic and immunologic disorders.

The disease is characterized by an insidious onset with headache, fever, and weakness. Slight pallor and, later, purpuric spots, spontaneous or related to trauma, may appear.

Oral Manifestations. Gingival bleeding is an early sign. Necrotic ulcers similar to those seen in agranulocytosis may develop, particularly in the buccal mucosa, palate, and gingiva.

Diagnosis. Bone marrow aspiration and biopsy, in addition to the white blood counts in peripheral blood, establish the diagnosis.

Differential Diagnosis. This includes cyclic neutropenia, agranulocytosis, acute leukemia, infectious mononucleosis, and thrombocytopenic purpura.

Treatment. Bone marrow transplantation is the therapy of choice.

21.3.6 Thrombocytopenic Purpura

Definition. This is characterized by a decrease in platelets in the peripheral blood. The disorder may be due to a primary failure of the bone marrow to generate platelets (idiopathic thrombocytopenic purpura) or it may be secondary to the use of a myelotoxic agent (drugs, radiation, etc.). The clinical picture is dominated by a purpuric rash on the skin and a bleeding diathesis [5].

Oral manifestations. Petechiae and ecchymosis usually occur, especially in the palate and buccal mucosa. Gingival bleeding is a frequent early sign.

Diagnosis. Bone marrow aspiration and a peripheral platelet count establish the diagnosis.

Differential diagnosis. This includes agranulocytosis, aplastic anemia, leukemia and polycythemia vera.

Treatment. Corticosteroids are often effective.

21.3.7 Myelodysplastic Syndrome

Definition. Myelodysplastic syndrome includes a heterogeneous group of refractory anemias often associated with thrombocytopenia, neutropenia, and/or monocytosis. The disease may be secondary to chemotherapy and radiotherapy. It is classified into five groups depending on hematologic disorders. Multiple bacterial infections and hemorrhage are characteristic.

Oral Manifestations. These are characterized by persistent and recurrent ulcerations, hemorrhage, and, rarely, candidosis and periodontitis.

Diagnosis. Bone marrow aspiration and a peripheral cell count establish the diagnosis.

Differential Diagnosis. The conditions that must be considered include agranulocytosis, aplastic anemia, leukemia, and thrombocytopenia.

Treatment. Treatment consists in transfusions and antibiotics.

References

1. Goldfarb A, Nitzan DW, Marmary Y. Changes in the parotid salivary gland of beta-thalassemia patients due to hemosiderin deposits. Int J Oral Surg 1983; 12: 115–118
2. Kostmann R. Infantile genetic agranulocytosis. A review with presentation of ten new cases. Acta Pediatr Scand 1975; 64: 362–366
3. Baehni PC, Payot P, Tsai C-C, Cimasoni G. Periodontal status associated with chronic neutropenia. J Clin Periodontol 1983; 10: 222–224
4. Sickles EA, Greene WH, Wiernik PH. Clinical presentation of infection in granulocytopenic patients. Arch Intern Med 1975; 135: 715–718
5. James WD, Guiry C, Grote W. Acute idiopathic thrombocytopenic purpura. Oral Surg 1984; 57: 149–152

CHAPTER 22

Metastatic or Secondary Carcinoma of Oral Mucosa

D. Ioannides

Definition. Metastatic or secondary carcinomas of the oral mucosa are rare. Nearly 1 % of all oral malignancies are metastases [1]. They are important since in 20 % [2] to 33 % [1] of cases, they may be the first clinical evidence of the primary malignancy elsewhere in the body.

Etiology. Metastatic cancer in the oral cavity results from hematogenous spread [1]. Nearly every type of cancer, including sarcoma, can give rise to oral metastasis, but it is the more common types of carcinoma – breast, kidney, lung, colon, and prostate cancer – that are usually seen. The incidence of metastasis from primary tumors to the oral cavity is shown in Table 22.1 [1, 3, 5–7]. Besides the metastatic tumors, infiltrates in the jaws are almost invariably demonstrated in patients with acute leukemia [1].

Oral Manifestations. Most metastatic carcinomas occur in the lower half of the oral cavity. The majority are located in the jaws [1–7], and especially in the premolar and molar areas of the mandible (70 % of cases) and the maxilla (20 %) [1–7]. The earliest sign may be the loss of sensation on the affected site or failure of an extraction site to heal.
A nodular or polypoid mass is then produced, which grows rapidly. The surface may be smooth and covered by intact mucosa. When the lesions become larger, they frequently develop a mucositis or an ulcerated surface as a result of chronic trauma from mastication [7]. Swelling, pain, pressure, loosening, or even extrusion of teeth can be noted as the lesions evolve [3, 5, 6]. In contrast, some types of cancer can induce new bone formation, resulting in an enlargement or deformity of the jaw. Spontaneous jaw fractures are rare, even in advanced cases [3].
The areas of involvement in the oral soft tissue are the tongue (5 % of cases), cheek (3 %), gingiva, and other oral tissues (2 %) (Fig. 22.1) [1, 9, 10]. Metastatic lesions may closely simulate benign reactive lesions, such as hemangioma, pyogenic granuloma,

Table 22.1 Metastases to the oral cavity

Primary disease site	Proportion of cases
Breast	20–30 %
Thyroid gland	6–16 %
Kidney	13–15 %
Lungs	12–17 %
Genitourinary system	6–10 %
Gastrointestinal tract	6– 9 %
Variety of other organs[a]	5–21 %

[a] Melanoma (scalp), lip (squamous cell carcinoma), parotid gland, submaxillary gland, liver, femur, knee neuroblastoma; and retinoblastoma in children

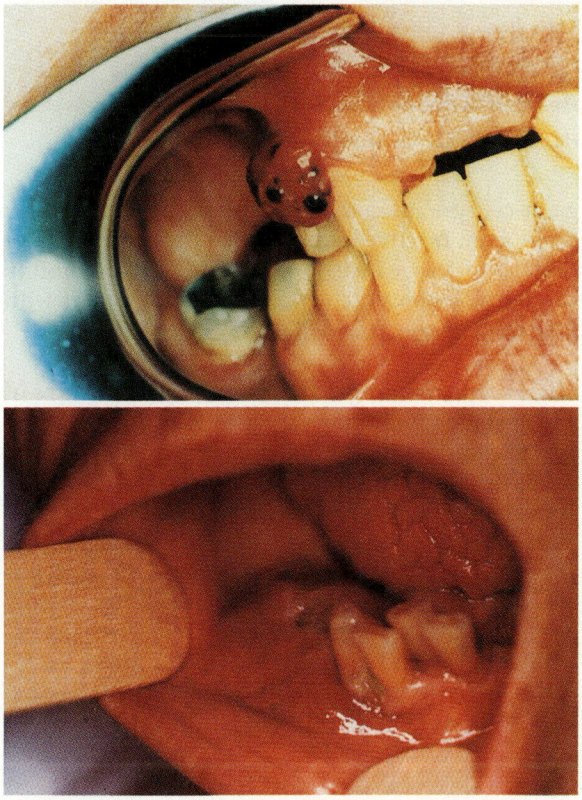

Fig. 22.1 a, b. Metastatic adenocarcinomas of the breast in the soft oral tissue. Courtesy of D. Antoniadis, D.D.S., Department of Stomatology, Aristotle University School of Medicine, Thessaloniki, Greece

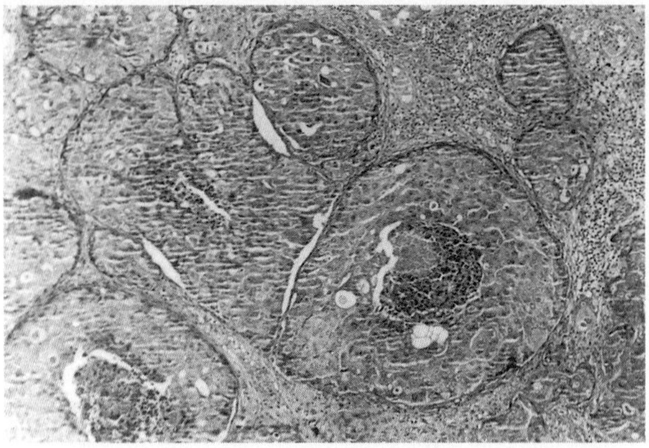

Fig. 22.2. Microscopic section of the tumor shown in Fig. 22.1. A glandular pattern is shown. Original magnification × 80

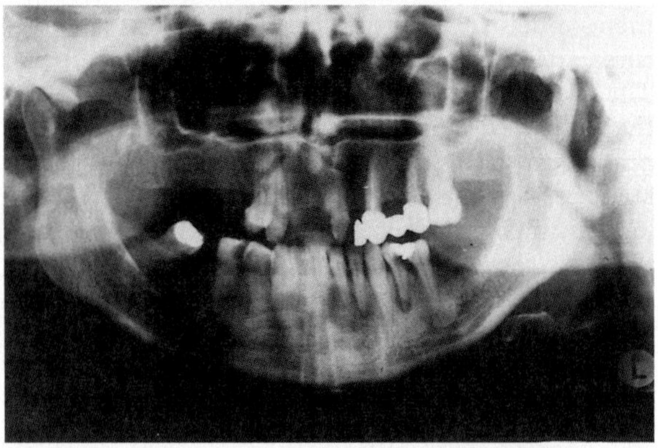

Fig. 22.3. X-ray of the same tumor as in Figs. 22.1 and 22.3

giant-cell granuloma, or peripheral fibroma. They differ from reactive lesions in that they demonstrate rapid and progessive growth [9]. This possibility should be seriously considered in any patient with known or suspected malignancy.

Microscopic Findings. The microscopic structure of a metastatic tumor may vary greatly from that of the parent tumor, or both tumors may have an identical microstructure. In addition, a secondary tumor may appear to be more or less malignant than the primary one. Most cases (70 %) are adenocarcinomas (Fig. 22.2). Sarcomas and epidermoid carcinomas are unusual [11]. The glandular pattern can usually be clearly demonstrated in these cases. Then, the examination should concentrate on the breast in females, the prostate in males, and the gastrointestinal tract, kidneys, and thyroid and parotid gland in both sexes [2, 11].

Diagnosis/Differential Diagnosis. The radiological appearance of these tumors is variable and may be simulated by a group of benign or malignant lesions. The majority of metastases are osteolytic (Fig. 22.3) and appear in the molar area [1, 7].
The differential diagnosis of metastatic tumors of the oral cavity includes osteomyelitis or bone infection, granuloma, cysts, benign tumors, primary malignant tumors, including minor salivary tumors and amelanotic melanomas, systemic diseases involving bone and/or soft tissues (histiocytosis X, etc.), as well as bone involvement in systemic malignancies (multiple myeloma, etc.) [2].

Treatment. Treatment of secondary carcinomas of the oral cavity aims to provide relief from pain and to prolong life. It consists in surgery, radiation, chemotherapy, hormone therapy, or a combination of any of these methods [2, 8]. The prognosis is poor, since the metastasis is indicative of disseminated disease. The 4-year survival rate is still low, at approximately 10 % [8].

Acknowledgement. The author thanks Dr. Elizabeth Lazaridou, a dermatologist at the Aristotle University School of Medicine, Thessaloniki, Greece, for her assistance in the preparation of this chapter.

References

1. Bhaskar SN. Synopsis of oral pathology. St Louis: Mosby, 1986: 355–358
2. Meyer I, Shklar G. Malignant tumors metastatic to mouth and jaws. Oral Surg 1965; 20: 350–362
3. Hirshberg A, Leibovich P, Buchner A. Metastases to the oral mucosa: analysis of 157 cases. J Oral Pathol Med 1993; 22: 385–90
4. Neville B, Damm D, White D, Waldron C. Color atlas of clinical oral pathology. Philadelphia: Lea and Febiger, 1991: 220
5. Castigliano SG, Rominger CJ. Metastatic malignancy of the jaws. Am J Surg 1954; 87: 496–507
6. McCarthy P, Shklar G. Diseases of the oral mucosa. Philadelphia: Lea and Febiger, 1980: 518–20
7. Wood N, Goaz P. Differential diagnosis of oral lesions. St Louis: Mosby Year Book 1991; 79–82, 187–194, 419–42
8. Batsakis J. Tumors of the head and neck – clinical and pathological considerations. Baltimore: Williams and Wilkins, 1974: 169–76
9. Ellis G, Jensen J, Reingold I, et al. Malignant neoplasms metastatic to gingivae. Oral Surg 1977; 44: 238–45
10. Hatziotis J, Constantinidou H, Panayotou P. Metastatic tumors of the oral soft tissues. Oral Surg 1973; 36: 544–50
11. Lumerman H. Essentials of oral pathology. Philadelphia: J.B. Lippincott, 1975: 85–7

CHAPTER 23

Oral Disease Prevention

B. Lorusso, P. Cortellini, and S. Parrini

Oral health may be defined as the absence of oral diseases and conditions that compromise or limit the functional, social, psychological, and economic well-being of an individual. Oral health may be maintained by preventing oral diseases.

Prevention of oral diseases can be divided into general prevention and local prevention (primary and secondary prevention).

23.1 General Prevention

General prevention is essentially based on education and information programs in order to generate awareness of the importance of oral health maintenance in the population.

Health education is defined by Green and Kreuter as "any planned combination of learning experiences designed to predispose, enable, and reinforce voluntary behavior conductive to health in individuals, groups or communities" [1]. Health education is required at all levels for all kinds of people when a health procedure is provided or implemented.

This kind of prevention is a whole-population preventive strategy.

23.2 Local Prevention

The most important areas for local prevention are: (1) soft tissue diseases of the oral cavity, (2) dental caries, and (3) periodontal diseases.

23.2.1 Prevention of Soft Tissue Diseases

Prevention of cancer and its precursor stages has the highest priority. Oral cancer and precancer (e.g., leukoplakia, erythroplakia, and submucous fibrosis) have been shown to be associated with excessive use of tobacco and alcohol [2]. Primary prevention and health promotion (Table 23.1) directed at the control of life-style factors (tobacco, alcohol, food, environment) are of critical importance to reduce the impact of oral precancer and cancer.

Secondary prevention aims at early recognition of oral cancer. Small lesions and precancerous lesions can be detected through a simple clinical screening examination and can be treated with conservative treatment [3].

To obtain good efficacy and efficiency in mass screening for oral cancer, the following strategies can be adopted: (1) include a specific soft tissue examination during adult dental mass screening; (2) concentrate on precancerous lesions as target disease; (3) restrict the range of subjects screened according to risk status, particularly age and tobacco smoking.

23.2.2 Prevention of Dental Caries

Some species of bacteria present in dental plaque are responsible for tooth decay and periodontal diseases. Studies from Western industrialized countries, as well as Africa, China, and Japan show that dental caries is the main cause of tooth loss and the most prevalent worldwide disease [4]. Dental caries prevention (Table 23.1) is based on diet, oral hygiene, and use of fluoride and dental sealants.

The importance of *diet* is based on chemical and physical properties of food. A diet rich in sugar promotes caries formation in the absence of proper oral hygiene. Soft, sticky food favors plaque formation and accumulation. A "clean tooth does not decay" has always been the very simple message upon which all the caries prevention strategies have been based.

Instructions for self-care to remove cariogenic factors and plaque bacteria should be enforced, along with a 6-month professional supportive care program for early diagnosis and professional *oral hygiene*.

Fluoride is another component of any preventive program. Both systemic (Table 23.2) and topical fluoride use provides benefits. The dramatic decrease in caries prevalence observed in some seg-

Table 23.1. Summary of the main methods of preventing oral diseases

Methods of disease prevention	Target population	Time-frame
Dental caries		
Fluorides		
Systemic		
– Community water fluoridation	Entire population	Lifetime
– Dietary fluoride supplement	Children	Birth to teens
– School water fluoridation	Children	School years
– Salt fluoridation	Entire population	Lifetime
– Milk fluoridation	Children	School years
Topical		
– Professionally applied: Fluorides, varnishes	AS	High-risk population
– Self-applied:		
Mouth rinses	According to need	Age 6 and older
Dentifrices	Entire population	Lifetime
Dental sealants	Children and youths	School years
Decreased frequency of:		
Ingesting carciogenic food and beverages	Entire population	Lifetime
Oral hygiene measures:		
Toothbrushing with fluoride dentifrices	Entire population	Lifetime
Periodontal diseases		
Oral hygiene measures		
By self-care: toothbrushing, flossing	Entire population	Lifetime
– Professional	Entire population	Lifetime
– Pharmacological agents	Periodontal patients	As needed
Oral Cancer		
Avoid use of tobacco, reduce alcohol, use sunscreen protection	Youths and adults	Lifetime
Early diagnosis		

ments of the population (more than 50 %) in the developed countries [5, 6] has been explained in terms of the widespread use of fluoridized toothpastes, changes in dietary patterns, and improvements in oral cleanliness. Two major mechanisms [7–9] of action of fluoride are known: (1) increasing enamel resistance in the pre-eruption stage and (2) promoting and enhancing the premineralization of porous enamel and initial carious lesions after eruption.

It is now well established that fluoride exerts its main role at the plaque/enamel interface. A low concentration of the fluoride ion prevents demineralization and promotes remineralization.

Pit and fissure *sealants* are plastic coatings [10, 11], which complement fluorides by protecting the occlusal and rough surfaces, especially of posterior teeth (Fig. 23.1). Sealant application should be scheduled for the times of the first and second molar eruption (ages 6–8 and 12–14).

Table 23.2. Fluoride supplements in parts per million

Fluoride in water (ppm)	0–2 years	2–3 years	3–14 years
< 0.3	0.25	0.50	1.00
0.3–0.7	0	0.25	0.50
> 0.7	0	0	0

23.2.3 Periodontal Disease Prevention

Prevention of periodontal diseases is based on bacterial plaque control by means of oral hygiene [12]. Oral hygiene consists in mechanical removal of food debris and plaque from dental surfaces.

Supragingival plaque control by personal oral hygiene and regularly repeated professional tooth cleaning has been shown to bring about the resolution and recurrence of gingival inflammation both in children [13] and in adults [14]. In addition, oral hygiene has been shown to be indispensable during both the active phase and the supportive phase of periodontal therapy [15]. Effective plaque control is achieved by self-care and/or professional care.

The most important condition for successful establishment of need-related tooth-cleaning habits is a well-motivated, well-informed, and well-instructed patient.

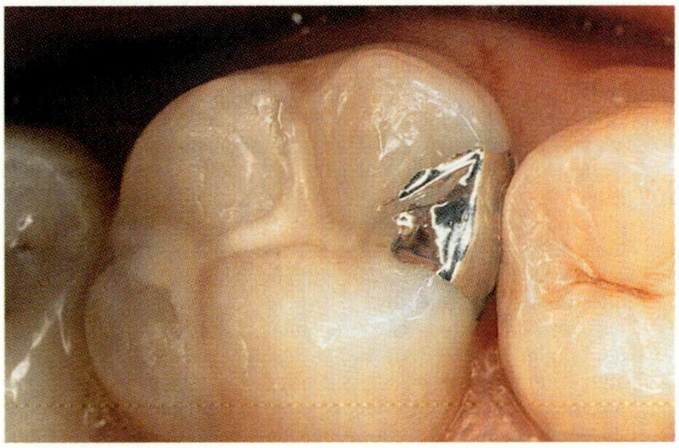

Fig. 23.1. Pits and fissures protected over time by sealants

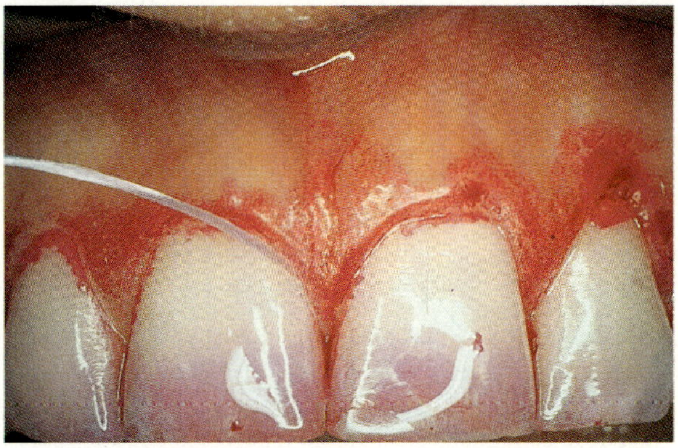

Fig. 23.3. Dental floss reaching the base of the interdental papilla

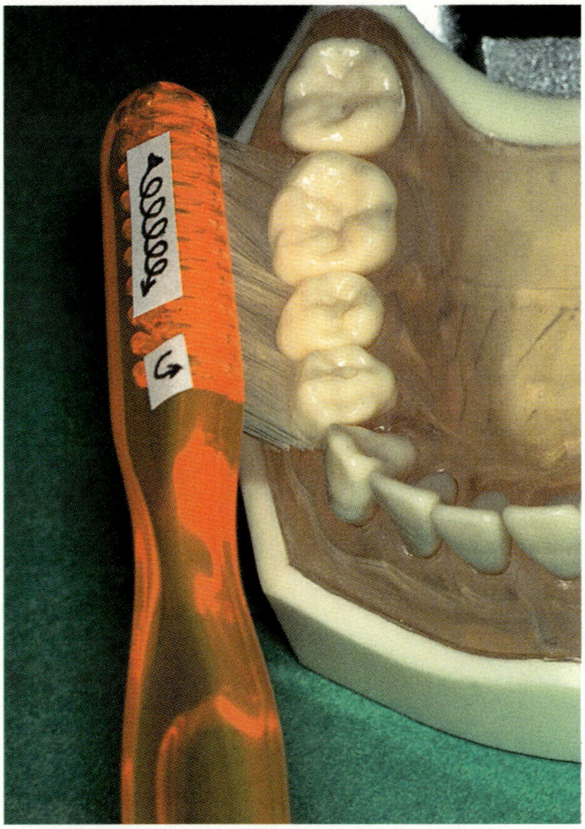

Fig. 23.2. Modified Bass technique applied to a model

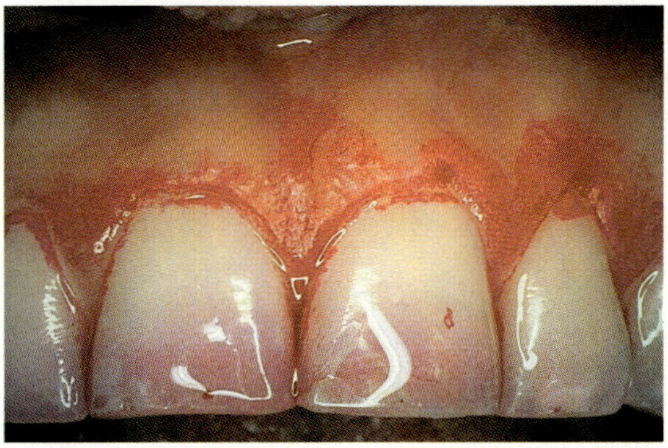

Fig. 23.4. Disclosing tablets pointing out dental areas not brushed

Patients should be motivated, informed, and given practical instruction on following a personal preventive program: the effectiveness of plaque control by self-care depends on this program. Home oral hygiene is commonly performed with toothbrush, dental floss or dental flat tape, pointed toothpicks, and interdental brushes.

The most effective and widespread technique of brushing is to put the end-bristles on the dentogingival sulcus at an angle of about 45° (Fig 23.2) to the long axis of the tooth and move it lightly to and fro. Afterwards, bristles are rotated coronally and the procedure repeated 3–4 times for each group of teeth. This procedure, called the Bass technique [16], which has been modified since first proposed, is applied to both lingual and buccal sides and followed by horizontal brushing of the masticatory surface. Interdental brushes can be used in the presence of wide open interdental spaces

The use of dental floss (Fig. 23.3) or dental flat tape is recommended for approximal tooth cleaning.

Disclosing tablets (Fig. 23.4) can be helpful for self-evaluation of plaque removal. Professional implementation of home measures for plaque control should be enforced at regular intervals. Ramfjord [17] has revealed that deficiencies in supragingival cleaning could apparently be compensated for by 3 monthly professional tooth cleaning in conjunction with any necessary subgingival instrumentation.

Probably the most important challenge for prevention is the identification of risk factors for the diseases. Such knowledge will in turn facilitate the identification of those individuals for whom dental caries and periodontal diseases will become a serious oral health problem, prior to the development of irreversible periodontal damage.

References

1. Green LW, Kreuter MW. Health promotion planning and education: an environmental approach. 2nd Ed. Mountain View: Mayfield, 1991
2. Pindborg JJ. Oral cancer and precancer. Bristol: John Wright, 1980
3. Zakrzewska JM, Hindle I, Speight PM. Practical considerations for the establishement of an oral cancer screening programme. Commun Dent Health [Suppl] 1993; 70–85
4. Chauncey HH, Glass RL, Alman JE. Dental caries. Principal cause of tooth extraction in a sample of US male adults. Caries Res 1989; 23: 200–205
5. Von der Fehr F, Schwartz E. Recording dental caries and health statistics in Europe. In: Thylstrup A, Fjerskov O (Ed). Textbook of clinical cariology. 2nd Ed. Copenhagen: Munksgaard 1994; 193–217
6. Marthaler TM. Caries status in Europe and predictions of future trends. Caries Res 1990; 24: 381–396
7. König KG. Role of fluoride toothpastes in a caries-preventive strategy. Caries Res 1993; 27 (Suppl 1): 23–28
8. Newbrun E. Current regulations and recommendations concerning water fluoridation, fluoride supplements, and topical fluoride agents. J Dent Res 1992; 71: 1255–1265
9. Newbrun E. Fluorides and dental caries. Springfield: Charles C. Thomas, 1986
10. Murray JJ. Efficacy of preventive agents for dental caries. Caries Res 1993; 27 (Suppl 1): 2–8
11. Ripa LW. Sealants revisited: an update of the effectiveness of pit- and -fissure sealants. Caries Res 1993; 27 (Suppl): 77–82
12. Lang NP, Cumming PR, Löe H. Toothbrushing frequency as it relates to plaque development and gingival health. J Periodontol 1973; 7: 396–405
13. Axelsson P, Lindhe J. The effect of a preventive programme on dental plaque, gingivitis and caries in schoolchildren. Results after one and two years. J Clin Periodont 1974; 1: 126–138
14. Axelsson P, Lindhe J. Effect of controlled oral hygiene procedures on caries and periodontal disease in adults. J Clin Periodont 1978; 5: 133–151
15. Lindhe J, Nyman S. Long-term maintenance of patients treated for advanced periodontal disease. J Clin Periodont 1984; 11: 504–514
16. Bass CC. An effective method of personal oral hygiene. J Louisiana Med Soc 1954; 106: 100–112
17. Ramfjord SP. Maintenance care for treated periodontitis patients. J Clin Periodontol 1987; 14: 433–437

CHAPTER 24

Surgical Procedures for the Lips and Oral Cavity

F. M. Camacho and R. M. Ortega

24.1 Introduction

This chapter is in two parts: First we shall discuss the surgical procedures to be applied for lips and commissures, which necessarily require special techniques; then we shall focus on the oral cavity: excision of the dermatosis or tumour (in any of its benign or malignant forms) and closure of the defect with direct suture, grafts and local flaps. At the end we treat surgery of the tongue.

24.2 Surgery of the Lips

The lips are a rather problematic area when a repair is needed, because of the cosmetic need to preserve the integrity of the vermilion border, the submucosal tissue, and because of the limited amount of oral mucosa [1]. All surgical procedures involving the lips must conform with the following fundamental rules:

1. Unaesthetic scars and lip line distortions must be avoided.
2. The vascular and nervous structures should be damaged as little as possible. Correct three-layered closure (mucosa-muscles-skin) is mandatory.
3. Scars must be buried in the natural folds: vermilion border, nasolabial fold and horizontal fold of the chin (mental crease).
4. Most parts of any incisions must be vertical, except in the vermilion and commissures, where they must be transversal.
5. For anesthetic purposes, nerve blockade must be sufficient: blockade of the infraorbitary nerve for upper lip surgery and of the mental nerves for lower lip surgery are necessary.

We divide the surgery of the lips into three types: (a) vermilionectomy; (b) upper and lower lip surgery and lip reconstruction; and (c) surgery of the oral commissures.

24.2.1 Vermilionectomy

When actinic cheilitis, glandular cheilitis or small squamous cell carcinomas have developed on the vermilion, a vermilionectomy may be necessary. This technique entails horizontal excision of the vermilion, which is also known as "lip-shave". The steps in this are (Fig. 24.1):

1. Blockade of the mental nerves with 2% mepivacaine.
2. Eliptical excision of the vermilion (Fig. 24.1 a).
3. The labial mucosa below the submucosa must be undermined and the salivary glands on the surgical surface removed.
4. Follicles arising on the lip's cutaneous surface must be cut out to prevent them from growing and producing traumatism on the surface of the upper lip (Fig. 24.1 b).
5. The labial mucosa must be moved anteriorly to cover the denuded surface.
6. The last step of this operation is the direct suture with 4-0 silk thread between the cutaneous surface and mucosa. With the aim of facilitating this suture we must provide three reference points (Fig. 24.1 c), one in the center and two in the commissural angles. The assistant must stretch these sutures to allow the surgeon to suture the vermilion border.

Final Considerations. The immediate results are good once the postoperative swelling has disappeared. The patient must be restricted to a liquid diet for the first 48 h and a soft diet for the next 2 days. The stitches can be removed after 4–7 days. Results appear excellent, at least from the cosmetic point of view; some patients report tenseness, pain and paresthesia, but these disappear in due course [2] (Fig. 24.1 d, e).

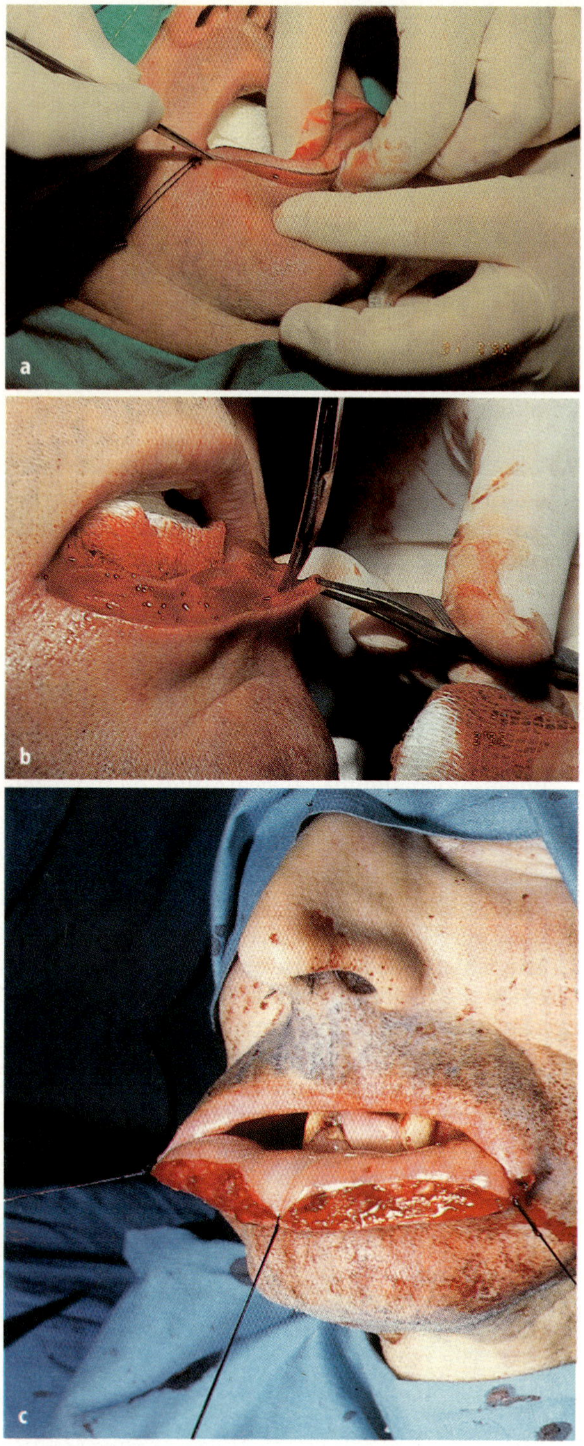

Fig. 24.1. **a** Vermilionectomy: elliptical excision of vermilion. **b** The follicles arising in the lip's cutaneous surface must be cut out to avoid traumatism in the upper lip. **c** Three reference points to facilitate the suture

24.2.2
Lip Surgery

The upper and lower lips are symmetrical structures located upon the orbicular oris muscle. For defects smaller than one third of the lips or less, the wedge-shaped excision is most suitable because it allows the vermilion border to be kept in the original position and the wound can be closed with direct sutures.

We discuss here the various techniques that can be applied when dealing with the upper and lower lip: procedures to repair defects of the cutaneous surface, the mucosal surface, the vermilion, and those involving the total lip thickness. Mention will be made of most of these procedures, but lack of space compels us to describe only the most relevant ones in detail.

24.2.2.1
Upper Lip Surgery

The upper part of the lip is bordered by the nose and nasolabial fold. It is a difficult area to reconstruct because of the cupid's bow in the center; when that disappears, the esthetic results are compromised [3].

When the defect is confined to the cutaneous surface, two types of flaps can be applied, depending on the location of the defect. If it is located in the middle of the lip near the cupid's bow, it is better to eliminate the total lip mass from the vermilion borderline towards the subnasal fold. This will leave a four-sided defect in the middle, which can be closed with a double advancement flap with Burow's discharge triangles in the nasolabial fold. If the defect is triangular and its base is on the vermilion border, two triangular A-T advancement flaps must be applied on the vermilion border. If the base of the defect is located in the nasal orifice, two V-T advancement flaps can be performed by means of discharge triangles or crescentic perialar excision.

If the defect is triangular and located in the lateral region of the lip, it can be closed with an A-T flap. If it is four-sided, a single-pedicle "advancement U-flap" with Burow's discharge triangle in the perialar region will be useful. Another possibility is the crescentic perialar advancement flap.

Transposition flaps are unsuitable, as are rotation flaps, at least in male patients, as they transfer hairless skin to a pilary area. The most frequent procedure is use of the nasolabial flap (Fig. 24.2 a,b).

When the defect is in the labial mucosa, it can be closed by direct suture, although a transposition flap of the adjacent endobuccal mucosa may be needed. Skin grafts may also be applicable, providing the skin of the donor area is hairless.

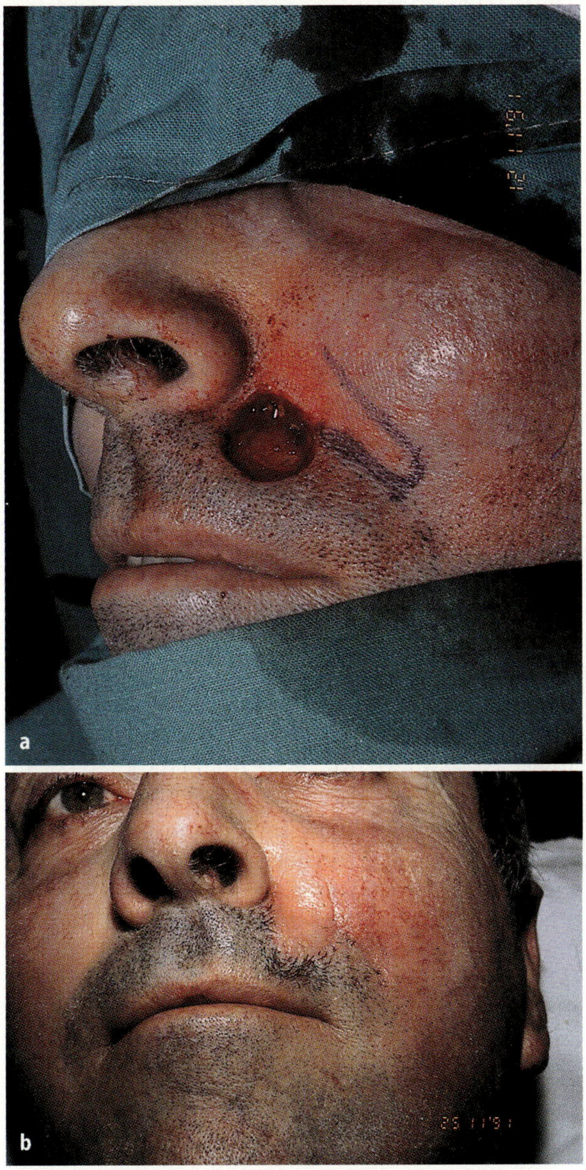

Fig. 24.2. a Basal cell carcinoma on the upper lip: once it was removed, it left a cutaneous defect. Nasolabial flap design is indicated. **b** Once the flap was transposed, the hairless skin was too evident in the moustache area

There are three different techniques for repairing defects of the vermilion: advancement flaps taken from the vermilion itself, Abbé's apron-shaped flap of endobuccal mucosa, and the lingual flap [4].

When the defect involves the total lip thickness, there are several possibilities, which, again, depend on the location. If the defect is lateral and smaller than one third of the lip, the through-and-through suture can be used. When the excision reaches the nasolabial fold, an advancement flap combined with a W-Y-plasty can be used in the outer side, and an advancement flap of endobuccal mucosa will close the inner defect.

On other occasions, when more than one third of the upper lip has been removed, the defect can be closed with an advancement flap of the cheek with a crescentic perialar discharge or with an advancement U-flap, which involves cutting out Burow's triangles from the cheek. If the defect is located in the middle of the lip, a double advancement flap or bilateral U-plasty can be designed; in this case, two different types of flap will be needed, because the inner surface of the flap must be lined with mucosa. In the outer part, a skin-muscle flap with four Burow's triangles must be performed. Once they are sutured to each other, the suture line will be placed along the nasolabial fold.

When there is a large defect in the center of the lip, the Sabattini-Stein-Estlander-Abbé flap (a rotation-transposition flap from the lower lip, also known as cross-V-lip flap or V-flap lip-lip) can be used and kept in position for 3 weeks, time enough to allow the flap to receive a blood supply from the new bed. The pedicle can then be closed and the vermilion and lip reconstructed.

The most extreme difficulty is reconstruction following radical upper lip excision. Bilateral fan flaps or Gillies's flaps (which are full-thickness cheek flaps with an inferior, medial pedicle based on the labial artery of the commissure) may be useful from the surgical joint of view, but they are less adequate from the esthetic standpoint since this technique does not permit reconstruction of the cupid's bow [5] (Fig. 24.3 a–c).

24.2.2.2
Lower Lip Surgery

The lower lip is bordered by the mental crease. When the defect comprises skin only, it can be repaired with advancement flaps with discharge triangles in the mental crease. Occasionally, instead of the triangle, we may perform a perimental crescentic excision or use an advancement flap in step-plasty form, for which small rectangles are eliminated on both sides of the chin.

If the defect involves the vermilion, it can easily be repaired with an advancement flap from the vermilion itself, with a flap from the labial mucosa of the upper lip or from the adjacent endobuccal mucosa, and even with the tongue flap technique described below [4].

If the defect involves the labial mucosa, it can be repaired with a lateral advancement flap from the remaining labial mucosa and the adjacent endobuccal mucosa.

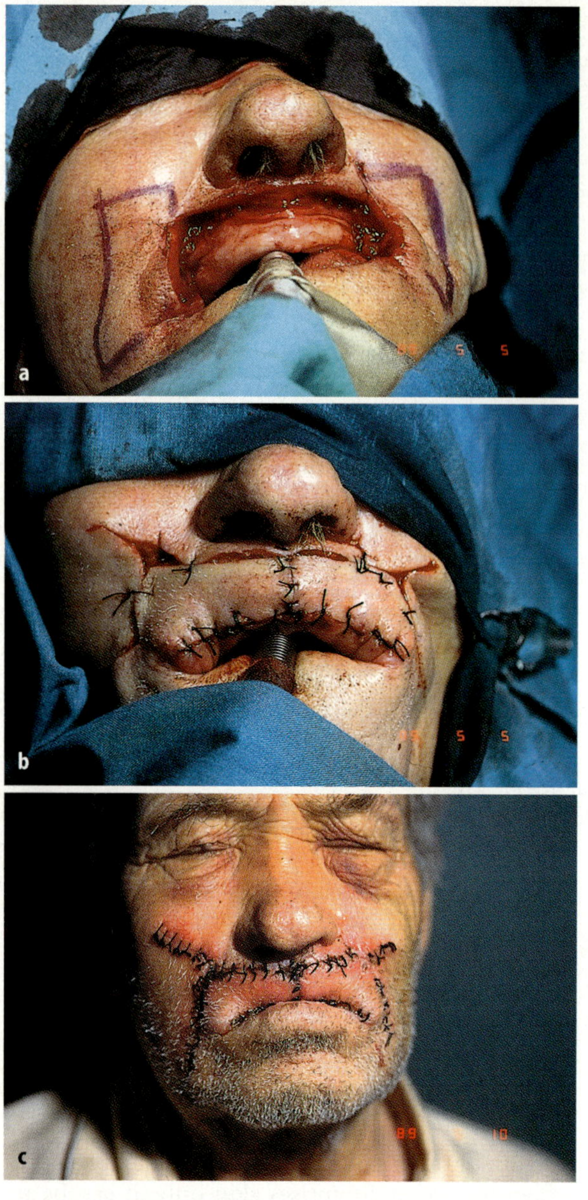

Fig. 24.3. **a** Bilateral fan flaps (Gillies' flaps): once the lip is removed, the bilateral fan flaps are designed. **b** The flaps are transposed, placed in position and sutured to each another. **c** Final appearance after surgery

Far more problematic is the reconstruction of the entire lower lip. As mentioned before, if a small tumor is removed, the wedge-shaped excision is best: when the defect is smaller than one third of the lip it can be closed by direct suture. The only problem is the mental crease: the final excision *must not* cross it. To avoid this we can perform either a triangular excision or a Z-plasty ending in the crease. In this fashion, once the two flap tips are transposed, the suture will remain in the crease. Another possibility is to perform an M-plasty distally, avoiding this area.

When the tumor is large and a large proportion of the lower lip has been removed, a rectangular excision can be performed. In this situation, we may design either an advancement flap in step-plasty form (Fig. 24.4 a–d), or unilateral/bilateral trapezoid flaps on one/both sides of the chin, with their corresponding discharge triangle(s), or crescentic perimental excision(s) on one (Figs. 24.5) or both sides.

In cases in which the vermilion loss is very extensive, the combination of a crescentic perimental excision and a triangular excision reaching the nasolabial fold may also be suitable, but it is important to bear in mind that the nasolabial triangle must not be totally cut out, as a portion of mucosa will have to be advanced and applied to the skin advancement flap to repair the vermilion. This is the so-called Bernard's technique.

The Sabattini-Stein-Estlander-Abbé flap should not be used to repair large defects of the lower lip, because it is better for the upper lip, except for the the lateral reconstruction that requires posterior surgery to repair the commissure (Figs. 24.6). When use of this type of flap to repair a central defect is planned, it is first necessary to raise an advancement flap from the remainder of the lip towards the commissure, so as to obtain a lateral defect. This is the so-called Grabb's technique.

When tumor excision involves total loss of the lower lip, the reconstruction may be performed with two innervated myocutaneous flaps: one is a rotation flap from the orbicularis oris muscle of the cheeks, which is lined with endobuccal mucosa (Karapandzic's technique); the second comprises the depressor anguli oris muscle and is performed by means of two fan flaps similar to those employed in the upper lip. It is essential that the whole of the vascular and nervous pack is contained in the pedicle (Gillies' technique).

24.2.3 Surgery of the Commissure

Whenever the Sabattini-Stein-Estlander-Abbé method is applied to reconstruct the upper or lower lip, the commissure needs to be reconstructed after a period of 3 weeks, during which the flap must stay in place, before the pedicle is cut out. Some authors [6] have carried out the "commissuroplasty" several weeks after the first procedure, incising three triangles and rotating them into specific positions.

Although there are many techniques involving cutaneous flaps (inverse bilateral transportion flap, and rhomboid bilateral transposition flaps) or mucosal flaps (endobuccal mucosa flap, lingual flap, and endobuccal and vermilion flap), the aim of this chapter is to explain different surgical tech-

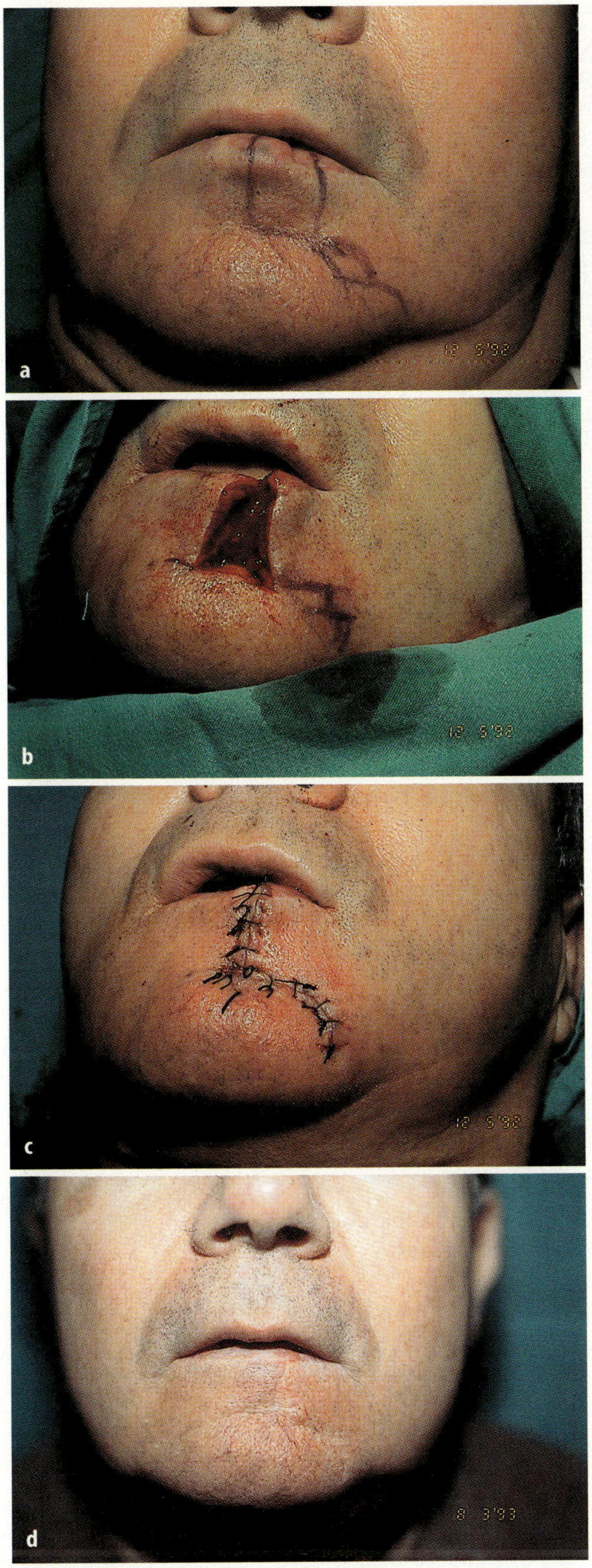

Fig. 24.4. **a** Step-plasty (advancement flap): squamous cell carcinoma on the lower lip. The advancement flap in step-plasty form is designed. **b** The quadrangular defect is sutured. The mucosa is approximated, and the cutaneous side will be closed with an advancement flap. **c** Final appearance just after surgery. The mental crease is bordered by stitches. **d** Appearance of the patient 1 year later

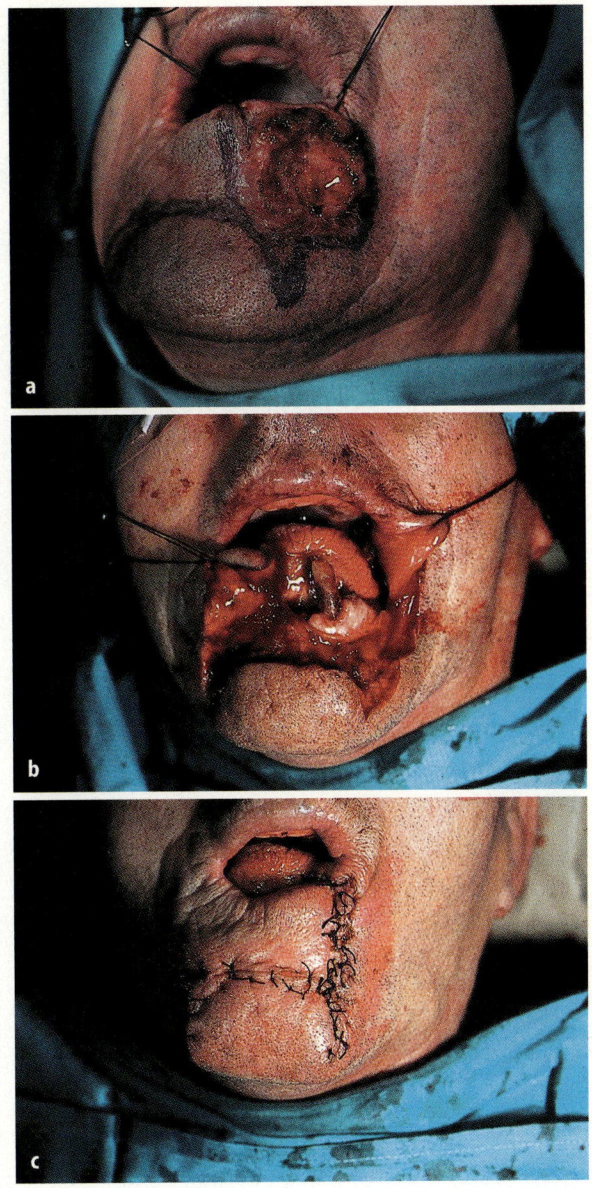

Fig. 24.5. **a** Large squamous cell carcinoma on the left side of the lower lip. The crescentic perimental discharge excision is designed on both sides of the chin. **b** The carcinoma has been removed and the crescentic perimental discharge excision performed. **c** Final appearance just after suturing of the perimental advancement flap

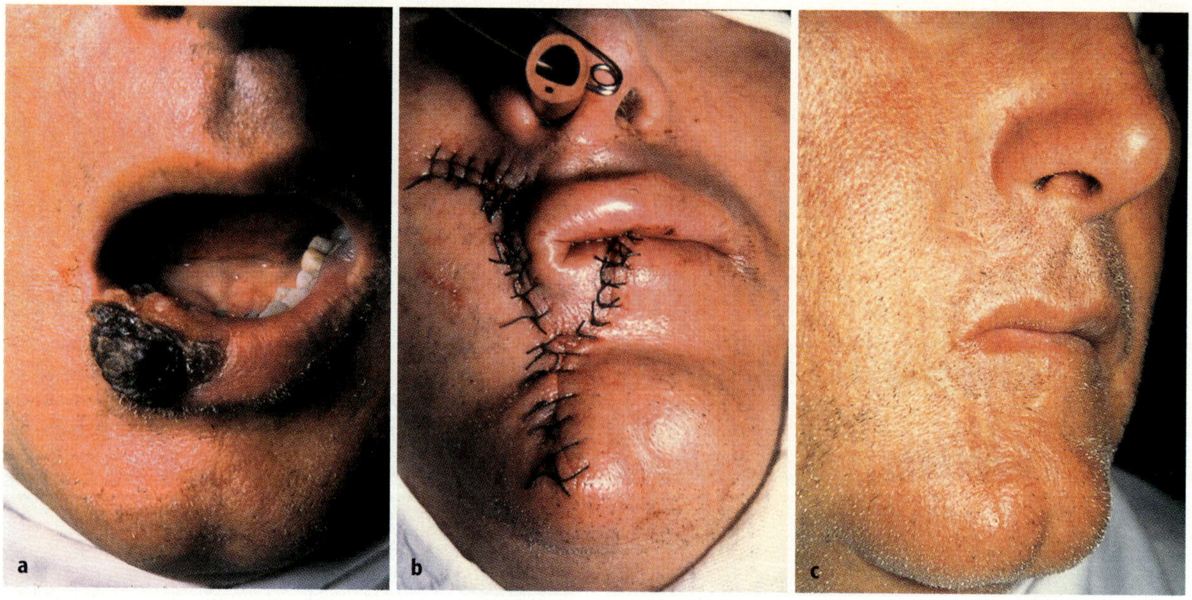

Fig. 24.6. a Squamous cell carcinoma on the right side of the lower lip. **b** After removal of the carcinoma by a wedge-shaped excision in the lateral lower lip, the triangular defect was closed with a Sabattini's flap. **c** Appearance 6 months later. The patient refuses commissuroplasty

niques rather than reconstructive surgical procedures.

24.3 Surgery of the Oral Cavity

Successful surgery or the oral cavity presupposes profound knowledge of its anatomy [7]. It comprises the palate, tongue, lingual and sublingual region (mouth floor or base of tongue), the gingivodentary and endobuccal area, and the lips. We shall only discuss the surgical procedures used for the palatal area, the endobuccal surface, the mouth floor, and the tongue.

24.3.1 Features of Surgery of the Oral Cavity [8]

1. The exceptional vascularization of the oral cavity allows the performance of large-scale reconstructions which never necrose.
2. Since the turnover of the mucosa is faster than that of the skin, healing is far more rapid and does not leave hypertrophic scars or keloids.
3. The antibacterial agents of the saliva prevent infections, although it is also a damp medium that tends to macerate electrocoagulation wounds.
4. In the postoperative period, a liquid diet is mandatory. In extreme cases, a nasogastric tube and thorough hygiene of mouth and wound are needed.

24.3.2 Surgery of the Palate

Although the most common surgical procedure of the palate is repair of a cleft, we shall not describe that in this chapter, as it lies halfway between the field of dermatological surgery and that of reparative plastic surgery. Suffice it to say that we usually employ the Veau-Wardill technique of two anterior and two posterior flaps [8]. Occasionally, we observe leiomyomas, mixed tumors of the salivary glands, palatal nicotinic leukokeratosis, oral florid papillomatosis, and other benign and malignant tumors.

24.3.3 Surgery of the Endobuccal Mucosa and Mouth Floor

Both the endobuccal mucosa and the mouth floor can be the sites of various benign and malignant processes, such as white sponge nevus, cysts of the upper maxilla, hemangiomas, lymphangiomas, lipomas, schwannomas, tumors of the salivary glands, leukoplakia, erythroplasia, and carcinomas. Only epulis, ranulae, and Sutton's granuloma fissuratum are specific to the mouth floor; they can all be removed by excision and the wound closed by direct suture. In some isolated cases, double advancement flaps are necessary. The donor areas are left to secondary healing.

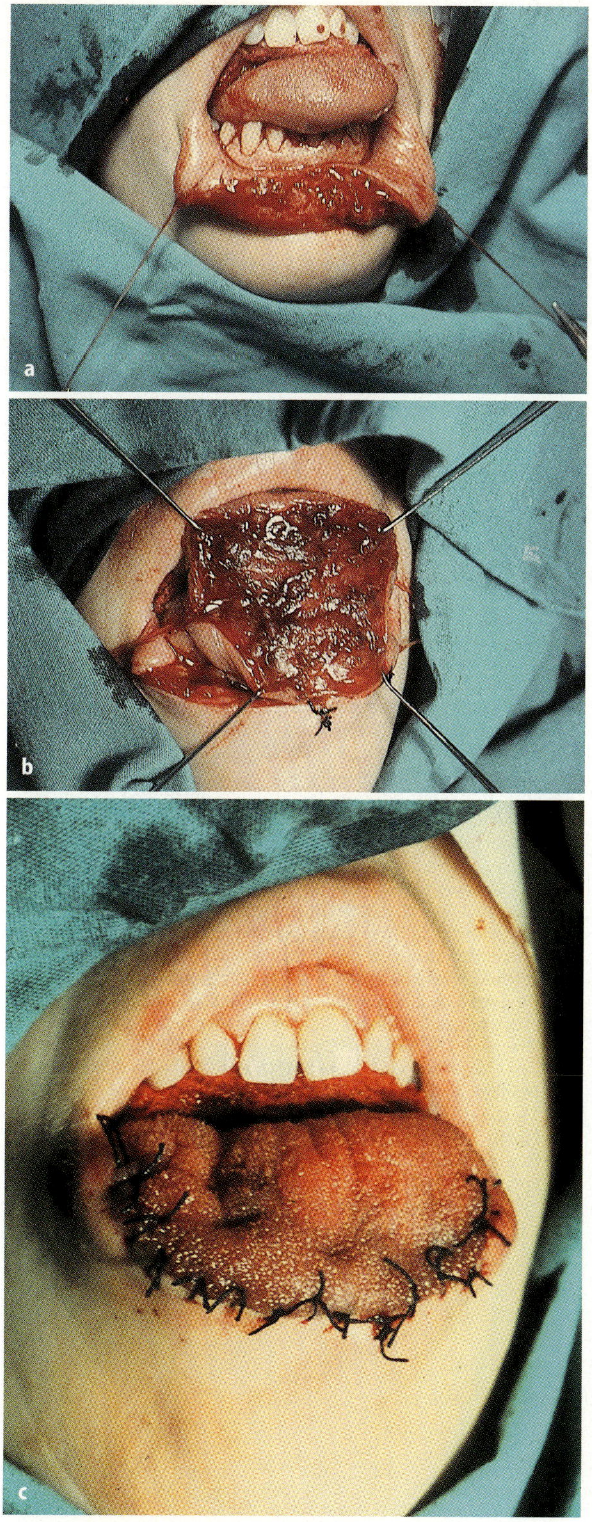

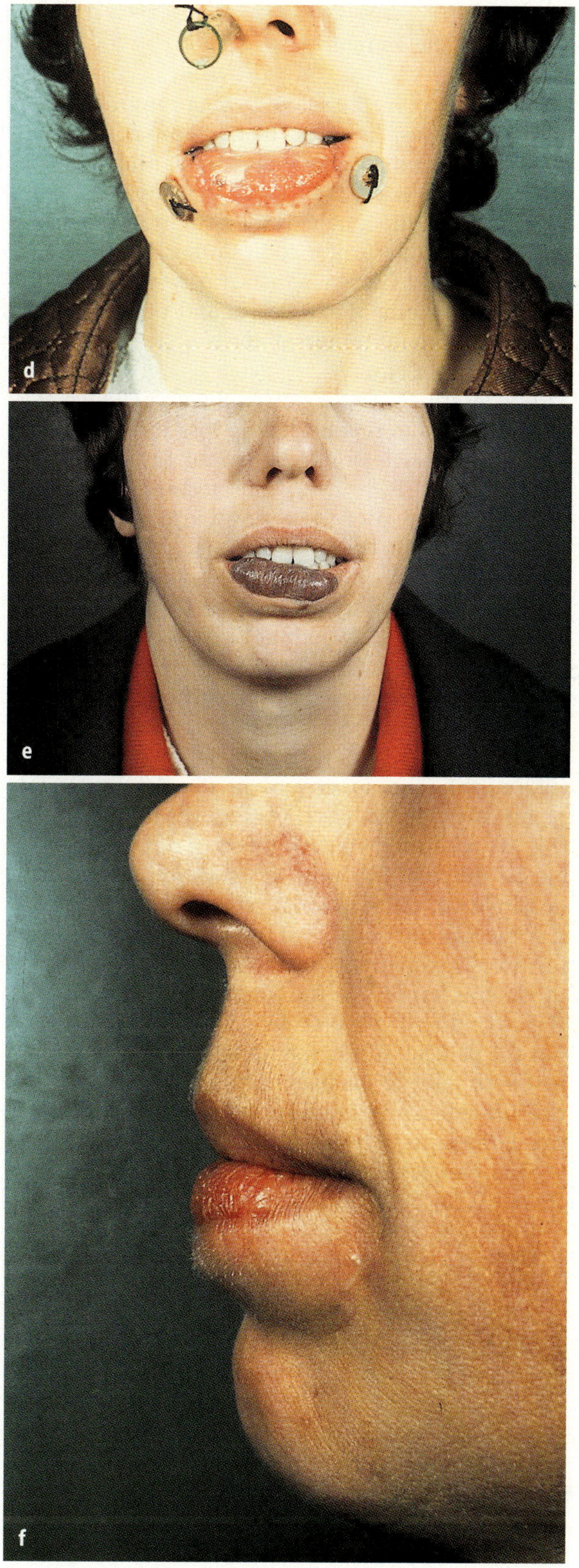

Fig. 24.7. **a** Lingual flap (Camacho-Dulanto technique). After removal of a large hemangioma invading skin, vermilion, muscle, and gingivodental mucosa, this large defect was observed. **b** The tip of the tongue is cut in "sandwich" form. **c** The upper part of the lingual flap is covering the defect on the skin and the vermilion area. **d** Approximation sutures with buttons are located between tongue and commissures. **e** Preoperative appearance of the patient. **f** Appearance 1 year after surgery

24.3.4 Surgery of the Tongue

The tongue can be the site of benign tumors, such as lymphangiomas, lipomas, hemangiomas, leiomyomas, schwannomas, and leukoplakia. Malignant tumors can also affect the tongue, but the most common tumor of the tongue is the benign Abrikossov's tumor or granular cell myoblastoma. All these neoplasms usually resolve satisfactorily with excision and direct suture. Macroglossia and other centrally located malignant tumors of the tongue require central hemiglossectomy.

We describe here the personal technique we have used for years to repair total lip loss including skin, vermilion, muscle, and mucosa up to the gingivolabial groove (Fig. 24.7a). This technique employs a "sandwich" flap of the tip of the tongue.

24.3.5 Lip Reconstruction by Means of a Lingual Flap (Camacho-Dulanto Technique)

This technique is carried out by cutting the tip of the tongue in the form of a sandwich, reaching the muscular layer where a direct catgut suture is performed (Fig. 24.7b). The upper part of the flap is used to repair the semimucosa of the vermilion border (Fig. 24.7c), and the inferior part to repair the endobuccal mucosa. Since, in this position, there is the possibility of unintentional retraction, which would tear the flap out of its position, it is advisable to perform approximation sutures with buttons between the lateral borders of the tongue and commissures (Fig. 24.7 d). After 14–21 days, it is possible to cut out the pedicle, suture the tip of the tongue and adjust both flaps at the back. At first there will be noticeable edema and venous congestion, which will cause the patient to use camouflage cosmetics.

One year later the results can be considered excellent from both functional and esthetic points of view: the lingual mucosa has adapted to its new function and the papillae and rugosities typical for this area have completely disappeared with time (Fig. 24.7e, f). Furthermore, speech ability is totally recovered, even the pronounciation of the letter "r".

Other types of dermatological operations for restoration of the oral cavity and pharyngeal function following ablative surgery remain outside the field of dermatological surgery; nevertheless, we would like to point out here the neurosensory radial forearm flaps as the technique of choice for reconstruction of a variety of oral cavity and pharyngeal defects [9, 10].

References

1. Moy RL, Rivlin D. Flaps and grafts in the repair of facial defects. Curr Opin Dermatol 1996; 3: 158–162
2. Sánchez Conejo-Mir J, Pérez Bernal AM, Moreno Giménez JC, Camacho Martínez F. Follow up of vermilionectomies: evaluation of the technique. J Dermatol Surg Oncol 1986; 12: 180–184
3. Camacho F, Dulanto F. Cirugía del cáncer de labio. Reconstrucciones de labio superior, inferior y comisuras. In: Camacho F, Dulanto F (Eds). Cirugía dermatológica. Madrid: Grupo Aula Médica, 1995: 447–468
4. Dulanto F, Armijo M, Camacho F, Sánchez Muros J. Hemangioma de labio inferior. Tratamiento quirúrgico con colagajo pediculado lingual. Actas Dermosifiliogr 1977; 68: 75–84
5. Camacho F, Moreno JC, Sanchez-Conejo-Mir J. Total upper lip reconstruction with bilateral fan flaps. J Dermatol Surg Oncol 1992; 18: 627–628
6. Ono I, Ariga K, Gunji H, Hasegawa T, Sato M, Kaneko F. A method with three triangular flaps as a secondary operative procedure after reconstruction of the lower lip by Estlander's method. Plast Reconstr Surg 1992; 90: 700–706
7. Jimenez-Castellanos Ballesteros J. Embriología y anatomía del macizo facial. Monogr Dermatol 1997; 10: 1–14
8. Ortega R, Serrano S. Curugía de la cavidad oral y cuello. In: Camacho F, Dulanto F (Eds). Cirugía dematologica. Madrid: Grupo Aula Médica, 1995: 415–430
9. Moscoso JF, Urken ML. Radial forearm flaps. Otolaryngol Clin North Am 1994; 27: 1119–1140
10. Bodin IK, Lind MG, Arnander C. Free radial forearm flap reconstruction in surgery of the oral cavity and pharynx: surgical complications, impairment of speech and swallowing. Clin Otolaryngol 1994; 19: 28–34.

Subject Index

Printing and binding: Druckerei Triltsch, Würzburg